Global Malnutrition

Global Malnutrition: Pathology and Complications addresses various types of malnutrition including deficiencies (undernutrition), excesses (overnutrition), and imbalances in a person's intake of nutrients. Malnutrition is considered a global health crisis causing various types of chronic diseases in humans. Malnutrition is very serious when affecting children as the result can be a lifetime of serious health problems. This book addresses the importance of combating undernutrition and overnutrition. It discusses the prevalence of nutritional disorders and epidemics, and nutritional requirements for various populations, and focuses on special populations most affected by nutritional disorders.

Features:

- Covers various diseases caused by poor diet and nutrition
- Provides suggestions on preventing malnutrition by improving diet and nutrition
- Discusses nutritional disorders and epidemics
- Presents information on nutritional requirements in special populations
- Contains clinical case studies with critical thinking questions and answers, clinical treatments, and costs

Featuring an engaging writing style and excellent flow of material, *Global Malnutrition: Pathology and Complications* contains practical applications for use in clinical practice. It includes suggestions about improving diet and nutrition in order to prevent malnutrition. Figures enhance content, and questions at the end of chapters with corresponding answers at the end of the book reinforce the subject matter.

Global Malnutrition
Pathology and Complications

Jahangir Moini, Oyindamola Akinso, and Raheleh Ahangari

CRC Press
Taylor & Francis Group
Boca Raton London New York

CRC Press is an imprint of the
Taylor & Francis Group, an **Informa** business

Cover credit: Shutterstock

First edition published 2024
by CRC Press
6000 Broken Sound Parkway NW, Suite 300, Boca Raton, FL 33487-2742

and by CRC Press
4 Park Square, Milton Park, Abingdon, Oxon, OX14 4RN

CRC Press is an imprint of Taylor & Francis Group, LLC

Library of Congress Cataloging-in-Publication Data
Names: Moini, Jahangir, 1942- author. | Akinso, Oyindamola, author. |
Ahangari, Raheleh, author.
Title: Global malnutrition : pathology and complications / edited by
Jahangir Moini, Oyindamola Akinso, and Raheleh Ahangari.
Description: First edition. | Boca Raton, FL : CRC Press, 2024. |
Includes bibliographical references and index. | Summary: "Global Malnutrition:
Pathology and Complications addresses various types of malnutrition
including deficiencies (undernutrition), excesses (overnutrition), and
imbalances in a person's intake of nutrients. Malnutrition is considered
a global health crisis causing various types of chronic diseases in
humans. Malnutrition is very serious when affecting children as the
result can be a lifetime of serious health problems. This book addresses
the importance of combatting undernutrition and overnutrition.
It discusses the prevalence of nutritional disorders and epidemics;
nutritional requirements for various populations; and focuses on special
populations most affected by nutritional disorders"— Provided by publisher.
Identifiers: LCCN 2023018221 (print) | LCCN 2023018222 (ebook) |
ISBN 9781032295343 (hardback) | ISBN 9781032295350 (paperback) | ISBN 9781003302032 (ebook)
Subjects: LCSH: Malnutrition. | Malnutrition—Complications. |
Malnutrition—Pathophysiology. | Malnutrition—Prevention. |
Nutritionally induced diseases.
Classification: LCC RC623 .M65 2024 (print) | LCC RC623 (ebook) | DDC
362.1963/9—dc23/eng/20230817
LC record available at https://lccn.loc.gov/2023018221
LC ebook record available at https://lccn.loc.gov/2023018222

ISBN: 9781032295343 (hbk)
ISBN: 9781032295350 (pbk)
ISBN: 9781003302032 (ebk)

DOI: 10.1201/b22969

Typeset in Times
by codeMantra

Dr. Moini:

I am dedicating this book to my new precious granddaughter, Anastasia Pearl Kihm.

Dr. Akinso:

I am dedicating this book to my daughter, Oluwatamilore Soremekun.

Dr. Ahangari:

This book is dedicated to my husband and my precious daughter.

Contents

PART II Implications of Nutrition for Special Populations

PART III Nutritional Disorders

About the Authors

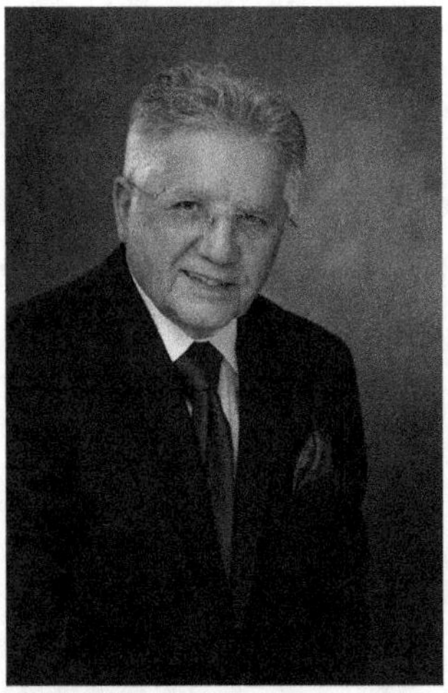

Dr. Jahangir Moini was an Assistant Professor at Tehran University, Medical School, Department of Epidemiology and Preventive Medicine, for 9 years and Director of Epidemiology for the Brevard County (Florida) Health Department for 18 years. He was the Director of Science and Health for Everest University in Melbourne, Florida, for 15 years as well as a Professor of Science and Health at Everest for a total of 24 years. For 6 years, he was a Professor of Science and Health at Eastern Florida State College but is now retired. Dr. Moini has been actively teaching for 39 years, and for 24 years, has been an international author of 56 books. His *Anatomy & Physiology for Healthcare Professionals* was translated and released in Japan and South Korea in 2020. Also, his *Complications of Diabetes Mellitus* was translated and released in Spanish in 2023.

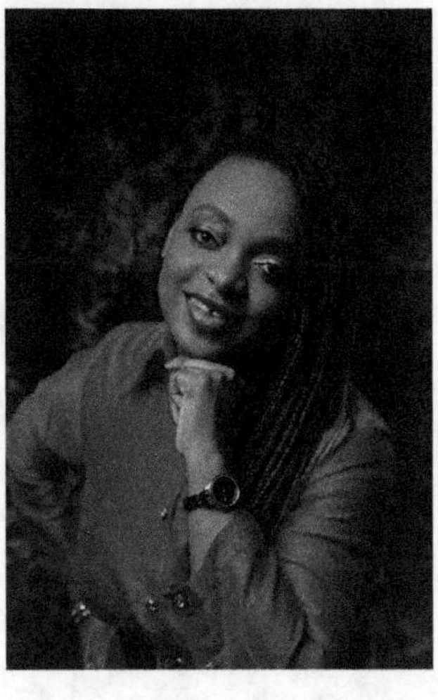

Dr. Oyindamola Akinso is a Public Health Professor at Wingate University in North Carolina. She is a global health specialist with over a decade of experience in public health practice and research. While in Nigeria, Oyindamola was deeply involved in global health practice, including working in nonprofit and international development organizations, to improve maternal and child health in underserved populations. She is extensively involved in work on women and children's health, adolescent sexual and reproductive health, gender-based violence and trauma in marginalized populations, and communicable disease control in the sub-Saharan African region.

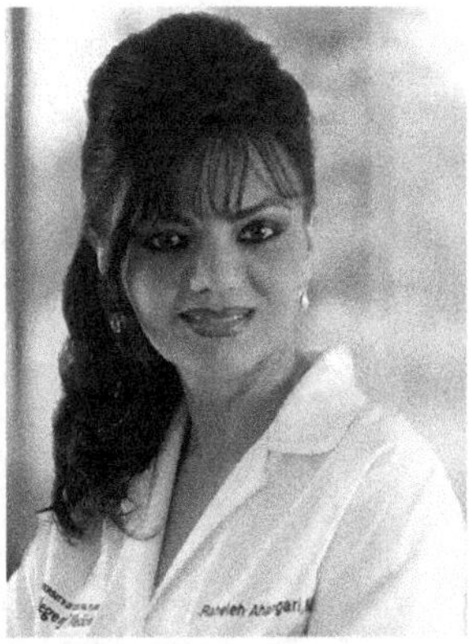

Dr. Raheleh Ahangari is an Associate Professor of Medicine and coordinator of the Biomedical Sciences master assessment program, as well as coordinator of the Biotechnology master assessment program in the Burnett School of Biomedical Sciences at the UCF College of Medicine. She is currently teaching Human Physiology, Clinical Embryology, and Clinical Endocrinology. She received her Doctor of Medicine (MD) degree from Carol Davila Medical University, Bucharest, Romania. She then moved to a post-doc position in Wuerzburg, Germany, in 2000. Her studies focused on immunology, looking for signal transduction mechanisms in apoptosis and T-cell proliferation in the Department of Immunology-Virology of Wuerzburg University. In 2003, she received an Assistant Professor position in Anatomy at the Saba University School of Medicine in the Netherlands-Antilles. She joined UCF as a teaching faculty in 2005. Dr. Ahangari is a graduate faculty scholar and has directed several independent studies in endocrine and metabolic disorders and chaired a number of honors in major thesis works as well as several master's capstone projects. She has 49 publications and abstracts, and is the coauthor of three books.

Preface

Global Malnutrition: Pathology and Complications is a comprehensive and easy-to-read resource that addresses the importance of combating undernutrition and overnutrition, which affect more than one billion people worldwide. Malnutrition is responsible for more than 50% of all childhood deaths, and its effects also include many types of chronic diseases as well as decreased economic productivity. Overnutrition has become a serious global threat to overall health, with more than 35% of the world's population being overweight. In the United States, nearly 70% of the population is overweight. All types of people are affected by malnutrition worldwide, and when it affects children under age five, it can result in poor growth and development, and lifelong health problems. Pregnant women suffering from malnutrition are more likely to have premature births and serious health complications, and their babies have more incidence of birth defects. Malnutrition is a worldwide health crisis that must be addressed seriously by all healthcare professionals.

There is no other book currently on the market similar to this one. Therefore, there is a widespread need for this book to fill a missing gap in available resources. It contains detailed information about the prevalence of nutritional disorders and epidemics. There is discussion of nutritional requirements and focus on special populations most affected by nutritional disorders, as well as individual nutritional effects upon various body systems. There is also focus on clinical treatments and costs. The issues of malnutrition are globally significant for people of all ages, from infants to the elderly. The book provides detailed information about how poor nutrition causes a variety of health problems for people throughout the world, which are often serious and life threatening.

Global Malnutrition: Pathology and Complications is written in a highly engaging writing style, offering excellent material flow that is broken up by numerous, interesting figures and tables. Each chapter begins with an outline of the text headings, followed by learning objectives and an overview. There are "Focus On" boxes that highlight important points to be remembered. Each section ends with "Test Your Knowledge" questions about the most essential information. The text features practical applications for use in clinical practice. Additionally, there are "You Should Remember" boxes about specific topics that should be retained. This book covers major pathophysiologies and diseases caused by poor diet and nutrition, offering suggestions on preventing malnutrition by improving diet and nutrition. This book's color printing makes images more effective and improves the experience of the reader. The text also includes bullet-pointed lists and key terms. Actual clinical case studies are included, which feature critical thinking questions. The answers to these questions are within a separate section at the end of the book. At the end of each chapter, there are multiple-choice Study Questions, and their answers are also listed at the end of the book. The final part of each chapter is a "References" section that lists additional sources of information on the topics within this book.

Acknowledgments

The authors appreciate the contributions of everyone who assisted in the creation of this book, Randy Brehm, Tom Connelly, and Greg Vadimsky. The authors also wish to acknowledge Dr. Morvarid Moini for contributing artwork. The authors would also like to thank "Kokila Devi" for her assistance in the creation of this book.

Part I

Introduction

1 Nutrition and Health

OUTLINE

Nutritional Requirements
Nutrition in Clinical Medicine
  Surgical Nutrition
  Nutrition in ICU
  Nutrition in Burn Patients
  Nutrition in Trauma Patients
  Nutrition in Patients with Cachexia
Nutrient–Drug Interactions
Food Additives and Contaminants
Key Terms
Clinical Case Studies
Study Questions
Further Reading

LEARNING OBJECTIVES

After study of the chapter, readers should be able to:

1. Describe six classes of nutrients.
2. Explain three functional categories of nutrients.
3. Describe complex carbohydrates and give an example for each.
4. Explain the differences between cholesterol and triglyceride.
5. List essential amino acids.
6. Describe the body mass index.
7. Explain electrolyte imbalances in severe burn patients.
8. Discuss nutrient–drug interactions.
9. Explain why food additives are used.
10. List some common food additives.

OVERVIEW

Good nutrition throughout the lifespan helps prevent malnutrition as well as many noncommunicable diseases and conditions. Many people, however, do not eat a nutritious diet because of increased production of processed foods, increasing urbanization, and changing lifestyles. Today, people widely consume more foods that are high in energy, fats, sugar, and sodium, while eating insufficient quantities of fruit, vegetables, and whole grains. Though the basic principles of good nutrition and resultant good health are the same for everyone, the exact makeup of a person's required diet varies based on age, gender, lifestyle, and the amount of physical activity.

NUTRITIONAL REQUIREMENTS

Nutrition is the science of food, nutrients, and related substances, as well as how they act, interact, and are balanced in relation to health and disease. The human body ingests, digests, absorbs, transports, utilizes, and excretes food substances so that all body cells can be energized, constructed, and maintained. The six classes of **nutrients** in foods are carbohydrates, lipids, proteins, vitamins, minerals, and water. Nutrients are essential for health and cannot be made at all or in enough quantities to support health. *Essential nutrients* have certain biological functions, cause a decline in normal biological function if they are removed from the diet, and restore normal function when returned to the diet prior to any permanent damage occurring.

There are nutrients that yield energy and those that do not. The energy-yielding nutrients are carbohydrates, lipids, and proteins. Carbohydrates consist of glucose, glycogen, and starch. Lipids include linoleic acid (omega-6) and alpha-linolenic acid (omega-3). Proteins include amino acids. The non-energy-yielding nutrients include the water-soluble and fat-soluble vitamins, along with minerals. The water-soluble vitamins include thiamin, riboflavin, niacin, pantothenic acid, biotin, pyridoxine, cobalamin, and ascorbic acid. All of these are classified as "B vitamins" except for ascorbic acid (vitamin C). The fat-soluble vitamins include vitamins A, D, E, and K. The major minerals consist of calcium, chloride, magnesium, phosphorus, potassium, sodium, and sulfur. The trace minerals include chromium, copper, fluoride, iodide, iron, manganese, molybdenum, selenium, and zinc. There are also "questionable" minerals such as arsenic, boron, nickel, silicon, and vanadium. The final non-energy-yielding nutrient is water.

Nutrients have three functional categories. There are those that mostly provide energy, usually expressed in **kilocalories** (kcal); those that are needed for growth, development, and maintenance; and those that regulate processes while keeping functions occurring normally. There is some amount of overlap, and the energy-yielding nutrients plus water make up major portions of most foods. Since carbohydrates, lipids, and proteins are required in large amounts, they are known as **macronutrients**. Vitamins and minerals, needed in small amounts, are known as **micronutrients**. Most carbohydrates and most fats, along with all proteins, provide energy. Growth and development are promoted by proteins, lipids, some vitamins and minerals, and water. Body processes are regulated by proteins, some lipids, some vitamins and minerals, and water.

DOI: 10.1201/b22969-2

Carbohydrates are primarily made up of the elements called *carbon*, *hydrogen*, and *oxygen* (see Figure 1.1). The main dietary sources of carbohydrates are fruits, vegetables, grains, beans, and sugars. Primarily, carbohydrates are classified as *simple* or *complex*. The simple carbohydrates are small structures also called sugars. They include table sugar (sucrose) and blood sugar (glucose). Sugars such as glucose can bone chemically, forming large carbohydrates, known as complex carbohydrates or *polysaccharides*. Complex carbohydrates include **glycogen** (in muscles), starch (in grains), and fibers. The major source of cellular energy is glucose, which is derived from simple carbohydrates and starch. Glucose and the majority of other carbohydrates provide about 4 kcal/g. Since fiber cannot be broken down by digestive processes, it only provides a small amount of energy. When insufficient dietary carbohydrates are consumed, there is insufficient glucose, and the body must manufacture it from proteins.

Lipids, which include fats and oils as well as **cholesterol**, are compounds that are also mostly made up of carbon, hydrogen, and oxygen. *Fats* are lipids that solidify at room temperature. Oils remain liquid at room temperature. Lipids provide more energy than carbohydrates or proteins – about 9 kcal/g. Lipids are insoluble in water, but can dissolve in organic solvents such as benzene and ether. A **triglyceride** is a type of lipid that is the major form of dietary fat. It is also an important energy source. Triglycerides are the primary form of energy that is stored in the body. They consist of three fatty acids attached to one molecule of **glycerol** (see Figure 1.2). Fatty acids are long chains of carbon that are flanked by hydrogen, with an acid group attached to the end that is opposite to the glycerol. Based on the chemical structure of dominant fatty acids, most lipids are either **saturated** or **unsaturated**. This aids in determining if a lipid will be solid or liquid at room temperature, and influences how it affects human health. Nearly all foods have varieties of saturated and unsaturated fatty acids. However, plant oils usually contain primarily unsaturated fatty acids and are liquid at room temperature. Many animal fats are rich in saturated fatty acids, so they are solid at room temperature. In general, unsaturated fats are the healthier type, since saturated fat increases blood cholesterol, which is able to block the arteries and lead to cardiovascular disease. The unsaturated fatty acids called *linoleic acid* and *alpha-linolenic acid* are essential diets that must be part of the diet. They act as structural cell membrane components and aid in regulating blood pressure and nerve transmissions. Enough of the essential fatty acids can be supplied by only a few tablespoons of daily vegetable oil and consuming fish two or more times per week. Unsaturated fats that have been processed so that their structures change from the common *cis* form to the *trans* form are known as **trans fatty acids**. These are most common in foods that are deep-fried, such as French fries

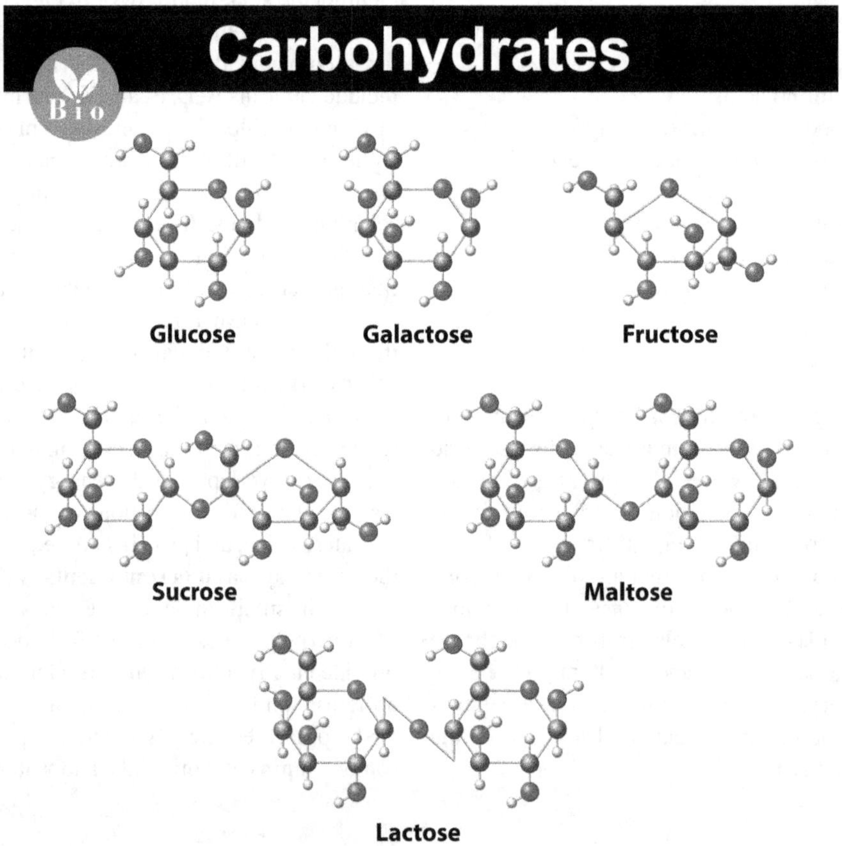

FIGURE 1.1 The structure of various forms of carbohydrates.

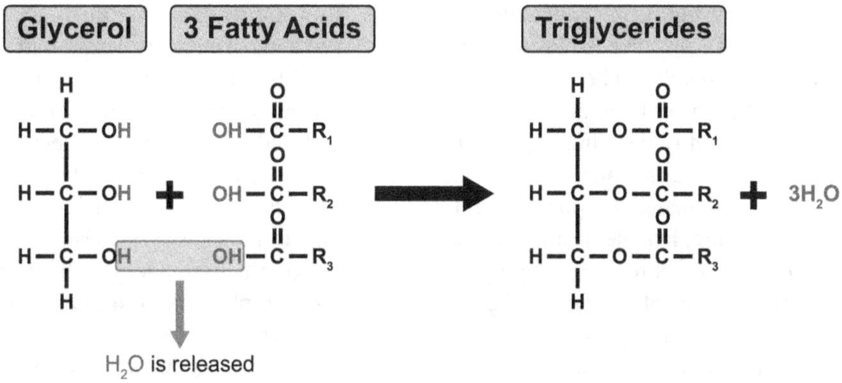

FIGURE 1.2 The structure of glycerol, which combines with three fatty acids, to form a triglyceride.

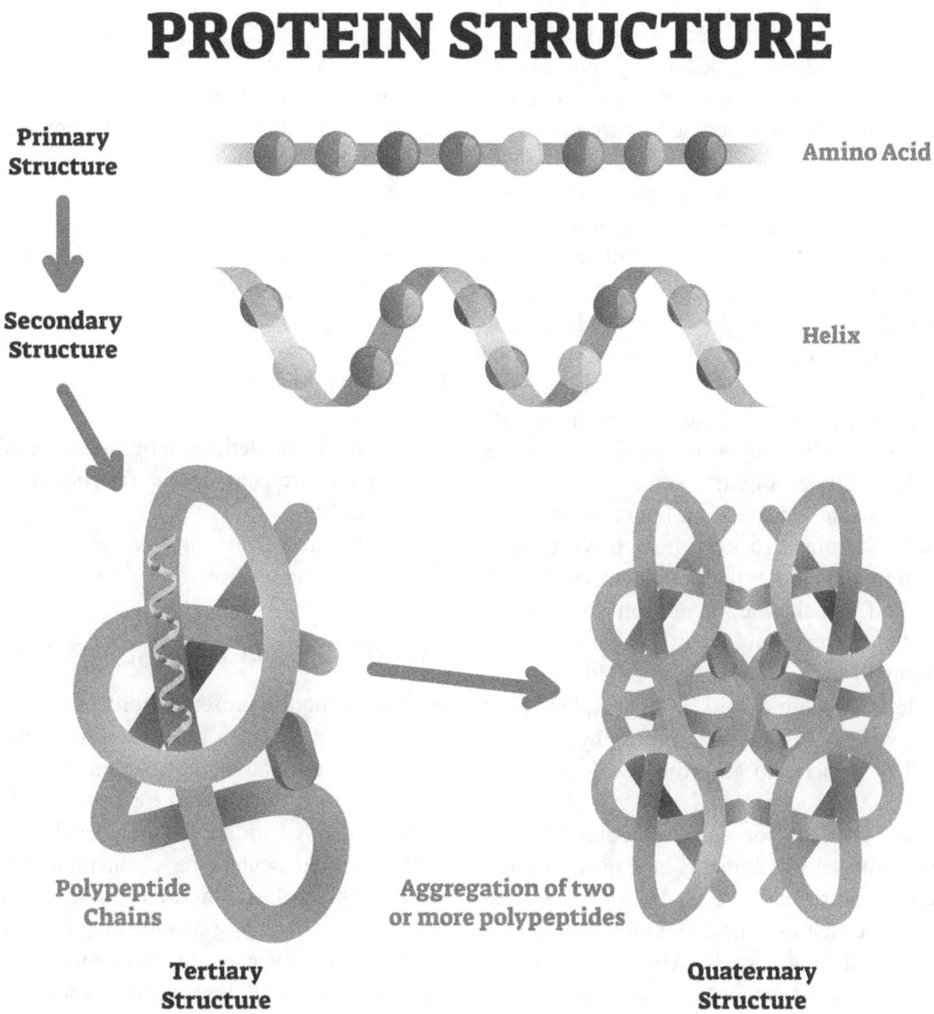

FIGURE 1.3 The structure of a protein.

or donuts, baked snacks such as cookies or zcrackers, and solid fats such as the stick form of margarine, or in shortening. When there are large amounts of *trans fats* in the diet, a person's health is at risk. Therefore, trans fats along with saturated fat must be avoided or minimized.

Proteins are also made up of carbon, hydrogen, oxygen, and nitrogen (see Figure 1.3). They are the primary structural materials of the human body. They make up major parts of bones and muscles, and are also present in blood, cell membranes, enzymes, and immune factors. Proteins provide about 4 kcal/g of energy, but the body usually does not use much protein for its energy needs. Proteins are formed when amino acids bind together. There are 20 common amino acids in food, with nine of them being essential adult nutrients, and one other amino acid being essential for infants. The 20 common amino acids are alanine, arginine, asparagine, aspartic acid, cysteine, glutamine, glutamic acid, glycine, histidine, isoleucine, leucine, lysine, methionine, phenylalanine, proline, serine, threonine, tryptophan, tyrosine, and valine. The nine essential amino acids for adults are histidine, isoleucine, leucine, lysine, methionine, phenylalanine, threonine, tryptophan, and valine. The one essential amino acid for infants is histidine. The primary function of vitamins is to enable chemical reactions in the body, some of which help to release the energy from carbohydrates, lipids, and proteins. Minerals usually function as groups of similar atoms or as parts of mineral combinations, and are required for normal body functions – especially in the nervous system, skeletal system, and in water balance. Vitamins are discussed in greater detail in Chapter 10, while minerals are discussed in greater detail in Chapter 11.

The final class of nutrients consists of water, which like minerals, is inorganic. Water is actually the nutrient that is needed in the largest quantity out of all of them. It is made up of two molecules of hydrogen and one molecule of oxygen, hence its abbreviation as "H_2O". Water has many vital functions, acting as a solvent, lubricant, and a mode of transport of nutrients in the body. Water also helps in the regulation of body temperature. Many foods, along with beverages, supply water. The body also manufactures some water as a byproduct of **metabolism**.

Plant components that are found in fruits, vegetables, legumes, and whole grains are known as **phytochemicals**. Animal components are called **zoochemicals**. Both phytochemicals and zoochemicals are physiologically active compounds, but are not essential dietary nutrients. Even so, many of them provide good health benefits. People that regularly consume fruits and vegetables have reduced risks for developing cancer. Some phytochemicals are believed by experts to stop the development of cancer. Also, some phytochemicals and zoochemicals are linked to reduced risks for cardiovascular disease. Multivitamin and mineral supplements lack most of these benefits. Therefore, nutritionists and dietitians suggest that the diet should be rich in fruits, vegetables, legumes, and whole-grain breads and cereals. Also, foods of animal origin such as fatty fish provide ample quantities of omega-3 fatty acids, which are highly beneficial zoochemicals, and fermented dairy products provide **probiotics**. Phytochemicals and zoochemicals are further classified as *functional foods* since they provide health benefits that are more than are supplied by the traditional nutrients found in them. These functional foods offer more features that can decrease disease and promote good health. There are four categories of functional foods, which are summarized as follows:

- Conventional (unmodified whole) foods – dairy products, fish, fruits, herbs, nuts, spices, vegetables
- Modified (fortified, enriched, enhanced) foods – breakfast bars containing ginkgo biloba, calcium-fortified orange juice, cheese made with plant sterols, omega-3-enriched breads
- Medical foods, formulas, or supplements (used under medical supervision) – flavocoxid (for osteoarthritis), phenylalanine-free baby formulas (for **phenylketonuria**), VSL#3 probiotic (for ulcerative colitis)
- Special foods that meet certain dietary needs – gluten-free foods (for **celiac disease**), infant formula for certain infants, lactose-free foods (for lactose intolerance), sugar-free foods (for weight loss)

FOCUS ON NUTRITIONAL LABELING

On packaged foods and drinks, the "nutrition facts label" has been updated in recent years, making it easier to make informed choices. The "daily value" is the recommended amount of nutrients to consume or not exceed per day. The "percent of daily value" is how much a nutrient in a single serving contributes to the daily diet.

Test Your Knowledge

1. What is the definition of an "essential nutrient"?
2. What are the three functional categories of nutrients?
3. Why must *trans* fats and saturated fat be avoided or minimized?

NUTRITION IN CLINICAL MEDICINE

With or without a present disorder, nutritional deficiencies often make a patient's health worse. Malabsorption is one example of a disorder that causes nutritional deficiencies. Older patients hospitalized for acute conditions often have undiagnosed nutritional deficiencies that require treatment. Many medical centers have nutrition support teams that combine physicians, dietitians, nurses, and pharmacists. They help clinicians prevent, diagnose, and treat hidden nutritional deficiencies. Overnutrition contributes to many chronic disorders. These include cancer, hypertension, diabetes mellitus, obesity, and coronary artery disease. For galactosemia, phenylketonuria, and other hereditary metabolic disorders, dietary restrictions are required.

A patient requires nutritional evaluation if he or she has suspected deficiencies or toxicities of essential nutrients, or undesired body weight or composition. An infant or child with insufficient growth or development also requires an evaluation of nutritional status. These types of evaluations are regularly done as part of clinical examinations in older people, those taking multiple medications, those with psychiatric disorders, and those with systemic disorders that last for more than several days. General nutritional status is evaluated via patient history, physical examination, and, for some people, tests. For suspected undernutrition, laboratory tests (such as albumin levels) and skin tests (for delayed hypersensitivity) may be needed. Body composition analysis requires skinfold measurements and bioelectrical impedance analysis. These are used to estimate the percentage of body fat in the evaluation of obesity.

Patient history includes assessment of dietary intake, weight changes, risk factors for deficiencies, and a careful review of systems. A more detailed dietary history is obtained by a dietitian, usually using a list of foods eaten over the previous 24 hours and a food questionnaire. Food diaries can be used to record all foods that are eaten. The most accurate record is the **weighed ad libitum diet**. The patient records daily weight and all foods that are consumed. A complete physical examination includes measurements of height, weight, and distribution of body fat. **Body mass index** (BMI) is more accurate than using height and weight tables. It is calculated by the patient's weight per kg, divided by height in square meters (m^2). This adjusts weight for height. For infants, children, and adolescents, there are standards for growth and weight gain. Disproportionate **truncal obesity** is linked to cardiovascular disorders, cerebrovascular disorders, diabetes mellitus, and hypertension more often than fat that is located elsewhere on the body. Truncal obesity is assessed by measuring waist circumference in patients with a BMI of less than 35 inches. This may help predict risks for cardiovascular disorders, diabetes, hypercholesterolemia, and hypertension. Risks are increased if the waist circumference is more than 40 inches (102 cm) in men or more than 35 inches (88 cm) in women.

Surgical Nutrition

Nutrition after surgery is very important, with protein being extremely essential. Protein helps repair body tissues, form antibodies to fight infections, and synthesize collagen so that scars can form. Good protein sources include fish, lean poultry, seafood, legumes, nuts, and seeds. Fatty red meats should be limited since they may trigger inflammation. Supplemental protein may come from beans, tofu, and vegetarian foods such as textured vegetable protein. Dairy products, though another source of protein, must be moderately used because they can cause constipation. Foods that help reduce pain and inflammation after surgery include the following:

- Canola, extra virgin olive oil, and soybean oils
- Dark-colored fruits (blueberries, cranberries, eggplant, red apples, red grapes)
- Fatty fish (flounder, halibut, salmon, sardines, sole, trout, tuna)
- Flaxseed meal or oil
- Green and black tea
- Onion, garlic, and green leafy vegetables
- Soy products (edamame, soy milk, tempeh, tofu, whole soy beans)
- Turmeric
- Walnuts, almonds, peanuts

Vitamins that reduce inflammation and accelerate wound healing include vitamin A (cantaloupe, carrots, leafy greens, red bell pepper, sweet potato), vitamin C (bell peppers, broccoli, kiwi, oranges, potatoes, strawberries, tomatoes), and vitamin D (egg yolk, fortified milk, salmon, tuna, plus from direct exposure of the skin to sunlight for 10 minutes, two times per week). The mineral *calcium* is essential for bone repair, soft tissue healing, normal blood clotting, muscle contraction, and normal heartbeat. It is highly present in milk, milk products, and dark green leafy vegetables. The minerals zinc and copper are also important. Zinc is found in fish, lean meats, legumes, oysters, poultry, and whole-grain breads or cereals. Copper is highly present in dark leafy greens, legumes, nuts, oysters and other shellfish, potatoes, and whole grains.

To avoid constipation after surgery, it is important to drink enough water and eat enough fiber. It is important to limit foods that are refined or include extra fat, salt, and sugar. To increase the insoluble fiber intake, choose cereals, fruits, darkly colored vegetables, and whole-grain breads. If possible, exercise and activity should be attempted as much as possible, since this helps stimulate the intestine. Foods that can cause constipation include the following:

- Cheese
- Dried or dehydrated foods (beef jerky, dried fruits [except for prunes], potato chips)
- Milk and dairy products
- Red meat
- Refined or processed foods (packaged high-calorie foods such as cookies and pork rinds), boxed meal mixes, white bread, and white rice
- Sweets (cakes, candies, pastries)

To treat constipation, a high-fiber cocktail can be used, which combines applesauce, wheat bran, and prune juice. Just one tablespoon is used per day to start, but this is slowly increased each day until the correct amount is found. Some patients have a lack of appetite after surgery, but this usually passes over a few days. Nutritious foods must be consumed as early in the recovery process as possible since failing to eat enough after surgery delays the healing process. If there is no constipation but the appetite remains poor, calorie-dense foods such as avocado, potatoes, or smoothies with dairy, fruit, and a protein powder should be consumed.

FOCUS ON NUTRITION AFTER SURGERY

After surgery, an individual has a higher risk of infections, falls, pneumonia, and decreased mobility. The ten best foods to eat that help promote healing after surgery include berries, vegetables, fats (fish, nuts, oils), dark leafy greens, meats or other alternatives, eggs, probiotics, brightly colored fruits, whole grains, and water.

Test Your Knowledge

1. How is body mass index (BMI) calculated?
2. Which foods help reduce pain and inflammation after surgery?
3. Which foods accelerate wound healing after surgery?

Nutrition in ICU

When a patient is in the intensive care unit (ICU), nutrition is obviously important. Though it can vary widely, there are some generalized rules. Nutritional goals are determined on an individual basis. If available, **indirect calorimetry** is used or estimated based on 25 kcal/kg of body weight per day. There is no single predictive equation that is better than any others. Enteral nutrition is preferred initially unless it is contraindicated. Enteral nutrition is started within 48 hours at 30 mL per hour and then escalated in most cases. There is no strong evidence that meeting 100% of the energy goals will improve mortality, and there is weak evidence that this can actually be harmful for well-nourished patients. It is believed that the 100% goal rate is more appropriate during the recovery stages of a critical illness. Earlier in an acute illness, 33%–66% of the goal rate may be appropriate if the patient is premorbidly well-nourished.

Interruptions of enteral nutrition should be minimized, and higher makeup rates should be used, so that higher gastric aspirates that generally are comfortable can be returned. The patient should be sat up to a 45-degree angle. Pro-kinetic agents such as metoclopramide and erythromycin should be started. If the goals of the patient's nutrition are unmet after approximately 48 hours, parenteral nutrition should be added as a supplement. A well-nourished patient can actually wait for seven days without enteral nutrition or **total parenteral nutrition** (TPN). A malnourished patient cannot wait, so nutritional treatment should start immediately. It should begin at an 80% rate and begin preoperatively for any malnourished patients that are surgical candidates. Parenteral nutrition should be added to inadequate enteral nutrition intake to make up for lost nutrition.

Nutrition in Burn Patients

Severe burns cause significant metabolic abnormalities, making nutritional support extremely important and challenging. Burns cause a continuing **hypermetabolic** state and increased **catabolism**, resulting in increased muscle wasting and **cachexia**. The metabolic rates of burn patients can be more than twice the normal rates. Failure to fulfill needed energy requirements causes impaired wound healing, organ dysfunction, and increased susceptibility to infection. Burn patients need adequate assessment and provision of nutrients.

Severe burns may cause varying amounts of electrolyte imbalances. Initially, sodium is low because it exits the extracellular space, due to increased vessel permeability. Children are at increased risk of dilutional **hyponatremia**. After resuscitation, potassium may be high since fluids containing sodium, plus sodium itself, returning to the extracellular space. This is worsened by an acute kidney injury, resolution of edema (which concentrates the sodium), and a free-water deficit.

Hyperkalemia initially occurs due to potassium leaks from cell lysis and tissue necrosis. With third degree burns, the entire epidermis and dermis have been severely damaged and nerve endings have been destroyed. Without the natural barrier against water loss, fluid seeps from the burned area, resulting in dehydration and electrolyte imbalance. Unless fluids are replaced, there will be kidney failure and hypovolemic shock. Hypophosphatemia, **hypoproteinemia**, and hypocalcemia are also seen. The hypoproteinemia and hypocalcemia are related to the importance of the burned body surface.

Most clinicians recommend early enteral nutrition with high-carbohydrate formulas, though nutritional support is individualized, monitored, and adjusted throughout recovery. Carbohydrates are the preferred energy source since high-carbohydrate diets promote wound healing and result in a protein-sparing effect. Care is needed, since glucose given in excess of what the patient can utilize leads to **hyperglycemia**, conversion of glucose to fat, **glucosuria**, and dehydration. Many patients need supplemental insulin in order to maintain satisfactory blood glucose. Insulin also promotes muscle protein synthesis and wound healing. Severely burned patients receiving insulin along with a high-carbohydrate, high-protein diet have better donor site healing, lean body mass, bone mineral density, and shorter hospitalizations.

Burn patients have special dietary needs to provide sufficient nutrients so that they can heal. Even though the appetite may be poor, it is also important that a diet high in calories and protein be consumed. If this is not possible, a feeding tube may be required. Most burn patients become able to eat regular food by the time they are discharged from a hospital. A *burn dietitian* and the hospital kitchen staff will ensure that the burn patient receives adequate nutrition. Healthy eating for burn patients means eating small meals, five to six times per day. High-protein foods include meat, eggs, beans, milk, yogurt, cheese, nuts, peanut butter, and tofu.

FOCUS ON ENERGY INTAKE FOR BURN PATIENTS

Recommended daily energy intake for burn patients is different between adults and children. Adults should receive 25 kcal/kg, plus 40 kcal per each percent of burn area. For children, the intake should be 1,800 kcal plus 2,200 kcal per square meter of burn area, per day. Individualized nutrition assessments are needed for patients with burns on more than 20% of total body surface area.

Nutrition in Trauma Patients

Trauma is any physical damage to the body and includes an immediate cardiovascular response plus an inflammatory response that occurs several hours after the injury. Finally, there is a metabolic response that must be considered, especially during recovery. These responses are broken down as follows:

- *Cardiovascular response* – hemorrhage, tissue damage, pain, anxiety
  - Heart rate and total peripheral vascular resistance increase to maintain blood pressure
  - Once 33% of blood volume is lost, the BP falls and is accompanied by bradycardia and syncope
  - Once 44% of blood volume is lost, the heart rate greatly increases
- *Inflammatory response* – **cytokine** production, swelling
  - The change in cytokine production can lead to multiple organ failure
  - The "one-hit" insult involves multiple organ failure occurring immediately after severe trauma
  - The "two-hit" insult involves multiple organ failure being triggered by a secondary insult such as surgery, infection, and/or ischemia over a few days after the trauma
- *Metabolic response* – hypermetabolism, insulin resistance, hyperglycemia, increased protein breakdown, wound healing

A trauma patient's nutritional state is highly influential upon wound healing. Moderate or severe protein energy malnutrition impairs or delays this. Protein deficiency interferes with formation of new capillaries, proliferation of **fibroblasts**, **proteoglycan** production, and synthesis of **collagen**. Of the amino acids, arginine is known to improve wound healing and immune function. Other needed nutrients include vitamins A, C, and E, plus zinc, copper, selenium, and manganese. Iron also plays a part in wound healing.

One of the most important types of trauma is severe head injury, which causes patients to suffer hypermetabolism, hypercatabolism, hyperglycemia, acute-phase response, and alterations of the immune system. The next most important type of trauma is abdominal and torso trauma.

Energy expenditure in these patients equals 135%–165% of the basal metabolic rate – a very high increase. It is related to increased **catecholamine** levels, and possibly, hyperactivity of the autonomic nervous system. These levels are highest the first three days after injury. Hyperglycemia is common during the first 24 hours after the head trauma, aggravates ischemia, and is positive related to the severity of any head injury. The acute-phase response includes fever, increased white blood cells (even without any infection), increased **alpha1-antitrypsin**, **C-reactive protein**, and decreased serum albumin. About 60% of patients with severe head injury have immune system alterations that lead to infections. Trauma patients are at risk of aspiration pneumonia because of reduced vomiting reflex.

Nutritional support is only initiated after intracranial pressure and peripheral **hemodynamics** have been stabilized. For other traumas, early nutrition is preferred over delayed nutrition since it improves outcome and decreases the rate of infections. The enteral route is preferred over the parenteral route, though enteral feeding has little effect upon infectious complications. Parenteral nutrition is considered if enteral nutrition cannot be started within 48 hours after hospitalization. GI motility may be reduced due to phenobarbital-induced coma. Overfeeding must be avoided since conversion of excess nutrients to glycogen or lipid requires energy, increasing oxygen consumption and leading to increased carbon dioxide production plus dilation of brain arteries. This raises intracranial pressure.

Early nutritional support, within 72 hours, is more beneficial than delayed feeding if the patient has blunt or penetrating trauma, since it leads to three times lower chances for **sepsis**. Total enteral nutrition (TEN) is preferred over TPN since it allows for better use of nutrients, prevents **atrophy** of the GI mucosa, preserves GI flora, reduces stress response, and maintains immunocompetence. Small bowel feeding is indicated in cases of severe trauma or less severe trauma with flail chest, spinal cord injury, severe pelvic fracture, major soft tissue injury, or closed head injury. Gastric feeding may be poorly tolerated, due to gastroparesis, during three to four days after trauma. If **laparotomy** is indicated, a fine-bore **jejunostomy** is preferred over a nasogastric tube. Small bowel feeding is contraindicated with full-blown shock, sepsis, and incomplete resuscitation that causes reduced splanchnic blood flow. This may result in non-occlusive bowel **necrosis**. The small bowel needs an increased blood flow in order to absorb nutrients, which cannot occur during shock. TPN is given if the patient has had prolonged GI dysfunction, such as high-output **fistulae**, massive small bowel resection, intolerance to enteral feeding, and a high risk of non-occlusive small bowel necrosis.

YOU SHOULD REMEMBER

Trauma results in combined cardiovascular, inflammatory, and metabolic responses. Nutritional support is useful during the inflammatory and metabolic phases and improves outcomes. Total enteral nutrition is preferred over total parenteral nutrition. For patients with head trauma, close attention must be paid to controlling intracranial pressure, so overfeeding must be avoided.

Test Your Knowledge

1. How do severe burns affect metabolism?
2. What are the three responses that occur in trauma patients, and what do they cause?
3. What are the effects of the most important type of trauma?

Nutrition in Patients with Cachexia

Cachexia is the development of widespread muscle wasting because of chronic starvation. The conversion of amino acids into glucose requires the muscles to be robbed of stored glucose. Cachexia is further defined as a complicated **metabolic syndrome** characterized by loss of muscle with or without a loss of fat mass. The prominent clinical features in adults are weight loss and in children, growth failure, excluding any endocrine disorders. Related features include anorexia, inflammation, and increased muscle protein breakdown. Cachexia is often related to a stress response in which the **fight-or-flight** reaction is amplified. There is an increase in stress hormones – especially catecholamines and cortisol. Levels of human growth hormone and testosterone simultaneously begin to decrease. A catabolic and hypermetabolic state results. In catabolism, the body breaks down components to release energy for increased demands. The metabolic rate and body temperature increase. An increased supply of glucose is needed. This can come from **gluconeogenesis** or the fast breakdown of lean body mass. Over an extended period of time, there is significant weight loss as well as the loss of lean body mass (see Figure 1.4). Wound healing slows since the body has insufficient energy and nutritional substrate. To build new tissue, proteins must be available to fuel **anabolism**. The patient with cachexia does not have these proteins available.

The first response to the condition is often a *hypercaloric diet*. However, the patient with cachexia does not usually respond to additional calories well, since the metabolic machinery is not functioning normally. In cancer patients with cachexia, consuming more calories does not result in weight gain. For patients with any form of cachexia, diet intervention instead focuses on providing the following:

- 55%–60% of total calories as complex carbohydrates
- 20%–25% of total calories as protein
- 20%–25% of total calories as fat

NUTRIENT–DRUG INTERACTIONS

While medications often improve health and quality of life, some of them have negative affects upon certain nutrients. This is most common in older people that take multiple medications. The actual needs for certain amounts of nutrients may be altered

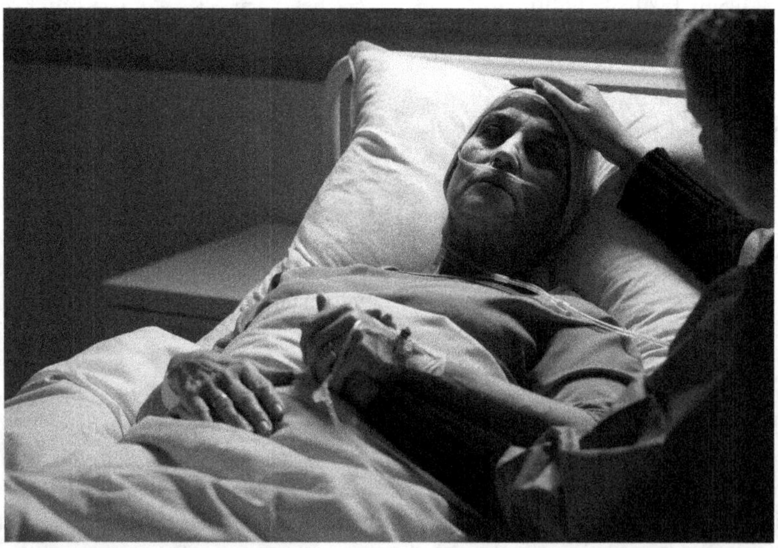

FIGURE 1.4 A patient with cachexia.

by medications. Aspirin increases chances for stomach bleeding, so long-term use may increase the need for iron and other nutrients. Antibiotics may cause the body to become deficient in vitamin K because they can destroy normal flora in the large intestine. Some medications such as diuretics and laxatives impair nutrient use by resulting in excess excretion of water and minerals. Supplements can also affect nutritional status. Large doses of iron supplements can interfere with zinc and copper function in the body. Folate supplements can make a vitamin B12 deficiency less obvious. Therefore, people taking medications must eat foods that are dense in nutrients. Any food or supplement that interferes with the function of the medications must be avoided. Vitamin K can reduce function of oral anticoagulants. Aged cheeses can interfere with drugs used for hypertension and depression. Grapefruit can interfere with tranquilizers and some cholesterol-lowering medications. Patients should always consult physicians, pharmacists, or registered dietitians about restrictions on food or supplements. Table 1.1 summarizes nutrient–drug interactions for common medications.

Test Your Knowledge

1. What are the features of cachexia in adults and children?
2. In which group of people are nutrient–drug interactions most common?
3. What nutrient and drug may interact to cause anemia, due to blood loss?

FOOD ADDITIVES AND CONTAMINANTS

The variety and availability of food in the world today has been expanded by food preservation, processing, additives, and production practices. It is affected by refrigeration, canning, irradiation, conventional farming, organic farming, and biotechnology. There are still concerns that remain about food and water safety. Common foods such as fresh produce and beef may become contaminated with harmful bacteria, resulting in foodborne illness. There is much debate on use of pesticides, antibiotics in animals intended for consumption, biotechnology that genetically modifies animals and plants, and food additives that are listed on container labels. Food additives are often used to improve, thicken, preserve, and flavor various foods. Examples include the following:

- *Ethoxylated monoglycerides and diglycerides* – to improve dough characteristics in bread products

TABLE 1.1
Nutrient–Drug Interactions for Common Medications

Affected Nutrients	Examples of Drugs	Use	Possible Mechanism
Calcium, iron, vitamin B12	Antacids (such as aluminum hydroxide/magnesium hydroxide suspension)	Reduction of stomach acidity	Decreased absorption because of altered gastrointestinal pH
Vitamin K	Anticoagulants (such as warfarin)	Prevention of blood clots	Interference with utilization
Iron	Aspirin	Anti-inflammatory and pain-relieving agent	Anemia because of blood loss
Calcium, potassium	Laxatives (cathartics)	Induction of bowel movements	Poor absorption
Vitamins A, D, E, K	Cholestyramine	Reduction of blood cholesterol	Poor absorption
Vitamin B12	Cimetidine	Treatment of ulcers	Poor absorption
Carotenoids, magnesium, vitamin B12	Colchicine	Treatment of gout	Decreased absorption due to intestinal mucosa damage
Calcium, zinc	Corticosteroids (such as prednisone)	Anti-inflammatory agents	Poor utilization of calcium, poor absorption of zinc
Potassium, sodium	Furosemide (a potassium-wasting diuretic)	To decrease blood pressure	Increased loss
Magnesium, potassium	Hydrochlorothiazide (a thiazide diuretic)	To decrease blood pressure	Increased loss, decreased absorption
Tyramine (in aged foods such as cheeses and wine)	Tranylcypromine (an Tranylcypromine (a monoamine oxidase inhibitor [MAOI]) inhibitor)	An older antidepressant	High BP due to limited tyramine metabolism
High-fiber diets	Amitriptyline	Tricyclic antidepressant	Weight gain due to appetite stimulation

- *Salt, alcohol, and vinegar* – to preserve and flavor foods
- *Xanthan gum* – to thicken foods such as salad dressings

There are more than 10,000 food additives, found mostly in processed foods that are transported over long distances and stored for long periods before being purchased. They help keep the food products appealing, fresh, nutritious, and safe. Food additives are classified as *intentional* or *incidental.* Intentional food additives are added to achieve a goal, such as greater nutritional value, longer shelf life, or better color or flavor. The most common food additives are flavors or flavor enhancers, with over 2,600 used today. Common food additives also include preservatives, food colorings, wax, emulsifiers, sweeteners, and texture enhancers. Table 1.2 summarizes common food additives.

Incidental or indirect additives are not intentionally added. They become part of foods through factors in cultivation, packaging, processing, storage, or transport. They have no function in the finished food product, and they are not listed on labeling. However, some incidental additives have safety concerns. Pesticide residues and arsenic are present in some foods. Another additive, **bisphenol A** (BPA), is a compound found in the lining of certain metal cans, plastic food containers, and water bottles. Nearly everyone in the United States consumes BPA, which is excreted in the urine. However, BPA is an *endocrine disrupter*, altering normal metabolism. It may be linked to damage to the liver and pancreas, thyroid dysfunction, and increases changes for cardiovascular disease, diabetes mellitus, and obesity. Exposure to BPA is most troublesome during fetal development. While the Food and Drug Administration (FDA) considered BPA safe to use, experts do not all agree. Additional research is needed. Today, maybe BPA-free products are available.

Most food additives are synthetic compounds, but this does not ensure they are less safe than natural compounds. Toxicity is determined by an additive's effects in the body, and the amount of the additive that is present. Many plants contain natural toxins that are stronger and present in higher amounts than intentional food additives. Some cancer research reveals that humans ingest 10,000 times more, by weight, natural toxins from plants than in synthetic additives or pesticides. Regulation of food additives is the job of the FDA, according to the 1958 Food Additives Amendment of the Federal Food, Drug, and Cosmetics Act. Color additives were regulated under a 1960 amendment. Food manufacturers must test and prove the safety of new additives, and receive FDA approval, before using them in food products.

Some additives are exempt from this process, such as those called *prior-sanctioned substances*, and other that are on the *Generally Recognized as Safe (GRAS) List.* Prior-sanctioned substances are additives that were approved by the FDA and the US Department of Agriculture (USDA) before 1958. They include preservatives used in processed meats, such as sodium nitrate and sodium nitrite. A GRAS additive is one that can be used safely, according to scientific data, a history of safe use, and the knowledge of experts. Because of safety concerns, some food additives as well as color additives have been removed from the food supply after 1958. An example is *safrole*, a natural flavoring that is used to be used in root beer. Beginning in 1998, the FDA allowed food companies to use a qualified panel of experts to determine their own GRAS guidelines. They are encouraged to report their findings to the FDA, but this is not mandatory. Thousands of GRAS additives, such as spices and vitamins, have many years of history of safe use. Even so, about 3,000 GRAS additives that include 1,000 already determined to be "safe" additives have never been reviewed by the FDA. This is considered a public health concern.

Consuming artificial sweeteners may change the gut microbiota, increasing risks for hyperglycemia and metabolic syndrome. In rodent studies, long-term exposure to the artificial sweetener *aspartame* is linked to increased risks of certain cancers, but research in humans is lacking. The sodium nitrite that is added to cured meats can be converted to carcinogenic **nitrosamines** in the stomach. Therefore, adding ascorbic acid or erythorbic acid to cured meats limits nitrosamine production. Some artificial colors have caused allergic-type reactions in children, increased hyperactivity, and, in animals, have caused cancer. With additional study, many food additives are likely to be reduced or banned.

In sensitive people, some food additives cause adverse symptoms. Sulfites are sulfur-based chemicals used as antioxidants and food preservatives. They cause about one of every 100 people, especially if they have asthma, to have shortness of breath or GI symptoms. Therefore, sulfites are prohibited on salad bars and other raw vegetables. They are used in frozen or dehydrated potatoes, beer, and wine, and are indicated on food labels. Monosodium glutamate is a flavor enhancer that has caused some people to experience chest pain, flushing, dizziness, hypertension, rapid heartbeat, headache, and nausea. Many food companies are reducing the amount of additives based on consumer requests. A good rule of thumb is to always read food labels and remember that more highly processed foods usually have more additives.

YOU SHOULD REMEMBER

While growing, rice plants take in more arsenic from soil than other plants do. This occurs via the irrigation water used when rice is grown in flooded fields, and from farming chemicals. Rice must be repeatedly flush with fresh hot water to remove stored arsenic. Over time, arsenic causes skin pigment changes, lesions, and hyperkeratosis. It can also lead to skin, bladder, and lung cancers, diabetes mellitus, and pulmonary or cardiovascular disease.

TABLE 1.2
Common Food Additives

Type	Example	Uses
Acidic agents	Acetic, ascorbic, lactic, and phosphoric acids	To add tartness; inhibit growth of microorganisms (in beverages, candies, frozen desserts, pickles, processed meats, salad dressings, and salsas)
Alternative sweeteners	Aspartame, sucralose	To sweeten baked goods, beverages, yogurt
Anti-caking agents	Ammonium citrate, calcium silicate, magnesium stearate	To keep powdered mixes and other foods free-flowing
Antimicrobial agents	Calcium propionate, sodium benzoate, sorbic acid	To inhibit growth of bacteria, fungi, and molds in baked goods, beverages, jams, jellies, processed meats, and salad dressings
Antioxidants	Alpha-tocopherol, ascorbic acid, butylated hydroxyanisole (BHA), butylated hydroxytoluene (BHT), erythorbic acid, sulfites	To control negative effects of oxygen, prevent fats from spoiling; used in breakfast cereals, chewing gum, nuts, processed meats; also to prevent discoloration of light-colored foods (fruit, sliced potatoes, white wine)
Certifiable color additives	Citrus Red #2, multiple FD&C colors (Blue #1 and 2, Green #3, Red #3 and 40, Yellow #5 and 6), Orange B	Human-made dyes that are certified by the Food and Drug Administration (FDA) for use in food; found in many different food products
Color additives	Annatto, beet coloring, beta-carotene, caramel coloring, cochineal	Natural colors from animal, mineral, or plant sources; they are exempt from FDA certification, and used in many different foods
Curing agents	Sodium nitrate, sodium nitrite	To prevent growth of *Clostridium botulinum* in cured meats such as bacon, ham, hot dogs, salami; they contribute to the pink color
Emulsifiers	Egg yolks, diglycerides, monoglycerides, soy lecithin	To prevent separation of baking mixes, frozen desserts, margarine, peanut butter, salad dressings
Enzymes	Chymosin, lactase, pectinase, rennet	To affect carbohydrates, fats, or proteins; chymosin and rennet are needed for cheese making, lactase makes milk more digestible, and pectinase improves clarity of some fruit juices and jellies
Fat replacers	Cellulose, modified food starch	Used in low-fat salad dressings and reduced-fat ice cream
Flavors and spices	Include herbs, salts, sugars	Such as fruit flavorings in popsicles
Flavor enhancers	Guanosine monophosphate (GMP), monosodium glutamate (MSG)	To enhance flavor or contribute a savory flavor to foods such as noodle mixes, rice, and soups
Humectants	Glycerol, sorbitol	To retain flavor, moisture, texture; used in energy bars, marshmallows, soft candies
Leavening agents	Baking powder, baking soda, yeast	To add carbon dioxide and other leavening gases for improved texture of baked products (including baking mixes, breads, cakes, and cookies)
Stabilizers and thickeners	Gelatin, gums (carrageenan, guar, xanthan), pectin	To add creaminess and thickness to dairy products, frozen desserts, gelatin mixes, pudding, salad dressings, yogurt
Vitamins, minerals, protein	Folic acid, niacin, riboflavin, thiamin, vitamin A, iodine, iron, various proteins	To add nutrients (to fortify food products and replace nutrients lost in processing)

YOU SHOULD REMEMBER

Types of foods that usually have higher quantities of food additives include precooked, prepackaged, canned, frozen, and instant foods, as well as mixes and snack foods. It is important to limit consumption of highly processed foods, and replace them with fruits, vegetables, whole grains, meats, and dairy products.

Food and water contamination is most common from viruses and bacteria. Less common contamination is from fungi and parasites. Illness can occur when microorganisms directly infect cells of the GI tract or other organs, or secrete a toxin. Foodborne intoxication can occur without a living pathogen to be present in the food, unlike a foodborne infection. Toxin-producing bacteria only have to infuse the food with the toxin they carry. Most pathogenic microorganisms that result in foodborne illness come from an infected human or animal, reaching food via these routes:

- *Fecal contamination* – from being excreted out of infected humans or animals. In areas of poor sanitation, water sources may be contaminated with raw sewage. In the United States, pathogens may spread by fecal contamination of soil and irrigation water from farm and wild animals. It also occurs when food is handled by someone who has had contact with feces or sewage and has not thoroughly performed hand washing. Bacteria can be carried by insects from sewage, onto food. Foodborne illnesses from fecal matter are transmitted by the *fecal-oral route*.
- *Contamination by an infected person* – transferred to food directly from the contaminated person, via open wounds, coughing, or sneezing. Pets can also be a source of foodborne pathogens, if a food preparer comes in contact with them and then does not perform adequate hand washing.
- *Cross-contamination* – when an uncontaminated food touches a food or object that is contaminated – including cutting boards, knives, or plates. Though proper cooking can kill bacteria present on many types of foods, any foods that are not cooked, such as lettuce, easily transfer the bacteria from the kitchen to any person that eats them.

Any food can transmit pathogenic bacteria. The most common sources are meats that are raw or insufficiently cooked, eggs, poultry, fish, shellfish, fresh produce, and unpasteurized dairy products. The most common bacterial causes of foodborne illnesses in the United States are *Salmonella* species, *Clostridium perfringens*, *Campylobacter jejuni*, *Escherichia coli*, *Shigella* species, and *Staphylococcus aureus*. In developing countries, *Vibrio cholerae* is a more common cause. Table 1.3 summarizes the common bacteria that cause foodborne illnesses.

FOCUS ON *SALMONELLA*

There are approximately 2,500 different strains of *Salmonella*. It is a Gram-negative bacteria. Infections are more common in summer months. The bacterium is not killed in the freezing process. The best way of avoiding illness from *Salmonella* is to cook food thoroughly and perform correct hand washing, especially when preparing raw eggs, chicken, and seafood.

Test Your Knowledge

1. What is the difference between intentional and incidental food additives?
2. What can artificial sweeteners do to human gut microbiota?
3. Which foods most commonly transmit pathogenic bacteria?

Most bacteria grow fastest in temperatures between 41°F and 135°F (5°C and 57°C). Though high temperatures can kill toxin-producing bacteria, they may not inactivate the toxins. Most pathogenic bacteria require oxygen for growth, but some *Clostridium* species only grow in oxygen-free environments. In the **spore** state, bacteria can be viable for months to years, proliferating once conditions improve.

Regarding viruses and foodborne illnesses, prevention requires sanitary food preparation practices and cooking food thoroughly. The most common viral causes of foodborne illness are summarized in Table 1.4. Nearly 50% of all foodborne illnesses are caused by *noroviruses*, which are extremely contagious. The *stomach flu* is an example of a foodborne illness caused by a norovirus. Outbreaks are most common on cruise ships, or in hotels, restaurants, and hospitals. A type of norovirus called a *rotavirus* is a significant cause of diarrhea in children. The hepatitis A virus causes liver disease, is spread via contaminated food or water, and can be prevented by hand washing and the hepatitis A vaccine. Immunoglobulin given within one week to exposed individuals can also decrease infection.

Parasites that cause foodborne illnesses are most prevalent in tropical countries with poor sanitation. They appear to be increasing in industrialized countries such as the United States. For example, over 400,000 people were infected by a *Cryptosporidium* outbreak, via a contaminated water supply, in Milwaukee, Wisconsin. There are over 80 foodborne parasites that affect humans. Parasites include **protozoa**, which are unicellular, such as *Cryptosporidium* and *Toxoplasma gondii*. **Helminths** are worm-like parasites. They include tapeworms, anisakis roundworm, *Trichinella spiralis*, and *Cyclospora cayetanensis*. Parasitic infections spread from person-to-person contact as well as through contaminated food, water, and soil. Table 1.5 summarizes parasitic causes of foodborne illness.

TABLE 1.3
Common Bacteria that Cause Foodborne Illnesses

Bacteria	Food Sources	Symptoms	Incidence
Salmonella species	Peanut butter, produce (usually raw sprouts), raw and undercooked eggs, fish, meats, poultry; unpasteurized milk	Onset: 6–72 hours; Symptoms: fever, nausea, abdominal cramps, headache, diarrhea, vomiting, possible death (in infants, elderly, immunocompromised); Illness lasts 4–7 days	Estimated 1.027 million infections per year (about 2,000 strains of the bacteria cause disease, but just three strains cause nearly 50% of cases)
Clostridium perfringens	Beef, gravy, Mexican food, poultry	Onset: 8–24 hours; Symptoms: abdominal pain, diarrhea; Illness lasts 1 day or less, but longer in elderly or infants	Estimated 966,000 infections per year
Campylobacter jejuni	Contaminated water, raw and undercooked meat and poultry, unpasteurized cheese and milk	Onset: 2–5 days; Symptoms: abdominal cramping, muscle pain, diarrhea that may be bloody, fever; Illness lasts 2–7 days	Estimated 845,000 infections per year
Escherichia coli	Produce (lettuce, spinach, sprouts), undercooked ground beef, unpasteurized juice and milk	Onset: 1–9 days; Symptoms: abdominal cramps, and in children under age 5 and the elderly, hemolytic uremic syndrome (which can lead to kidney failure and death); Illness lasts 2–10 days in most cases	Estimated 265,000 infections per year
Staphylococcus aureus	Cream-filled custards and pastries, salads made with chicken, egg, ham, potatoes, tuna; whipped cream	Onset: 1–6 hours; Abdominal cramps, diarrhea, nausea, vomiting; Illness lasts 1–3 days	Estimated 241,000 infections per year
Shigella species	Fecal-oral transmission from foods contaminated by handlers; also from produce and water supplies	Onset: 1–3 days; Abdominal cramps, diarrhea that is often bloody, fever; Illness lasts 5–7 days	Estimated 131,200 infections per year
Listeria monocytogenes	Raw meats and vegetables, ready-to-eat deli meats and hot dogs, refrigerated smoked fish, unpasteurized ice cream, milk, and soft cheeses	Onset: 9–48 hours (for early symptoms) but 3 days to 3 months (for severe symptoms); Symptoms: fever, headache, muscle aches, vomiting; can cause confusion, stiff neck, convulsions, loss of balance, premature birth, stillbirth	Estimated 1,600 infections per year, with 255 being fatal
Vibrio species (the *vulnificus* species causes most cases, with the parahaemolyticus and *cholerae* species being much less common)	Raw and undercooked shellfish (especially oysters), contaminated food and water, human carriers	Onset: 1–2 days; diarrhea, abdominal pain, vomiting; in more severe cases, sepsis with chills, fever, blistering skin lesions, hypotension; Illness lasts 3 or more days	Estimated 95 infections per year, mostly in summer; if sepsis develops, 35% of cases are fatal
Clostridium botulinum	Poorly canned fish, meats, vegetables, herb-infused oils, bottled garlic, honey, potatoes baked in foil and kept at room temperature	Onset: 18–36 hours, or between 4 hours and 10 days; Symptoms: double and blurred vision, drooping eyelids, difficulty swallowing, slurred speech, muscle weakness, paralysis of face, arms, respiratory muscles, trunk, legs; is fatal in some cases; Illness lasts for days to weeks	Estimated 55 cases per year, with 5%–10% being fatal
Yersinia enterocolitica	Oysters, raw or undercooked pork (especially intestines), tofu, water	Onset: 1–11 days; Symptoms: abdominal pain, fever, diarrhea that is often bloody; Illness lasts 1–3 weeks or more	Relatively rare; most common in children under age five (can lead to reactive arthritis, and infections of the heart and kidneys)

TABLE 1.4
Most Common Viral Causes of Foodborne Illness

Virus	Food Sources	Symptoms	Incidence
Norovirus (Norwalk and Norwalk-like viruses), human rotavirus	Any foods prepared by infected handlers; contaminated shellfish, fruits, vegetables	Onset: 1–2 days; Symptoms: severe diarrhea, nausea, vomiting, stomach cramping, fever, chills, muscle aches; Illness lasts 1–2 days or more, but patients should not return to work until 2 or 3 days after total remission	Estimated 5.5 million infections per year (for the norovirus, as little as 10–100 particles can cause infection)
Hepatitis A virus	Any foods prepared by infected handlers; especially uncooked foods, or those touched after cooking (pastries, sandwiches, salads), contaminated shellfish, fruits, vegetables	Onset: 15–50 days; Symptoms: anorexia, nausea, vomiting, fever, dark urine, jaundice, fatigue; may lead to liver damage and death; Illness lasts for weeks up to 6 months	Estimated 1,600 infections per year (children and young adults most susceptible)

TABLE 1.5
Parasitic Causes of Foodborne Illness

Parasite	Food Sources	Symptoms	Incidence
Tapeworms	Raw or undercooked beef, pork, or fish from areas with poor sanitation	Onset: 2–4 months after ingestion of live cysts; Symptoms: abdominal discomfort, diarrhea, malaise	Estimated 20 million cases globally per year, but rare in the United States
Cryptosporidium	Water, or any food contaminated by a handler or the environment	Onset: 2–10 days; Symptoms: severe watery diarrhea, abdominal pain, fever, nausea, vomiting, weight loss; more severe in immunocompromised patients; Illness lasts 2 days to 2 weeks in those that are otherwise healthy	Estimated 748,000 infections per year
Toxoplasma gondii	Raw or undercooked seafood, beef, lamb, pork, or venison; unwashed fruits and vegetables; also from handling cat litter, leading to contamination of foods	Onset: 5–20 days; Symptoms (if they occur): fever, headache, diarrhea, muscle soreness; can spread to the brain, eyes, heart, and other muscles; can be fatal to fetus of pregnant woman; Illness lasts for several weeks	Estimated 86,700 infections per year
Trichinella spiralis	Pork and wild game	Onset: 1–4 weeks; Symptoms: GI problems, muscle weakness, fluid retention in the face, fever, flu-like symptoms; Illness is long since larvae can live in muscles for years	Estimated 40–340 infections per year (greatly decreased because of better pork handling)
Cyclospora cayetanensis	Water, contaminated imported fresh produce, basil, raspberries, snow peas	Onset: 7 days; Symptoms: watery diarrhea, vomiting, muscle aches, anorexia, fatigue, weight loss; Illness lasts 10–12 weeks	Estimated 100–200 infections per year, mostly in warmer regions
Anisakis roundworm	Raw or undercooked fish	Onset: 12 hours or less; Symptoms: violent stomach pain, nausea, vomiting (due to worms entering the wall of the stomach or intestine)	Number of cases is unknown; most common where raw fish is regularly consumed

Molds are fungi that can be carried by the wind or animals. They mostly grow in dark, wet places that have no air circulation. They can grow by sending out *threads* that resemble roots into their food sources, plus the formation of endospores on the outside of the food. The endospores cause the mold to have a colorful, fuzzy appearance, and allow the mold to move to new locations. Foods that are most likely to have mold include breads, cheese, and fresh produce. There are thousands of types of foodborne molds. Some cause allergies or respiratory conditions, and a few fungi produce **mycotoxins** that cause *invasive candidiasis*, nervous system disorders, and damage to the kidneys and liver. The most severe mycotoxins are *aflatoxin*, *ergot*, and those that are produced by the fungi called *Fusaria*. The **aflatoxin** produced by the mold that affects peanuts, walnuts, pecans, corn, and cottonseed can cause liver cancer. Ergot comes from a dark purple-colored mold growing on poorly stored grains such as rye. Several forms of *Fusaria* grow on grains stored for long periods of time, producing deadly mycotoxins. In most industrialized nations, mycotoxins are not a serious problem since food production minimizes the growth of molds. Foods are closely monitored for molds and destroyed if they have them. In other areas of the world, mycotoxin poisonings may occur in Kenya, Africa, where in 2004 an aflatoxin poisoning caused many people to have liver damage and death. Table 1.6 summarizes types of toxins in food sources.

TABLE 1.6
Types of Toxins in Food Sources

Toxin	Food Sources	Symptoms	Comments
		Mycotoxins	
Aflatoxin *(Aspergillus flavus, Aspergillus parasiticus)*	Corn, nuts, peanuts, rice, spices, wheat (especially due to disease or drought)	Acute toxicity: impaired immune function, liver damage or failure, malaise, malnutrition; sometimes fatal; Chronic toxicity: abdominal pain, vomiting, liver failure or cancer; can be fatal	Aflatoxin B-1 is the most common fungal toxin in grains and nuts, causing significant disease; there have been zero human illness outbreaks due to aflatoxins in the United States
Ergot *(Claviceps purpurea)*	Poorly stored grains (usually rye)	Hallucinations, severely constricted blood flow to limbs leading to gangrene, spontaneous abortion, burning and tingling, muscle twitching and contractions	Rare today due to inspections and agricultural procedures; it may have caused the odd behaviors during the Salem witch trials
		Fish and Shellfish Toxins	
Ciguatera toxin	Fish that have ingested a toxin-producing algae (amberjack, barracuda, grouper, hogfish, moray eel, scorpion fish, snapper, surgeonfish, triggerfish)	Onset: 6 hours; Symptoms: nausea, vomiting, temperature reversal, weakness; Illness can last days to years	Unknown number of cases
Shellfish poisoning (amnesic, diarrheic, neurotoxic, paralytic)	Clams, cockles, crabs, lobster, mussels, oysters, scallops	Paralytic onset: 15 minutes to 10 hours (numbness, tingling, respiratory paralysis, death); Diarrheic onset: minutes to hours (nausea, vomiting, diarrhea, abdominal pain, chills, fever, headache); Neurotoxic onset: 30 minutes to 3 hours; (mouth and throat tingling and numbness, muscle aches, dizziness, temperature reversal, diarrhea, vomiting); Amnesic onset: 24–48 hours; (diarrhea, vomiting, abdominal pain, confusion, disorientation, memory loss, seizures, coma, death)	Cases unknown; infection not inactivated by cooking or freezing

(Continued)

TABLE 1.6 (*Continued*)
Types of Toxins in Food Sources

Toxin	Food Sources	Symptoms	Comments
Scombroid poisoning	Anchovy, amberjack, bluefish, mahi-mahi-sardine, tuna	Onset: 2 to several hours (diarrhea, rash, flushing, headache, sweating, difficulty breathing, vomiting) though symptoms resolve quickly	Bacterial decomposition of the fish causes histamine production and symptoms; actual cases unknown but one of the most common seafood-related illnesses
Tetrodotoxin	Pufferfish (fugu) gonads, intestines, liver, skin	Onset: 20 minutes to 3 hours (headache, mouth numbness, nausea, vomiting, diarrhea, paralysis, respiratory distress)	Unknown cases, however, this fish is a Japanese delicacy that is only prepared by licensed chefs
		Plant Toxins	
Safrole	Mace, nutmeg, sassafras	Cancer (if consumed in high doses)	Used to be a food additive, but is now banned
Solanine	Green spots on potato skins, and in potato sprouts	Onset: 8–12 hours (diarrhea, nausea, vomiting, hallucinations, loss of sensation, paralysis)	Preventable, by storing potatoes in dark areas, discarding sprouts, peels, bruised or cut areas, and green spots
Mushroom toxins	Amanita and other species	Onset: minutes up to 3 days; dizziness, hallucinations, other neurological symptoms stomach upset (the most lethal varieties cause kidney and liver failure, coma, death)	Illness is usually from wild mushrooms, occurring worldwide, estimated to affect hundreds of people per year
Herbal teas	Those that contain comfrey or senna	Onset is based on dose and may take weeks to develop (abdominal pain, diarrhea, nausea, vomiting, liver damage)	Though used in folk medicines they are no safe for consumption
Lectins	Usually kidney beans or other raw or undercooked legumes	Onset: 1–3 hours (abdominal pain, diarrhea, nausea, vomiting)	Illness is from lectin proteins (as few as 4–5 raw beans); outbreaks occur when beans are not sufficiently cooked

Test Your Knowledge

1. What are the most common viral causes of foodborne illness?
2. What are the symptoms of infection with the parasite called *Cryptosporidium*?
3. Which aflatoxin can cause liver cancer?

KEY TERMS

Aflatoxin

Alpha1-antitrypsin

Anabolism

Atrophy

Bisphenol A

Body mass index

Cachexia

Carbohydrates

Catabolism

Catecholamine

Celiac disease

Cholesterol

Collagen

C-reactive protein

Cytokine

Fibroblasts

Fight-or-flight

Fistulae

Flaccid

Glasgow Coma Score
Glucosuria
Glycogen
Helminths
Hemodynamics
Hyperglycemia
Hyperkalemia
Hypermetabolic
Hyponatremia
Hypoproteinemia
Indirect calorimetry
Jejunostomy
Kilocalories
Laparotomy
Lipids
Macronutrients
Metabolic syndrome
Metabolism
Micronutrients
Mycotoxins
Necrosis
Nitrosamines
Nutrients
Phenylketonuria
Phytochemicals
Probiotics
Proteins
Proteoglycan
Protozoa
Saturated
Sepsis
Total parenteral nutrition
Trans fatty acids
Triglyceride
Truncal obesity
Unsaturated
Weighed ad libitum diet
Zoochemicals

CLINICAL CASE STUDIES

Clinical Case Study 1

A 31-year-old woman with no significant prior medical history was hospitalized because of severe right upper quadrant pain. She underwent surgery for an intraperitoneal hemorrhage caused by the rupture of a liver hematoma. The patient was then put into the intensive care unit. Even though she was not hypertensive, she was diagnosed with hemolysis, elevated liver enzymes, and low platelet count, based on abnormal blood test results. While in the ICU, the patient was given total parenteral nutrition and enteral nutrition for 19 days, because oral feeding was not practical. Early on, TPN was not sufficient to meet her increased nutritional demand (because of the disease and surgery). Continuous nutritional support enabled sufficient enteral nutrition therapy, and soon, oral feeding. The patient recovered fully and was discharged.

CRITICAL THINKING QUESTIONS

1. In the intensive care unit, how is indirect calorimetry used?
2. When is enteral nutrition usually started in the ICU?
3. How long can a well-nourished patient actually wait in the ICU without enteral nutrition or total parenteral nutrition?

Clinical Case Study 2

A 33-year-old man was hospitalized with multiple injuries from a motorcycle accident. Most of the damage was to the left side of his body: an ischemic left arm from the axilla downward, a left compound femur fracture, and top skin layers torn away from the muscles of the lower left leg. A laparotomy revealed an ischemic right colon and proximal third transverse colon secondary to a possible injury of the right colic and ileocolic vessels. The patient underwent a right hemicolectomy, end ileostomy with mucous fistula, left arm amputation, plus debridement, and insertion of metal rods into various parts of his left leg. The patient was transferred to ICU, intubated, and ventilated. The patient's initial BMI was 34 kg/m^2 (class 1 obesity), but this was adjusted after the arm amputation. Initially, the patient had a nasogastric tube inserted, but he became nauseous soon after and vomited, so parenteral nutrition was started instead. Over time, the patient started to deteriorate, developing uremic encephalopathy, causing reintubation to be needed. His kidney function worsened, and hyperkalemia developed. Eventually, he had a seizure (attributed to uremia). Careful management was able to resolve the issues, though hypernatremia and hypophosphatemia both occurred temporarily. Though it took about seven weeks in all, the patient eventually was able to eat normally.

CRITICAL THINKING QUESTIONS

1. What are the three responses that occur because of trauma to the body?
2. How does a trauma patient's nutritional state influence wound healing?
3. With blunt or penetrating trauma, what type of nutritional support is preferred?

Clinical Case Study 3

A 48-year-old man with chronic myelogenous leukemia is undergoing intravenous chemotherapy and has cancer-related cachexia. Because he has developed sores in his mouth, related to the chemotherapy, it is difficult for the patient to eat. He states that it hurts too much when he chews. The patient is given a medication for his mouth pain plus a mouthwash that contains an analgesic. His diet is changed to be high-protein and high-calorie (though still healthy). He is taught to avoid dry, crunchy, acidic, spicy, and salty foods as much as possible. Many of his foods are cut into small pieces or pureed, and he is encouraged to drink protein-rich smoothies.

CRITICAL THINKING QUESTIONS

1. What are the prominent clinical features of cachexia in adults and children?
2. With cachexia, what occurs over an extended period of time?
3. What does diet intervention focus on for patients with cachexia?

Clinical Case Study 4

An 83-year-old woman had a hip replacement surgery after falling at home. Prolonged rehabilitation will be necessary. The patient has mild dementia, so feeding herself with help is not possible. Her current weight is 80% of the ideal weight for her height. She has moderate wasting of skeletal muscle and fat. Her skin has numerous petechiae, and her hair falls out easily when combed. Since her operation, the patient has been receiving IV fluids with electrolytes. Her laboratory tests reveal low levels of blood urea nitrogen, creatinine, and albumin. Her serum calcium and phosphorus are in the low-normal range.

CRITICAL THINKING QUESTIONS

1. Why is protein so essential after surgery?
2. What foods help reduce pain and inflammation after surgery?
3. Which vitamins and minerals are important to accelerate wound healing after surgery?

Clinical Case Study 5

A 71-year-old man was admitted to a local burn unit after an accident at home. He had burns over 17% of his body. There were partial thickness burns on the lower abdomen, hands, and forearms. The patient's family reported he had developed a chest infection about one week before the accident. Formal IV fluid resuscitation was required at the burn unit. The burns were managed with dressings, plus full medical and nursing care. Any surgical intervention was decided not to be appropriate because of the patient's age, the type of injury, and the chest infection. The patient's nutritional status, energy level, protein and fluid intake, and important biochemical and hematological results were all evaluated to determine the type of nutritional support required.

CRITICAL THINKING QUESTIONS

1. How do severe burns affect metabolism?
2. Why are carbohydrates the preferred energy source for burn patients?
3. What does healthy eating for burn patients mean?

STUDY QUESTIONS

1. Which of the following are NOT energy-yielding nutrients?
   A. Vitamins
   B. Proteins
   C. Lipids
   D. Carbohydrates

2. Which of the following is the source of linoleic acid?
   A. Proteins
   B. Amino acids
   C. Lipids
   D. Carbohydrates

3. Which of the following nutrients is a macronutrient?
   A. Vitamin K
   B. Calcium
   C. Vitamin B12
   D. Protein

4. Triglycerides consist of three fatty acids attached to one molecule of:
   A. Glycerol
   B. Trans fatty acid
   C. Nitrogen
   D. Probiotic

5. Gluten-free foods are used to meet certain dietary needs in which of the following?

A. Phenylketonuria
B. Celiac disease
C. Truncal obesity
D. Cachexia

6. Overnutrition may contribute to all of the following, EXCEPT:
   A. Diabetes mellitus
   B. Cancer
   C. Hyperkalemia
   D. Obesity

7. Which of the following can prevent constipation?
   A. Cheese
   B. Prune juice
   C. Red meat
   D. White rice

8. Nutrition–drug interactions most commonly occur in which of the following individuals?
   A. Elderly
   B. Pregnant
   C. Infant
   D. Toddler

9. Which of the following vitamins may interact with folate supplements?
   A. Vitamin B1
   B. Vitamin B3
   C. Vitamin B9
   D. Vitamin B12

10. Which of the following food additives may be used to thicken salad dressings?
   A. Salt
   B. Xanthan gum
   C. Vinegar
   D. Ethoxylated monoglyceride

11. Which of the following incidental additives found in the lining of certain metal cans may be linked to liver and pancreas damage?
   A. Bisphenol A
   B. Arsenic
   C. Lead
   D. Iron

12. Which of the following additives may change the gut microbiota and increase risks for metabolic syndrome and hyperglycemia?
   A. Sodium nitrite
   B. Sulfite
   C. Artificial sweeteners
   D. Sodium nitrate

13. Which of the following is classified as protozoa?
   A. *Trichinella spiralis*
   B. *Toxoplasma gondii*
   C. Anisakis roundworm
   D. *Cyclospora cayetanensis*

14. The aflatoxin produced by which of the following microorganisms can cause liver cancer?
   A. *Salmonella*
   B. *Trichinella spiralis*
   C. Mold
   D. *Toxoplasma gondii*

15. Which of the following is the food source of anisakis roundworm?
   A. Raw or undercooked fish
   B. Water and snow peas
   C. Pork and wild game
   D. Raw or undercooked beef

FURTHER READING

1. Barth, M., Bell, R.A., and Grimmer, K. (2020). *Public Health Nutrition: Rural, Urban, and Global Community-Based Practice.* Springer Publishing Company.
2. Bender, D.A. (2014). *Introduction to Nutrition and Metabolism*, 4th Edition. CRC Press.
3. Bender, D.A., and Cunningham, S.M.C. (2021). *Introduction to Nutrition and Metabolism*, 6th Edition. CRC Press.
4. Bernstein, M., and McMahon, K. (2022). *Nutrition Across Life Stages*, 2nd Edition. Jones & Bartlett Learning.
5. Biedermann, S., and Olson, D. (2014). *Introduction to Health Information Management.* Paradigm / Kendall Hunt Publishing.
6. Contento, I.R., and Koch, P.A. (2020). *Nutrition Education: Linking Research, Theory, and Practice*, 4th Edition. Jones & Bartlett Learning.
7. DeBruyne, L.K., and Pinna, K. (2019). *Nutrition for Health and Health Care*, 7th Edition. Cengage Learning.
8. Digate Muth, N., and Murphy Zive, M. (2019). *Sports Nutrition for Health Professionals*, 2nd Edition. F.A. Davis.
9. Dunford, M., and Doyle, J.A. (2021). *Nutrition for Sport & Exercise*, 5th Edition. Cengage Learning.
10. Edelstein, S. (2022). *Community and Public Health Nutrition*, 5th Edition. Jones & Bartlett Learning.
11. Frazier, K. (2015). *Nutrition Facts: The Truth About Food.* Rockridge Press.
12. Hayden, J. (2017). *Introduction to Health Behavior Therapy*, 3rd Edition. Jones & Bartlett Learning.
13. Lanham-New, S.A., Hill, T.R., Gallagher, A.M., and Vorster, H.H. (2019). *Introduction to Human Nutrition (The Nutrition Society Textbook)*, 3rd Edition. Wiley Blackwell.
14. Mukherjee, J.S. (2017). *An Introduction to Global Health Delivery – Practice, Equity, Human Rights.* Oxford University Press.
15. Neff, R. (2014). *Introduction to the U.S. Food System–Public Health, Environment, and Equity.* Jossey-Bass.
16. Rawson, E.S., Branch, J.D., and Stephenson, T.J. (2017). *Williams' Nutrition for Health, Fitness and Sport*, 12th Edition. McGraw-Hill.

17. Reeder, A., and Couey, R. (2014). *Nutritional Manual – Discover the Answers to All Your Health Questions (Treasures of Health)*. Designed Publishing.
18. Rosenthal, J., and Chopra, D. (2019). *Integrative Nutrition: A Whole-Life Approach to Health and Happiness*, 5th Edition. Integrative Nutrition LLC.
19. Schmid, R., Fallon Morell, S., and Gedgaudas, N.T. (2015). *Primal Nutrition: Paleolithic and Ancestral Diets for Optimal Health*, 3rd Edition. Healing Arts Press.
20. Schneider, M.J. (2020). *Introduction to Public Health*, 6th Edition. Jones & Bartlett Learning.
21. Sizer, F., and Whitney, E. (2022). *Nutrition: Concepts & Controversies*, 16th Edition. Cengage Learning.
22. Snelling, A.M. (2015). *Introduction to Health Promotion.* Jossey-Bass.
23. Spano, M.A., Kruskall, L.J., and Thomas, D.T. (2017). *Nutrition for Sport, Exercise, and Health.* Human Kinetics.

2 Global Issues with Nutrition

OUTLINE

LEARNING OBJECTIVES

After study of the chapter, readers should be able to:

1. Describe how BMI is used to classify people as overweight or obese.
2. Explain the higher rates of obesity in the United States.
3. Discuss the risk factors for obesity.
4. Describe the primary cause of global hunger.
5. Explain the global prevalence of nutritional problems.
6. Describe protein-energy malnutrition.
7. Discuss the distribution of malnutrition by age and gender.
8. Explain the effects of malnutrition on the quality of life.
9. Describe the impact of malnutrition on the global economy.
10. Discuss the effects of politics on food advertising.

OVERVIEW

There is more than enough food produced to feed the global population, hundreds of millions of people still have issues with proper nutrition or malnutrition. Global hunger is once again increasing, with the number of undernourished people increasing by approximately 50 million per year. This is linked to issues with wars, other conflicts, environmental issues, and the COVID-19 pandemic. Poor nutrition is widely associated with poverty and implicates many social, political, demographic, and societal factors. Poverty-level living conditions often result in food insecurity, poor healthcare measures, unsafe environments, poor sanitation, contaminated food and water, and lack of education.

GLOBAL PROBLEMS WITH NUTRITIONAL ISSUES

Malnutrition in all of its forms is linked to major causes of death and disability, on a global scale. This applies to perinatal, infections, and chronic diseases. While hundreds of millions of children under age five are underweight and many more are stunted, being overweight or obese is also a global problem. Globally as of 2021, one in every nine people has problems with hunger, while one in every three is overweight or obese. More countries today experience a double burden, with undernutrition coexisting with being overweight or obese, plus other diet-related non-communicable diseases. Also, being overweight or obese is a problem in wealthier countries, at rates of as much as five times higher than in poorer countries. The global food crisis is being driven to **famine** levels because of wars affecting the lack of grain exports.

Obesity

Obesity is an abnormal increase in the proportion of **adipocytes**, primarily in the viscera and subcutaneous tissues. It may be **exogenous** or **endogenous**. Hyperplastic obesity is caused by an increase in the number of fat cells. Hypertrophic obesity results from an increase in the size of fat cells. The term *overweight* signifies a BMI of 25–29.9 kg/m^2, and *obesity* is determined by a BMI of 30 kg/m^2 or higher. Body fat distribution can be assessed by waist-to-hip ratios. A ratio above 1.0 (for men) and above 0.8 (for women) signals an increased risk of obesity. Body mass index is the suggested approach for categorizing weight relative to height for adults. Weight in kilogram is divided by height in square meters. The formula can also be calculated in weight in pounds divided by the height in square inches, multiplied by 703. Table 2.1 summarizes the classification of overweight and obesity by using BMI.

People who are classified as *overweight* may or may not appear to be excessively fat. Some adults are overweight due to increased muscle mass. Generally, risks for fat-related health problems increase continuously as BMI exceeds 25. New guidelines recommend the use of waist circumference measurements for a more accurate understanding. For people in the overweight and *class*

DOI: 10.1201/b22969-3

TABLE 2.1
Classification of Overweight and Obesity by BMI

Classification	Class	BMI in kg/m²	BMI in lb/inches²
Underweight	N/A	Less than 18.5	Less than 1605.7
Normal	N/A	18.5 to 24.9	1605.7–2161.2
Overweight	N/A	25.0 to 29.9	2169.9–2595.2
Obesity	I	30.0 to 34.9	2603.8–3029.1
Obesity	II	35.0 to 39.9	3037.8–3463.1
Extreme Obesity	III	40 or higher	3471.8

I obese categories, with a high-risk waist circumference, there must be lifestyle changes to improve health and result in weight loss. Some patients with a BMI of 27.0–29.9 develop extreme metabolic complications, though these improve with weight loss. These patients are candidates for pharmacotherapy and other more aggressive treatments. For example, Asians are at risk for metabolic complications of obesity at lower BMI and waist for circumferences than Caucasians, Hispanics, African Americans, and Pacific Islanders. The guideline for at-risk BMI in Asians is 23–24.

Comorbidities and future **morbidity** are of higher incidence when the BMI is more than 30. The US Food and Drug Administration (FDA) currently recommends that pharmacotherapy be used as an adjunct treatment for all obesity classifications, even without any medical complications. Extreme obesity (a BMI over 40) prompts consideration of **bariatric surgery** after medical treatments have failed. For class II obesity, bariatric surgery may be done if medical treatments fail, and if severe and possibly life-threatening complications exist. Waist circumference should be measured in overweight and class I obese adults. When it exceeds the BMI cutoff points, there must be additional evaluation to detect other risk factors for cardiovascular disease. Class II or class III obese adults have a high-enough risk that makes waist circumference not that important.

Obesity is a global pandemic and a serious threat to public health. Over the past four decades, the number of overweight and obese adults has increased dramatically. Today, the increase in **prevalence** is slowing and becoming more consistent. In the most recent study (2017–2018) by the US Centers for Disease Control and Prevention (CDC), the prevalence of obesity for men and women was broken down as follows:

- Women (20–39) – 39.7%
- Men (20–39) – 40.3%
- Women (40–59) – 43.3%
- Men (40–59) – 46.4%
- Women (60 and over) – 43.3%
- Men (60 and over) – 42.2%

As of 2016, a collection of studies revealed that the global population added an average of 1.5 kg of weight per year, definitely signaling an obesity epidemic. It is estimated that there are now more than 650 million obese people around the world. This is higher than ever before in history and has surpassed the number of dangerously underweight people. As of 2022, there are a total of 53 countries that have populations with obesity rates that are 25% or more. However, the top ten most obese countries have much higher obesity rates than this. The top ten are as follows: the island of Nauru (61%), the Cook Islands (55.9%), the islands of Palau (55.3%), the Marshall Islands (52.9%), the islands of Tuvalu (51.6%), the island of Niue (50%), the islands of Tonga (48.2%), the islands of Samoa (47.3%), the atolls and island of Kiribati (46%), and the islands of Micronesia (45.8%). Figure 2.1 shows the 53 countries of the world with obesity rates of 25% or more.

YOU SHOULD REMEMBER

In the United States, more than four in ten adults are obese. This makes up 41.9% of the adult population or about 139.5 million people. Approximately one out of every five deaths is linked to obesity.

Differences in overweight or obese African Americans, Mexican Americans, and European Americans are very widespread. The highest rates are seen in African American women and Mexican Americans of both sexes. However, this information must include the inverse relationship between socioeconomic status and obesity – especially in women. Females of lower socioeconomic classes are more likely, compared to those in higher socioeconomic classes, to be obese. This relationship reduces the racial differences in obesity prevalence. It is not known if other racial differences in obesity prevalence are because of genetic factors, social factors, or constitutional body makeup.

Obesity is a direct result of a sedentary lifestyle and chronic ingestion of excess calories. However, genetics

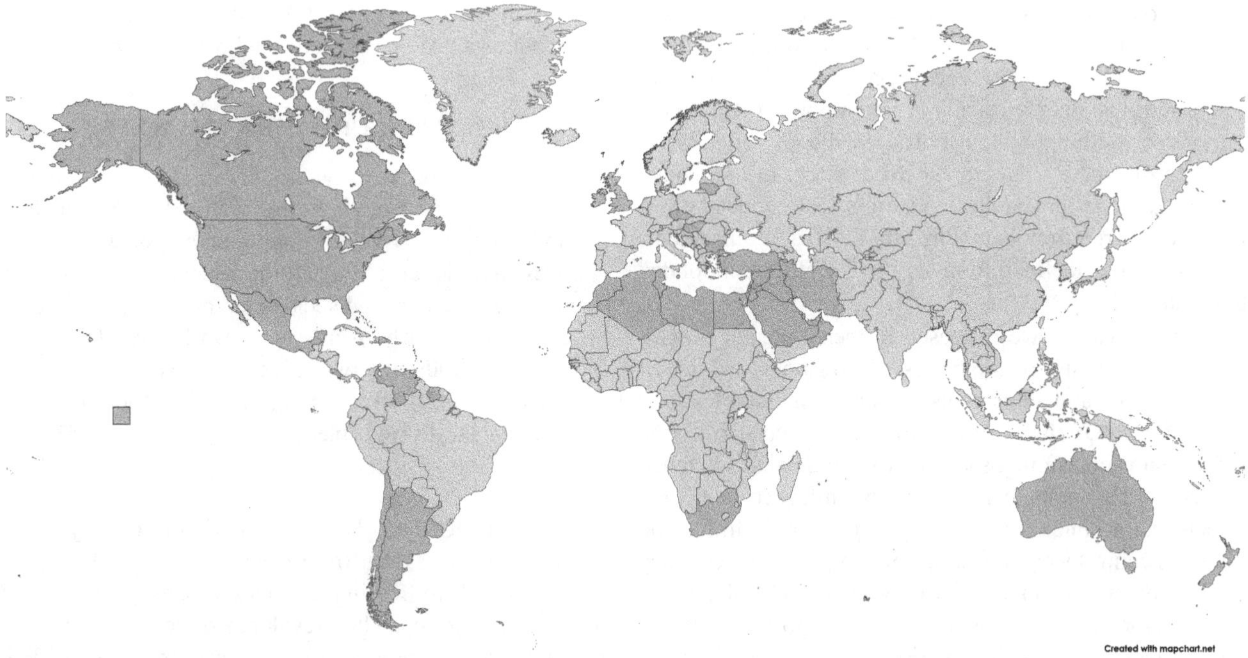

FIGURE 2.1 Countries of the world with obesity rates of 25% or more.

TABLE 2.2
Risk Factors of Obesity

Modifiable	Non-modifiable	Environmental
Energy input Excess calories – from diets that are high in fats and sugars, and also energy-dense	Aging, ethnicity, gender, genetics, menopause, prenatal and postnatal effects, physiologic factors, psychological factors	Built environment Motorized transportation, automation, and mechanization
Energy output Sedentary lifestyle – with low exercise and low physical activity		Food policy Access, availability, cost, marketing, and quality

influence about 40%–70% of obesity cases. Research has mostly focused on social and environmental factors, referring to components influencing dietary intake and physical activity. Other possible contributors include food choices, age, gender, ethnicity, maternal influences during the perinatal period, stress, depression, sleep disturbances, adiposity rebound, food access and marketing, **automation**, mechanization, urbanization, pollutants that disrupt endocrine function, and effects of pharmaceuticals. Weight-causing drugs include corticosteroids, lithium, certain antidepressants, benzodiazepines, anticonvulsants, thiazolidinediones, beta-blockers, and some other antipsychotic drugs.

The risk factors of obesity also include modifiable and non-modifiable components. Therefore, obesity results from behavioral, environmental, genetic, and sociocultural factors. Table 2.2 summarizes the risk factors of obesity.

Environmental factors influence energy intake and expenditure directly or indirectly. Therefore, obesity is linked to food marketing strategies (especially to children) and the round-the-clock availability of cheap foods that are convenient to consume. These foods contain usually high in fat and sugar, extremely processed, contain large portions, and are ready to eat. Excess calorie consumption and obesity have developed from increases in fast-food portion size over history. In the 1970s, in Westernized countries such as the United States, portion sizes increased dramatically but then became even more excessive in the 1980s with the advent of fast-food chains offering huge amounts of food in each "meal". Total energy intake increases with larger portion sizes. "Super-sized" portions have developed mostly because of the public wanting "more for their money". Larger portions mean more calories. A typical 32-ounce soft drink contains nearly 400 calories.

Environmental factors influence physical activity and the expenditure of energy. Our **built environments** either discourage or less often, encourage physical activity. In urban settings, people usually rely more on cars and other motorized methods of transportation. People often drive for long distances to get to and from work. In most businesses, automation and mechanization have reduced physical activity requirements. Physical activity requirements in school have declined from about 45% of the school day to about 25%.

Our behaviors have increased in their sedentary qualities, such as the use of computers, video games, and television. Children and adolescents are simply moving less and sitting more. Often, as these activities are occurring, the individual is consuming snack foods and drinks sweetened beverages. Psychological factors also influence how food affects energy intake. Some people consciously limit food intake to control weight, feelings of hunger, or the tendency to overeat at certain times. Between individual people, these factors modify how varieties and portion sizes of foods affect eating. Social situations in which food is eaten, and emotional states, can also affect food intake.

As of 2010, more than 43 million children were overweight throughout the world. This is more than double the amount (20 million) in 2005 – just five years. Rates of obesity in developed countries are double that of developing countries, but developing countries have many more children affected. It is estimated there are more than 35 million overweight or obese preschoolers in developing countries, but only over eight million in developed countries. In the United States, the sharp rise in childhood obesity resembles the increase in adult obesity. In 1990, the prevalence of childhood obesity was not greater than 15% in any participating state, but by 2010, no state had a prevalence of less than 20%. Figure 2.2 shows the CDC's figures on childhood obesity in the United States for different age groups, and also contrasts differences between boys and girls.

FOCUS ON CHILDHOOD OBESITY

The childhood obesity crisis is preventing many children from having a future healthy life. No one is immune to the risks of growing up as overweight or obese individual. The condition affects children of all races, ethnicities, and socioeconomic levels. Obesity often strikes early in life (ages two to five). Obesity rates for children between six and eleven have more than quadrupled over the past 40 years, and for adolescents, they have tripled.

Recent CDC data show that childhood obesity in the United States has risen from nearly 14% in 1999 to more than 18% in 2016. During this period, obesity rose 33% in the 2–19 age group. The prevalence of severe obesity has remained consistently high in the past ten years (6.3% in males and 4.9% in females during 2015–2016). Childhood obesity is more common in African Americans, Hispanics, and American Indians when compared with Caucasians. In the 12–19 age group, African American adolescent girls had the highest prevalence of obesity (28%), followed by Hispanic girls (20%) and Caucasian girls (15%). For boys, the highest obesity was in Hispanics (22%), followed by African Americans (19%) and Caucasians (17%).

In multi-ethnic four-year-olds born in the United States, 18.4% were obese. The highest obesity prevalence was in Native American children (31.2%), followed by Hispanics (22%), African Americans (20.8%), Caucasians (15.9%), and Asians (12.8%). Childhood obesity also varies by socioeconomic status (see Figure 2.3).

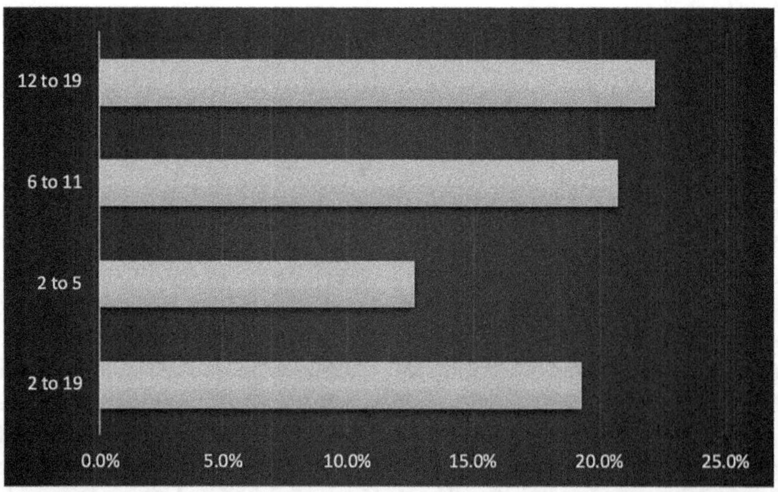

FIGURE 2.2 Prevalence of obesity in children 2–19 years of age, in the United States 2017–2020.

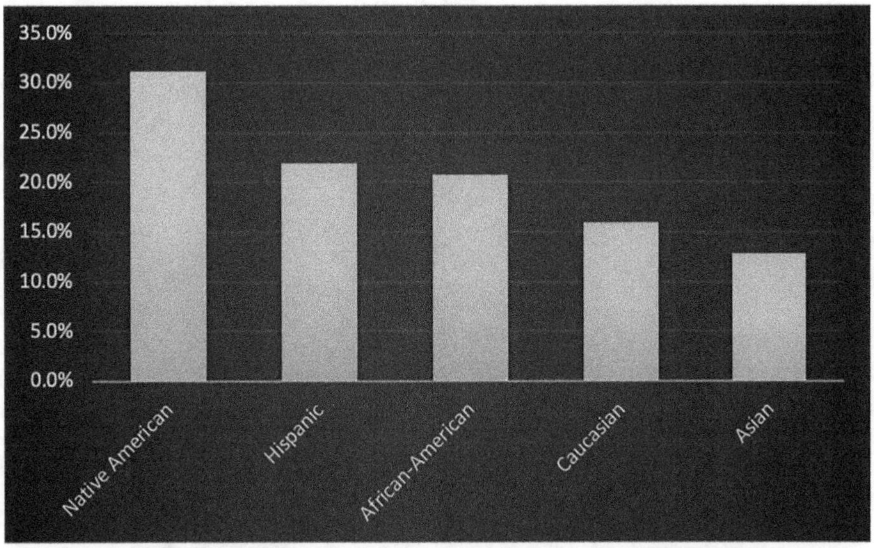

FIGURE 2.3 Obesity in four-year-old children of different racial/ethnic groups in the United States.

FOCUS ON MEAT IN THE DIET

Recent studies recommend that red meat, bacon, or sausage should only be consumed once per week, to reduce the likelihood of heart disease. Other meat sources, such as fish and chicken, are healthier choices.

Test Your Knowledge

1. What is the difference between intentional and incidental food additives?
2. What can artificial sweeteners do to human gut microbiota?
3. Which foods most commonly transmit pathogenic bacteria?

Famine

Up to 811 million people face issues with hunger every day, on a global scale. Between 2019 and 2020, the number of undernourished individuals grew by up to 161 million, largely driven by wars and the COVID-19 pandemic. Also, about 690 million people are undernourished. Fortunately, the rate of stunting in children fell from 33% under age five in the year 2000 to 21.3% under age five in 2019. As of 2022, four areas had the highest rates of famine: South Sudan, Yemen, and the northern parts of Ethiopia and Nigeria. Other areas with significant levels of famine include the Central African Republic, the Democratic Republic of the Congo, Myanmar, Somalia, and the Central Sahel region (see Figure 2.4).

It is important to understand that the primary cause of global hunger is war and other conflicts, which tear families apart, force communities out of their homes, destroy infrastructure, and disrupt food production. For example, because of the war between Russia and Ukraine in 2022, and the fact that Ukraine is a major producer of about 40% of the world's grain, exports of grain have been blocked by the Russians, affecting the entire world. The ten countries or territories with the highest number of people in crisis include the following:

- The Democratic Republic of the Congo – 20.5 million people – decades of civil war have resulted in millions being dead or displaced
- Afghanistan – 14.1 million – about 95% of Afghans do not have enough food
- Nigeria – 12.8 million, with the famine mostly located in the northeast due to food shortages and increasing attacks by the Boko Haram terrorist group
- Ethiopia – 12.1 million – due to the Tigray War brought on by the Tigray People's Liberation Front, which has been labeled a terrorist group
- Yemen – 11 million – more than 2 million children are severely malnourished, with 500,000 at risk of dying without treatment
- Syrian Arab Republic – 9.5 million – up to 6.5 million people live in overcrowded camps, with another 5.7 million have fled to other countries
- Republic of Sudan – 7.1 million
- South Sudan – 4.7 million – the famine is prevalent because of a combination of civil war, widespread flooding with some areas of severe drought, and increasing violence
- Pakistan – 3.6 million – in 2021 and 2022, an acute food insecurity situation hit three provinces of the country (Balochistan, Khyber Pakhtunkhwa, and Sindh)

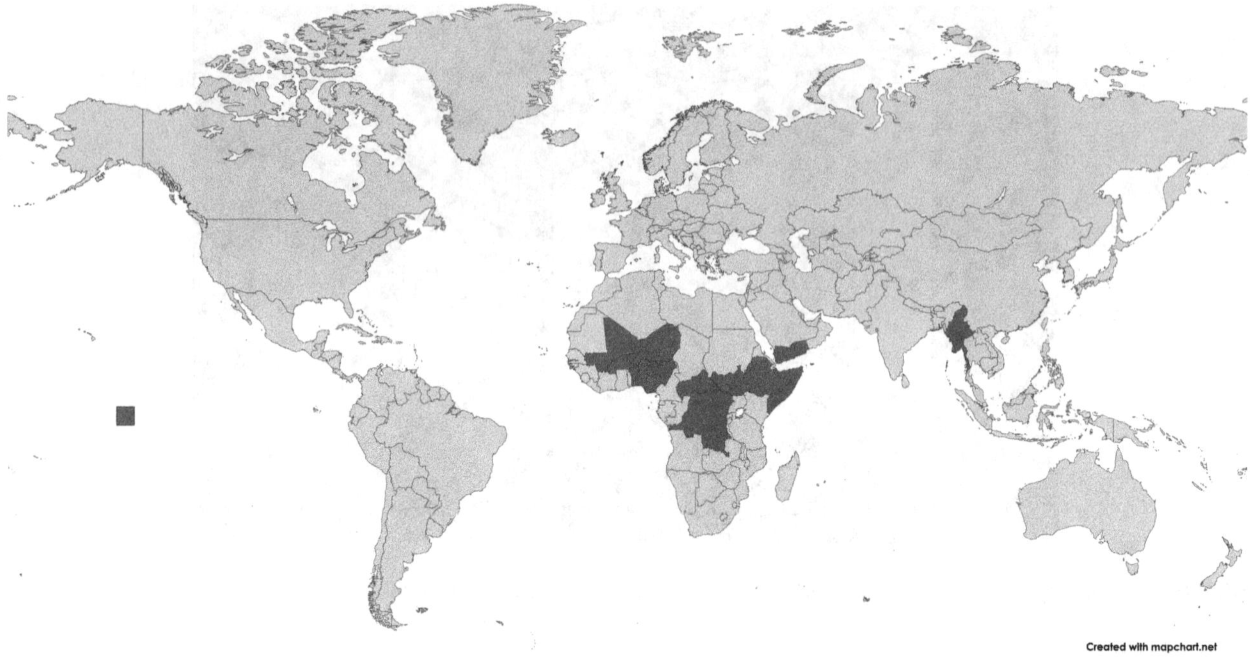

FIGURE 2.4 Areas of the world with significant rates of famine in 2022.

- Haiti – 3.2 million – famine has been heavily influenced by extreme weather events that occurred between 2000 and 2019

Globally, levels of hunger are exceedingly high. Hundreds of millions of people require urgent assistance across a total of 53 countries or territories. This is an increase of almost 40 million people compared to the previous levels recorded in 2020. By 2021, over 39 million people faced "emergency or worse" hunger conditions, in over 36 countries.

FOCUS ON GLOBAL HUNGER

Undernutrition, with less than 1,800 calories per day, has resulted in many cases of hunger throughout the world. *Food insecurity* means a lack of food availability, access, and utilization. Without food security, undernutrition also signifies deficiencies in energy, protein, vitamins, and minerals. Global hunger is increasing and will affect 10% of the earth's population soon. Largely based on the COVID-19 pandemic, the number of undernourished people increased by up to 161 million.

GLOBAL PREVALENCE OF NUTRITIONAL PROBLEMS

A variety of nutritional problems exist around the world. The most common of all is iron deficiency, which affects a total of approximately two billion people. The World Health Organization (WHO) estimates that there are approximately 469 million women of reproductive age, and about 600 million preschool or school-age children that are anemic, and 50% of these cases are caused by iron deficiency. This may lead to increased perinatal mortality, delayed mental and physical development, negative behavioral outcomes, and reduced physical performance.

Following iron deficiency, global iodine deficiency is still extremely prevalent, with nearly two billion people affected. Children and lactating women are most vulnerable. About 50 million people that are iodine deficient present with clinical manifestations. Universal salt iodization programs have only reached about 71% of the global population. The countries with the highest prevalence of iodine deficiency include Madagascar, Cambodia, Lebanon, Mali, Norway, Tajikistan, Haiti, Vanuatu, Burundi, Israel, Iraq, Vietnam, Samoa, Germany, Nicaragua, South Sudan, Finland, Democratic People's Republic of Korea (North Korea), Mozambique, Burkina Faso, and the Russian Federation. Figure 2.5 illustrates these countries.

In developing countries, protein-energy malnutrition is still a significant problem. When malnutrition occurs during pregnancy and lactation, it may result in a negative impact on fetal development. There can be long-term health risks, including risk of obesity, metabolic dysregulation, and abnormal neurobehavioral development. **Kwashiorkor** is most common where there are limited food supplies (see Figure 2.6). It mostly affects children and infants in sub-Saharan Africa, Southeast Asia, and Central America. The most common age group that is affected includes children from the time of weaning off of breast milk until age five. **Marasmus**

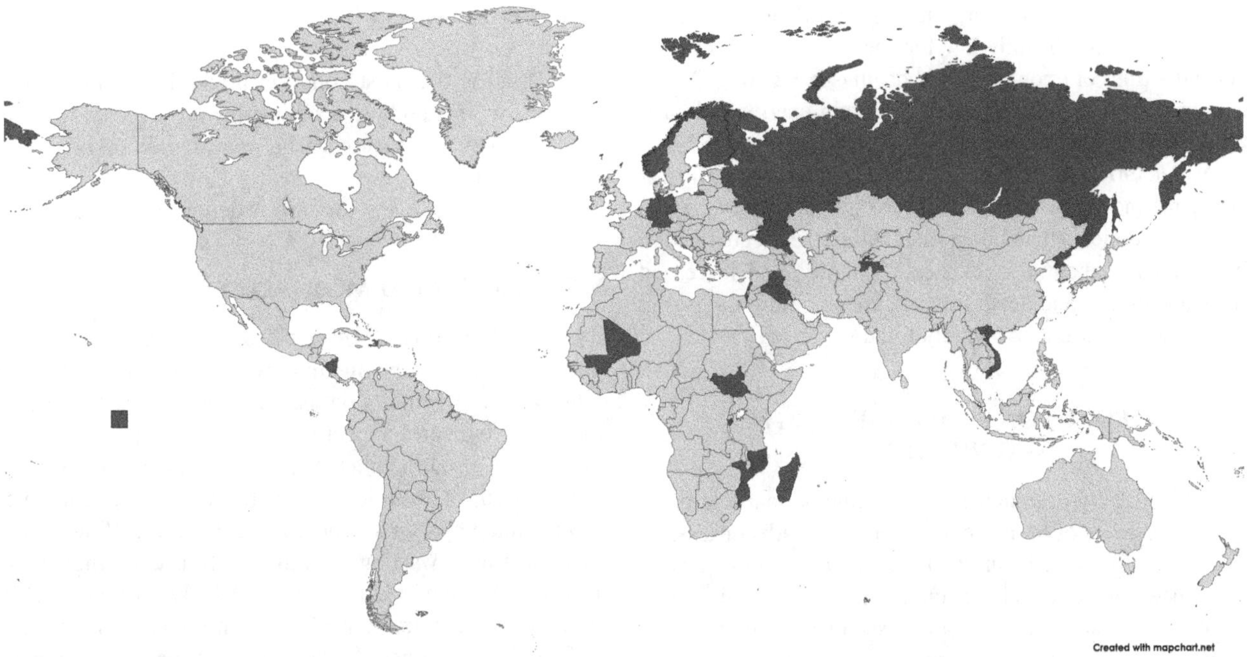

FIGURE 2.5 Countries with the highest prevalence of iodine deficiency.

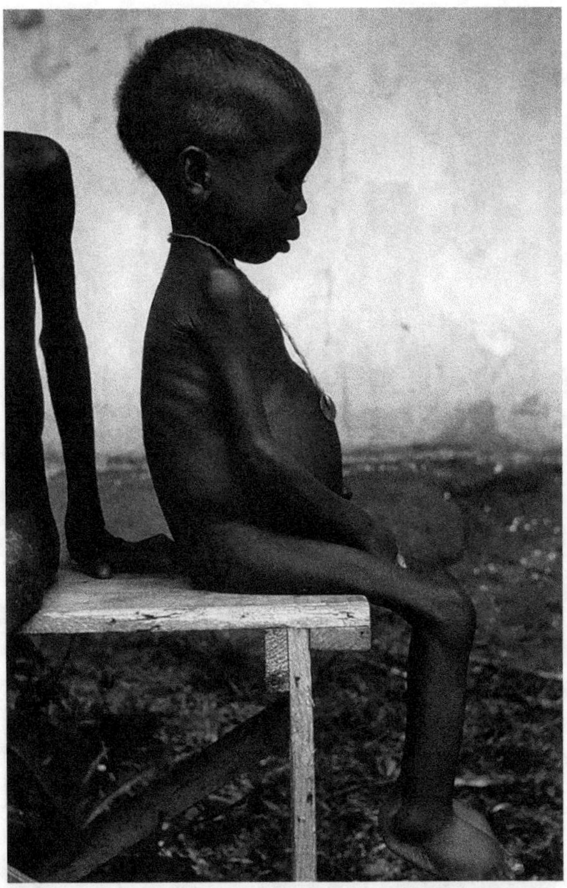

FIGURE 2.6 Kwashiorkor.

is severe undernourishment causing an infant's or child's weight to be significantly low for age, often below, 60% of normal – this commonly leads to death (see Figure 2.7). The countries with the highest rates of protein-energy malnutrition (kwashiorkor and marasmus) are shown in Figure 2.8.

About 190 million children under age five are vitamin A deficient, and about 5.2 million have night blindness. Severe vitamin A deficiency in infants and children can cause visual impairments, anemia, weakened immunity, and increased risks for disease and death from measles or diarrhea. About 9.8 million are affected by night blindness as well.

FOCUS ON PROTEIN-ENERGY MALNUTRITION

Protein-energy malnutrition, an unintentional loss of 10% or more of body weight over six months or less, results in reduced muscular size and strength, plus reduced work capacity or endurance. It is composed of many biological disorders caused by a lack of food. In children, it leads to impaired growth and bony deformities. The condition becomes life-threatening when susceptibility to infectious diseases increases, and normally non-lethal diseases become fatal.

Test Your Knowledge

1. What is the most common mineral deficiency in the world and how many people are affected?
2. What is the difference between kwashiorkor and marasmus?
3. What does severe vitamin A deficiency cause?

MORBIDITY AND MORTALITY

Global malnutrition is still not under control and results in wasting, shunting, being underweight, and micronutrient deficiencies. *Wasting* is defined as "low weight-for-height" and often indicates recent, severe weight loss. However, wasting can also last for a long time, usually because of poor-quality food, or insufficient quantities of food, sometimes accompanied by frequent or chronic illnesses. Without adequate treatment, wasting in children is linked to a higher risk of death. Wasting affected about 7.3% (49 million) of children under five years of age in 2018 throughout the world.

Stunting is defined as "low height-for-age" and results from chronic or recurrent undernutrition. This is usually due to poverty, poor health and nutrition of the mother, frequent illnesses, plus inappropriate feeding and care early in life. Stunted children cannot reach their physical or

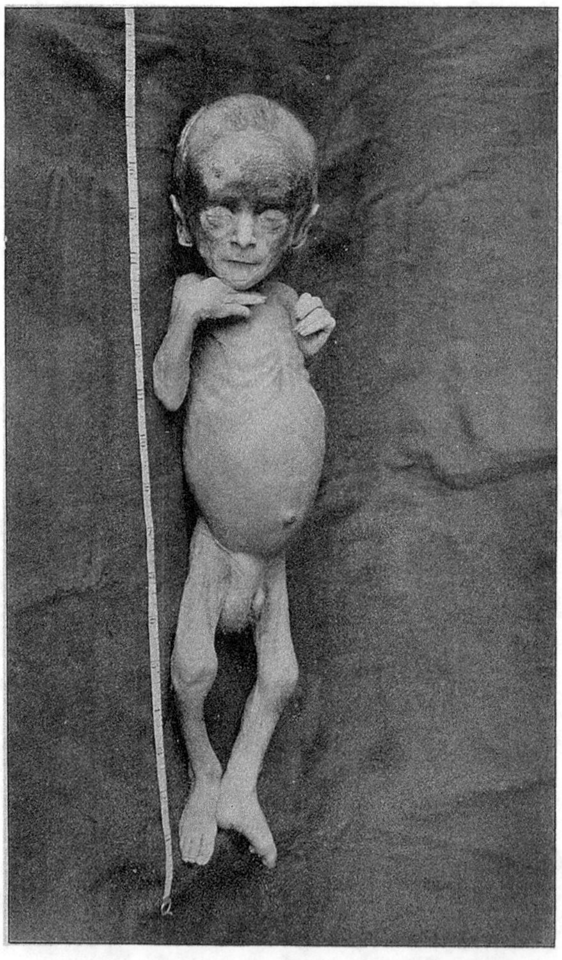

FIGURE 2.7 Marasmus.

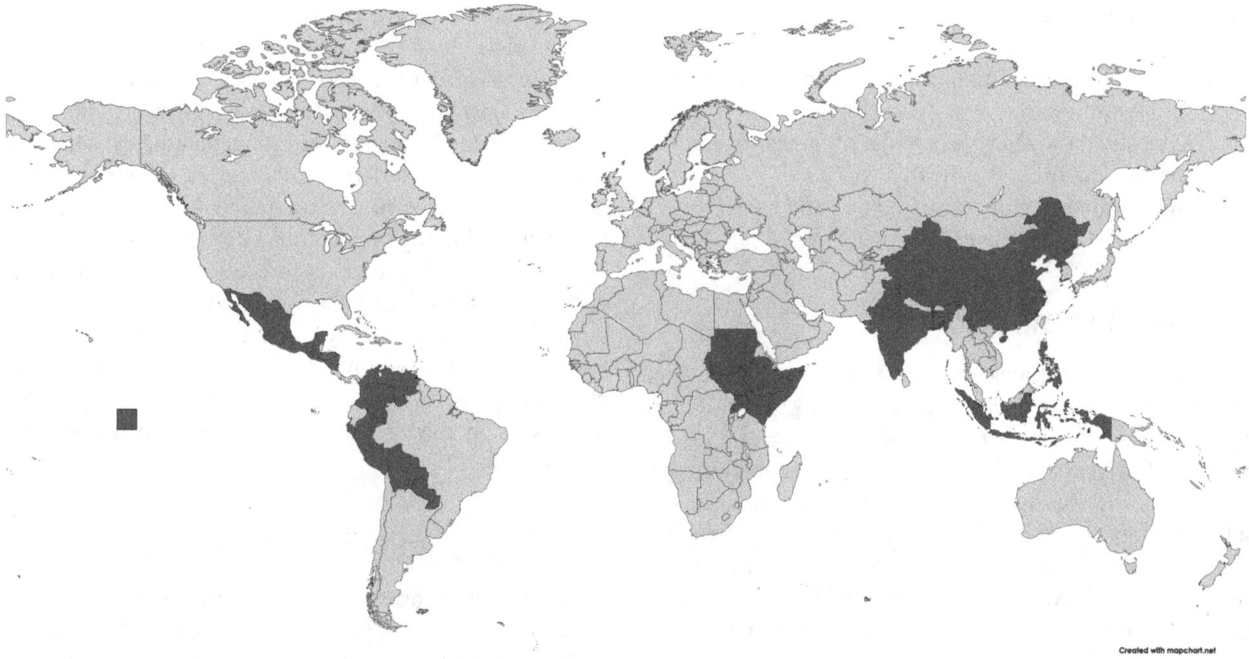

FIGURE 2.8 Countries with the highest rates of protein-energy malnutrition.

cognitive potential. Stunting affected about 22% (149 million) of children under five years of age in 2018.

Underweight is defined as "low weight-for-age", but it may also be stunted, wasted, or both. About 45% of deaths in children under five years of age are linked to some form of undernutrition. This is most common in low- and middle-income countries. Concurrently, rates of childhood overweight and obesity in these countries are increasing. To combat these forms of malnutrition, the WHO has set Sustainable Development Goals to eradicate all forms by 2030. This will require universal access to nutritional interventions and healthy diets. As of 2022, about nine million people die annually of hunger or hunger-related diseases. This is more than from AIDS, malaria, and tuberculosis *combined.*

FOCUS ON THE HIGHEST RISK OF MALNUTRITION

Forms of malnutrition affect every country in the world. Women, infants, children, and the elderly are at the highest risk of malnutrition. Poverty increases the risks for malnutrition and also increases poorer outcomes once it has occurred. Poor people are more likely to be affected by different forms of malnutrition, which increases healthcare costs, reduces productivity, and slows down economic growth.

URBAN VERSUS RURAL DIFFERENCES

In general, people that live in urban locations have better nutritional status than those that live in rural locations. In most countries, urban areas offer greater availability of food, better housing, closer health services, and more variety in types of employment. Utilities such as electricity, water, and sanitation are also more readily available. Even though this is true, recent studies show that urban malnutrition is increasing. In a study of 36 countries, factors that were evaluated concerning less urban malnutrition in comparison to rural malnutrition included women's education and status, available safe water and sanitation, and higher household incomes. In one comparison of rural and urban areas of African countries, focusing on severe acute malnutrition in children under five years of age, the following interesting data were revealed:

- Out of a total of 34 countries, 26 of them had more malnutrition in their rural areas than in their urban areas
- The countries with the largest differences between rural and urban area malnutrition included Ethiopia, Mozambique, Cameroon, the Democratic Republic of the Congo, Namibia, and Guinea
- The differences in percentages of malnourished young children were much smaller in urban areas that had higher percentages than in rural areas; in other words, when rural areas had more malnutrition, the differences in percentages between these areas and urban areas were much larger than the other way around

When Central, Southern, and Western Asian countries were studied for the same data, a reverse situation occurred. Of the countries with severe acute malnutrition in young children, the percentages between rural and urban areas were much more balanced. This may be because the urban areas are much more overpopulated in these countries compared to Africa.

Test Your Knowledge

1. What are the definitions of the terms "wasting" and "stunting"?
2. Globally, how many people die of hunger or hunger-related diseases annually?
3. Which areas (rural or urban) generally have more problems with malnutrition, and why?

ACCESS TO NUTRITION

Though the global prevalence of moderate to severe food insecurity has been increasing since 2014, in 2020, the increase was so large that it equaled the increase of the previous five years combined. Almost one in three people throughout the world (2.37 billion) did not have access to adequate food in 2020. This is an increase of nearly 320 million people within one year. Moderate food insecurity is most prevalent in Africa (33.7%), followed by Latin America and the Caribbean (26.7%), Asia (17.2%), and Northern America and Europe (7.4%). Severe food insecurity follows the same patterns, but with lower percentages: Africa (25.9%), Latin America and the Caribbean (14.2%), Asia (10.2%), and Northern America and Europe (1.4%). Healthy diets are expensive. Coupled with continuing high levels of income inequality, healthy diets cannot be obtained by billions of people – primarily poorer individuals – in all global regions.

The goals of improving access to nutrition involve six general areas, according to the Food and Agriculture Organization of the United Nations. These include the following:

- Integration of humanitarian, development, and peace-building policies in areas where there are wars and other conflicts
- Improving food systems that can better survive in harsh climates
- Strengthening the resilience of the most vulnerable people to economic problems
- Making interventions throughout food supply chains to lower the costs of foods that are high in nutrients
- Solving poverty and structural inequalities to ensure interventions that help poorer individuals
- Promoting dietary patterns that have better impacts on human health

It will be essential to ensure not only access to nutrition on a global scale but to lower costs for nutritious foods as well. Costly, unaffordable healthy diets are linked to increased food insecurity and all forms of malnutrition. Food supply disruptions and interrupting income, because of COVID-19, mean that people across the globe have more difficulties in accessing nutritious foods. It has become more difficult for poorer, vulnerable populations to have access to healthy diets. More than 1.5 billion people cannot afford a diet that meets the recommended levels of essential nutrients. Over three billion cannot even afford the least expensive healthy diet. People that are moderately food insecure do not have regular access to nutritious foods in large-enough amounts, even when they are not necessarily suffering from hunger. Countries that are in food crises have more extreme challenges in accessing nutrition – primarily in countries in which these crises have been long-term. Key barriers to accessing nutrition include distances to food marketplaces, and available time in busy schedules to prepare healthy meals. It will be important in the future to promote healthy, safe food environments, provide physical access to nutritious foods, reduction of unhealthy ingredients in food products, and promote better nutrition education for all.

FOCUS ON FOOD ACCESS

As of 2020, nearly one in every three people did not have access to enough food. This equaled about 2.37 billion people. It was an increase of nearly 320 million people since 2019. The most severe conditions exist in African countries, with 33.7% of the population having moderate food insecurity and 25.9% having severe food insecurity. Food access is most severely restricted in poorer areas, and the lowest socioeconomic levels are unable to afford healthy diets.

DISTRIBUTION OF MALNUTRITION BY AGE, GENDER, AND ETHNICITY

The distribution of malnutrition varies between age groups, gender, and ethnicities. For children in 2020, 22% of all children, globally, under five years of age were stunted, while 13.6 million were wasted, and 5.7% were overweight. For adolescents, the prevalence of stunting was 10.2%, underweight was 5.5%, and overweight or obesity was 21.4%. Approximately 462 million adults are underweight while more than 1.9 billion are overweight or obese. In many countries, including the United States, malnutrition is a hidden epidemic in elderly people, with 50% of older adults being at risk. Malnutrition in people over age 65 is often unrecognized and insufficiently treated. Between 60% and 80% of the elderly that are hospitalized have some level of malnutrition.

In general, women are more vulnerable to malnutrition than men. They usually have smaller, less muscular bodies and require about 25% less energy per day. Even so, they need the same amount of nutrients, so they must eat more nutrient-rich foods than men. However, foods rich in nutrients such as vegetables and protein are often the most expensive. While pregnant or breastfeeding, women need foods that are even richer in nutrients to maintain energy and nutrition levels. Around the world, women and girls represent 60% of all undernourished people. The United Nations estimates that 70% of the people in poverty globally (a total of 1.3 billion) are females. Over 120 million women in developing countries are underweight. In some areas such as South Asia, 60% of the women are underweight while the remainder is not.

The African community is most affected by malnutrition. People from Africa or with African heritage have consistently faced hunger at higher rates than other racial or ethnic groups due to social, economic, and environmental challenges. In the United States in 2020, about 24% of African American people had some level of food insecurity – over three times higher than Caucasian Americans of European background. This is in part related to poverty. The United States has an overall poverty rate of about 11.4%, but in the African American community, the poverty rate is 19.5%. In the non-Hispanic, Caucasian community, the poverty rate is 10.1%.

Test Your Knowledge

1. Where is severe food insecurity most prevalent?
2. In which group of people is malnutrition a "hidden epidemic"?
3. Which continent is most affected by malnutrition?

MALNUTRITION AND QUALITY OF LIFE

Malnutrition has an extremely negative effect on the quality of a person's life. It also doubles the risk of mortality in hospitalized patients and triples it in elderly patients after they are discharged from a hospital. Malnutrition has significantly negative effects on all organ systems, with primary effects on the musculoskeletal, cardiovascular, respiratory, gastrointestinal, endocrine, and central nervous systems. It also has an extreme psychosocial effect. Lack of nutrition also reduces the quality of life because the immune system is depressed, and the likelihood of infections and disease is increased.

Malnourished individuals have reduced muscle function, a loss of cardiac muscle that results in reduced cardiac output, and negative effects regarding renal function. They experience poor diaphragmatic and respiratory muscle function, increased risks for hypothermia, and more episodes of falling and injuries. Malnourished patients recover more slowly from fractures as well. Early stages of malnutrition result in a loss of digestive enzymes, so lactose can no longer be tolerated. As the colon becomes unable to absorb liquids, electrolytes, and normal secretions, diarrhea results.

The complications of malnutrition lead to psychosocial issues because of changes in a variety of social and work aspects, impacting the quality of life. Malnutrition negatively affects daily functioning, and cognitive functioning, and makes frailty syndrome more severe. For people in poorer communities, their quality of life is impacted by malnutrition even more severely, because of a lack of resources and services. Malnutrition relates to social determinants of health that include poverty, economic instability, low health literacy, and less access to affordable healthcare. As well as with undernutrition, being overweight or obese may significantly increase risks for chronic diseases such as heart disease and diabetes mellitus, decreasing the quality of life.

ECONOMICS AND CULTURE

Malnutrition has a huge impact with regard to costs. The estimated impact on the global economy is up to $3.5 trillion every year, which is equivalent to $500 per person. The costs result from lost economic growth and investments in human capital related to preventable child deaths and premature adult mortality. Additional costs come from impaired learning potential, poor performance in school, reduced adult labor productivity, and increased expenses for health care. Direct costs of undernutrition, overweight-related, or obesity-related conditions are estimated to be between $1 trillion and $2 trillion every year. The complete therapy needed to save the life of one severely wasted child is between $100 and $200. Just looking at four African countries, the potential costs to treat child undernutrition alone are staggering, as follows:

- Uganda – $254 million per year
- Egypt – $213 million per year
- Ethiopia – $155 million per year
- Swaziland – $7 million per year

Food habits are examples of old, deeply specific aspects of many cultures. They are not easily changed since they focus on a source of emotional associations. Foods are often ceremonial or social within specific cultures. In relation to nutrition or malnutrition, it is important to understand each patient's cultural beliefs. Food beliefs may have good or bad effects on health status.

Test Your Knowledge

1. Which body systems are most affected by malnutrition?
2. What is the impact of malnutrition on the global economy every year?

SOCIOECONOMIC ISSUES IN DEVELOPING COUNTRIES

In developing countries, socioeconomic impacts are being felt that have long-term consequences that can reverse decades of progress in the eradication of poverty and malnutrition. Exports in developing Asian countries are falling. Population growth in Africa needs to be slowed by as much as 50%. In Latin American countries, 30 million people are close to crossing the poverty line. Global growth, global value chains, international trade, and investment activities are suffering, which will likely have lasting socioeconomic implications.

In nearly all developing countries, wasting and stunting affect the poor much more often than people with higher incomes. In about 33% of developing countries, however, socioeconomic inequality in wasting is limited and not significant. Therefore, socioeconomic inequality in childhood malnutrition in developing countries does not appear to be related to the average malnutrition rate. It is important to take into account the prevalence of childhood malnutrition across all socioeconomic groups.

EFFECTS OF POLITICS ON FOOD ADVERTISING

Due to large financial and political resources, corporations and government agencies that regulate them have a huge influence on food choices and food advertising. Large food companies easily push their products into various cultures and even our thoughts about food choices – usually in an unhealthy manner. Government agencies are often concerned with protecting these companies rather than public health. For example, the US Department of Agriculture promotes the meat and dairy industries while simultaneously giving the public "good nutrition guidelines". Food marketing to children is generally toward products that are unhealthy. The use of cartoon characters on packaging persuades them to want to eat those products regardless of how unhealthy they may be.

FOOD EDUCATION

Schools play an important role in educating students about good food choices to improve healthy eating behaviors. Nutrition education is a crucial part of comprehensive health education. Unfortunately, most school children receive less than 8 hours of nutrition education every school year. Health education and health promotion programs that focus on nutrition and diet are essential for the parents of schoolchildren. Suggested methods for nutritional education include learning counting by using pictures of fruits and vegetables, learning fractions by measuring recipe ingredients, studying how plants grow, and learning about cultural food traditions. Students should also be educated about agriculture, food sources, health, and nutrition. Hands-on learning can include gardening, farm field trips, and cooking lessons. These activities increase their knowledge and prompt them to want to try more new foods as well as eat more fruits and vegetables. Gardening teaches them how to prepare the soil, plant seeds, and harvest fruits and vegetables, and then prompts them to want to taste what they have grown. Healthy eating messages can be incorporated into morning announcements, activities, printed materials, and parent–teacher meetings.

FOCUS ON MALNUTRITION

About 45% of all countries that have submitted data have current undernutrition and overweight problems. Malnutrition is responsible for more health problems than any other cause in the world. More than 200 million children under five years of age are stunted or wasted. Nearly 88% of all countries experience more than one form of malnutrition.

Test Your Knowledge

1. What are the negative socioeconomic issues occurring in developing countries?
2. How does food advertising directed at children result in unhealthy eating?
3. What are the suggested methods of food education for children?

KEY TERMS

Adipocytes

Automation

Bariatric surgery

Endogenous

Exogenous

Famine

Kwashiorkor

Malnutrition

Marasmus

Morbidity

Prevalence

CLINICAL CASE STUDIES

Clinical Case Study 1

A 46-year-old man is concerned because of his excessive weight, which is 40 pounds more than he weighed in college. His family history is troublesome: his father died of a heart attack, his brother has already had one heart attack, and his sister has high cholesterol. Both his parents and all of his grandparents had problems with high cholesterol. His physician encourages him to start a new diet and exercise program, which he agrees to. The dietitian that implements the new diet advises him to eat smaller meals during the day, but more often, to help balance his glucose and avoid him becoming "starved" by the time he gets home from work. The patient's new exercise program starts slowly so that he can adjust to making time for walking and swimming. Over time, it increases in intensity as he begins to lose weight and feel much better.

CRITICAL THINKING QUESTIONS

1. What are the risk factors for obesity?
2. Why has decreased physical activity become so prevalent?
3. What is the prevalence of obesity in men of different ages?

Clinical Case Study 2

A 31-year-old mother of two girls lived with them in an old trailer in a rural section of Florida. She had been employed as a certified nursing assistant for ten years, a job that she enjoyed but that did not pay very well. The woman continued to search for a better-paying job so that she and her girls could move to a better living situation. From time to time, the woman had to skip meals to feed her daughters. She received some assistance from a local food bank, but constantly worried about where their next meals were coming from.

CRITICAL THINKING QUESTIONS

1. What does food insecurity mean?
2. In malnourished children, what does "wasting" mean?
3. Is access to nutrition becoming better or worse?

STUDY QUESTIONS

1. An increase in the number of adipocytes is referred to as:
   A. Hypertrophic obesity
   B. Subcutaneous obesity
   C. Hyperplastic obesity
   D. Famine

2. Comorbidities of being overweight have a higher incidence when the BMI is more than:
   A. 20
   B. 24
   C. 27
   D. 30

3. The highest rates of being overweight, in women in the United States, are seen in the:
   A. Mexican Americans
   B. African Americans
   C. Asian Americans
   D. European Americans

4. Which of the following is NOT a direct cause of obesity?
   A. Genetic influence
   B. Sedentary lifestyle
   C. Excess physical activity
   D. Chronic ingestion of excess calories

5. Childhood obesity is less common in which of the following ethnic groups?
   A. Caucasians
   B. African Americans
   C. Hispanics
   D. Native Americans

6. Which of the following is the most common of all nutritional deficiencies around the world?
   A. Protein
   B. Calcium
   C. Iron
   D. Vitamin B12

7. The most common age group affected by kwashiorkor is from:
   A. Birth to one year
   B. One to three years
   C. One to four years
   D. One to five years

8. Which of the following causes marasmus?
   A. Lipid energy malnutrition
   B. Protein-energy malnutrition
   C. Iodine deficiency
   D. Vitamin B12 deficiency

9. Protein-energy malnutrition leads to impaired growth, and which of the following?
   A. Bone deformity
   B. Fatty liver
   C. Kidney failure
   D. Hypertension

10. Iron deficiency may to all of the following, EXCEPT:
    A. Increased perinatal mortality
    B. Delayed mental development
    C. Hypothyroidism
    D. Negative behavioral outcomes

11. Which of the following terms is used when an individual's BMI is 16?
    A. Normal
    B. Underweight
    C. Overweight
    D. Underline obesity

12. Which of the following BMI numbers may mean that bariatric surgery is necessary?
    A. 25
    B. 29
    C. 32
    D. 42

13. Which of the following drugs will not cause a person to become overweight?
    A. Ibuprofen
    B. Corticosteroids
    C. Lithium
    D. Benzodiazepine

14. A typical 32-ounce soft drink contains about how many calories?
    A. 400
    B. 250
    C. 180
    D. 120

15. Which of the following age groups of children in the United States has the highest prevalence of obesity?
    A. 2 to 5
    B. 6 to 11
    C. 12 to 14
    D. 12 to 19

FURTHER READING

1. Andrews Henningfeld, D. (2009). *Famine (Global Viewpoints)*. Greenhaven Press.
2. Armstrong-Mensah, E.A. (2019). *Global Health: Issues, Challenges, and Global Action – Lecture Notes*. Wiley Blackwell.
3. Barilla Center for Food & Nutrition, and Nierenberg, D. (2018). *Nourished Planet – Sustainability in the Global Food System*, 2nd Edition. Island Press.
4. Barth, M., Bell, R.A., and Grimmer, K. (2020). *Public Health Nutrition: Rural, Urban, and Global Community-Based Practice*. Springer.
5. Eaton Dyer, J., and Falsani, C. (2019). *The End of Hunger: Renewed Hope for Feeding the World*. IVP Books.
6. Fanzo, J., and Davis, C. (2021). *Global Food Systems, Diets, and Nutrition: Linking Science, Economics, and Policy*. Palgrave Macmillan.
7. Food Forum, Food and Nutrition Board, Health and Medicine Division, and Medicine National Academies of Sciences, Engineering, Pray, L. (2016). *Food Literacy: How Do Communications and Marketing Impact Consumer Knowledge, Skills, and Behavior? Workshop Summary*. National Academies Press.
8. Gaimard, M. (2014). *Population and Health in Developing Countries – Demographic Transformation and Socio-Economic Development 2*. Springer.
9. Haerens, M. (2011). *Obesity (Global Viewpoints)*. Greenhaven Press.
10. MacDonald, R., and Reitmeier, C. (2017). *Understanding Food Systems – Agricultures, Food Science, and Nutrition*. Academic Press.
11. McLaren, S.W. (2022). *Nutrition and Global Health*. Wiley Blackwell.
12. Ndayizigamiye, P., Barlow-Jones, G., Brink, R., Bvuma, S., Minty, R., and Mhlongo, S. (2020). *Perspectives on ICT4D and Socio-Economic Growth Opportunities in Developing Countries*. IGI Global.
13. Nestle, M., and Pollan, M. (2013). *Food Politics: How the Food Industry Influences Nutrition and Health* (Volume 3). University of California Press.
14. Parker, C. (2014). *Nutrition & Science (Nutrition: A Global View)*. Village Earth Press.
15. Rahman, A. (2020). *Malnutrition: Prevalence, Risk Factors, and Outcomes*. Nova Science Publishers Inc.
16. Simone, J. (2014). *Nutrition and Politics (Nutrition: A Global View)*. Village Earth Press.
17. Simons, R. (2014). *Nutrition and Poverty (Nutrition: A Global View)*, 2nd Edition. Village Earth Press.
18. Stein, N. (2014). *Public Health Nutrition: Principles and Practice in Community and Global Health*. Jones & Bartlett Learning.
19. Sturtz Sreetharan, C., Brewis, A., Hardin, J., Trainer, S., and Wutich, A. (2021). *Fat in Four Cultures: A Global Ethnography of Weight*. University of Toronto Press.
20. Walker, I. (2016). *Nutrition and You (Nutrition: A Global View)*. Village Earth Press.

Part II

Implications of Nutrition for Special Populations

3 Newborns and Premature Infants

OUTLINE

LEARNING OBJECTIVES

After study of the chapter, readers should be able to:

1. Discuss daily fluids and calories needed for newborns.
2. Describe the basal metabolic rates of infants.
3. Explain physical growth during adolescence.
4. Describe body composition during growth in children.
5. Explain the effects of parental diet upon offspring.
6. Describe the purpose of growth charts.
7. Explain the advantages of breastfeeding.
8. Discuss alternative feeding and its disadvantages.
9. Explain baby bottle syndrome and its prevention.
10. Describe failure to thrive.

OVERVIEW

Major advances in medical and nutritional care have enormously reduced the nutritional problems and improved the survival rates of high-risk preterm and sick newborn infants. Research has shown that babies born prematurely have poor postnatal growth. Very early prematurity usually means that the impairment will be more severe and will persist for a longer time. Adequate nutrition is often difficult or impossible to achieve in these infants. In most immature infants, growth retardation continues for months. It is possible that the catch-up growth can deviate from the normal percentiles on the growth chart and the ability to achieve a near-normal percentile could be delayed and incomplete. Preterm infants are shorter and lighter than full-term infants. Reduced stature and head size may result in lower intelligence. Though better growth is linked to improved neurodevelopmental outcomes, this can be achieved with dietary manipulation. There also may be a link between increased postnatal growth and increased morbidity and mortality in childhood and adult life. This chapter provides an overview of the current understanding of growth impairment in infants and the effects in later life.

NEWBORNS

A *newborn* is considered to be a baby between birth and one to two months of age. Successful breastfeeding is improved by allowing the newborn to nurse as soon as possible after delivery. Many infants spit up mucus after feeding because the gastroesophageal smooth muscle are slack, although this normally stops within two days. If mucus continues to be brought up, vomiting occurs past two days, or the vomit is **bilious**, a thorough evaluation of the upper gastrointestinal (GI) and respiratory tracts is required, to find any congenital anomalies.

Daily fluid and calorie needs are varied with age but are proportionately greater in newborns than in older children and adults. Newborns must be fed on demand, which is usually 8–12 times per day. The average intake for each feeding in the first few days is often 15–30 mL. After two days, feeding is adequate when the infant appears to be satisfied after each "meal", with six to eight wet diapers and regular bowel movements per day, adequate sleep, staying alert while awake, and gaining weight. Nutritional recommendations are usually not based on evidence. Vitamin needs are based on breast milk versus standard infant formula, the mother's diet, and daily intake. Undernutrition is signified by a loss of 5%–7% of weight in the first week. Birthweight should be regained by two weeks if the infant is breastfed, but early if given formula.

A review of demographic and health survey data in 54 countries revealed a high prevalence of infants at risk of malnutrition under six months of age, as follows:

- 21.3% of infants are **wasted**
- 20.1% of infants are underweight
- 17.8% of infants were born with a low birthweight
- 17.6% of infants are stunted

DOI: 10.1201/b22969-5

PREMATURE INFANTS

Premature birth is defined as a baby born before the 37th week of pregnancy. Prematurity is defined by the **gestational age** at birth. In previous years, any infant weighing less than 5.5 lbs (2.5 kg) was called premature. Though premature infants are usually smaller, this definition, based on weight, is not correct. Many infants that weigh less than this are mature or *post-term and postmature* as well as being *small for gestational age*. They have different appearances and problems. As of 2020, approximately 10% of births are premature, which is higher than in previous years. About 27% are called *early term*, which has also increased. Premature infants, including late preterm infants that may be the size of some full-term infants, have higher rates of morbidity and mortality compared to full-term infants. Categories of premature infants include the following:

- *Extremely preterm* – less than 28 weeks of gestation
- *Very preterm* – 28 weeks to 31 weeks, 6 days
- *Moderately preterm* – 32 weeks to 33 weeks, 6 days
- *Late preterm* – 34 weeks to 36 weeks, 6 days

A precise assessment of growth versus gestational age is given by the **Fenton growth chart** (see Figure 3.1). Premature infants are categorized by birthweight as the following:

- *Extremely low birthweight* – less than 2.2 pounds (1,000 grams)
- *Very low birthweight* – 2.2 to 3.3 pounds (1,000 to 1,499 grams)
- *Low birthweight* – 3.31 to 5.5 pounds (1,500 to 2,500 grams)

The risks for prematurity include having previously delivered a premature baby, multiple-birth pregnancies, use of tobacco or alcohol, substance abuse, and a period of less than 18 months between pregnancies. With premature births, there is an increased risk of complications. These include **jaundice**, kidney problems, infections, breathing problems, heart and brain problems, cerebral palsy, vision and hearing problems, dental abnormalities, behavioral conditions, impaired cognitive function, and chronic health conditions. In premature babies, the most common type of jaundice is referred to as *exaggerated physiologic jaundice*, in which the liver is unable to remove bilirubin from the body. The skin takes on a yellowish tint. If the bilirubin level is too high, it can cause bilirubin toxicity and brain damage (**kernicterus**). Phototherapy is generally started before the level gets too high. This involves placing the baby under bright lights, which helps break down the bilirubin, for less than a week.

Kidney problems include fluids, electrolytes, and wastes often occur within the first four to five days after delivery, especially if the baby was born less than 28 weeks into gestation. A neonatal intensive care unit will carefully record the amount of urine the baby produces, and blood levels of **creatinine**, potassium, and urea. Care is taken if antibiotics are required because it must be ascertained whether the medications will be properly excreted. Sometimes, fluid intake must be restricted or enhanced so that blood substances do not become overly concentrated. Generally, fluid and salt restriction is effective as the immature kidneys of the baby improve and being to function normally.

Premature babies may develop infections anywhere in the body. They are difficult to treat because there is less immune system development and fewer antibodies from the mother, compared to full-term infants. Also, premature infants often require a variety of medical procedures, including insertion of a catheter, IV line, endotracheal tube, and ventilator – each of these increases the chance of infections. Signs of infection include lack of alertness or activity, difficulty feeding, poor muscle tone, body temperature fluctuations, jaundice, pallor, spotting of the skin color, bradycardia, and apnea. Treatments include antibiotics, IV fluids, mechanical ventilation, and oxygen. Most infants respond well to treatments, but the earlier treatment begins, the better the chance of recovery from the infection.

Breathing problems are common in premature infants because the lungs often lack **surfactant**. Without this liquid, the lungs cannot expand and contract normally, increasing the risks for **respiratory distress syndrome**. Some infants also develop apnea, with breathing pauses lasting for 20 seconds or more. A ventilator may be required, but being on a ventilator for a long time increases the risk of **bronchopulmonary dysplasia**. Even though long-term use of a ventilator can injure the lungs, the infant may still require continued oxygen therapy and ventilator support. **Patent ductus arteriosus** is the most common heart condition in premature infants. Indomethacin can be used, which causes the ductus arteriosus to close.

Cerebral palsy may occur in premature infants. It affects muscle tone and coordination, movement, and balance. Regarding vision problems, premature infants are at risk for *retinopathy*, which can cause gradual retinal scarring and detachment. This increases the risk of vision loss or blindness. Hearing problems range from a minor loss to deafness and may be of unknown cause in premature infants. Hearing tests are done in the hospital or an outside facility after discharge. Later signs of hearing loss include not being startled by loud sounds, not imitating sounds by the age of six months, not babbling by the age of one year, and not turning to face parents when their voices are heard. Treatments for hearing loss include ear tubes, hearing aids, surgery, and cochlear implants.

Dental problems can affect premature infants later in life and include tooth discoloration, delayed tooth growth, and improper alignment. Fortunately, these can be corrected by a pediatric dentist. Children born prematurely are also more likely to have behavioral or psychological problems. Chronic health problems that affect premature infants include asthma, feeding difficulties, and **sudden infant death syndrome** (SIDS).

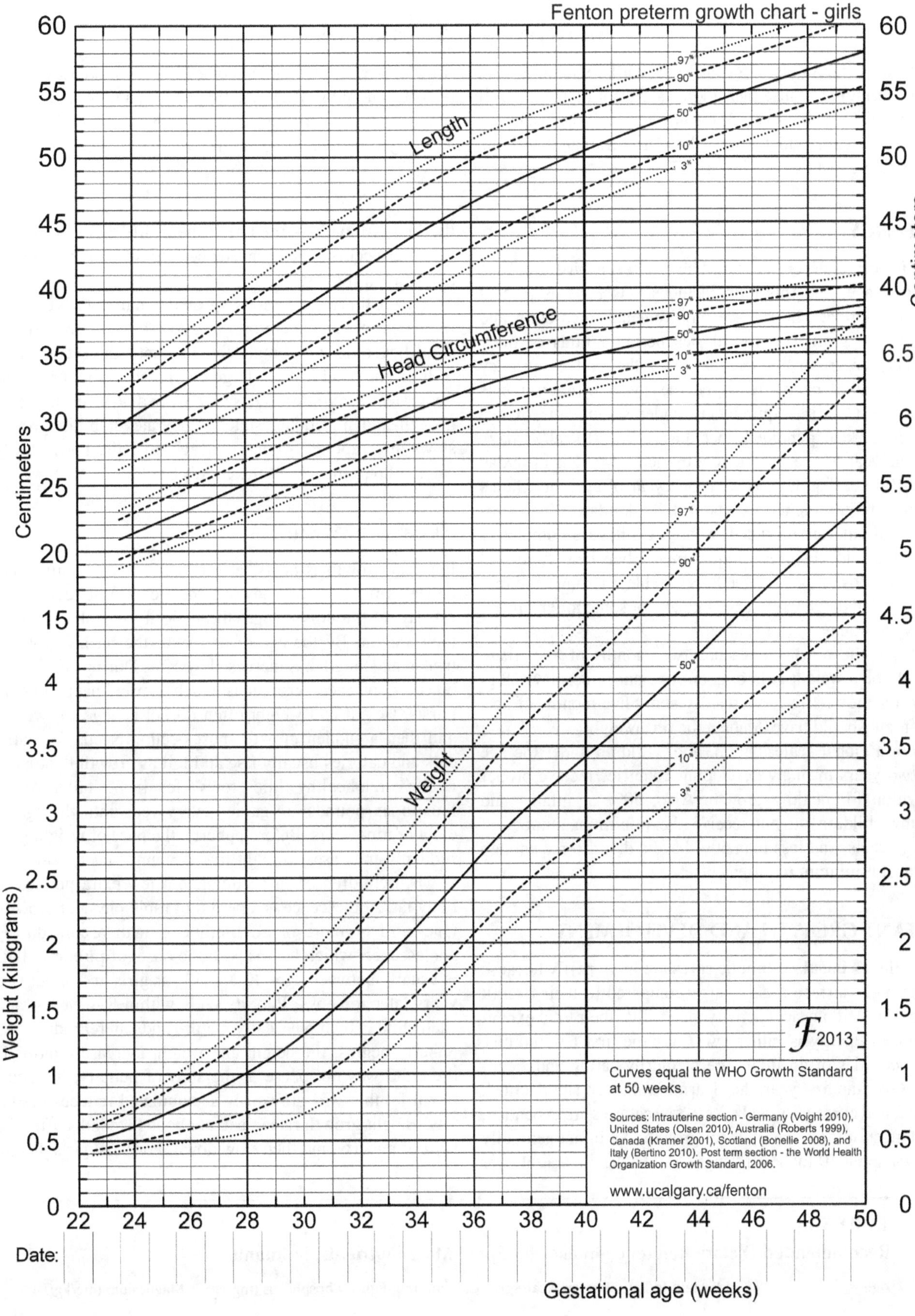

FIGURE 3.1 The Fenton growth charts for girls and boys.

FOCUS ON INFANT NUTRITION

Infants should not be given water until six months after birth. Their hydration should come only from breast milk or formula because their kidneys are not mature until the age of six months. Their small stomachs and developing kidneys put them at risk for nutrient loss and water intoxication. Water intoxication results in excess water in the bloodstream, which lowers the concentration of sodium, potentially causing hyponatremia, which can lead to brain swelling and death.

INFANCY

An **infant** is described as a baby between birth and one year of age, and this term includes *newborns* as part of its description. The relative requirements for protein and energy, in grams or kilocalories per kilograms of body weight, progressively decline from the end of infancy through adolescence. However, the absolute requirements increase. Calorie requirements under six months of age are 50–55 kcal per pound per day (110–120 kcal/kg/day). At one year of age, calorie requirements are 45 kcal/lb/day (95–100 kcal/kg/day). Also at one year of age, an infant's protein requirements are about 1.2 g/kg/day. When protein and calories provided by breast milk are completely digested and absorbed, requirements between three and nine months of age may be lower. Table 3.1 shows the recommended dietary reference intakes for some **macronutrients**, in infants.

Once the newborn reaches two months of age, there should be a weight gain of about one ounce per day (28 g/day) for the first few months. By about five months of age, an infant should have doubled the birthweight.

On a global scale, only 33% of children under the age of two years in many developing countries receive proper nutrition for healthy growth. Also, 50% of infants and young children do not receive the minimum number of daily meals, and less than 50% have a diet diverse enough to meet minimum requirements.

INFANT GROWTH AND DEVELOPMENT

An infant's **basal metabolic rates** are high, partly because their body surface area is large compared to their overall size. Limited physical activity means that their total expenditure of energy is rather low. Over the first few months, the activities of an infant are primarily eating and sleeping. Over the first year, they learn to roll over, sit up, crawl, stand, and eventually, walk. Very few calories are expended, and most of their energy is for growth. An infant generally grows about 10 inches in length and triples in weight over the first 12 months – the only time in life this fast growth rate ever occurs. Energy needs per unit of body weight are also at their highest.

During this rapid period of growth, an infant's brain also increases in size. Therefore, to allow for this growth, the skull bones do not completely fuse until the second year of life. The head is quite large compared to the rest of the body. Head circumference is used by pediatricians to assess growth and nutritional status. The rate of brain growth slows after about 18 months of age, and the body slowly catches up to the size of the child's head.

HEIGHT AND WEIGHT

Physical growth is at its fastest in infancy, meaning that nutrients per unit of body weight are also at their highest. By six months of age, the majority of babies double their weight. By the age of one year, the birthweight has tripled and length has increased by 50%. During childhood, however, physical growth is much slower, happening in bursts. Height and weight often do not change for weeks, and then a sudden growth spurt occurs. Needs for nutrients and calories usually rise and fall as growth fluctuates. Each year, a healthy child grows a few inches taller. About four to six pounds are gained every year until the age of eight or nine years. Before puberty, the pace of weight gain suddenly increases to eight to ten pounds each year, and is when children often accumulate a few extra pounds of body fat. Adolescence is a period of rapid physical growth. One-third or more of all lifetime growth occurs during adolescence, which begins with the onset of **puberty**. This is usually between ages 10 and 13 for girls and about two years later for boys. Puberty ends within 8–10 years, and each child is then physically mature and can reproduce. As puberty begins, the height and weight increase rapidly. If the child was not obese at the start of puberty, the additional fat that was previously accumulated reduces gradually. Height growth rates peak at about 18 months after the start of puberty and then slow down. For most girls, height

TABLE 3.1
Recommended Dietary Reference Intakes for Some Macronutrients, in Infants

Age	Protein (g/kg)	Energy (kcal/kg)	Calcium (mg/kg)	Phosphorus (mg/kg)	Magnesium (mg/kg)
Birth to six months	2.2	108.3	66.7	50.0	6.7
Six months to one year	1.6	94.4	66.7	55.6	6.7

increase is at its fastest at the age of 11 years. It slows down gradually until the adult height is reached, at ages 14 or 15. Menstruation usually starts during this particular growth spurt, and a slight amount of additional height is gained two years after **menarche**. Most boys have their fastest growth increase between ages 13 and 14, attaining adult height at approximately age 18. Girls and boys sometimes continue growing taller as they enter their 20s. In adolescence, females grow about 10 inches taller (25 cm), while boys grow about 12 inches taller (30 cm). Once growing stops, teenagers weigh 45%–85% more than when puberty started.

Body Composition

Body composition also changes during growth, affecting nutrient requirements. Body water declines during the first two or three years of life, reaching levels very close to those of adults. Lean body tissue increases as infants and children grow. Boys and girls enter adolescence with similar amounts of lean body tissue. During adolescence, boys secrete testosterone, causing a gain in muscle mass, a heavier skeleton, and more red blood cells than girls. By the end of adolescence, girls have 66% as much lean body tissue as boys.

Body fat increases from birth to one year, then declines slowly up to age seven. Then, it starts to gradually increase yet again. In adolescence, body fat increases in girls but declines in boys. The reason is that girls produce estrogen, which stimulates the growth of subcutaneous fat, which is necessary for sexual maturity. When a girl's body fat makes up 16%–17% of her body weight, and she reaches the weight of 100 pounds (46 kg), the menstrual cycle starts. It becomes regular once she reaches a level of about 22% body fat. The increasing regularity of menstruation is an indicator that a girl is nearing the adult amounts of body fat, and that growth is getting close to ending. Once adolescence ends, girls have two times as much body fat, as a percentage of overall weight, as boys.

It used to be believed that overfeeding in infancy would increase the number of adipose cells. However, we now know that the number of adipose cells can increase even in adulthood. If energy intake is limited in infancy, the growth and development of other organ systems – especially the brain and nervous system – may also be extremely restricted. Most obese infants become preschoolers of normal weight without any major diet restrictions. It is not wise to greatly restrict an infant's dietary intake, or that of a child or teen, due to the risks of stunted growth and development.

Body Organs and Systems

There is a multitude of changes that occur within the human body. For instance, the kidneys of newborn infants become twice as large and become more efficient in eliminating waste during infancy. The stomach slowly enlarges and begins secreting digestive enzymes. By four to six months of age, the digestive tract has greatly matured. An infant can then eat more food and metabolize nutrients from larger amounts of foods than human milk or infant formula.

The organs grow and develop during childhood, with many of them reaching their adult size and function. Growth of the brain is 75% complete by the age of two years. By the age of nine, the heart is almost at the adult size and the respiratory system is nearly at the adult level of function. The digestive tract is fully functional late in childhood. These systems are able to grow and mature to suit the needs of the child. Maturity of the digestive system means that it absorbs nutrients more fully. A mature circulatory system can effectively bring nutrients and oxygen required by the body for growth. Nutrient absorption that is more complete means that a child can start building stores of nutrients needed for adolescence. About 50% of the peak adult bone mass is reached during adolescence. The most important changes are the maturation of the reproductive system and the development of secondary sexual characteristics.

GROWTH CHARTS

Infant growth is assessed by the use of growth charts that measure changes in height and weight. Different growth charts are used for boys and girls. There is a general correlation between height and weight over time, though every infant has a unique growth *percentile*. One to three years are required for the percentile to develop, though premature infants may move up several percentiles (mostly regarding length-for-age) because of *catch-up growth*, in which they reach the size they would have been earlier if they had been full-term. Consistency in height and weight over time must be considered. An infant that suddenly drops far below the established profile for his or her weight may be underfed or sick. Generally, healthy children with good nutrition maintain approximately the same percentile curves from year to year. The growth rate of a child reveals the intake of calories and nutrients. A good indicator of recent nutritional status is the body mass index (BMI)-for-age or the weight-for-length of children under the age of two years. If the diet has recently been insufficient, there is a drop in BMI since weight decreases as the height stay the same. Excessive calorie intake causes increased BMI since weight increases with no increase in height. Stature-for-age reveals long-term nutritional status because undernutrition usually must be long-term until stature is noticeably affected.

Small growth spurts and lags are normal. If a child overeats, the BMI-for-age may jump several percentile curves. The length-for-age and weight-for-age percentiles (for boys) are shown, from birth to 36 months, in Figure 3.2. The percentiles for girls of these ages are very similar and are not shown. When a child's access to food is restricted, the BMI-for-age may drop excessively, and if this continues severely, stature-for-age may also drop to a lower percentile. If this goes below the 5th percentile and the child does not have short parents, growth stunting is probably occurring. Special growth charts are also available that include the 3rd and 97th percentiles for children. They are used to assist with proper care.

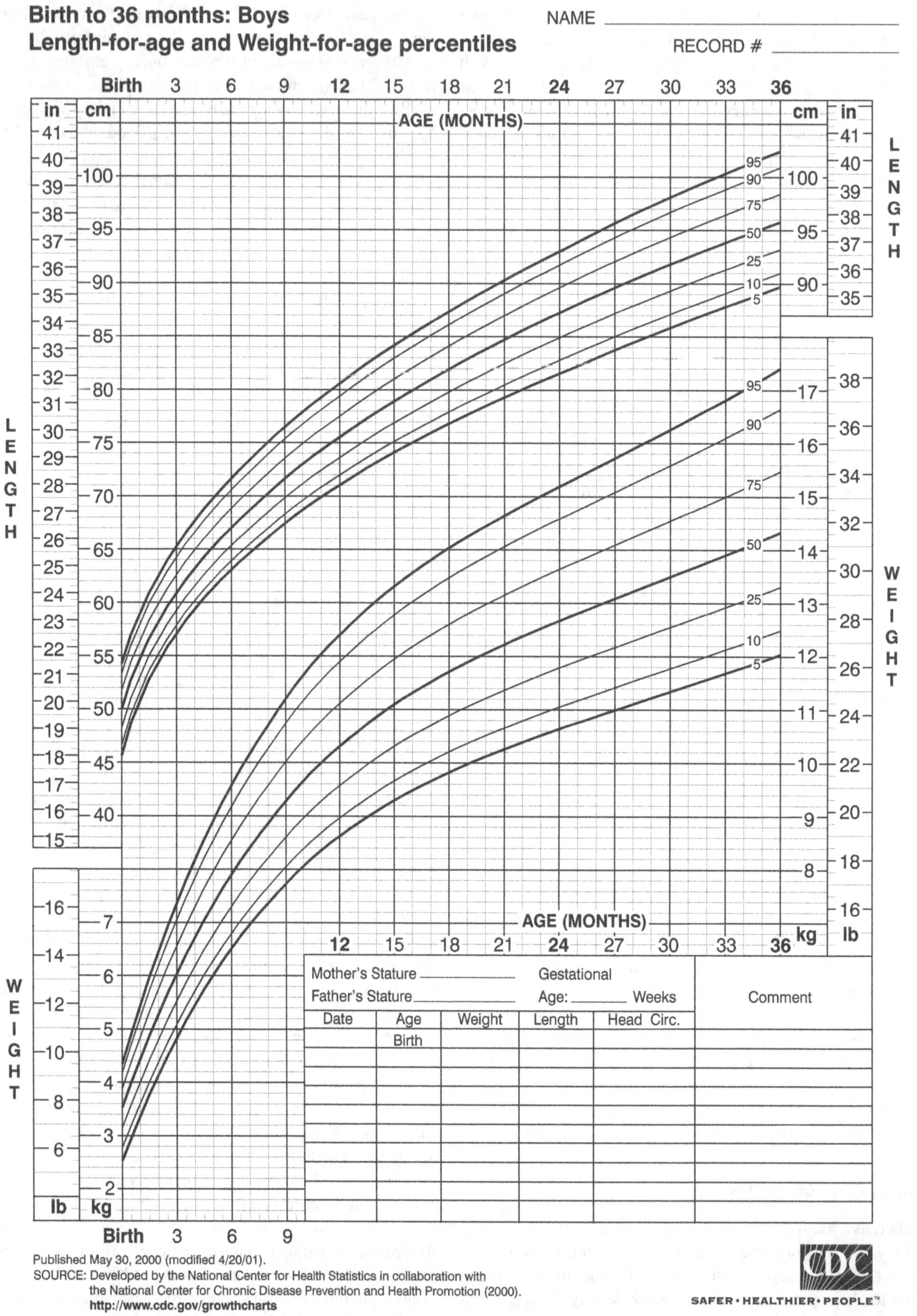

FIGURE 3.2 Birth to 36 months: Boys – Length-for-age and weight-for-age percentiles.

Early physical examinations usually involve measuring the child's head circumference to assess overall growth as well as brain growth. The brain grows more quickly during infancy than in any other time of life. The fast growth of the brain ends when the child is about 18 months old. Nutritional status and its effects on brain development and **intelligence quotient** (IQ) is hard to measure. It is believed that breast milk contains the essential fatty acids called *docosahexaenoic acid* and *arachidonic acid*, which promote brain and nervous system development. However, companies that make infant formula now add these essential fatty acids, but it is unknown if the effects are the same as when they are present in breast milk.

FOCUS ON CHILDHOOD BODY MASS INDEX

A child is overweight if the BMI-for-age reaches the 85th percentile. The child is obese if it reaches the 95th percentile. At this point, obesity is diagnosed when a physical examination indicates that the child is *overfat*, meaning that the excess body fat impairs health. A child is underweight if the BMI-for-age drops to below the 5th percentile.

Test Your Knowledge

1. What is the meaning of extremely low birthweight?
2. What are the risks of prematurity?
3. What is the reason that metabolic rates in infants are high?

EFFECTS OF PARENTAL DIET UPON OFFSPRING

When parents eat low-protein or high-fat diets, it can lead to metabolic disorders in their adult offspring. The Developmental Origins of Health and Disease is a school of thought that focuses on how prenatal factors such as stress and diet impact the development of diseases when children reach adulthood. Experimental evidence indicates that environmental factors that affect parents do play a role in reprogramming the health of their offspring throughout their lifespan. In particular, parental low-protein diets are known to be related to metabolic disorders in their children, such as diabetes.

Underweight infants also have a greater risk of heart disease. An important question involves where the "memory" of early nutrition is located in the body. A promising possibility is **epigenetic** changes, which involve chemical changes to DNA, which influence the genes that can be turned on or silenced. Because the pathways that regulate a child's metabolism, growth, and eating behaviors are sensitive to in utero influences, childhood weight disorders may begin during pregnancy. A *pregnancy diet* with higher inflammatory potential is linked to faster BMI growth rates in children between ages 3 and 10. Less adherence to a Mediterranean-styled diet during pregnancy is linked to higher BMI through adolescence. This diet is rich in fruits, vegetables, nuts, legumes, and extra virgin olive oil. The food choices that a woman makes during pregnancy may be related to the food choices they later offer their children. Maternal nutrition during pregnancy may be related to long-term weight issues in offspring. Healthcare providers must be extremely alert to children at high risk for weight gain based on maternal dietary habits during pregnancy. They should encourage healthy, nutritious food choices that will support a healthy weight throughout infancy, childhood, and adolescence.

BREASTFEEDING

For infants, breast milk is the best type of nutrition. Breastfeeding should continue for a minimum of six months, with solid foods being introduced from that time up to one year. After one year, breastfeeding can continue for as long as the mother and infant desire, but it should be a complement to a full diet of solid foods and fluids. When a mother's diet is diverse enough, a breastfed infant does not need any dietary or vitamin supplementation. In some cases, however, oral vitamin D supplements (once per day) that start during the first two months are given to prevent rickets caused by deficiency of this vitamin. Infants with the highest risk of vitamin D deficiency include premature infants, those with darker skin, and those that live in northern climates and receive less sunlight exposure. After six months, breastfed infants in locations where the water supply does not have enough natural or supplemental fluoride should be given fluoride drops. Local fluoride content information is available from dentists and health departments. Infants under six months of age should not be given additional water because of the risks of developing hyponatremia.

The position used during breastfeeding should be comfortable for the mother and infant. The mother should support the breast with her hand to make sure it is centered in the infant's mouth, which will reduce soreness. The center of the infant's lower lip is stimulated with the nipple so that the **rooting reflex** occurs and the mouth opens widely. The infant is encouraged to take in as much of the breast and areola as possible, with the lips placed about 1–1½ inch (2.5–4 cm) from the base of the nipple. The infant's tongue will compress the nipple against the hard palate. At first, it takes two or more minutes for the **let-down reflex** to occur. Milk volume increases with infant growth and stimulation from suckling. The duration of a feeding is usually determined by the infant.

The infant should continue to nurse on one breast until it softens, or the infant's suckling slows or stops. The mother can break the suction with one finger before removing the infant from one breast and offering the other one. Over the first few days, the infant may nurse only on one side, but then the mother should alternate sides with each feeding. If the infant often falls asleep before finishing nursing, the mother can remove the infant when suckling slows down, burp the infant, and switch the infant to the other breast. This switching keeps the infant awake for feedings while stimulating milk production in both breasts. Mothers are encouraged to feed infants on demand, or about every 1½–3 hours (meaning 8–12 feedings per day). This frequency gradually decreases. Some newborns under 5.5 pounds (2,500 grams) may need to feed more often to prevent hypoglycemia. For the first few days, the infant may need to be awakened and stimulated to nurse. Small or late preterm infants should not be allowed to sleep for long periods at night. Large full-term infants that feed well, as proven by the number of stools, can sleep for longer times. Over time, a schedule that allows the infant to sleep as long as possible is usually best for everyone in the family.

Whenever possible, a woman that is breastfeeding her infant should avoid all drugs. If drug therapy is required, it should not include any contraindicated drugs or those that suppress lactation, such as bromocriptine, levodopa, or trazodone. Drugs that should be avoided are listed in the *LactMed database* of the U.S. National Library of Medicine.

For all breastfeeding women, when a drug is needed, the safest option must always be chosen. They are usually taken immediately after breastfeeding or before the infant's longest sleep period. This is not very helpful, however, when an infant nurses often. Common drugs that are known to be safe during breastfeeding include acetaminophen, penicillin, cephalosporins, ibuprofen, and insulin. Drugs with a long history of use are generally safer than newer drugs that have not been widely tested and their effectiveness and safety cannot be fully evaluated. Weaning an infant from breastfeeding can occur whenever the mother and infant desire. Usually, this does not occur until the infant is at least one year old. Slow weaning over weeks or months as solid food is introduced is the most common method. Some mothers and infants can stop breastfeeding quickly with no problems, but others continue breastfeeding once or twice per day for 18 months or longer. No breastfeeding schedule is absolutely correct – it is highly individualized and experts recommend that babies be breastfed exclusively without formula, water, juice for the first six months.

FOCUS ON BREAST PUMPS AND MILK STORAGE

Sometimes, a breast pump is required to increase or maintain milk production. For most mothers, a total of 90 minutes per day of breast pumping, broken up into six to eight sessions, will produce enough milk for an infant that is not directly breastfed. Mothers that have jobs can pump breast milk to maintain milk production while away from the infant. Its frequency should match the infant's feeding schedule. Pumped breast milk is immediately refrigerated if it will be used within two days, or immediately frozen if it will be used after two days. Refrigerated milk not used within four days is discarded because of possible bacterial contamination. The container of frozen milk is placed in warm water and it should not be microwaved.

ADVANTAGES OF BREASTFEEDING

Practitioners encourage breastfeeding, starting before the infant's birth, and discuss the following advantages:

- Breast milk enhances nutrition, cognitive development, and protection against allergies, infections
- Women that breastfeed have reduced fertility while lactating and more quickly return to their normal conditions that existed before delivery; the uterus returns to normal and weight loss occurs; the mother is also protected against obesity, osteoporosis, ovarian cancer, and premenopausal breast cancer

Milk production is completely established after delivery of a single infant within 72–96 hours, but even earlier when there are multiple births. The first milk that the mother's body produces is **colostrum**, which is high in calories and protein. It is thin and yellow in color, providing immunoprotection because it is rich in antibodies, lymphocytes, and macrophages. Colostrum additionally stimulates the passage of **meconium**. After colostrum, the breast milk that is produced has a variety of features, which include:

- High lactose content – this provides a quick source of energy that is compatible with neonatal enzymes
- Large amounts of vitamin E – this important antioxidant can help prevent anemia by causing red blood cells to survive longer
- Twice the amount of calcium compared to phosphorus – this prevents calcium-deficiency tetany
- Effects on the stool and intestinal flora PH – this protects against bacterial diarrhea
- Transfer of protective antibodies – from mother to infant
- Cholesterol and taurine – are important for brain growth regardless of the maternal diet
- Omega-3 and omega-6 fatty acids – along with their very long-chain polyunsaturated derivatives, may contribute to better visual and cognitive outcomes in comparison with formula feeding

Most commercial formulas today are supplemented with arachidonic acid (ARA) and docosahexaenoic acid (DHA) – these are the very long-chain polyunsaturated derivatives supplied by omega fatty acids. These additives to formula make it closer to actual breast milk while reducing possible development differences caused by using formula.

FOCUS ON EARLY SWITCHING FROM BREASTFEEDING TO FORMULA

Switching from breastfeeding to formula too early is bad for an infant and can also cause painful breast engorgement in the mother. Making a switch such as this quickly without a slow transition is not suggested by medical professionals. It can take from two to six weeks for an infant to fully transition to formula. Signs that formula is not being well-tolerated include excessive crying or fussiness after feeding, extra gas, and loose or watery stools.

Test Your Knowledge

1. Why is breastfeeding important?
2. What is the rooting reflex?
3. Why should a newborn be breastfed immediately after birth?

COMPLICATIONS OF BREASTFEEDING

The primary complication of breastfeeding is underfeeding, which can lead to the infant becoming dehydrated or developing **hyperbilirubinemia**. Risk factors include the infant being small or premature, the mother having her first delivery, being ill, or following a difficult or operative delivery. Feeding adequacy is roughly determined by daily diaper counts. By the age of five days, a normal newborn wets at least six diapers and soils at least four diapers per day. If this count is lower, underhydration and undernutrition are suggested. Stools should change from dark meconium at birth to light brown, and then yellow. Weight is another consideration, and not meeting **growth landmarks** suggests undernutrition. If the infant is always irritable before six weeks of age, underfeeding is indicated. **Colic** is signified by irritability that develops around six weeks of age that is unrelated to hunger or thirst. Dehydration is suspected if the intensity of the infant's crying decreases or the skin becomes **turgid**. Extreme signs of dehydration include lethargy and sleepiness, requiring testing for hypernatremia.

For mothers that are breastfeeding, common complications include breast engorgement, nipple soreness, plugged ducts, mastitis, and anxiety. Breast engorgement occurs early during lactation and can last for one to two days. This may be reduced by early, frequent feeding. A comfortable nursing bra, worn 24 hours per day, can be helpful. Cool compresses after breastfeeding and mild analgesics such as ibuprofen. Just before breastfeeding, the mother may have to massage the breasts or use warm compresses, expressing breast milk manually to allow the infant to get the swollen areola into the mouth. When breastfeeding is done, cool compresses help reduce engorgement and provide more relief. Excessive milk expression between feedings encourages engorgement, so expression is only done enough to relieve discomfort.

If nipples become sore, the infant's position may need to be changed. Sometimes, an infant draws in one lip and sucks it, which will irritate the nipple. The mother can use her thumb to ease out the infant's lip. After breastfeeding, she can express a small amount of milk and let it dry on the nipples. Then, cool compresses can be used for additional relief. Plugged ducts are signified by slightly tender lumps that develop when there are no other signs of systemic illness. Continued breastfeeding results in adequate breast emptying. Warm compresses and massage of the area of a plugged duct before any additional breastfeeding may help with breast emptying. Breastfeeding positions can be alternated because various areas of the breast empty better based on the infant's position. A good nursing bra helps by not contributing to milk stasis that would be caused by regular bras with wires or constrictive straps.

Mastitis is common, signified by warm, tender, swollen, and wedge-shaped breast areas. It is caused by blocking, plugging, or **engorgement**. There can be a secondary infection, mostly with penicillin-resistant *Staphylococcus aureus*, and less often with *Streptococcus* species or *Escherichia coli*. With a mastitis infection, there may be flu-like aches, chills, and/or a fever of 101°F (38.5°C) or higher. Mastitis is diagnosed by history and physical examination. Infectious mastitis can be distinguished from noninfectious mastitis based on white blood cell counts of 10^6/mL or higher and cultures of breast milk indicating the presence of bacteria at 10^3/mL or higher. When symptoms of mastitis are mild and present for less than 24 hours, conservative management may be sufficient for treatment. This includes milk removal by breastfeeding or pumping, compresses, analgesics, a supportive bra, and stress reduction. When symptoms do not improve within 12–24 hours, or the mother has an acute illness, antibiotics that are safe during breastfeeding are started. These include oral cloxacillin, dicloxacillin, or cephalexin, four times per day for 7–14 days. If the mother's condition does not respond quickly or there is an abscess, community-acquired methicillin-resistant *Staphylococcus aureus* must be considered. However, breastfeeding can be continued during treatment. The mother's anxiety, frustration, and feelings of inadequacy can be caused by insufficient experience with breastfeeding, difficulties holding the infant or getting the infant to suckle, fatigue, problems determining if nourishment has been adequate, and physiologic changes after delivery. These are the most common reasons that a mother decides to stop breastfeeding. Early follow-up should occur with a pediatrician or lactation specialist and can help stop the early termination of breastfeeding.

ALTERNATIVE FEEDING

Though natural breast milk is the best method of feeding an infant during the first year, *infant formula* is an acceptable alternative. No other option is nutritionally complete. Formula feeding allows for controlled nutrition. Commercial infant formulas are available in the form of concentrated liquids, powders, and prediluted liquids that are ready to use right out of the container. Each type contains vitamins and most contain iron supplementation. Infant formula, when preparation is required, involves the use of fluoridated water. If fluoridated water is unavailable, oral fluoride drops must be given after the age of six months. The choice of the formula is based on each individual infant's needs. A formula based on cow's milk is the most popular choice unless the infant has any of the following:

- Spitting up after feeding
- Diarrhea, with or without blood
- Hives
- Poor weight gain (which suggests a sensitivity to cow's milk, or lactose intolerance, though this is very rare in infants)

All formulas based on soy milk in the United States do not contain lactose. Even so, some infants that are allergic to cow's milk protein are also allergic to soy protein. In these cases, a hydrolyzed formula is required. These are derived from cow's milk, but the proteins are broken down into smaller chains. This makes them less allergenic. For the rare cases of infants allergic to hydrolyzed formula, true *elemental formulas* are available, made from free amino acids.

Bottle-fed infants are also fed on demand. However, the formula is digested more slowly than breast milk, meaning that these infants can be fed every 3–4 hours. The initial formula volumes are 0.5–2 ounces (15–60 mL), which are slowly increased during the first week up to 3 ounces (90 mL), about six times per day. This supplies approximately 120 kcal/kg (2.2 pounds) at one week for an infant that weighs 3 kg (6.6 pounds).

BABY BOTTLE SYNDROME

Baby bottle syndrome is also referred to as *nursing caries* and *bottle mouth caries.* There is a pattern of caries in which the deciduous upper incisors and molars are more severely affected. The lower incisors are usually only mildly affected, or completely healthy. Baby bottle syndrome is caused by the frequent exposure of a child's teeth for long periods to liquids containing sugar. These include milk, formula, fruit juice, and other sweetened liquids. Bacteria in the mouth feed on the sugar, increasing and generating acid as a waste product. Baby bottle syndrome can destroy the teeth of an infant or young child (see Figure 3.3). Potential problems of baby bottle tooth decay include:

- Infection, if tooth decay is left untreated, may be serious
- Poor speech problems or poor eating habits if baby teeth do not develop properly because of deterioration
- Adult teeth that may cause crowding or grow in crookedly
- Chronic pain
- Pain or difficulty chewing

To prevent baby bottle syndrome, the following steps are suggested:

1. Give your child water to drink when thirsty.
2. Clean your child's teeth daily.
3. Do not allow your child to sip on a bottle filled with milk, formula, or juice for long periods.
4. Ensure that your child does not fall asleep with a bottle filled with milk, formula, or juice.

SOLID FOODS

Solid foods are best introduced after the infant is six months of age, with breastfeeding or bottle-feeding continuing as well. Solid food is not needed for nutrition any earlier than four months of age and can result in food allergies and celiac disease. The **extrusion reflex** makes feeding solid

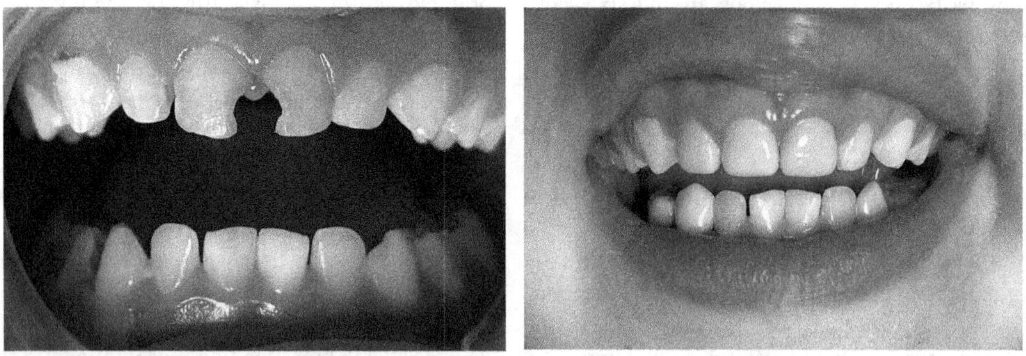

(A) (B)

FIGURE 3.3 Baby bottle syndrome: (A) the effects of sugar in milk, and (B) after being corrected by dental procedures. (Courtesy: Morvarid Moini DMD, MPH; Pearl Pediatric Dental.)

foods difficult. Other experts argue about solid foods are acceptable to be started between four and six months of age. Some food allergies, such as those to peanuts or eggs, are of reduced risk of occurrence if they benefit from an earlier introduction to the foods rather than a later introduction.

It is best to breastfeed or bottle-feed an infant first, followed by solid food so that adequate nourishment is received. The first solid food is usually an iron-fortified rice cereal. It is non-allergenic, easy to digest, and supplies a good amount of iron. Generally, only one new single-ingredient food should be introduced per week to identify food allergies. There is no specific order of foods required, but they are generally introduced with textures that increase in coarseness. For example, after the rice cereal, soft table foods can be tried, followed by chopped table foods. Pureed meat can be given since this process prevents it from being aspirated. It is a good source of iron and zinc, making it a good early solid food. If the parents are vegetarian, sufficient iron and zinc can be supplied via iron-fortified cereals and grains, green leafy vegetables, dried beans, and yeast-fermented whole-grain bread. Homemade meals are as good as commercial food products, though commercial preparations of beets, carrots, collard greens, spinach, and turnips are better before the infant is one year of age because they have appropriately low levels of nitrates. High nitrate levels can cause methemoglobinemia in young children. These levels are found in vegetables grown with water supplies that have been contaminated by fertilizers.

At one year of age or later, children can start drinking whole cow's milk, but reduced-fat milk cannot be given until at least two years of age. Milk intake should be limited to 16–24 ounces per day in young children, because higher intake can reduce the intake of other good nutritional sources, leading to iron deficiency. Juice is a poor source of nutrition and leads to dental caries, so it is limited to four to six ounces per day at a maximum. Ideally, it should be avoided completely. By about 24 months of age, the child's growth rate usually slows down, and less food is required. Some children even refuse to eat some meals. It is important to assess food intake over one week, and not during one meal or over one day. Underfeeding solid food is only important if the child does not achieve his or her expected weight at the normal rate.

FOCUS ON SOLID FOODS TO AVOID

Any foods that could be aspirated and block the airway must be avoided. These include round candies, whole nuts, hot dogs, and any meat that is not pureed, popcorn, and grapes (unless they are cut into very small pieces). Whole nuts are avoided until two or three years of age since they do not completely dissolve when chewed and small pieces can be aspirated, leading to pneumonia or other complications.

FOCUS ON HONEY DURING INFANCY

For infants younger than one year of age, honey must be avoided, since botulism is a risk. Both raw and regular honey may contain small amounts of the bacterium called *Clostridium botulinum*, which can cause botulism. An infant's digestive tract has not yet developed sufficiently to fight off the bacteria.

HEALTHY FEEDING GUIDELINES

Generally, infants should be fed whenever they seem hungry. However, for premature infants or those with certain medical conditions, scheduled feedings advised by a pediatrician are best. A hungry baby will often cry, but this is a late sign of hunger. Typical hunger cues to watch for include licking the lips, sticking the tongue out, the rooting reflex, putting one hand to the mouth repeatedly, opening the mouth, fussiness, and sucking on anything close to the mouth. All infants are different regarding feeding. The following are general guidelines for healthy infant feeding:

- Most newborns eat every two to three hours, meaning eight to twelve times every day – they may only take in 0.5 of an ounce of breast milk or formula per feeding for the first one or two days, but later will usually drink one to two ounces per feeding; this increases to two to three ounces per feeding by two weeks of age
- At about two months of age, infants usually take four to five ounces per feeding, every three to four hours
- At four months, infants usually take four to six ounces per feeding
- At six months, infants may take up to eight ounces every four to five hours

Most infants increase the amount of the drink by an average of one ounce per month, eventually leveling off at seven to eight ounces per feeding. Bottle-fed infants are more likely to overfeed than those that breastfeed. This is partly because drinking from a bottle can require less effort than breastfeeding.

When an infant is overfed, common problems include stomach pain, gas, and spitting up or vomiting. Overfed infants also have a higher risk for obesity later in life. It is better to offer less since more milk or formula can always be given if the infant wants it. Giving less also allows infants time to realize when they are full. If an infant appears to want to eat all the time, even when full, the pediatrician must be consulted. Health-weight infants that like to suckle for comfort rather than nutrition can be given a pacifier to soothe them. For breastfed infants, it is best to start offering a pacifier at three to four weeks of age. Most infants will double their birthweight by five months of age and triple it by twelve months of age. If an infant is having trouble gaining weight, the time between feedings should not be too long, even if the infant must be awoken to feed. Diaper counts and growth charts help in determining whether an infant is receiving adequate feedings or is being underfed or overfed.

FEEDING PROBLEMS DURING INFANCY

For infants, minor variations in daily food intake are common. Parents are often worried, but they can be reassured by practitioners that these variations are not significant unless there are signs of disease or changes in growth progress – especially weight. The most important changes are in the child's percentile rank on standard growth charts, which are more important than absolute changes. An infant with a feeding problem or disorder will continue to have problems that can affect overall health and development. Feeding problems include difficulty swallowing, aspiration, refusal to drink or eat, arching the back or stiffening while feeding, crying or fussiness while feeding, taking more than 30 minutes for each feeding, lack of alertness or falling asleep while feeding, avoiding foods with certain textures, extreme drooling, coughing or gagging while feeding, difficulty breathing while feeding, frequent spitting up or vomiting, or vocal hoarseness during or after feeding.

Poor feeding can be due to illnesses such as ear infections and colds, stress, pain from teething, and the adverse effects of medications. Causes of infant feeding and swallowing problems include prematurity, low birthweight, **cerebral palsy**, asthma, heart disease, muscular dystrophy, **autism**, cleft lip, and **cleft palate**. If untreated, feeding problems can result in malnutrition, dehydration, lung infections, and later problems with speech, cognition, and behavior. Treatments for feeding problems may require a team approach including the pediatrician, dietitians, and speech-language pathologists (since they can suggest techniques for feeding that may improve swallowing problems). There may be a need for medications to treat reflux, trying different foods or differently textured foods, changing food temperature, eating smaller and more frequent meals, changing the infant's position while eating, switching feeding methods, and sometimes, feeding tubes. Warning signs of feeding problems include insufficient amounts of wet diapers per day, infrequent or hard stools during the first month, and increasing signs of jaundice.

FOCUS ON EMERGENCY WARNING SIGNS

When an infant develops a fever over 100°F (38°C), wheezing, bloody vomit or stool, or constant crying, immediate medical attention is required. Signs of an allergy or digestive disturbance include vomiting after feeding, frequent watery or loose stools, or severe skin rashes.

FAILURE TO THRIVE

Failure to thrive is a term used to describe an infant or child's weight being consistently below the third to fifth percentile for age and gender, a progressive weight decrease to below the third to fifth percentile, or a decrease in two major growth percentiles over a short period. It may be due to a known medical condition, or because of environmental factors. Either way, nutrition is inadequate. Failure to thrive may be organic, nonorganic, or mixed in most cases. In the mixed form, organic and nonorganic causes overlap. Children with organic disorders also have non-healthy environments or parental interactions that are dysfunctional. Children with severe undernutrition due to nonorganic failure to thrive can also develop organic medical problems. Growth failure is caused by an acute or chronic disorder, and interferes with the intake of nutrients, absorption, metabolism, or excretion. There may also be a disorder present that increases energy requirements, including illness of any organ system.

Nonorganic failure to thrive is because of insufficient calorie intake, usually manifesting as an inability to gain weight. Lengthwise growth and head circumference increases are normal for a while until they are impacted by a lack of sufficient calories. There is a psychosocial form in which growth failure is concurrent with or precedes poor weight gain. This may be caused by mental stress, resulting in increased levels of hormones such as catecholamines and corticosteroids, which oppose the effects of growth hormones. As many as 80% of children with growth failure do not have an organic disorder. Growth failure is due to a lack of food and/or stimulus deprivation. Lack of food may be because of poverty, insufficient understanding of proper feeding techniques, **overdilution** of formula to make it last longer because of financial problems, and an inadequate supply of breast milk due to maternal stress, poor nutrition, or exhaustion.

With the nonorganic failure to thrive, there is usually a set of disordered interactions between the child and parents or caregivers. Sometimes, **hospitalism** is present, in which the infant has depression that is caused by stimulus deprivation. The infant becomes apathetic and eventually anorexic. The stimulation may be insufficient because the parent or caregiver is also depressed or apathetic, lacks good parenting skills, has anxiety about providing care or feels unfulfilled by it, has hostility toward the child, or is responding to actual or perceived stressors. These may include marital problems, significant losses, financial problems, or demands of other children if the family is very large. Not all cases of nonorganic failure to thrive are due to poor caregiving. Each child's temperament, abilities, and responses help to form the nurturing patterns of the caregiver. The child may be difficult concerning feeding. In some cases, there is simply a mismatch between the child's needs and the caregiver's abilities.

The prevalence of failure to thrive, globally, depends on risks such as low income, presence of infectious diseases, poverty, and insufficient nutrition. Higher rates occur in economically disadvantaged rural and urban areas. For example, in Guatemala, based on different reference standards, 19% and 34% of weight deficits in growth-restricted young children were attributed to failure to thrive during the first three months of life. Children that are malnourished at three to five years of age often had deficits by the end of their first year of life. Malnutrition or undernutrition represents the most common cause of failure to thrive globally.

Test Your Knowledge

1. When should solid foods be started for infants?
2. What are some examples of feeding problems during infancy?
3. What is the meaning of failure to thrive?

KEY TERMS

Baby bottle syndrome

Bronchopulmonary dysplasia

Cerebral palsy

Cleft palate

Colic

Colostrum

Creatinine

Engorgement

Epigenetic

Epiphyses

Fenton growth chart

Gestational age

Growth landmarks

Hospitalism

Hyperbilirubinemia

Intelligence quotient

Jaundice

Kernicterus

Let-down reflex

Mastitis

Meconium

Menarche

Overdilution

Patent ductus arteriosus

Puberty

Respiratory distress syndrome

Rooting reflex

Sudden infant death syndrome

Surfactant

Turgid

CLINICAL CASE STUDIES

Clinical Case Study 1

Oliver is a ten-month-old baby boy that has been completely breastfed, with no formula feeding. He has been started on solid foods three to four times per day and loves peaches, pears, and watermelon, as well as some cooked vegetables and avocado. Currently, Oliver is not receiving any vitamin or mineral supplements. The baby's mother does not give him infant meats because she does not like the look of them, and feels that table meat are too tough for his system. It is suggested that Oliver be given formula and infant cereal to increase his iron intake because his hemoglobin is lower than normal. This is likely because he is not consuming any significant sources of iron or zinc. The pediatrician suggests some information for Oliver's mother to read about how other women include iron-rich foods for their babies as they are transitioning to solid foods from breast milk.

CRITICAL THINKING QUESTIONS

1. How long should breastfeeding continue?
2. What important features are found in breast milk?
3. What are good early sources of iron for infants?

Clinical Case Study 2

Amy was born prematurely at 25 weeks and has a chronic lung disease. After birth, she was intubated immediately and given positive pressure ventilation because of prematurity. In about one month, she was able to be extubated and placed on 40% oxygen via nasal cannula. She was started on parenteral nutrition. Once medically stable, Amy's mother started breastfeeding her, slowly increasing feedings as needed, even though the infant had trouble breathing occasionally while suckling. Over time, Amy was able to be given only breast milk, and the parenteral nutrition was tapered off. After a few months, her health status improved greatly.

CRITICAL THINKING QUESTIONS

1. What defines a premature infant?
2. What are common feeding problems during infancy?
3. What problems occur from early switching from breastfeeding to formula?

Clinical Case Study 3

A newborn boy was gaining weight over the first two weeks very well, but at nine weeks he had lost 6 lbs and was now below his birthweight. His mother reported regular spitting up after feeding. The mother had switched from breastfeeding to formula, which may have been related to the problem. Everything else about the infant was normal except for loose skin folds handing off of his legs. This failure to thrive prompted a search for metabolic abnormalities, and profound hypochloremia plus severe alkalosis were found. The infant also had severe hyponatremia and hyperkalemia. An ultrasound revealed that the pylorus, which connects the stomach to the duodenum had enlarged to the point that food could not empty of the stomach. This pyloric stenosis, a gastric outlet obstruction, results in projectile vomiting. A minor surgical procedure was done, with an incision made along the pylorus sphincter to relax the canal and allow food to pass. It was immediately successful.

CRITICAL THINKING QUESTIONS

1. What is "failure to thrive"?
2. What is the organic form of this condition?
3. What are infants' basal metabolic rates high early in life?

STUDY QUESTIONS

1. The Fenton growth chart assesses growth versus which of the following?
   A. Gestational weight
   B. Gestational age
   C. Gestational length
   D. Age of the mother

2. Which of the following is a complication of exaggerated physiologic jaundice?
   A. Cerebral palsy
   B. Kidney failure
   C. Arrhythmia
   D. Kernicterus

3. Which of the following may cause respiratory distress syndrome in a premature baby?
   A. Lack of surfactant
   B. Deficiency of folic acid
   C. Hypoglycemia
   D. Lack of creatine

4. Which of the following is the most common heart condition in premature infants?
   A. Enlargement of the right ventricle
   B. Mitral valve stenosis
   C. Patent ductus arteriosus
   D. Atrial septal defect

5. Which of the following is the average growth, in length during an infant's first 12 months?
   A. 5 inches
   B. 10 inches
   C. 15 inches
   D. 20 inches

6. Which of the following substances in breast milk promotes brain development?
   A. Folic acid
   B. Vitamin C
   C. Vitamin B12
   D. Arachidonic acid

7. Premature newborns under 5.5 pounds may need to feed more often in order to prevent which of the following?
   A. Hypoglycemia
   B. Hypocalcemia
   C. Hypokalemia
   D. Hypernatremia

8. The advantages of breastfeeding include all of the following, except which one of these answer choices?
   A. Cognitive development
   B. Protection against infection
   C. Protection against allergies
   D. Reduced development of hydrocephalus

9. Soy milk does not contain which of the following?
   A. Glucose
   B. Lactose
   C. Essential proteins
   D. Essential fatty acids

10. Which of the following may cause baby bottle syndrome?
    A. Exposure to liquids containing sugar
    B. Exposure to liquids containing iron
    C. Exposure to liquids containing vitamin C
    D. Exposure to liquids containing zinc

11. Breastfeeding should continue for a minimum of how many months?
    A. 3
    B. 6
    C. 12
    D. 16

12. Growth of the brain is 75% complete by which age?
    A. Two years
    B. Three years
    C. Five years
    D. Ten years

13. Body fat increases between which of the following ages?
    A. Birth to one year
    B. One to three years
    C. Three to five years
    D. Five to seven years

14. The lack of which of the following substances in premature infants may cause breathing problems?
    A. Meconium
    B. Creatinine
    C. Colostrum
    D. Surfactant

15. Which of the following terms is used to describe an infant or child's weight below the fifth percentile for age and gender?
    A. Hospitalism
    B. Failure to thrive
    C. Sufficient nutrition
    D. Growth landmark

FURTHER READING

1. American Academy of Pediatrics (AAP). (2020). *Newborn and Infant Nutrition: A Clinical Decision Support Chart.* American Academy of Pediatrics.
2. Brown, J.E. (2019). *Nutrition Through the Life Cycle*, 7th Edition. Cengage Learning.
3. Erlich, K., and Genzlinger, K. (2018). *Super Nutrition for Babies, Revised Edition – The Best Way to Nourish Your Baby from Birth to 24 Months.* Fair Winds Press.
4. Fett, R. (2019). *Brain Health from Birth: Nurturing Brain Development During Pregnancy and the First Year (It Starts with the Egg).* Franklin Fox Publishing LLC.
5. Jana, L.A., and Shu, J. (2020). *Heading Home with Your Newborn: From Birth to Reality*, 4th Edition. American Academy of Pediatrics.
6. Kleinmann, R.E., and Greer, F.R. (2019). *Pediatric Nutrition*, 8th Edition. American Academy of Pediatrics.
7. Koletzko, B., Poindexter, B., and Uauy, R. (2014). *Nutritional Care of Preterm Infants – Scientific Basis and Practical Guidelines (World Review of Nutrition and Dietetics*, Volume 110). S. Karger.
8. Konek, S.H., and Becker, P.J. (2019). *Samour & King's Pediatric Nutrition in Clinical Care*, 5th Edition. Jones & Bartlett Learning.
9. More, J. (2021). *Infant, Child, and Adolescent Nutrition – A Practical Handbook*, 2nd Edition. CRC Press.
10. Pediatric Nutrition Practice Group, Steele, C., and Collins, E. (2018). *Infant and Pediatric Feedings: Guidelines for Preparation of Human Milk and Formula in Health Care Facilities*, 3rd Edition. Academy of Nutrition and Dietetics.
11. Pediatric Nutrition Practice Group. (2011). *Infant Feedings: Guidelines for Preparation of Human Milk and Formula in Health Care Facilities*, 2nd Edition. American Dietetic Association.
12. Porto, A., and DiMaggio, D. (2016). *The Pediatrician's Guide to Feeding Babies and Toddlers.* Clarkson Potter/Ten Speed.
13. Sears, W., Sears, R., Sears, J., and Sears, M. (2004). *The Premature Baby Book (Sears Parenting Library).* Little, Brown, and Company.

4 Children and Adolescents

OUTLINE

LEARNING OBJECTIVES

After study of the chapter, readers should be able to:

1. Discuss influences on childhood food habits and intake.
2. Describe the most common food allergies.
3. Explain malnutrition and hunger in children and related effects upon health.
4. Describe the effects of decreased gastric intrinsic factor upon the blood.
5. Explain factors of malnutrition in development of attention-deficit/hyperactivity disorder.
6. Describe how vegetarianism can be implemented in childhood.
7. Explain avoidant/restrictive food disorder.
8. Discuss physical growth and development in adolescence.
9. Explain growth spurts in both genders.
10. Describe nutrition-related concerns for adolescents.

OVERVIEW

Physical development is the most readily visible area of child development. Height and weight increase along with development of fine motor and gross motor skills. During the first few years, a baby's brain produces so many connections that they actually have more of them than in an adult brain. Parents should encourage and teach specific skills, and promote a healthy lifestyle for their children. This includes helping them to get sufficient sleep, eat a well-balanced diet, and be physically active. Parents must model behaviors and encourage these very important health habits. Teaching safety and maintaining a safe home environment (especially in the early years) is very important. Have regular child health check-ups and keeping immunizations up to date is important as well. Another large transition awaits every child: adolescence, which brings about the physical development of puberty, plus cognitive, social, and emotional changes. Adolescence is the period of development, generally beginning around age 12, which ends at emerging adulthood (about age 18), or into the mid- to late 20s. In the United States, adolescence is a time in which independence from parents develops, while still remaining connected to them.

CHILDHOOD

Childhood is the period of being a child, from the end of infancy until the adolescent years. Generally, it is believed that childhood ends once puberty begins. In infancy, toddlerhood, and early childhood, the body's physical development is rapid. During infancy and childhood, growth does not occur at a steady rate. Growth slows between four and six years old. The size of our brains increases rapidly. For example, the brain of a two-year-old is 55% of its adult size, and by six years old, the brain is about 90% of its adult size. During early childhood (ages three to six), the frontal lobes grow rapidly. There is a large variety of disorders and conditions that occur during childhood that may influence childhood health and development. These include various infections, food allergies, congenital disorders, and cancers.

INFLUENCES ON CHILDHOOD FOOD HABITS AND INTAKE

Childhood food habits and intake are influenced by food availability, eating routines, food marketing, emotions, and the cultural and social meanings of food. Eating habits are affected by biological, economic, physical, and social determinants. Biological determinants include appetite, hunger, and taste. Economic determinants include availability, cost, and income. Physical determinants include access, education, cooking skills, and available time. Social determinants include culture, family, meal patterns, and peers. Factors that drive food choices include, taste, texture, appearance, early food experiences, habit, culture,

DOI: 10.1201/b22969-6

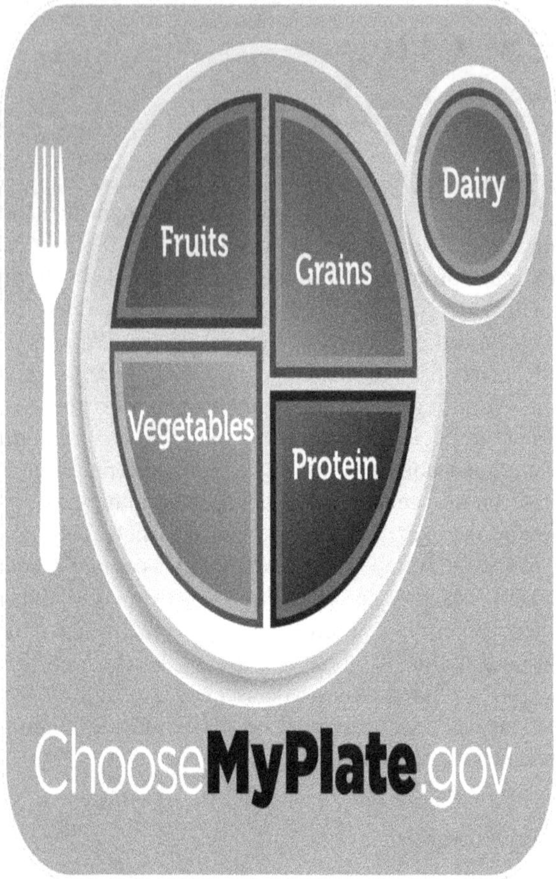

FIGURE 4.1 The MyPlate.gov meal choice image.

geography, advertising, social factors, health concerns such as food allergies, and emotions.

Childhood food intake is influenced by participation in family meals, which usually means better food choices and lower risks for becoming overweight. Children that eat in front of a television usually make poorer food choices. Factors that influence how much a child eats include nutrition, hunger, appetite, personal taste, availability, time, convenience, geography (climate and environment), family, and culture. Parents play a strong role in childhood eating behaviors since they provide genes as well as environment. They influence children's preferences and eating behaviors by making some foods available instead of others, and by acting as models of eating behavior.

MyPlate.gov is a website that encourages good nutrition for people of all ages, and features the popular plate graphic that shows how much of each meal should be divided between the various food groups (see Figure 4.1). It also has a special section called *MyPlate.gov/Life-Stages/Kids* that encourages children to learn and remember important information about healthy eating. It includes a variety of facts and fun suggestions for children. These suggestions are as follows:

- *Eat more fruits and vegetables* – make half of your plate contain fruits and vegetables every day
- *Try whole grains* – ask for oatmeal, whole-wheat breads, or brown rice
- *Think about your drink* – choose water and low-fat or fat-free dairy milk (or if needed, lactose-free or fortified soy milk)
- *Mix up your proteins* – include different items like seafood, beans, lentils, nuts, eggs, meats, and poultry
- *Get involved* – help by putting away groceries, stirring ingredients, peeling fruits, assembling salads, or setting the table
- *Be active your way* – find ways to be active and move your body for at least one hour per day, by walking to school, riding your bike, or playing sports with friends

FOCUS ON TRENDS IN CHILDREN'S DIETS

Regardless of standards of dietary recommendations, trends in total energy intake in children have increased over the past decades. Total caloric intake and the consumption of fruits, fruit juices, sweetened beverages, poultry, and cheese have increased. Total intake of milk, vegetables, soups, and eggs have decreased. About 16% of children in the United States do not meet any food group recommendations, and only 1% consume recommended amounts for all food groups.

Test Your Knowledge

1. What factors affect the eating habits of children?
2. What are the recommendations of MyPlate for children?

FOOD ALLERGIES

A food allergy is an abnormal response of the body to a specific food. Food allergies affect the immune system. They are similar to food intolerance, but this condition does not affect the immune system. Before a food allergy occurs, a sensitive child must have been exposed to the food at least once prior, or could be sensitized to it via the breast milk. The second time the child eats that food, the allergic symptoms may happen. As immunoglobulin E (IgE) antibodies react, histamines are released, causing hives, asthma, mouth itching, difficulty breathing, stomach pains or cramps, swelling, eczema, throat tightness, **wheezing**, hypotension, vomiting, or diarrhea. The symptoms range from uncomfortable to life-threatening.

Anaphylaxis is a severe allergic reaction that is life-threatening. The symptoms include difficulty breathing, shortness of breath, wheezing, a feeling as if the throat is closing, hoarseness, trouble talking, swelling of the face, lips, tongue, and throat, skin changes (coolness, moistness, pallor, or a blueish color), faintness, lightheadedness, confusion, nausea, vomiting, diarrhea, tachycardia or bradycardia, hypotension, loss of consciousness, and seizures. Anaphylaxis is a medical emergency that requires someone to call 911 immediately. If an epinephrine autoinjector is available, it must be used. A child with severe allergies of any type, including food allergies, should always have two epinephrine autoinjectors with them wherever they are. There are eight food types that cause about 90% of all food allergies. These include the following:

- Eggs (protein group)
- Milk (dairy group)
- Peanuts (protein group)
- Wheat (grain group)
- Soy (protein group)
- Tree nuts (fruit group)
- Fish (protein group)
- Shellfish (protein group)

The most severe reactions are usually caused by peanuts, tree nuts, fish, and shellfish. About 5% of children under five years of age have food allergies. The majority of children eventually outgrow their food allergies, but the allergies to peanuts, tree nuts, fish, and shellfish may last throughout life. Allergic symptoms of food allergies begin with minutes to 1 hour after ingesting the food. For most children, only a very small amount of the food that provokes an allergic reaction is required. In a severely allergic child, 1/44,000 of a peanut kernel can cause the allergic reaction.

Food allergies can be prevented by avoiding the foods that cause the signs and symptoms. There is no medication that prevents food allergies. It is very important to also avoid foods that are in the same group. For certain foods that must be avoided, the child may require vitamin or mineral supplementation to replace what is present in the food they cannot eat. Some children, as guided by a healthcare provider, can be given certain foods again after three to six months to see if the allergy has been outgrown. Many food allergies are short-term and the food can be eventually tolerated after the age of three or four years. Milk and soy allergies are most common in infants and younger children. The signs and symptoms may be different, including colic, blood in the stool, and poor growth. For milk and soy allergies, the pediatrician must be contacted.

The diagnosis of a food allergy begins with a physical examination and complete health history, including a list of foods eaten before the allergic symptoms occurred. Tests include a skin **prick test**, to measure if there is IgE antibody to a specific **allergen**. A small amount of diluted allergen is put on the skin and the area is scratched. If the test positive a small raised wheal will appear after about 15 minutes. Testing for many allergens can be done at the same time. Skin prick testing is not often done if the child or adolescent has recently had a severe allergic reaction. Blood tests can also be done when a skin prick test cannot be done or there are additional questions about a food allergy. Neither a skin nor blood test can determine how severe an allergic reaction will be. A food challenge test is performed by an allergist who gives the patient a very small amount of an allergen by mouth or inhalation. The patient is watched closely for a reaction. Food challenges are most commonly done if an allergist believes the patient will be able to eat a food again without a reaction.

The goal of treatment for food allergies is to stay away from foods that cause the symptoms. It is extremely important to avoid those foods and anything else in the same food group. When a child or adolescent cannot eat certain foods, vitamin supplements may be needed. Some individuals outgrow food allergies during childhood or adulthood. Some food allergies are so severe that even touching the specific food can cause a skin reaction.

Test Your Knowledge

1. What are the symptoms of anaphylaxis?
2. What are the most severe food allergy reactions in children?
3. What is the skin prick test?

NUTRITIONAL CONCERNS OF CHILDHOOD

During preschool and school-age years, the activities of children increase while their growth rate slows. They grow slowly and steadily, averaging two to four inches per year until adolescence, in which growth rapidly increases. Until age eight or nine, nutrient needs for boys and girls are not different. Therefore, the Dietary Reference Intake (DRI) values for macronutrients, micronutrients, and fiber are grouped together for children between ages four and eight.

Estimated energy requirements (EERs) vary based on each child's age, weight, and level of activity – which can vary widely. All children should be encouraged to engage in play that utilizes their muscles. The diet should support normal growth and appropriate physical activity, minimizing risks for excessive weight gain. Therefore, the United States Department of Agriculture (USDA) has created a Daily Food Checklist for preschoolers (see Figure 4.2).

In the preschool years, total dietary fat intake should be slowly reduced to a level that is closer to that of an adult: 25%–35% of total energy. Saturated fats can be reduced by serving lean proteins, lower-fat dairy products (1%–2% milk), and minimal intake of fried foods. The diet for children should not provide less than 25% of calories from fats because they are growing, developing, and maturing. Children that are highly impressionable or easily influenced by their peers are likely to categorize foods as good or bad, resulting in incorrect views of food choices and inappropriate eating habits.

For carbohydrates, children should have 130 g/day (about 45%–65% of total daily energy intake). The best choices are *complex carbohydrates*, from fruits, vegetables, whole grains, and legumes. Simple sugars should be

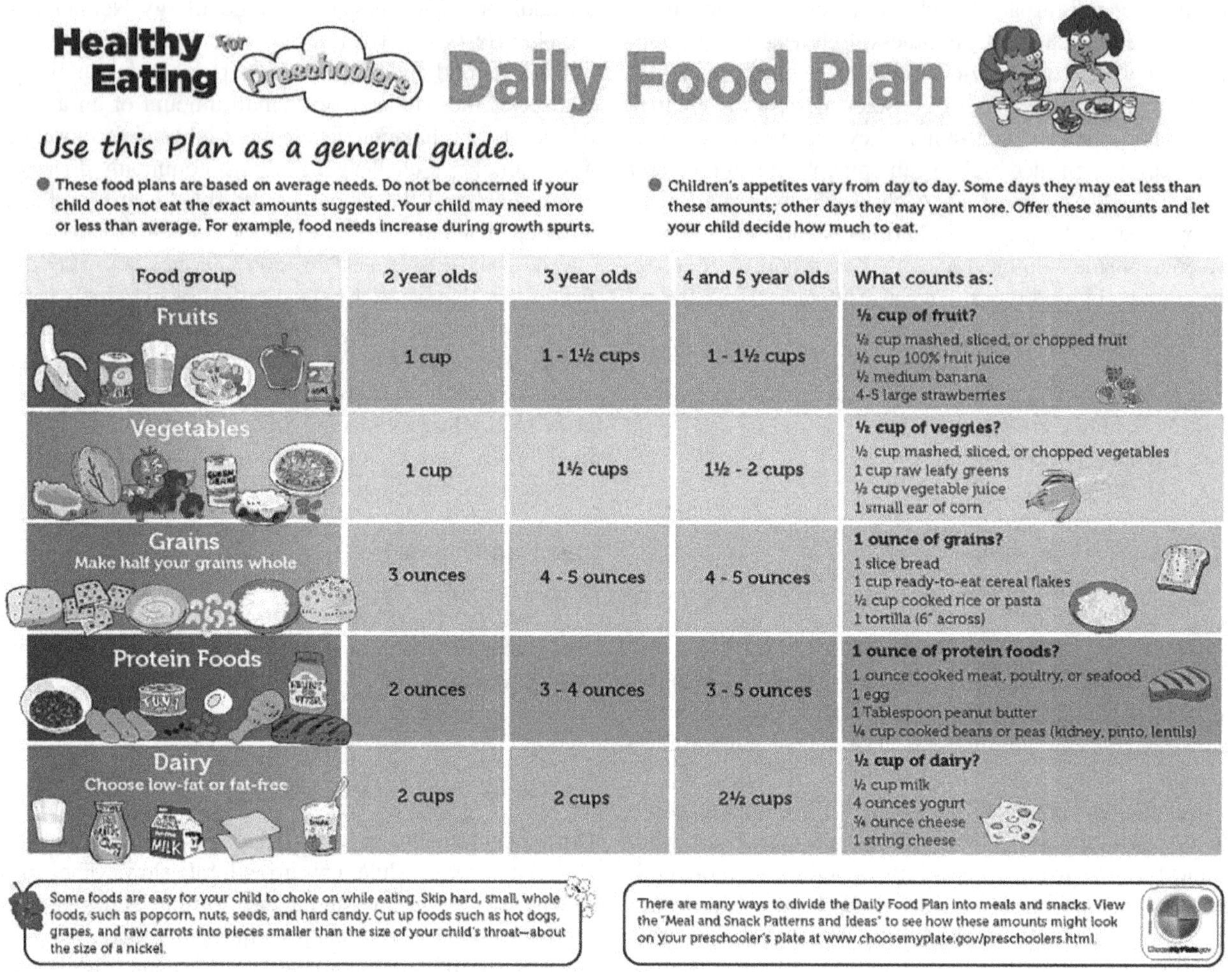

Healthy Eating for Preschoolers Daily Food Plan

Use this Plan as a general guide.

- These food plans are based on average needs. Do not be concerned if your child does not eat the exact amounts suggested. Your child may need more or less than average. For example, food needs increase during growth spurts.
- Children's appetites vary from day to day. Some days they may eat less than these amounts; other days they may want more. Offer these amounts and let your child decide how much to eat.

Food group	2 year olds	3 year olds	4 and 5 year olds	What counts as:
Fruits	1 cup	1 - 1½ cups	1 - 1½ cups	**½ cup of fruit?** ½ cup mashed, sliced, or chopped fruit; ½ cup 100% fruit juice; ½ medium banana; 4-5 large strawberries
Vegetables	1 cup	1½ cups	1½ - 2 cups	**½ cup of veggies?** ½ cup mashed, sliced, or chopped vegetables; 1 cup raw leafy greens; ½ cup vegetable juice; 1 small ear of corn
Grains Make half your grains whole	3 ounces	4 - 5 ounces	4 - 5 ounces	**1 ounce of grains?** 1 slice bread; 1 cup ready-to-eat cereal flakes; ½ cup cooked rice or pasta; 1 tortilla (6" across)
Protein Foods	2 ounces	3 - 4 ounces	3 - 5 ounces	**1 ounce of protein foods?** 1 ounce cooked meat, poultry, or seafood; 1 egg; 1 Tablespoon peanut butter; ¼ cup cooked beans or peas (kidney, pinto, lentils)
Dairy Choose low-fat or fat-free	2 cups	2 cups	2½ cups	**½ cup of dairy?** ½ cup milk; 4 ounces yogurt; ¾ ounce cheese; 1 string cheese

Some foods are easy for your child to choke on while eating. Skip hard, small, whole foods, such as popcorn, nuts, seeds, and hard candy. Cut up foods such as hot dogs, grapes, and raw carrots into pieces smaller than the size of your child's throat—about the size of a nickel.

There are many ways to divide the Daily Food Plan into meals and snacks. View the "Meal and Snack Patterns and Ideas" to see how these amounts might look on your preschooler's plate at www.choosemyplate.gov/preschoolers.html.

FIGURE 4.2 USDA Daily Food Checklist for preschoolers.

obtained from fruits or 100% fruit juices. Foods that are high in refined sugars (candies, cakes, cookies) should only occasionally be consumed. Too much fiber can be harmful since it can make a child feel full quickly, interfering with sufficient food intake and absorption. Daily protein intake is 0.95 grams per kilogram of body weight, per day. The most nutritious sources of protein include lean meats, fish, poultry, lower-fat dairy products, soy-based food products, and legumes. Table 4.1 summarizes nutrient recommendations for toddlers and children.

For children up to age eight years, the need for most micronutrients increases slightly as they grow. If a child is not receiving enough nutrients because of skipping breakfast, trading lunches, or because of low-income households, any deficits may be corrected with pediatric vitamin and mineral supplements that provide no more than 100% of the Daily Value for micronutrients.

Daily fluid recommendations are about five to eight cups of beverages that include drinking water. Exact requirements vary based on the child's level of physical activity and the environment. Children should be reminded, especially with more physical activity, to drink fluids sufficiently to stay hydrated, especially in hot weather. The negative effects of peers with poor diets must be addressed. A "cool" kid that drinks soda and eats potato chips is, on a dietary level, much worse off than another child who eats fruit, whole-wheat peanut butter sandwiches, or drinks low-fat milk. Parents can educate their children about famous athletes and entertainers that consume highly nutritious diets.

Parents should model healthy diets to their children. A great idea is to teach children how to grow foods, shop, plan, and prepare meals. Children with input into their diet may be more likely to play an active role in decision-making about foods. Families that prepare and eat meals together usually have a better diet and healthier weights. Family meals encourage conversations and closeness with each other.

Attending school often requires busy morning schedules, but children should never skip breakfast or eat insufficient quantities of food. Hunger during school increases risks for behavioral and learning problems. In school, many children eat whatever they want, or in excessive amounts. They often trade items in home-packed lunches that they don't really like for other items that are preferred, even though they may be poorer in nutritional value. Sometimes, a proper lunch is not consumed in order to have more time for recess with friends.

TABLE 4.1
Nutrient Recommendations for Children

Nutrient	Toddlers	Children (4–8)	Children (9–12)
Fat	No recommended dietary allowance (RDA)	No RDA	No RDA
Protein	1.10 g/kg of body weight per day	0.95 g/kg of body weight per day	0.95 g/kg of body weight per day
Carbohydrate	130 g/day	130 g/day	130 g/day
Vitamin A	300 micrograms/day	400 mcg/day	600 mcg/day
Vitamin C	15 mg/day	25 mg/day	45 mg/day
Vitamin E	6 mg/day	7 mg/day	11 mg/day
Calcium	700 mg/day	1,000 mg/day	1,300 mg/day
Iron	7 mg/day	10 mg/day	8 mg/day
Zinc	3 mg/day	5 mg/day	8 mg/day
Fluids	1.3 liters/day	1.7 liters/day	Boys: 2.4 liters/day; Girls: 2.1 liters/day

Schools in many locations have adjusted to this by scheduling recess before lunch so that children are hungrier and thirstier when it is time to eat and drink. Another thing many schools have done is to stop having vending machines that offer poor food choices that are high in calories and low in nutrition.

FOCUS ON LIMITED FOOD CHOICES IN CHILDHOOD

Sometimes, a child will develop what is known as a *food jag*, in which he or she only wants to eat a small range of foods. Parents and teachers can help by educating the child about each food containing different types of nutrients, and then offer substitute food choices that contain extra nutrients, allowing the child to choose between them. Over time, food jags diminish in most children, and the child starts eating a wider variety of foods.

Test Your Knowledge

1. What are the most nutritious sources of protein?
2. How can parents model healthy diets to their children?

MALNUTRITION AND HUNGER IN CHILDHOOD

Malnutrition and hunger jeopardize children's health, development, and education. Over one of every six children lives in households that have some amount of food insecurity, with inconsistent access to sufficient food. African-American children have 25.6% food insecurity, while Hispanic children have 24.3%. Some children benefit well from food programs in school, but during the summer months, when there is no school, the food programs do not continue. Participation in the federally funded School Breakfast Program has been shown to improve academic achievement – especially in children at risk for malnutrition and hunger. Calories and portion sizes must be appropriate for the ages of the children participating. Table salt and saturated fat must be reduced to specific levels. Vending machines must meet specific nutrient guidelines.

Globally, undernutrition contributes to stunting and affects more than 149 million children under the age of five years. One-third of them live in India. More than 49 million children are wasted. There are also 40 million children in the world that are overweight. Undernutrition – especially stunting, wasting, and micronutrient deficiency – occurs more often today along with children that are overweight, but accurate statistics on incidence and prevalence over various countries is not well documented.

During childhood, there are a variety of concerns related to poor nutrition. **Dental caries** occur when bacteria in the mouth consume carbohydrates that are on the teeth. Acid is secreted by the bacteria, staring to erode tooth **enamel** and resulting in tooth decay. It is important to limit intake of sweets in children, along with drinks that contain large amounts of sugar. One additional serving of a sugar-sweetened drink per day can increase incidence of cavities by more than 20%. Frequent brushing helps eliminate sugars on teeth, along with the bacteria feeding on them. Fluoride prevents the development of cavities. It is important to keep primary and permanent teeth healthy and strong. Primary teeth guide permanent teeth into position, so problems with them can result in lifelong dental conditions. A child's first pediatric dental visit should occur at six months of age, or the first two teeth have erupted (see Figure 4.3). As soon as there are teeth, cavities are possible.

Intake of calcium is another concern, since it is needed for adequate **bone density** and many critical body and cellular functions. Inadequate calcium intake during childhood and adolescence can result **rickets**. Dairy products supply the largest amount of calcium in children in the United States. Even so, almost 60% of children have less than two servings of dairy per day. In early life and in the preschool years, milk consumption is mostly monitored by parents and caregivers. Older children, however, often consume

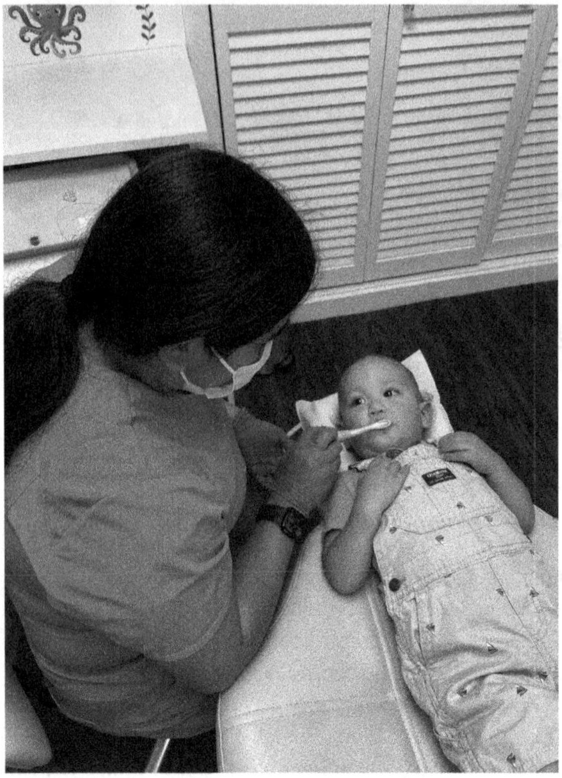

FIGURE 4.3 A child's first pediatric dental visit.

excessive amounts of sodas, sports beverages, fruit punch, and other sweetened drinks – instead of milk. This results in lower protein, calcium, magnesium, phosphorus, potassium, and vitamin A intake, increasing risks for poor bone health. Over four million households with children have issues with food insecurity and hunger in the United States.

NEURODEVELOPMENTAL DISORDERS

Neurodevelopmental disorders are disabilities that mostly affect the brain and neurological system. In children, examples of these disorders include attention-deficit/hyperactivity disorder (ADHD), autism, intellectual disabilities, learning disabilities, and impairment of hearing and vision. Children with neurodevelopmental disorders may have difficulties with language, speech, behavior, motor skills, learning, and memory. Symptoms and behaviors may change with growth and development, or remain permanent. Diagnosis and treatment may be difficult and often requires combinations of experts.

ADHD is the most common neurodevelopmental disorder in childhood and affects about 5% of children globally. Though genetics is a major risk factor, new evidence suggests that diet and child nutrition in early life influences the risk of developing ADHD during childhood, affects its severity, and determines its prognosis. The **gut microbiota** undergoes a dynamic, non-random maturation process until two to three years of age. Breastfeeding plays a protective role against ADHD. Chronic deficiencies of zinc, magnesium, iron, and iodine, plus deficiencies of polyunsaturated fatty acids, greatly impacts development and symptoms of ADHD.

Children with feeding and eating disorders have higher risks for clinically diagnosed emotional and behavioral disorders of childhood onset. These include ADHD, **autism** spectrum disorder (ASD), and intellectual disability. However, girls with feeding and eating disorders have higher risks for emotional or behavioral disorders, but not ADHD or ASD.

FOCUS ON SPECIAL NEEDS CHILDREN

Some physical and mental impairments can affect the nutrition of children. These impairments may require adaptive equipment and unique eating strategies to overcome limitations and ensure proper nutrition.

Test Your Knowledge

1. What are the signs and symptoms of children with neurodevelopmental disorders?
2. What are examples of neurodevelopmental disorders in children?

GENETIC CONDITIONS WITH SPECIFIC DIETARY INFLUENCES

Genetic conditions may affect vitamin and mineral absorption. An example is increased iron absorption in **hemochromatosis**, in which iron levels build up and overload. People with hemochromatosis have a gene variant on the short arm of chromosome 6. The absorption of vitamin B12 can be negatively affected by the genetically determined absence of gastric **intrinsic factor**, resulting in **pernicious anemia**. The ability to absorb vitamins A, E, and D is widely varied. The body does not produce these vitamins itself. The **bioavailability** of vitamin E via the diet is regulated by single **nucleotide polymorphisms**. These are controlled by genes involved in intestinal uptake and transport of the fat-soluble vitamins. Lactase is an intestinal enzyme that digests lactose, a sugar found in the milk of most mammals. Some people lose the ability to absorb lactose after being weaned off of breast milk. They are called **lactose malabsorbers**.

The diet has a profound effect upon how we express possibilities within our DNA. Diet can turn genetic markers on or off that play major roles in health. In animal studies, future generations of test subjects given high-fat diets experienced cardiovascular symptoms, even if their own diets were not high-fat. An **epigenetic marker** made future generations more likely to accumulate fat cells in the heart. Reducing the instance of this marker via dietary interventions protected future generations from heart disease. Perhaps changes to the current generations' diet, by increasing vegetables known to protect against certain cancers, can have long-term generational positive effects.

VEGETARIANISM IN CHILDHOOD

Vegetarian diets are beneficial to people of all ages. For children, a healthy vegetarian diet can be planned by working with physicians and registered dietitians that will meet nutritional needs and offer health benefits. Diets rich in fruits and vegetables as well as fiber, which are low in fat, improve heart health. Vegetarians are less likely to be overweight, have hypertension, or develop type 2 diabetes mellitus. However, children and teenagers on vegetarian diets must receive enough vitamins and minerals. The ways to get enough of the following vitamins and minerals are explained as follows:

- Vitamin B12 – dairy products, eggs, and vitamin-fortified breads, cereals, milk alternatives, and nutritional yeast
- Vitamin D – milk, vitamin D-fortified orange juice, other vitamin D-fortified products
- Calcium – dairy products, broccoli, dark green leafy vegetables, calcium-fortified cereals, milk alternatives, and orange juice; additionally supplied in dried beans
- Iron – dried beans, eggs, dried fruits, green leafy vegetables, whole grains, iron-fortified bread and cereals
- Protein – dairy products, eggs, and soy products, dried beans, nuts

For infants of **vegan** mothers, soy formula is important during the first six months, and vitamin B12 supplements may be required. Vitamin D recommendations are identical for vegetarian and non-vegetarian infants. Introduction of solid foods is also the same. Breastfed infants six months or older should receive enough iron from iron-fortified infant cereals. Once eating solids, protein-rich vegetarian foods include eggs, cottage cheese, pureed tofu, pureed and strained legumes (beans, chickpeas, lentils, split peas), and soy yogurt.

For toddlers, it is important to offer iron-fortified cereals and other foods. Toddlers are usually quite choosy about their diet. Toddlers that only like to eat vegetables may feel full before they actually get enough of needed calories and nutrients, since the amount of vegetables may be too bulky for their stomachs. Snack time can boost nutrition by offering healthy foods as snacks between meals. A pediatrician must assess whether a toddler needs vitamin or mineral supplements.

For older children and adolescents, a meat-free diet can be an excellent choice, prompting them to eat more fruits and vegetables. The best choice for growing teens is a lacto-ovo diet, which includes dairy products and eggs. Today, many schools offer vegetarian meal choices. It is important for parents to discuss healthy eating with their children, especially if they consume a vegetarian diet.

FOCUS ON ADOLESCENT EATING DISORDERS

It is important that parents monitor any self-imposed, restrictive diets. Adolescents with eating disorders often greatly reduce calories or cut out all fat or carbohydrates, saying they are on a "vegetarian diet". Preteens or teenagers must be instructed about understanding nutrients that may be missing from their diets. A good way to help monitor the situation is for the entire family to have at least one vegetarian meal together every week.

Test Your Knowledge

1. What is the genetic condition that causes increased iron absorption?
2. Which vegetarian foods are extremely rich in iron and calcium?

AVOIDANT RESTRICTIVE FOOD ISSUES

Avoidant/restrictive food intake disorder (ARFID) is an eating disorder. In children, it results in extremely choosy food intake and often, little interest in eating. By eating only a limited variety of the foods they will accept, poor growth and nutrition can result. This disorder usually begins earlier in life than other eating disorders. Children with ARFID may not feel hungry, or are repelled by food odors, tastes, textures, or colors. Some affected children have a fear of choking, pain, or vomiting while they eat. They are usually underweight, but some are of normal weight or even overweight because they only eat "junk food". Affected individuals are more likely to have anxiety, **obsessive-compulsive disorder**, ADHD, ASD, and problems at home or school because of their eating habits.

This disorder may cause affected children to not get enough minerals, protein, or vitamins. Some of them require tube feeding and nutritional supplements. Growth is usually poor and puberty may be delayed. Lack of nutrition can cause dehydration, hypotension, amenorrhea, and weakening of the bones and muscles. It is believed that ARFID is caused by combinations of genetic, psychological, and triggering events such as choking. Sometimes, gastroesophageal reflux disease (GERD) is present, which leads to feeding problems.

Diagnosis of avoidant restrictive food issues such as ARFID is based on physical examination, medical history, eating and exercise habits, and emotional issues. There is assessment of any significant weight loss, serious nutritional deficiencies, poor appetite, lack of interest in eating, or food avoidance. Testing may involve blood or urine tests or an electrocardiogram (ECG). Dealing with the condition early is the best way to treat it. Treatments involve physicians, dietitians, and eating disorder therapists. There may be nutrition counseling, medical care, and feeding therapy. If choking has occurred, a speech-language pathologist can perform a swallowing and feeding evaluation.

The primary goals of treatment are to achieve and maintain a healthy weight and eating patterns, increase food variety, and instruct how to eat without fear of choking, pain, or vomiting. Medications can be used to increase appetite or treat anxiety. The condition is usually treated at home, but hospitalization is sometimes required. The affected child is helped successfully when the entire family works together to change mealtime behaviors. Parents should serve and eat a variety of foods, schedule regular meals and snacks, have regular meal times together, encourage trying new foods without force, rewarding positive eating behaviors, and teach children to take a few deep breaths before eating, or encouraging participation in yoga, meditation, music, art, dance, writing, or spending time with friends.

FUNCTIONAL DISORDERS AND HYPERMOBILITY

Functional disorders and joint hypermobility-related disorders are etiologically and clinically heterogeneous groups of childhood pathologies. For example, ASD is seen in psychiatry, while musculoskeletal disciplines and genetics are implicated in hypermobility-related disorders. Both conditions are concurrent in more cases than would occur with chance. Hypermobility is often a sign of hereditary connective tissue disorder such as **Ehlers-Danlos syndrome** or **Marfan syndrome**. Joint hypermobility is an exaggerated increase in the range of a joint's mobility. This is more common in infancy, decreases with age, and affects females more than males. Just one hypermobile joint may suffer consequences of laxity, including tendencies for dislocation, traumatic **synovitis**, premature **osteoarthritis**, or pain without an obvious cause.

Young children with autism display manifestations such as hypotonia, clumsiness, joint laxity, **apraxia**, and toe walking (see Figure 4.4). There are genetic syndromes that link autism and hypermobility of the joints. **Fragile X syndrome** is the most common genetic comorbidity of ASD, with underlying connective tissue problems signified by soft skin, **scoliosis**, flat feet, and **pectus excavatum**. There are also clinical comorbidities between Marfan syndrome and neuropsychiatric conditions such as ASD, which had not been previously been documented. Ehlers-Danlos syndrome, in 80%–90% of cases, involves hypermobility.

Test Your Knowledge

1. What are the symptoms of avoidant/restrictive food intake disorder?
2. What are the manifestations of autism?

ADOLESCENCE

Adolescence is generally the period from when puberty begins (mostly around age 12–13) up to the age of 18, which is considered to be when an individual is physically an adult. It is a very unique stage of development and important for developing healthy routines that will greatly impact future life. Adolescents undergo rapid physical, cognitive, and psychosocial growth. There is more autonomy than in childhood, but the full rights and responsibilities of adulthood are not yet in place. Adolescents that engage in sexual activity and become parents are, in most cases, not sufficiently mature to handle the requirements of raising a child. Perhaps the most significant changes of adolescence are growth spurts, primary sex characteristics (changes in the reproductive organs), and secondary sex characteristics (signs of sexual maturity throughout the body that do not directly involve the reproductive organs).

PHYSICAL GROWTH AND DEVELOPMENT

At the beginning of sexual maturation, there is a dramatic impact upon nutritional requirements. Because of

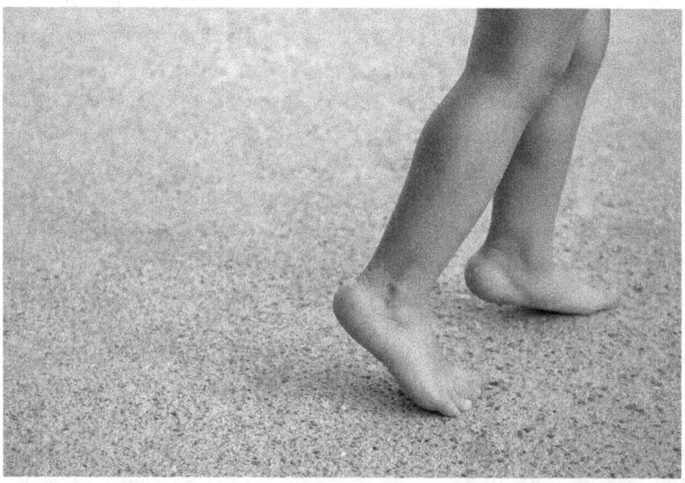

FIGURE 4.4 An autistic child toe-walking.

gender-specific hormones, the bodies of boys and girls develop differently. The changes begin between ages eight and nine, so DRI values are separately defined for boys and girls between nine and thirteen years of age. Hormonal changes control most of the growth that occurs during adolescence, with increased testosterone in boys and increased estrogen in girls. Both genders have growth spurts, which are fluctuating, accelerated increases in height during later childhood and adolescence. Growth spurts vary by factors such as gender, nutritional status, and race. Also, African-American girls enter puberty earlier and reach menarche earlier than girls from other races. African-American boys also are more likely to enter puberty earlier than boys from other races. The earliest stage of puberty has been found in African-American boys between nine and ten years of age.

There are large changes in weight and body composition. Girls gain about 35 pounds and boys gain about 45 pounds. This is highly varied, based on energy intake, genetics, and physical activity. Girls usually gain much more body fat around the buttocks, hips, breasts, thighs, and upper arms. Though these changes can be embarrassing, they are natural. Boys gain much more muscle mass than girls, with increases in muscle definition. Wide variances in physical activity levels result in individualized needs for energy. Even though much energy is required during rapid growth and maturation, adolescence is often when being overweight first manifests.

Diet

Nutrition for children and adolescents is similar as for adults, but in different quantities. Nutrient-rich foods include the following:

- **Proteins** – seafood, lean meat, poultry, eggs, beans, peas, soy products, unsalted nuts and seeds
- *Fruits* – fresh, canned, frozen or dried – for fruit juice, only drink 100% juice with no added sugars, and in limited servings; canned fruit that is "light" or packed in its own juice is better than other choices because it is low in added sugar; also, overconsumption of dried fruits adds extra calories
- *Vegetables* – fresh, canned, frozen, or dried – a variety should be supplied, including dark green, red, and orange colors, including beans, peas, starchy and non-starchy; for canned or frozen vegetables, choose low-sodium options
- *Grains* – whole grains such as whole-wheat bread, oatmeal, popcorn, quinoa, and brown rice; however, white bread, pasta, and white rice should be limited
- *Dairy* – fat-free or low-fat products including milk, yogurt, cheese, or fortified soy beverages

It is extremely important to limit added sugar, table salt, high-sodium foods, and saturated fats. Too much sugar can cause dental caries, obesity, and diabetes. Excessive table salt or high-sodium foods increases blood volume and leads to hypertension. Added sugars include brown sugar, corn sweetener, corn syrup, and honey. Soda and sports/energy drinks should be extremely limited or avoided altogether. Saturated fats mostly come from fatty meat and full-fat dairy products. They lead to obesity and cardiovascular disease. Vegetable and olive oils should replace saturated fats. Healthier fats are present in avocados, nuts, olives, and seafood.

The United States Food and Drug Administration banned trans fats in 2018, though products manufactured before that year could still be distributed until 2021. Since this ban, many manufacturers reformulated their products to use other ingredients such as *fully hydrogenated oil*, which contains no trans fats, but contains the saturated fatty acid known as **steric acid**. Trans fats may still be present in foods such as snacks, frozen pizza, fast food, margarine, and coffee creamer. Even when the product label says there is zero grams of trans fats per serving, there can still be up to 0.5 grams of trans fats per serving. Trans fats can be limited by avoiding any foods with *partially hydrogenated oil*.

FOCUS ON TRANS FATS

Trans fats are the worst type of fats to consume, and are also known as *trans fatty acids*. They increase LDL (bad) cholesterol while lowering HDL (good) cholesterol. The banning of trans fats by the United States and some other countries will prevent thousands of heart attacks and related deaths annually. Trans fats also increase the risks for stroke and type II diabetes because of their effects on cholesterol that encourage atherosclerosis.

Most children have way too much sodium in their diets, so they should be encouraged to snack on fruits and vegetables instead of cookies or chips. Low-sodium options are widely available. Daily guidelines for girls and boys of various ages are listed in Table 4.2, and Table 4.3 summarizes nutrient recommendations for children and adolescents.

In adolescence, there is a sharp increase in the need for micronutrients due to sexual maturation beginning and to ready the body for the adolescent growth spurt. If a teenager does not consume the recommended four cups of fruits and vegetables per day, deficiencies of vitamins A, C, and E may result. Fresh fruits and vegetables also increases intake of potassium and fiber, which may be low in the diets of children in lower-income households. Calcium, iron, and zinc are very important, but mostly are found in animal-based foods. The recommended dietary allowance (RDA) for iron is based on the fact that most girls do not begin menstruation until age 13 or later.

TABLE 4.2
Daily Guidelines for Girls and Boys of Various Ages

Ages	Girls	Boys
Two to four years	1,000 to 1,400 calories based on growth and activity levels; Protein – 2 to 4 ounces Fruits – 1 to 1.5 cups Vegetables – 1 to 1.5 cups Grains – 3 to 5 ounces Dairy – 2 to 2.5 cups	1,000 to 1,600 calories based on growth and activity levels; Protein – 2 to 5 ounces Fruits – 1 to 1.5 cups Vegetables – 1 to 2 cups Grains – 3 to 5 ounces Dairy – 2 to 2.5 cups
Five to eight years	1,200 to 1,800 calories based on growth and activity levels; Protein – 3 to 5 ounces Fruits – 1 to 1.5 cups Vegetables – 1.5 to 2.5 cups Grains – 4 to 6 ounces Dairy – 2.5 cups	1,200 to 2,000 calories based on growth and activity levels; Protein – 3 to 5.5 ounces Fruits – 1 to 2 cups Vegetables – 1.5 to 2.5 cups Grains – 4 to 6 ounces Dairy – 2.5 cups
Nine to thirteen years	Calories – 1,400 to 2,200 based on growth and activity levels; Protein – 4 to 6 ounces Fruits – 1.5 to 2 cups Vegetables – 1.5 to 3 cups Grains – 5 to 7 ounces Dairy – 3 cups	Calories – 1,600 to 2,600 based on growth and activity levels; Protein – 5 to 6.5 ounces Fruits 1.5 to 2 cups Vegetables – 2 to 3.5 cups Grains – 5 to 9 ounces Dairy – 3 cups
Fourteen to eighteen years	1,800 to 2,400 based on growth and activity levels; Protein – 5 to 6.5 ounces Fruits – 1.5 to 2 cups Vegetables – 2.5 to 3 cups Grains – 6 to 8 ounces Dairy – 3 cups	2,000 to 3,200 based on growth and activity levels; Protein – 5.5 to 7 ounces Fruits – 2 to 2.5 cups Vegetables – 2.5 to 4 cups Grains – 6 to 10 ounces Dairy – 3 cups

TABLE 4.3
Nutrient Recommendations for Adolescents

Nutrient	Adolescents (13–18)
Fat	No recommended dietary allowance (RDA)
Protein	0.85 g/kg body weight per day
Carbohydrate	130 g/day
Vitamin A	Boys: 900 mcg/day; Girls: 700 mcg/day
Vitamin C	Boys: 75 mg/day; Girls 65 mg/day
Vitamin E	15 mg/day
Calcium	1,300 mg/day
Iron	Boys: 11 mg/day; Girls: 15 mg/day
Zinc	Boys: 11 mg/day; Girls: 9 mg/day
Fluids	Boys: 3.3 liters/day; Girls: 2.3 liters/day

FOCUS ON HEALTHY EATING

Healthy eating is simply not good enough for children of all ages. Studies that analyzed child and adolescent food consumption show that only 61% of children eat healthy foods most of the time, and this is the *best* score for all age groups. The results continue to decrease with continued aging and growth. Only 55% of children between five and eight eat healthy, and the same is true for 52% of children aged nine to thirteen, and 51% of those aged 14–18.

Test Your Knowledge

1. Why sugar and table salt only be used in limited amounts in the diet?
2. Why should trans fats be limited in the diet?

PUBERTY

Puberty involves rapid growth, with the body eventually reaching reproductive maturity. There is rapid brain maturation and identity formation, plus a variety of emotional changes. Adjusting to puberty can be difficult for the adolescent and his or her parents. Most adolescents go through puberty effectively as long as there is good communication and support from family and friends. Hormonal changes start in the mid-primary school years, though puberty itself often starts at around 10 years for girls and 11 years for boys. All individuals are different and start and end puberty at different times, though girls usually start quite a while before boys.

For girls, the hips widen and the body shape gets "curvier" as height increases. **Acne** may develop, usually on the face, neck, shoulders, upper back, and chest. The first stage of breast growth is *budding*, and the breasts may sometimes be of different sizes. Tenderness of the breasts is common, though a pediatrician should be consulted if it seems excessive. Hair begins to grow in the pubic area and under the arms. Hair on the arms and legs gets darker. A clear or white discharge may occur from the vagina, which is a normal, self-cleaning process. The menstrual periods begin, in which the lining of the uterus thickens in preparation for pregnancy. Once a month, the lining is shed if a pregnancy has not occurred, which takes a few days. Each month, the menstrual period can slightly be longer or shorter, with 28 days being most common. These irregular periods are very common, especially within the first few years after they begin. Pain or cramps may occur before or at the start of the menstrual period. Exercise, use of a hot-water bottle against the abdomen, or over-the-counter pain medications may help.

With puberty, boys get taller, stronger, and more muscular. Acne may develop, and the voice will deepen, sometimes called *voice breaking* because of changes in tone. Hair grows in the pubic area, legs, under the arms, and on the face. It is fine in appearance at first, but then gets thicker and darker. The testicles and penis get larger, and one testicle may be larger than the other. Sexual function has no relationship to penis size. Wet dreams may occur, in which there is ejaculation while asleep. Erections can happen from nervousness, excitement, or for no obvious reason. They usually subside after a few minutes. Some young men experience breast growth and tenderness, which is a normal response to changing hormones, and will subside.

Emotional changes for girls and boys can occur before the physical changes. There may be a greater sense of "self", sexual interest in other people, and changes of energy, mood, and sleep patterns. There may be difficulty coping with the body changes, or self-consciousness about appearance. When an adolescent cannot achieve what he or she wants, there is often frustration or anger. These emotional changes are important, as the individual determines his or her own moral values and identity. Many adolescents describe feeling like a child and an adult at the same time. Exploration, risk-taking, and impulsive actions are also normal. The growing need for independence can result in arguments with parents or caregivers that only want the adolescent to be safe. It is important to work through these issues together. Clear rules and expectations should be set forth. It is very essential that adolescents and parents or caregivers communicate clearly about what is and is not acceptable to all.

Growth Spurts

Girls usually start having growth spurts between 10 and 11, while boys usually start between 12 and 13 – hence the reason why many girls of the same age as their male counterparts are taller, at least for a while. These are cartilage plates near the ends of long bones that provide for their longitudinal growth. Most girls reach full adult height by approximately age 18, though some continue to grow (but more slowly) after age 19. When closure of the **epiphyseal plates** occurs, skeletal growth ceases. Boys usually continue to grow up until age 21, though this process also slows eventually. Sometimes, the epiphyseal plates close early and the individual does not reach full height. This is most often due to malnutrition, because of an eating disorder or the use of anabolic steroids during this critical period of growth. Factors that increase or decrease the release of growth hormone including the following:

- *Factors that increase growth hormone release* – sufficient sleep, low blood glucose, regular exercise, stress; these are increased during puberty.
- *Factors that decrease growth hormone release* – insufficient sleep, age, gender, food, lack of exercise, fasting, circulating growth hormone, and insulin-like growth factor 1.

FOCUS ON GROWTH HORMONE

Throughout life, growth hormone regulates the fat, muscle, tissue, and bone in our bodies, as well as other aspects of metabolism. These include insulin action and blood sugar levels. Growth hormone levels naturally reduce from middle age onwards.

FOCUS ON GROWTH HORMONE DEFICIENCY

Growth hormone deficiency is also known as pituitary dwarfism, or simply, *dwarfism*. It is caused by insufficient amounts of growth hormone in the body, resulting in an abnormally short stature, though the body proportions are normal. It can be present at birth or developing later. Other signs and symptoms include delayed or even absent puberty, increased fat around the face and stomach, being overweight, and slow tooth development or hair growth.

Social Development

Adolescents experience significant social development as well as emotional development. The most important task they undergo is the search for their own identity, which may actually take an entire lifetime, but starts in adolescence. There is also a large struggle for independence from parents and caregivers. Strong social development is provided by parents that follow these guidelines:

- Undivided attention to adolescents when they want to talk
- Calm listening with concentration on the adolescent's point of view
- Speaking courteously and pleasantly with a friendly tone of voice
- Understand adolescent feelings with as little judgment as possible – be open and approachable to them

TABLE 4.4
Important Milestones during Childhood

Milestone	Approximate Age	Activities
Early object permanence	4 to 8 months	Following an object out of sight, searching for a partially hidden object
Object permanence	9 to 12 months	Searching for an object that is completely hidden from view
Cause and effect	9 months	Realizing his or her actions cause other actions or are linked to responses
Functional use of objects	12 to 15 months	Understands what objects are used for
Representational play	18 months	Pretends to use objects in a functional way on dolls or other people
Symbolic play	2 to 3 years	Using objects to symbolize something else during pretend play
Pre-academic skills	3 to 5 years	Knowing letters, numbers, shapes, colors, and counts
Logial thinking	6 to 12 years	Understanding conservation of matter, problem-solving requiring multiple steps, understanding different perspectives
Abstract thinking	13 or more years	Hypothesizing, thinking abstractly, and drawing conclusions

- Avoid anything that can cause humiliation or embarrassment concerning what they say or ask
- Listen carefully and offer parental views openly and honestly with love and mutual respect
- Encourage them to participate in activities they choose
- Give commendation often but do it appropriately – try not to focus on the bad – everyone needs appreciation
- Encourage adolescents to be part of family decision-making and work together – they need to sometimes challenge your opinions and methods in order to achieve normal separation, to develop their own adult identity

There are also guidelines that adolescents need to consider when interacting with parents on a variety of levels. These include the following:

- Parents are not the "enemy" even when there is a difference of opinion
- We all have our own feelings, needs, and insecurities – whether parent or adolescent
- Parents have experience and their point of view should be considered
- Feelings should be shared with parents – it helps them understand adolescents better
- Independence is more often granted when an adolescent lives up to his or her responsibilities at home and in school
- If an adolescent has criticisms of family, school, or government, practical improvements should be suggested
- Adolescents should always be as courteous and considerate to parents as they would be to their friends' parents

Cognitive Development of Intellectual Skills

Cognitive development is the forming of knowledge, skills, problem-solving, and disposition. It helps children think about and understand their environment. It occurs quickly over the first five years of live, in four primary areas: motor (physical), language/communication, cognitive, and social/emotional. Brain development is just one component. Fostering early cognitive development is essential for later success. Infants that learn from their parents how to distinguish sounds at six months of age are better able to read at four or five years of age. They should be allowed to "talk" with parents as common objects are named so that they can learn. The infant should be encouraged to explore toys and move around the room. Singing and reading are very good developmental activities. Books and puzzles help engage toddlers in early interest of reading. When a toddler shows an interest in anything specific, it is important to encourage that interest. All questions a young child asks about "why" something happens should be answered. Choices can be offered and the toddler can be asked to make a thoughtful decision. There should be guidance about exploring different ways of solving problems. Gentle guidance, encouragement, and patients, are very important in early cognitive and intellectual development. Cognitive and intellectual milestones are used to assess normal or abnormal development. Table 4.4 summarizes important milestones during childhood.

FOCUS ON PIAGET'S FOUR STAGES OF COGNITIVE DEVELOPMENT

Jean Piaget developed theories of cognitive development by observing children with experiments to discover how they learn, develop, and acquire skills at specific ages. His four stages of cognitive development are the sensorimotor stage (from birth to two years), preoperational stage (two to seven years), concrete operational stage (seven to twelve years), and formal operational stage (twelve years and older).

NUTRIENT NEEDS OF ADOLESCENTS

Around the age of 10 in girls and 12 in boys, there is often a greatly increased appetite which indicates that puberty is approaching. The body demands more calories in early adolescence than in any other time of life. Adolescents that are tall or highly active still have increased needs for energy into late adolescence. During middle and late adolescence, girls eat about 25% less calories per day than boys, so they are more likely to have vitamin and mineral deficiencies. Most adolescents get twice as much protein as they actually need. Complex carbohydrates are preferred over simple carbohydrates and should make up 50%–60% of an adolescent's caloric intake. Fat should make up no more than 30% of the diet. An adolescent that has a diet heavy in fats will put on weight regardless of activity levels. Fatty foods that contain cholesterol can lead to adult **atherosclerosis** and cardiovascular problems. Intake of saturated fat must be limited to no more than 10% of total daily calories. The other 20% of daily calories from dietary fat should come equally from monounsaturated fat and polyunsaturated fat. Packaged and processed foods must be extremely limited since they are loaded with fat, sugar, and sodium. A well-rounded diet helps adolescents to avoid common deficiencies, such as those of calcium, iron, zinc, and vitamin D. It is preferable to obtain nutrients from food sources and not supplements.

NUTRITION-RELATED CONCERNS FOR ADOLESCENTS

Since adolescence basically begins at puberty as secondary sexual characteristics develop and reproduction becomes possible, nutritional needs range widely. Adolescents have nutritional needs that are based on rapid height and weight increases, body composition changes, and their levels of physical activity.

During adolescence, fat redistributes differently in the body, between boys and girls. Boys gather fat centrally, around the waist, while girls usually collect fat **gluteally**, on the lower body. Adolescents, as well as children, have a higher prevalence of excessive body fat or obesity today than ever before. For example, in 1980, their obesity rates were about 6% of the population. Today over 20% are obese in the United States. There are racial, ethnic, and gender differences as well. African-American girls that are not Hispanic, and Mexican-American boys have the greatest risk of being overweight or obese than other groups. Being severely overweight or obese has increased more quickly than cases of being moderately overweight.

The causes of these nutrition-related concerns for adolescents include eating more snacks and meals away from home and adult supervision, larger food portions, higher calories in food choices, higher dietary fat, decreased physical activity, and more time spent sitting in front of a computer, video game, television, or using a cell phone. Intervention for overweight or obese adolescents must be done carefully and sensitively. One excellent method is to have them conduct a 24-hour food intake recall, which can then be discussed and evaluated to help them understand their eating behaviors. There can be discussion of the dangerous of obesity during adolescence leading to type II diabetes. A further example is that the racial or ethnic groups that have the highest rates of being overweight or obese also have the highest numbers of people with diabetes. Treatment of obesity must include the entire family of the affected adolescent.

FOCUS ON SUGAR-SWEETENED BEVERAGES

Soda, fruit drinks, and sports or energy drinks should be avoided in the diets of anyone, including children and adolescents. Average intake of added sugars is 11% in young children, and highest at 15%, in adolescents. Most of these beverages do not contribute to meeting any food group goals and usually contain high numbers of calories.

Test Your Knowledge

1. What emotional changes occur in adolescents?
2. What are the dietary fat recommendations for adolescents?
3. How prevalent is excessive body fat or obesity in adolescents?

KEY TERMS

Acne

Adolescence

Allergen

Apraxia

Atherosclerosis

Autism

Bioavailability

Bone density

Dental caries

Ehlers-Danlos syndrome

Enamel

Epigenetic marker

Epiphyseal plates

Fragile X syndrome

Gluteally

Gut microbiota

Hemochromatosis
Intrinsic factor
Lactose malabsorbers
Marfan syndrome
Nucleotide polymorphisms
Obsessive-compulsive disorder
Osteoarthritis
Pectus excavatum
Pernicious anemia
Prick test
Rickets
Scoliosis
Steric acid
Synovitis
Vegan
Wheezing

CLINICAL CASE STUDIES

Clinical Case 1

A four-year-old girl with cerebral palsy had experienced failure to thrive, associated with cardiac abnormalities, encephalitis, spasticity, and seizures. With treatment, the child now has stabilized heart function and no more seizures. After previously having been fed via nasogastric tube, the child's family have been able to maintain her weight via a normal, healthy diet. However, the girl is an extremely picky eater, and often chokes or gags when trying foods of new textures. She is now able to hold and drink from a cup, though her spasticity often causes her to spill her drink. The girl can pick up small pieces of food and eat them, and is able to use a spoon or fork though it is a little difficult for her. The girl's mother is a nurse who is interested in returning to work to help support the family, but she is concerned about her daughter's ability to do well in a preschool situation. Also, since the girl eats many small meals each day, her mother is concerned this may not fit in well with a preschool's meal schedule. She is worried about proper weight maintenance and continued normal growth for her daughter.

CRITICAL THINKING QUESTIONS

1. What are the recommended dietary (daily) allowances of nutrients for children between four and eight years of age?
2. What are the possible effects of school upon children's diets?
3. What common nutrient deficiencies may be related to neurodevelopmental disorders in children?

Clinical Case 2

A 15-year-old girl was seen by a physician because of breathlessness, pallor, and bradycardia. Her father accompanied her, and when asked about his daughter's diet, told the physician she had decided to become a vegetarian two years previously. Though most tests that were completed were within normal limits, the girl's B12 levels were very low, explaining her symptoms. She was also diagnosed with idiopathic autoimmune hemolytic anemia. The patient was started on daily vitamin B12 injections along with oral prednisolone for ten days. Her hemoglobin levels improved. The injections were gradually tapered to twice per week. Over five months, the girl had no more symptoms. Her diet was adjusted to increase iron content by adding more fortified breakfast cereals, green leafy vegetables (which previously she only consumed in small quantities), beans, and whole grains.

CRITICAL THINKING QUESTIONS

1. Which foods provide high levels of vitamin B12?
2. Which type of vegetarian diet is the best for growing teenagers?
3. What are the dangers that can occur if an adolescent chooses to reduce calories or cut out certain dietary items?

Clinical Case 3

A mildly autistic 12-year-old boy was treated for poor nutritional status, weight loss, and anemia. For years, he had only eaten a small variety of foods, refusing anything he perceived as "weird" – his term for foods of new textures or appearances. His diet, therefore, basically consisted of white bread, French fries, candy, chicken nuggets, pizza, noodles, crackers, and cereal. During his childhood, he had problems with constipation, abdominal pain, and nausea close to meal times. He also had a fear of choking on food or vomiting it back up immediately after eating. Basically, his mother described him as having a "fear of eating". The boy was diagnosed with avoidant/restrictive food intake disorder. He was treated for multiple vitamin and mineral deficiencies and enrolled in cognitive-behavioral therapy, family-based therapy, and two medications (sertraline and olanzapine). Over seven weeks, the boy learned to try new foods slowly, one by one. Within this time period he had already accepted six new types of foods, including fruits and vegetables, and his healthy began improving rapidly.

CRITICAL THINKING QUESTIONS

1. What is avoidant/restrictive food intake disorder (ARFID)?
2. How does a child with ARFID feel about eating?
3. What other conditions are more likely to be concurrent in a child with ARFID?

STUDY QUESTIONS

1. The size of a child's brain at age 6 is about which of the following percentages of the size of the adult brain?
   A. 40%
   B. 50%
   C. 60%
   D. 90%

2. All of the following may determine biological eating habits, EXCEPT:
   A. Hunger
   B. Education
   C. Taste
   D. Appetite

3. Which of the following is NOT a recommendation of MyPlate for children?
   A. Eat more fruit
   B. Drink whole milk
   C. Be more active
   D. Eat whole grains

4. Which of the following body systems is affected by food allergies?
   A. Cardiovascular system
   B. Respiratory system
   C. Immune system
   D. Nervous system

5. Which of the following foods may cause the most severe allergic reactions?
   A. Fish
   B. White bread
   C. Strawberries
   D. Salad dressings

6. All of the following are among the most nutritious sources of protein, EXCEPT:
   A. Fruits
   B. Soybeans
   C. Fish
   D. Legumes

7. How many children, globally, are suffering from undernutrition?
   A. 60 million
   B. 75 million
   C. 149 million
   D. 550 million

8. Dental caries in children occur when bacteria in the mouth consume which of the following food components?
   A. Carbohydrates
   B. Proteins
   C. Lipids
   D. Vitamins B and C

9. All of the following food deficiencies may increase risks for poor bone health, EXCEPT:
   A. Magnesium
   B. Potassium
   C. Vitamin A
   D. Sodium

10. Which of the following is an example of hypermobility?
    A. Marfan syndrome
    B. Hypothyroidism
    C. Iron deficiency anemia
    D. Renal failure

11. In which of the following ages does puberty usually begin?
    A. Ages 9 to 10
    B. Ages 10 to 11
    C. Ages 12 to 13
    D. Ages 13 to 15

12. The earliest stage of puberty has been found to occur in African-American boys between which ages?
    A. 9 and 10 years
    B. 10 and 12 years
    C. 13 and 14 years
    D. 15 and 16 years

13. Which of the following grains should be limited in an adolescent's diet?
    A. Brown rice
    B. Oatmeal bread
    C. Pasta
    D. Quinoa

14. All of the following factors increase growth hormone release, EXCEPT:
    A. Insufficient sleep
    B. Low blood glucose
    C. Regular exercise
    D. Stress

15. According to Jean Piaget's four stages of cognitive development, which of the following is Stage 3?
    A. Formal operational
    B. Concrete operational
    C. Sensorimotor
    D. Preoperational

FURTHER READING

1. Adams, F. (2021). *The Right to Food: The Global Campaign to End Hunger and Malnutrition.* Palgrave Macmillan.
2. Albers, S. (2018). *Eating Mindfully for Teens – A Workbook to Help You Make Healthy Choices, End Emotional Eating, & Feel Great.* Instant Help.
3. Berk, L. (2018). *Exploring Child & Adolescent Development.* Pearson.
4. Boyatzis, C., and Junn, E. (2019). *Annual Editions: Child Growth and Development*, 23rd Edition. McGraw-Hill.
5. Bryant-Waugh, R., and Higgins, C. (2020). *Avoidant Restrictive Food Intake Disorder in Childhood and Adolescence – A Clinical Guide.* Routledge.
6. Dorfman, K., and Layton, R.E. (2014). *Cure Your Child with Food: The Hidden Connection Between Nutrition and Childhood Ailments.* Workman Publishing Company.
7. Evans, Y.N., and Dixon Docter, A. (2020). *Adolescent Nutrition – Assuring the Needs of Emerging Adults.* Springer.
8. Hassan, A. (2016). *Food Security and Child Malnutrition: The Impact on Health, Growth, and Well-Being.* CRC Press.
9. Jha, R. (2021). *Hunger and Malnutrition as Major Challenges of the 21st Century.* World Scientific.
10. Kerksick, C.M., and Fox, E. (2016). *Sports Nutrition Needs for Child and Adolescent Athletes.* CRC Press.
11. Lonsdale, D., and Marrs, C. (2017). *Thiamine Deficiency Disease, Dysautonomia, and High Calorie Malnutrition.* Academic Press.
12. Maidenberg, M.P. (2016). *Free Your Child from Overeating: A Handbook for Helping Kids and Teens.* The Experiment.
13. Marotz, L.R. (2018). *Health, Safety, and Nutrition for the Young Child*, 10th Edition. Cengage Learning.
14. Meltzer Warren, R., and Chey, W.D. (2017). *A Teen's Guide to Gut Health – The Low-FODMAP Way to Tame IBS, Crohn's, Colitis, and Other Digestive Disorders.* The Experiment.
15. More, J. (2021). *Infant, Child and Adolescent Nutrition: A Practical Handbook*, 2nd Edition. CRC Press.
16. Nitzke, S., Riley, D., Ramminger, A., and Jacobs, G. (2014). *Rethinking Nutrition: Connecting Science and Practice in Early Childhood Settings (The Redleaf Professional Library).* Redleaf Press.
17. Resch, E. (2019). *The Intuitive Eating Workbook for Teens – A Non-Diet, Body Positive Approach to Building a Healthy Relationship with Food.* Instant Help.
18. Robertson, C. (2015). *Safety, Nutrition, and Health in Early Education*, 6th Edition. Cengage Learning.
19. Slomin, J. (2020). *Sports Nutrition for Young Adults – A Game-Winning Guide to Maximize Performance.* Rockridge Press.
20. Sorte, J., Daeschel, I., Amador, C., and Au, L. (2020). *Nutrition, Health, and Safety for Young Children – Promoting Wellness*, 4th Edition. Pearson.
21. Thomas, J.J. (2019). *Cognitive-Behavioral Therapy for Avoidant/Restrictive Food Intake Disorder – Children, Adolescents, and Adults.* Cambridge University Press.
22. Vargo, F.E. (2015). *Neurodevelopmental Disorders: A Definitive Guide for Educators.* W.W. Norton & Company.
23. Vickerstaff Joneja, J.M. (2013). *The Health Professional's Guide to Food Allergies and Intolerances.* Academy of Nutrition and Dietetics.
24. Williams, S.E., and Zahka, N.E. (2017). *Treating Somatic Symptoms in Children and Adolescents.* The Guilford Press.

5 Older Adults

OUTLINE

LEARNING OBJECTIVES

After study of the chapter, readers should be able to:

1. Explain the demographic trends of aging in the United States.
2. Describe changes in average life expectancy.
3. Discuss neurodegenerative processes.
4. Explain the changes in the digestive system due to the aging process.
5. Discuss the cognitive and psychological changes of older adults.
6. Describe the most common age-related changes in the skin and hair of older adults.
7. Discuss age-related changes in the male and female reproductive systems.
8. Explain the importance of nutrition for elderly people.
9. Identify the risks of sun exposure in older adults.
10. Discuss the role of the microbiome.

OVERVIEW

Older adults experience a variety of alterations in the body that may lead to nutritional status changes. Living along, poor health, multiple medications, lowered income, reduced senses of thirst, smell and taste, and problems chewing or swallowing are common issues that affect elderly nutrition. It is also extremely important for older adults to receive good hydration, which helps prevent a variety of negative health outcomes. Overall, good nutrition helps maintain health, and the nutritional and fitness choices made earlier in life greatly influence continued good health into the elderly years.

DEMOGRAPHIC TRENDS OF AN AGING SOCIETY

The number of people in the United States age 65 or older will more than double to reach 80 million by the year 2040. This is about 20% of the projected population. The number of adults 86 or older, which need the most assistance with basic personal care, will almost quadruple by the same year. Globally, the share of the population aged 65 years or over increased from 6% in 1990 to 9% in 2019. This is expected to rise to 16% by the year 2050, meaning that one in six people will be age 65 or older. The majority countries in the world are experiencing growth in the size and proportion of older people in the population. Aging has been fastest in Eastern and Southeastern Asia, Latin America, and the Caribbean. Throughout most of the world, survival beyond age 65 is improving. Population aging will put more financial pressure upon health care support systems.

Baby boomers, those individuals born between 1946 and 1964, are reshaping the elderly population. The current growth of the population aged 65 and older, largely driven by the baby boom generation, has never occurred before. This generation, in its older years, has challenged the economy, institutions, and infrastructure. This group of people is projected to nearly double from 52 million (in 2018) to about 95 million by the year 2060. It is also becoming more racially and ethnically diverse. Older adults are also working longer, which is a trend that is also predicted to increase. The average **life expectancy** has increased from 68 years in 1950 to 78.6 years in 2017. The gender gap in life expectancy is narrowing as well, from a seven-year gap in 1990 to a five-year gap today (76.1 years for men and 81.1 years for women). The demand for nursing homes and other forms of elder care will be impacted continually in the future. In the United States, Social Security and Medicare expenditures are expected to rise significantly.

By 2050, the world's population of people aged 60 years and older will double to more than 2.1 billion. The number of people aged 80 or older is expected to triple by 2050, reaching 426 million. Two-thirds of the global population over age 60 will live in low- and middle-income countries.

DOI: 10.1201/b22969-7

FOCUS ON THE FUTURE OF ELDERLY HEALTHCARE

Six important directions have been identified to prepare for high-quality healthcare for the booming elderly population. These include creating an adequately prepared workforce, strengthening the role of public health, remediating disparities and unequal treatment scenarios, developing new approaches to delivering care, allocating resources to palliative and end-of-life care, and redesigning long-term services and support systems.

Test Your Knowledge

1. What levels will the global population of adults aged 65 and over reach by 2050?
2. Which group of people is referred to as "baby boomers"?

THE PHYSIOLOGY AND PATHOLOGY OF AGING

The diseases related to aging are becoming more prevalent. Associated healthcare costs are increasing in all countries of the world. The mechanisms of cellular aging are better understood, at genetic, protein, and organelle levels. Systemic aging is also better understood today and possible biological advantages of aging are being studied. These advances are helping to improve prospects for targeted therapeutic interventions for aging and age-related disease. People over age 70 commonly have multiple chronic diseases. For example, the prevalence of benign prostate hyperplasias and prostate cancer in elderly men is nearly universal. Metabolic, immune, and cardiovascular dysfunction affects the majority of elderly people. Aging and disease appear to go hand-in-hand since aging is a key risk factor for chronic disease. Many treatments and interventions that target age-related diseases can increase lifespan, and some interventions delay diseases of aging.

NERVOUS SYSTEM

Neurodegenerative processes are strongly linked to loss of brain neurons. Cortical atrophy progresses as we age, with a 6%–11% loss of brain weight once a person passes the age of 80. There are decreases in cerebral hemisphere volume, the frontal region, the temporoparietal region, and the parieto-occipital region, along with increased lateral ventricle and third ventricle volume. Cortical atrophy precedes neurodegeneration if **dementia** has not developed. In patients with **Alzheimer's disease**, there is a 20%–25% greater cortical atrophy than in patients of the same age that do not have the disease (see Figure 5.1). Cerebral blood flow and oxygen consumption decrease, especially in areas with decreased gray and white matter. This heightens the risk for **stroke** with associated vascular disease. Smell, vision, auditory function, and vibrotactile sensation are also reduced.

The human brain starts to shrink when we are in age 30s or 40s, and the shrinkage rate increases even more by age 60. The frontal lobe and **hippocampus** experience the most shrinkage. As the cerebral cortex becomes thinner, its lower density leads to fewer connections, which may contribute to worsened cognitive processing. It is believed that the myelin in the white matter shrinks as well, reducing cognitive function. The brain also starts producing different levels of **neurotransmitters** and protein production.

CARDIOVASCULAR SYSTEM

Normal physiological changes occur in the cardiovascular system by aging. The myocardium and large blood vessels become stiffen, increasing **afterload** and impairing early diastolic filling. **Pacemaker cells** in the sinus node decrease with age. Myocardial contractility is of longer duration. The heart partially compensates for lower heart rate and maximal left ventricular contractility with exercise-induced dilatation of the left ventricle.

Left ventricular wall thickness progressively increases with age, independent of the presence of risk factors such as hypertension. This is accounted for by enlarging cardiac **myocytes**, though their actual number decreases over time. Local collagen concentration is altered. Collagen fibers increase. Though the myocyte to collagen ratio is relatively unchanged, this is mostly due to increase myocyte size, so hypertrophy is more prominent than hyperplasia. These changes contribute to increased myocardial stiffness and decreased compliance.

Increased contractility of the atrium leads to its hypertrophy and enlargement, indicated by an **atrial gallop** on auscultation. The **stroke volume** is unchanged, and is achieved in part by increasing end-diastolic volume. Resting heart rate does not change with aging, but the maximal heart rate that an 85-year-old person can achieve is about 70% of that of a 20-year-old person. The maximum cardiac output decreases, indicating that overall cardiac reserves diminish with age.

Normal aging affects the arteries as well, with **intimal hyperplasia** and thickening, and a decrease in vascular compliance and increased stiffness. The intimal thickness of the carotid artery increases two to three times between ages 20 and 90. Intimal thickening is a risk factor for **silent coronary artery disease** and is a component of subclinical vascular disease. The leg arteries after age 50 usually show calcifications and sclerosis. Dysfunctional endothelial vascular smooth **muscle tone** regulation results in stiffer arterial walls, which is independent of any atherosclerotic changes.

Increases in peripheral vascular resistance lead to increased systolic and diastolic pressure. Increases in

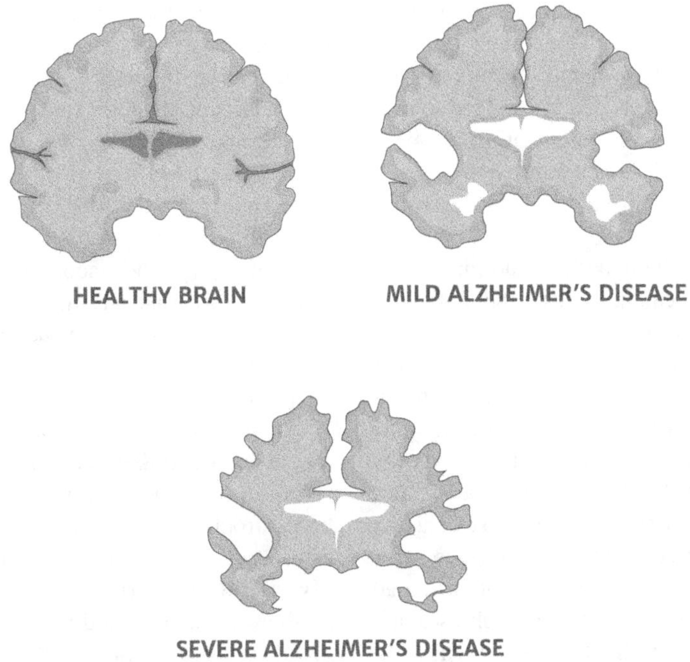

FIGURE 5.1 Cortical atrophy in relation to Alzheimer's disease.

central artery stiffness result in elevated systolic pressure, but reduced diastolic pressure. Central arterial stiffness becomes the main determinant of blood pressure. The most common form of hypertension after age 50 is **isolated systolic hypertension**. Increased **pulse pressure** is a better predictor of coronary disease than increased systolic pressure.

Respiratory System

In elderly people, the lung tissues, muscles, and bones change, which impact our ability to breathe. After age 35, the function of the lungs begins to decline. Breathing can slowly become more difficult year by year. The alveoli can lose their shape and become "baggy". The diaphragm may weaken, decreasing the ability to inhale and exhale. However, this change is only significant while exercising. The bones of the ribcage become thinner and change shape, meaning that the ribcage becomes less able to expand and contract with breathing. Nerves in the airways that trigger coughing become less sensitive to foreign particles, so when the particles increase in the lungs, they can damage the tissues. The immune system may weaken, increasing vulnerability to infections such as influenza and **pneumonia**.

Simple ways to protect the respiratory system and maintain better function throughout life include avoiding or quitting smoking, avoiding air pollution (including secondhand smoke, outdoor air pollution, chemicals, and radon), regular exercise, maintaining a healthy weight so that excess abdominal fat does not accumulate, not sleeping excessively (since too much bed rest allows mucus and fluid to settle in the lungs), having regular healthcare checkups, and getting annual vaccinations such the "flu" shot. During older adulthood, if lung capacity changes dramatically, or symptoms develop, a physician should be consulted.

Digestive System

With aging, there are many changes that affect the digestive system, beginning with a reduction in the senses of smell and taste. The gums recede, and there may be difficulty swallowing. **Peristalsis** in the esophagus decreases and the esophageal sphincters lose tension. The stomach walls lose elasticity. There is decreased production of bicarbonate and gastromucosal protection as well as delayed gastric emptying. The liver shrinks as **hepatocytes** are lost. There is a reduced ability of the liver to detoxify drugs and other substances, and the constitution of the bile changes. The pancreas experiences decreased secretion of pancreatic protease and lipase. In the small intestine, there is compromised gut-associated lymphoid tissue capacity. Peristalsis in the large intestine slows down. There is a decline in the rates of cell division and repair of the intestinal lining.

Food intake reduces with age because of a variety of reasons that result in reduced appetite, including physiological changes as well as altered psychosocial and pharmacological factors. Appetite is mainly regulated by sensors in the gastrointestinal tract (GIT), involving the hormones called *ghrelin*, *peptide tyrosine tyrosine (PYY)*, *cholecystokinin*, *insulin*, and *leptin*. The secretion of **ghrelin** and insulin increases, affecting appetite. When secretion of **cholecystokinin** and PYY increases, appetite is suppressed. **Leptin** is a hormone made by fat cells that decreases the appetite. About 50% of people aged 65–80 and about 75% of those over age 80 have a significant loss of the sense of smell. Accompanying this are age-related changes in taste cell membranes, which reduce the sense of taste. Diminished food intake can lead to weight loss and malnutrition, while the inability to taste and enjoy food can lead to anxiety. The ability to taste salty foods is reduced, and can lead to overconsumption of sodium-rich meals, aggravating hypertension and other conditions. Older adults are encouraged to use herbs or mild spices when cooking and eating, instead of salt, to increase flavor.

Age-related shrinkage of the maxillary and mandibular bones, and reduction in bone calcium causes the tooth sockets to slowly erode, leading to gum recession and a higher risk for tooth decay. People that are missing teeth or have poorly fitting dentures may find chewing difficult, resulting in them eating less, and the development of malnutrition. Some older people choose highly refined foods that are easy to chew, meaning that less dietary fiber is consumed. This affects bowel function and can cause constipation. **Xerostomia** is another common problem since saliva production decreases with age. This condition of dry mouth can also be due to medications or diseases such as diabetes mellitus. Xerostomia is more likely to occur when four or more prescription drugs are taken. Drug types that may cause xerostomia include diuretics, antihypertensives, antibiotics, bronchodilators, and antidepressants.

With age, the muscular contractions that initiate swallowing slow down, increasing transit time through the pharynx. This can lead to **dysphagia**, which may increase the risk of choking, or the feeling that food is stuck in the throat. As many as 27% of people aged 76 or older have dysphagia. In extremely old adults, impaired esophageal motility is common, and esophageal peristalsis definitely weakens with age. In some people, peristalsis is no longer triggered by every swallow. The upper and lower esophageal sphincters lose tension, with the lower sphincter having a greater reduction in pressure, leading to dysphagia, reflux, and heartburn. In 43% of older people, the gag reflex is absent.

Though most older adults continued to produce gastric acid at similar rates to those of younger adults, acid hyposecretion occurs in 10% of 20% of older people. This may compromise *bioavailability* of certain drugs as well as vitamin B12, leading to chronic atrophic gastritis. With aging, there is a reduction in the mucus-producing **goblet cells**, leading to reduced secretion of protective mucus and a weakened mucosal barrier. The stomach lining then is more likely to be damaged. A decline in gastric bicarbonate secretion means that the alkaline layer of the stomach, which protects it against gastric juices, is thinner. The **prostaglandin** content of mucus decreases, and lesions or ulcers are more likely, especially after taking non-steroidal anti-inflammatory drugs (NSAIDs), which many older people take regularly. Proton pump inhibitors (PPIs) suppress acid production, so they are often prescribed concurrently with NSAIDs. Since gastric emptying slows down, food remains in the stomach for a longer time, making the individual feel full longer and reducing appetite.

In the small intestine, there is an age-related decline in production of the enzyme called *lactase*, and individuals become more likely to be lactose intolerant. Certain bacteria increase over time, leading to bloating, pain, and decreased absorption of calcium, folic acid, and iron. Also, PPIs can provoke bacterial overgrowth, worsening NSAID-induced injury, and encouraging development of **inflammatory bowel disease**, diabetes, and autoimmune diseases. There is also a gradual reduction in the amount of **Peyer's patches** plus a slow loss of lymphoid follicles, which can result in uncontrolled growth of resident micro-flora.

An age-related slowing of transit in the large intestine is due to less **propulsive** activities, due to a reduction in neurotransmitters and neuroreceptors. This leads to constipation. Atrophy of the mucosa muscle layers of the colon also affects peristalsis. The walls start to sag, and pouches called **diverticuli** may form. Straining to defecate may increase pressure on weak blood vessel walls, leading to a **hemorrhoid** or several hemorrhoids. Cell division declines in the digestive epithelium and there is an age-related increase in colorectal cancer.

As populations of gastrointestinal (GI) microbes change, there is an increase in facultative anaerobes that include *streptococcus*, *staphylococcus*, *enterococcus*, and *enterobacteriaceae*, which thrive when there is inflammation. Aging has similar effects as those of inflammatory bowel diseases and obesity. As the single layer of epithelial cells becomes leaky with age, incidence of GI infections is higher, which is a primary cause of morbidity and mortality in the elderly. Infection with *Clostridium difficile*, which leads to a possibly fatal dehydrating diarrhea, is linked to two major risk factors: being age 65 years or older, and exposure to antimicrobial agents.

The pancreas decreases in weight and undergoes varying degrees of tissue fibrosis. There is impaired exocrine function, and reduced secretion of **chymotrypsin** and pancreatic lipase, which negatively affects digestion. The liver begins to lose its functional capacity and there is a decreased rate of protein synthesis and metabolism. The bile becomes thicker and has lower salt content, leading to higher plasma cholesterol – especially in women. Drugs are inactivated more slowly by the liver, so they can cause dose-related adverse effects. As a result, dosages for older people must be checked very carefully.

Test Your Knowledge

1. How and why does food intake reduce with aging?
2. What are the primary age-related changes in the stomach?
3. What is a primary digestive-related cause of morbidity and mortality in the elderly?

Immune System

Normally, the body's immune system defends against foreign or dangerous microorganisms (bacteria, viruses, and fungi), parasites such as worms, cancer cells, and transplanted organs and tissues. However, the immune system changes throughout life. As we age, it becomes less effective in a variety of ways. These are described as follows:

- There is less ability to distinguish between "self" and "nonself"; foreign **antigens** are not as easily identified; therefore, **autoimmune disorders** become more likely
- **Macrophages** destroy antigens such as bacteria and cancer cells more slowly, which may indicate why, for example, cancer is more common in older adults
- T-cells respond slower to antigens that they have previously encountered
- There are less white blood cells that can respond to new antigens; therefore, the body is less able to remember and defend against them
- There are fewer **complement proteins** produced in response to bacterial infections
- **Antibodies** become less able to attach to antigens, which partly explains why infectious diseases such as influenza and pneumonia are more common in older people and may result in death more often; also, these changes may help explain why vaccines are less effective in the elderly, and why they should receive any available booster shots

Musculoskeletal System

By aging, bone density begins to diminish. This process accelerates in women after they go through menopause. The bones become more fragile and likely to break – especially in people of older ages. The joints are also affected by changes in connective tissue and cartilage. As joint cartilage thins, components called *proteoglycans* are altered, and joints become less resilient, with more likelihood of being damaged. Therefore, joint surfaces often do not slide over each other which can lead to *osteoarthritis*. Joints also stiffen because connective tissue in the ligaments and tendons becomes more brittle and rigid. This results in a more limited range of joint motion.

Sarcopenia progresses continually. The amount of muscle tissue as well as the size and number of muscle fibers slowly decreases. This places more stress on joints (such as the knees), predisposing to arthritis or falls. Fortunately, regular exercise can partly overcome or delay losses in muscle mass and strength. The numbers of muscle fibers that undergo faster contraction decrease much more than the numbers of muscle fibers that undergo slower contraction.

Integumentary System

Among the most visible signs of aging are skin and hair changes. The skin becomes wrinkled and sagging, and the hair becomes gray or white. The greatest single factor influencing skin changes is sun exposure, which is seen by comparing areas of the body with regular sun exposure compared to areas that remain covered by clothing. People with lighter skin and blue eyes have more aging-related skin changes than those with darker and more heavily pigmented skin. The **epidermis** becomes thinner with aging and the number of **melanocytes** decreases as remaining melanocytes increase in size. Aging skin appears thinner, paler, and more translucent. In sun-exposed areas, pigmented age spots, also called "**liver spots**" may appear (see Figure 5.2). These are clinically known as *lentigos*. The connective tissue of the skin reduces in strength and elasticity, a condition known as *elastosis*, which produces a rougher skin appearance in people that spend a lot of time outdoors exposed

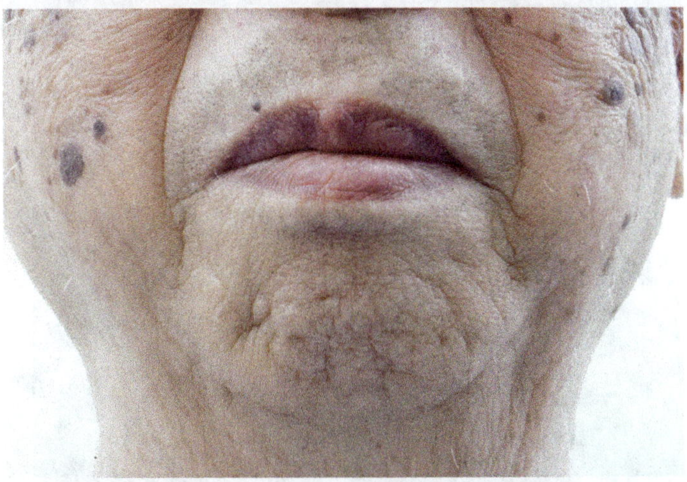

FIGURE 5.2 Liver spots.

to the sun (see Figure 5.3). As blood vessels of the dermis become more fragile, there can be easier bruising, bleeding under the skin, **cherry angiomas**, and similar conditions.

With aging, the **sebaceous glands** produce less oil, with men having the most decrease in this after age 80, while women slowly produce less oil after going through menopause. This makes it harder to keep the skin moist, and dryness or itchiness may occur. The subcutaneous fat layer thins, and has less insulation and padding, increasing risks of skin injury and reducing the capacity to regulate body temperature. Older adults often easily develop hypothermia in cold weather. The sweat glands produce less sweat and it is harder to stay cool. Risks for **heat stroke** are increased. Skin growths may include **skin tags**, warts, brown **seborrheic keratoses**, and other lesions (see Figure 5.4). Pink-colored **actinic keratosis** can develop, which have a slight change of becoming skin cancers.

Some people have less ability to sense touch, pressure, vibration, heat, or cold. Excessive friction against the skin is more likely to tear it. Fragile blood vessels can easily break. After even minor injuries, bruises, **purpura**, or **hematoma** can form. Pressure ulcers can be due to skin changes, thinning of the fat layer, less physical activity, poor nutrition, and illnesses. Sores are most obvious on the outside areas of the forearms but can occur anywhere. Older skin is repaired more slowly than younger skin, and wound healing can be as much as four times slower, contributing to pressure ulcers and infections. Healing is also affected by diabetes mellitus, blood vessel changes, and reduced immunity.

Since about 90% of older adults have some type of skin disorder, it is hard to differentiate them from normal age-related changes. Causes of skin disorders include nutritional deficiencies, obesity, arteriosclerosis, diabetes, heart disease, liver disease, medication reactions, and stress. Additional causes include allergies, climate, clothing, chemicals, and excessive indoor heating. Sunlight causes **elastosis**, non-cancerous skin growths, pigment changes, and skin thickening. Sun exposure is also linked to **basal cell carcinoma**, **squamous cell carcinoma**, and **melanoma**. Prevention must be a lifelong process, and involves preventing sunburn if possible, using a good quality sunscreen outdoors (even in winter), and wearing protective clothing and hats when needed. The most deadly of all skin cancers is melanoma, which has a poor prognosis. Good nutrition and adequate fluids are important since dehydration increases risks for skin injury. Minor nutritional

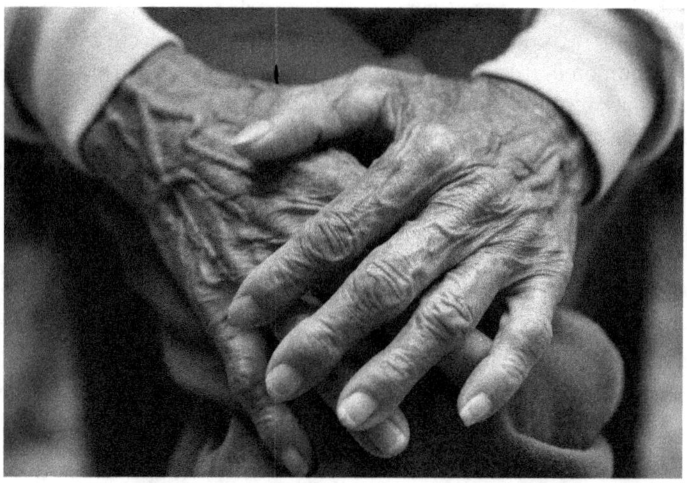

FIGURE 5.3 Elastosis of the skin of the hands due to sun exposure.

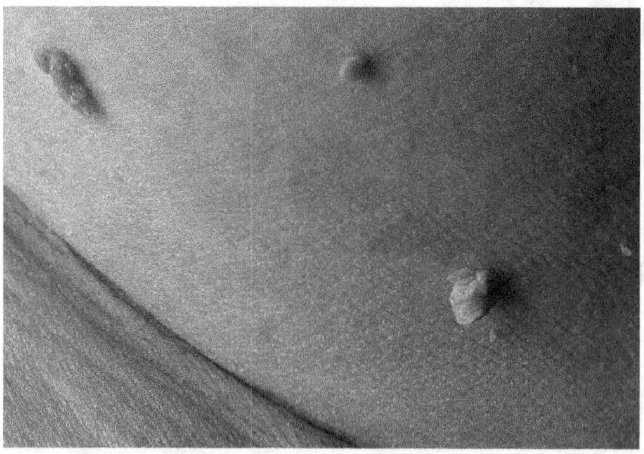

FIGURE 5.4 Skin tags.

deficiencies may cause rashes, lesions, and other skin changes. It is important to keep the skin moist with lotions and moisturizers, and avoid heavily perfumed soaps. Moist skin remains more comfortable and heals more quickly.

Urinary System

As we age, the kidneys and bladder also change and have reduced function. The number of nephrons decreases, so the ability to filter waste material from the blood is impacted. Therefore, kidney function diminishes. By age 70, there is a 30% reduction in the amount of nephrons. Blood vessels of the kidneys harden, causing the kidneys to filter blood more slowly. The bladder wall changes as its elastic tissue becomes stiffer so that it cannot stretch as easily, meaning that it cannot hold as much urine as earlier in life. Also, muscles of the bladder weaken. The urethra may become partially or totally blocked. In women, this can be cause by weakened muscles, which cause the vagina to **prolapse**. In men, the urethra can become blocked by an enlarged prostate gland. When an older adult is healthy, kidney function declines very slowly. However, illnesses, medications, and other conditions can significantly alter kidney function. **Urinary incontinence** and urinary retention are more common in elderly people.

Reproductive System

Age-related changes in the male reproductive system include effects upon testicular tissue, sperm production, and erectile function. These changes usually occur slowly. Some experts refer these changes as **andropause**. Most changes occur in the testes as testicular mass decreases. Levels of testosterone slowly decrease. Some men experience problems getting an erection, which is usually a general slowing and not a total lack of function. There may be sclerosis of the tubes that carry sperm. Though the testes continue to produce sperm, this occurs more slowly. The **epididymis**, **seminal vesicles**, and prostate gland lose some of their surface cells, yet continue to produce the fluid that helps carry sperm. The prostate gland enlarges as some tissue is replaced with a scar-like tissue. This is known as **benign prostatic hyperplasia** (BPH), and affects about half of all men. It may cause slowed urination and problems with ejaculation.

Fertility varies, and age does not predict male fertility, nor does prostate function affect it. Even if the prostate gland has been removed, a man can still father children, even in some cases into old age. While the volume of ejaculated fluid is usually close to the same, there are fewer live sperm in the fluid. However, the male *libido* may be reduced, and sexual responses can become slower and less intense. This may be due to decreased testosterone, or from psychological or social changes, illness, chronic conditions, or medications. Overall, aging alone does not prevent men from enjoying sexual relationships.

Erectile dysfunction (ED) may be a concern, and it is normal for erections to occur less often than in earlier life. Aging men often cannot have repeated ejaculations. However, 90% of cases of ED are due to a medical problem, and not just aging or a psychological problem. Medications used for hypertension, for example, can prevent the ability to achieve an erection or to maintain it for intercourse, and ED can also be caused by diabetes mellitus. If the condition is due to medications or illness, it is often successfully treated. Sometimes, BPH interferes with urination, increasing the likelihood for urinary tract infections and **prostatitis**. Prostate cancer becomes more likely with aging and early diagnosis is critical BPH to treat and decrees mortality.

As women age, most reproductive system changes are due to altered hormone levels, especially when menopause occurs and menstruation stops permanently. There will also be physical changes in the reproductive tract. Most women experience menopause around age 50 though it generally occurs anywhere between 45 and 55. The ovaries stop making estrogen and progesterone. They also stop releasing eggs, and pregnancy is no longer possible. Menopause is "official" once a woman has had no periods for one year. Any bleeding that occurs after one year without a period is not normal and requires assessment by a physician.

Other changes include thinning and drying of the vaginal walls, which become less elastic and more easily irritated. Sex may be painful because of these changes. Risks for vaginal yeast infections increase, and the external genital tissue decreases and thins, also becoming prone to irritation.

Hormone therapy with estrogen or progesterone (or both) can help reduce symptoms such as hot flashes, vaginal dryness, and pain with intercourse. It can be risky however, so hormone therapy is decided upon for each individual patient after risks and benefits are discussed. Topical estrogen can be applied inside the vagina to thicken the vaginal tissues and increase moisture and sensitivity. Overall, the effects of aging upon the female reproductive system can be somewhat improved with regular exercise, a healthy diet, and staying involved in activities with others.

FOCUS ON TESTOSTERONE AND HEART DISEASE

Testosterone levels decrease significantly after age 65, which is associated with an increase heart disease in men. Low testosterone may increase risks for coronary artery disease (CAD). Reduced levels in men with congestive heart failure (CHF) worsen prognosis and this is related to increased mortality. Testosterone replacement therapy can improve myocardial ischemia in men with CAD, and also improve exercise capacity in those with CHF.

Test Your Knowledge

1. How does good nutrition and hydration affect the integumentary system in older adults?
2. How does kidney function decline in the elderly?
3. What are the major male and female reproductive changes due to aging?

THE COGNITIVE AND PSYCHOLOGICAL CHANGES IN OLDER ADULTS

Today, we understand that adults continue to grow new brain cells throughout life – a fact which was not believed in earlier decades. Even so, this evidence only concerns the hippocampus and olfactory bulb. Factors that may alter **neurogenesis** include drugs, exercise, and stress. Sustained aerobic exercise appears to lead to more neurogenesis. Studies are ongoing concerning the grafting of neural stem cells to the hippocampus and other brain regions, in order to increase neurogenesis. Another factor is the stimulation of the brain by engaging in increased mental activities, which encourage more dendritic branching. Keep the brain engaged in regular challenging activities helps to slow the effects of aging.

Even during late adulthood, the brain can still repair and alter itself to adjust to age-related changes. *Lateralization* is the specialization of function in one brain hemisphere or the other. Via neuroimaging, researchers have discovered that brain activity in the prefrontal cortex is lateralized less in older adults engaging in mental tasks, compared to younger adults. This means that younger adults are able to complete many tasks using only one brain hemisphere, while older adults use both hemispheres. This decrease in lateralization may play a compensatory role as the brain ages. Use of both hemispheres may help maintain mental abilities as we reached an advanced age.

Though some areas of intelligence decline in late adulthood, others are maintained and can even increase. Usually, when the speed of processing information is needed to occur quickly, older adults perform more poorly than younger adults. This decline is often seen in middle-aged adults and becomes more obvious in older adults. The elderly also perform poorer in relation to memory. They take longer, in most cases, to remember knowledge they learned about the world, but usually can eventually retrieve it. Decline also occurs in working memory.

Certain areas of cognition improve with age, such as **wisdom**, which may increase because life experiences increase. Each individual has various levels of built-up wisdom. Though cognitive ability may lessen in older adults, there are training methods that help enhance memory. For example, physical fitness increases cognitive skills. Those that remain engaged in cognitive and physical activities are better able to maintain cognitive function during late adulthood. However, older adults are often less able to adapt than younger adults, limiting the amount of improvement in their cognitive skills.

Older adults generally evaluate previous life events and look for meaning in them. Via this process of evaluation, the older adult develops a sense of meaning or despair. They also have to adjust to thoughts of death, so if integrity has been established and life appears to have been meaningful, the fear of death is lower and the sense of meaning is improved. Without integrity, there is more despair and fear.

Most older adults enjoy good psychological health, but the number of them with mental or behavioral health problems will likely quadruple by 2030. Mental health disorders such as anxiety and depression cause reduced ability to function and poorer overall health in older adults. Problems that the elderly have to deal with often involve coping with health problems, caring for a spouse with dementia or disability, grief concerning loss of loved ones, and managing family conflicts. By addressing and treating mental health conditions, there can be lessened emotional suffering, better physical health, reduced disability, and an overall better quality of life – for the elderly and also for their families. Increased access to mental health services helps reduce expenditures by lowering amounts of required medications, and the need for more primary care visits or medical procedures.

The majority of people that provide psychological care have a good level of interest in working with older adults during their careers. Care may be provided in health care facilities, community-based private or group practices, patients' homes, and in long-term care, assisted-living, and hospice facilities. Care is given independently and as part of interdisciplinary terms. **Geropsychology** is devoted to the study of aging and provision of clinical services for older adults. The demand for mental health practitioners with elderly expertise will expand as the geriatric population continues to grow. It is estimated that, currently, nearly 66% of older adults with a mental disorder do not receive required services – especially in rural and underserved groups, including those in poverty as well as some ethnic and racial groups. Most older adults admit that they would prefer psychological services over taking antidepressants.

FOCUS ON GEROPSYCHOLOGY

Geropsychology is a specialty that applies the knowledge and methods of psychology to understanding and helping older persons and their families. It focuses on maintaining well-being, overcoming problems, and achieving maximum potential during later life. It addresses mental disorders, dementia, changes in decision making or everyday living abilities, chronic illnesses, behavioral health concerns, grief, loss, strains placed upon caregivers, adjustment to aging-related stressors, and end-of-life care.

Test Your Knowledge

1. Does remaining engaged in regular challenging activities slow the effects of aging?

2. What psychological factors do the elderly often have to deal with?
3. Is the field of geropsychology likely to grow in coming years?

NUTRITION AND AGING

Good nutrition throughout life helps prevent chronic disease. The elderly have a higher risk for chronic diseases such as cardiovascular diseases, diabetes, osteoporosis, and various cancers. Fortunately, certain elderly can reduce some risks by eating foods dense in nutrients and maintaining an active lifestyle. Generally, older adults have lower calorie needs, but the quality of nutrients is essential for them. Lower calorie needs in this group may be due to less physical activity, metabolic changes, or loss of bone and muscle mass. Nutrient needs are affected by chronic health conditions, multiple medications, and body composition changes. Following a healthy diet is extremely important.

Eating more fruits, vegetables, whole grains, and dairy products improves diet quality. It is important to reduce added sugars, sodium, and saturated fat. Good support from family, friends, and health professionals assists older people meet food group and nutrient recommendations. Sufficient protein helps prevent loss of lean muscle mass. Some elderly people eat less protein as they needed. Seafood, dairy products, fortified soy alternatives to dairy products, beans, peas, and lentils are excellent sources of additional protein. They also provide nutrients such as calcium, fiber, and vitamins B12 and D. The ability to absorb vitamin B12 may decrease with age and because of use of certain medications.

It is sometimes difficult for older adults to drink enough fluids to stay hydrated, because the thirst sensation declines with age. Drinking enough water prevents dehydration, aids in digestion, and adds zero calories. Unsweetened fruit juices, low-fat or fat-free milk, and fortified soy beverages are also helpful. Healthcare providers should remind older adults to drink beverages with meals and throughout each day. As for alcohol, older adults should only consume two drinks or less daily (for men) and one drink or less daily (for women). The older population may feel the effects of alcohol more quickly than younger adults. It may increase their risk of falls or accidents.

Sharing meals with family and friends helps increase enjoyment of food and provides an opportunity to interact as well as improve dietary patterns. Experimenting with different methods of cooking foods from all food groups helps identify acceptable, enjoyable, and appealing food textures – especially if chewing or swallowing is problematic. Good dental health is also important in order to chew. Safe food handling is very important since the risk of foodborne illness increases with aging because of a decline in immune system function.

Tube feeding is often used for chronically ill and dying patients. It may be needed to prevent aspiration pneumonia, to provide caloric support so that life is prolonged, and to enhance quality of life, such as when there is a proximal GI obstruction.

FOCUS ON ENERGY AND NUTRITIONAL REQUIREMENTS FOR OLDER ADULTS

The energy requirements for people aged 51 and older are 2,000–2,800 calories for men and 1,600–2,200 calories for women, each day, based on physical activity. The decrease in physical activity that usually happens with older adults influences nutrition requirements. However, the recommended intake of carbohydrates, proteins, and fat remain the same from middle age into old age. Older adults should substitute more unrefined carbohydrates such as whole grains for refine carbohydrates. Fiber is especially important to prevent constipation, diverticulitis, and colorectal cancer.

Test Your Knowledge

1. What is the recommended diet for older adults?
2. What are the limits on alcohol for older adults?
3. What are the important issues surrounding tube feeding for elderly patients with dementia?

THE ROLE OF THE MICROBIOME

The GI **microbiota** is an assembly of microorganisms in the intestines. Their genomes are known as the **microbiome**. Normal composition and function of the microbiome is required in order to maintain a healthy status. Aging is related to changes in the GI microbiota, which are often linked with physiological changes of the GI tract, plus changes in dietary patterns and declines in cognitive and immune function. All of these factors contribute to frailty. Nutritional strategies focus on restoring the microbiota in the elderly throughout the world, also taking into account other extra-intestinal targets of action.

The microbiota make up the greatest number and concentration of microorganisms in the human body, with *one hundred trillion* microbes in the colon. About 1,500 bacterial species exist in total, and each individual has about 150 different species present in the body. The microbiome contributes widely to our physiology and metabolism. After birth, the microbiota requires about three years to become diverse, complex, and stable. In a healthy adult, the dominant bacteria are **Firmicutes** and **Bacteroidetes**, making up 80%–90% of the total microbiota.

In the elderly, the GI microbiota shows less bacterial diversity, changes as to which species is dominant, less beneficial microorganisms present, increased facultative anaerobic bacteria, and decreased availability to total short-chain fatty acids. The levels of these fatty acids, which are the main bacterial metabolites in the colon, are reduced in the elderly. An altered microbiota is positively associated with frailty. Lifestyle and diet are the most important factors influencing changes in the microbiota, so healthy dietary habits in the elderly are vital. *Clostridium difficile* is an obligate anaerobic, gram-positive, spore-forming bacterium that is usually present in the large intestines of health adults. However, it can proliferate, producing toxins, and causing various disorders. Infection with this bacterium is the most common cause of **nosocomial** diarrhea. It mostly affects elderly hospitalized patients that have received broad-spectrum antimicrobial drugs. The most important risk factors for this condition are an age of 65 or older and exposure to antibiotics. Therefore, the increased susceptibility to disease in older adults, often related to malnutrition, impairment of the intestinal microbiota and pro-inflammatory status of the immune system prove that these individuals need proper nutrition and functional foods that will boost the microbiota and immune system.

FOCUS ON THE HUMAN MICROBIOME

The microbiome is the genetic material of all microbes that live inside and on the human body. The microbiome may weight up to five pounds. The bacteria in the microbiome help us digest food, regulate the immune system, protect against pathogenic bacteria, and produce vitamins B1, B2, B12, and K. Dysfunction of the microbiome is linked to autoimmune diseases, including diabetes mellitus, rheumatoid arthritis, muscular dystrophy, multiple sclerosis, and fibromyalgia.

Test Your Knowledge

1. What changes occur in the microbiota of older adults?
2. How does *Clostridium difficile* cause disease in the elderly?

KEY TERMS

Actinic keratosis
Afterload
Alzheimer's disease
Andropause
Antibodies
Antigens
Atrial gallop
Autoimmune disorders
Baby boomers
Bacteroidetes
Basal cell carcinoma
Benign prostatic hyperplasia
Cherry angiomas
Cholecystokinin
Chymotrypsin
Complement proteins
Dementia
Diverticuli
Dysphagia
Elastosis
Epidermis
Epididymis
Firmicutes
Geropsychology
Ghrelin
Goblet cells
Heat stroke
Hematoma
Hemorrhoid
Hepatocytes
Hippocampus
Inflammatory bowel disease
Intimal hyperplasia
Isolated systolic hypertension
Leptin
Life expectancy
Liver spots
Macrophages
Melanocytes
Melanoma
Microbiome
Microbiota
Myocytes
Neurogenesis
Neurotransmitters
Nosocomial
Pacemaker cells
Peristalsis
Pneumonia
Prolapse
Propulsive

Prostaglandin

Prostatitis

Pulse pressure

Purpura

Sarcopenia

Seborrheic keratoses

Seminal vesicles

Silent coronary artery disease

Skin tags

Squamous cell carcinoma

Stroke

Stroke volume

Urinary incontinence

Wisdom

Xerostomia

CLINICAL CASE STUDIES

Clinical Case Study 1

A 72-year-old woman began forgot recent conversations and had to start writing down daily tasks in order to remember to do them. She had smoked one pack of cigarettes per day for 30 years, but did not drink alcohol or use any medications except for acetaminophen. Her mental status did reveal anxiety and depression. A year later, she reported that her forgetfulness had gotten worse. Over a few more months, there were signs of early Alzheimer's disease.

CRITICAL THINKING QUESTIONS

1. How much cortical atrophy progresses as humans continue to age?
2. How significant is cortical atrophy with Alzheimer's disease?
3. After age 60, what are the features of brain shrinkage?

Clinical Case Study 2

A 69-year-old man developed a severe productive cough, with thick yellow sputum that contained streaks of blood. He was assessed by his physician and also found to have a fever, chills, and malaise. The patient described pain in the right side of his chest that he felt with each breath. He had lost 15 pounds over the past three months. Previous history revealed that the patient had smoked two packs of cigarettes per day over 50 years. His complexion was pale, and the coughing was nearly continuous. During percussion of the patient's chest, he was found to have dullness of the right mid-anterior and mid-lateral lung fields. Auscultation revealed bronchial breath sounds and crackles during breathing. The patient was diagnosed with acute pneumonia of the right middle lung lobe, and treatment was started with antibiotics in the hospital.

CRITICAL THINKING QUESTIONS

1. How can tissue damage in the lungs occur in elderly people?
2. What simple methods can protect the respiratory system and maintain better function throughout life?
3. What changes occur in the respiratory system after age 35?

Clinical Case Study 3

A 75-year-old woman is assessed because of losing 20 pounds over the previous six months, following a minor stroke that occurred a year before. She states that she eats two meals per day, that most foods have become tasteless to her, and that when she eats, she feels something "stuck" in her throat that causes her great discomfort and sometimes feels painful. The patient also has poorly fitting dentures that she does not wear very often. Her physician feels that she is at a risk of nutritional deficiency because of the involuntary weight loss and the problems with her dentures. Referred to a clinical nutritionist, the patient is educated about food choices that will be beneficial to her health status and that are easier to prepare and enjoy.

CRITICAL THINKING QUESTIONS

1. What are the common changes that affect the digestive system with aging?
2. Why do older adults often experience changes in the ability to taste?
3. How do teeth or denture problems affect nutrition in older adults?

STUDY QUESTIONS

1. Cherry angiomas are seen in which of the following?
   A. Brain
   B. Skin
   C. Stomach
   D. Spleen

2. Which of the following parts of the brain experience the most shrinkage by age 60?
   A. Frontal lobe
   B. Occipital lobe
   C. Parietal lobe
   D. Temporal lobe

3. Which of the following statements is false regarding the normal changes of the cardiovascular system?
   A. Pacemaker cells in the sinus node decrease
   B. Myocardial contractility is of shorter duration
   C. Left ventricular wall thickness increases
   D. The myocyte to collagen ratio is unchanged

4. Which of the following hormones increases appetite?
   A. Ghrelin
   B. Leptin
   C. Insulin
   D. Cholecystokinin

5. Which of the following cells secrete mucus in the digestive system?
   A. Lymphoid
   B. Goblet
   C. Stem
   D. Pacemaker

6. Why are older adults more susceptible to autoimmune disorders?
   A. There are fewer complement proteins
   B. Joints are affected by changes in connective tissue and cartilage
   C. Foreign antigens are not as easily identified
   D. Macrophages destroy antigens more slowly

7. With aging, as joint surfaces do not slide over each other, which of the following condition may develop?
   A. Sarcopenia
   B. Osteoporosis
   C. Faster contraction
   D. Osteoarthritis

8. The specialization of function in one brain hemisphere is called:
   A. Depolarization
   B. Neutralization
   C. Utilization
   D. Lateralization

9. Which of the following is most likely to take longer in elderly adults?
   A. Wisdom
   B. Memory
   C. Judgment
   D. Evaluation

10. The study of aging and provision of clinical services for older adults is referred to as:
    A. Neuropsychology
    B. Pathophysiology
    C. Genealogy
    D. Geropsychology

11. Which of the following cancers is the most deadly and has a poor prognosis?
    A. Squamous cell carcinoma
    B. Liver spots
    C. Melanoma
    D. Basal cell carcinoma

12. All of the following factors are linked in the gastrointestinal microbiota of the elderly, EXCEPT:
    A. Physiological changes of the GI tract
    B. Changes in dietary patterns
    C. Declines in cognitive and immune function
    D. An increased need to take fat-soluble vitamins

13. The genome of the GI microbiota is known as which of the following?
    A. Enterobacteriaceae
    B. Microbiome
    C. Firmicute
    D. Bacteroidete

14. All of the following factors may alter neurogenesis, EXCEPT:
    A. Stress
    B. Viral infections
    C. Exercise
    D. Some drugs

15. Nosocomial diarrhea mostly affects hospitalized elderly patients that receive which of the following?
    A. Broad-spectrum antibiotics
    B. Intravenous anticoagulants
    C. Intravenous normal saline
    D. Oral antihypertensive drugs

FURTHER READING

1. Erber, J.T. (2019). *Aging and Older Adulthood*, 4th Edition. Wiley-Blackwell.
2. Gasmi, A. (2020). *Nutrition for the Elderly – A Clinical Approach.* Gasmi.
3. Geirsdottir, O.G., and Bell, J.J. (2021). *Interdisciplinary Nutritional Management and Care for Older Adults – An Evidence-Based Practical Guide for Nurses (Perspectives in Nursing Management and Care for Older Adults).* Springer.
4. Hillier, S.M., and Barrow, G.M. (2014). *Aging, the Individual, and Society*, 10th Edition. Cengage Learning.
5. Hirsch, R.E. (2016). *The Human Microbiome – The Germs That Keep You Healthy.* Twenty-First Century Books (CT).
6. Keller, R.J. (2023). *Fitness for the Golden Years – Elderly Exercise and Nutrition – How to be More Active and Stay Healthy in Your Old Age.* Keller.
7. Kunkel, S.R., and Setterstein, Jr., R.A. (2021). *Aging, Society, and the Life Course*, 6th Edition. Springer.
8. Magnus, G. (2012). *The Age of Aging: How Demographics are Changing the Global Economy and Our World.* Wiley.

9. Martin, L., and Lecko, C. (2019). *Practical Nutrition and Hydration for Dementia-Friendly Mealtimes.* Jessica Kingsley Publishers.
10. Niedert, K.C. (2016). *Nutrition Care of the Older Adult – A Handbook of Nutrition throughout the Continuum of Care*, 3rd Edition. Academy of Nutrition and Dietetics.
11. Randall, L.O. (2007). *Aging and the Elderly: Psychology, Sociology, and Health.* Nova Science Publishers, Inc.
12. Ravdin, L.D., and Katzen, H.L. (2019). *Handbook on the Neuropsychology of Aging and Dementia (Clinical Handbooks in Neuropsychology)*, 2nd Edition. Springer.
13. Schiff, W. (2020). *Nutrition Essentials: A Personal Approach*, 3rd Edition. McGraw-Hill Education.
14. Seiler, W.O., and Stahelin, H.B. (2013). *Malnutrition in the Elderly.* Steinkopff / Springer.
15. Sorenson, M., Quinn, L., and Klein, D. (2018). *Pathophysiology: Concepts of Human Disease.* Pearson.
16. Taylor, A.W. (2021). *Physiology of Exercise and Healthy Aging*, 2nd Edition. Human Kinetics.
17. Watkins Bales, C., Locher, J.L., and Saltzman, E. (2015). *Handbook of Clinical Nutrition and Aging (Nutrition and Health)*, 3rd Edition. Humana Press.

6 Pregnant Women

OUTLINE

LEARNING OBJECTIVES

After study of the chapter, readers should be able to:

1. Explain the nutrient intake recommendations for pregnant women.
2. Identify risks that can occur because of obesity during pregnancy.
3. Discuss the acceptable target body mass indexes for pregnant women if they were of normal weight, underweight, and overweight or obese before pregnancy.
4. Compare the features of morning sickness with those of hyperemesis gravidarum.
5. Define and compare preeclampsia and eclampsia.
6. Explain the outcomes of consuming alcohol during pregnancy.
7. Describe the outcome of human immunodeficiency virus in pregnant women.
8. Identify the symptoms of gestational diabetes and explain its possible outcomes.
9. Discuss the dangers of extreme hypertension during pregnancy.
10. Summarize mental disorders during pregnancy.

OVERVIEW

Pregnancy is the period in which an egg cell is fertilized by a sperm to form a new cell that eventually develops into a new human being and is delivered. The period of human pregnancy is 40 weeks from the date of the last menstrual period, or 38 weeks from the time of conception, on average. Most pregnancies last for a total of 37–42 weeks. Energy requirements increase during pregnancy, especially after the first trimester. Complications may occur during pregnancy that can involve the mother's health, the baby's health, or both. Some women have health problems that arise during pregnancy, and other women have health problems *before* they become pregnant, which can lead to complications. It is very important for women to receive health care before and during pregnancy to decrease the risk of pregnancy complications. Nutritional issues during pregnancy include excessive of insufficient weight gain, both of which can result in harm to the baby. During gestation, a fetus is extremely susceptible to nutrient availability and energy balance, which are essential for optimal growth and development. An adequate diet during gestation contributes to preventing problems such as intrauterine growth retardation, excess or low birthweight, neonatal and maternal morbidity and mortality, plus complications at the time of delivery.

PRECONCEPTION NUTRITION

A healthy diet consumed by a woman, before becoming pregnant, is essential to the future health of her baby. Certain deficiency-related problems develop very early during pregnancy, often before the mother even knows she is pregnant. The preconception diet must be varied and sufficiently nutritious. A healthy preconception diet includes avoiding alcohol, illegal drugs, and any teratogens (which cause birth defects). Women must consult healthcare providers about the amounts of caffeine, herbs, medications, and supplements that they consume. A woman who smokes tobacco products must quit.

A healthy diet and appropriate physical activity before pregnancy help to achieve and maintain an optimal body weight. The best chance of a successful pregnancy is attained when the preconception body weight of the mother is between 19.8 and 26.0 kg per square meter. Any woman

DOI: 10.1201/b22969-8

that is underweight or overweight has a higher risk for infertility or pregnancy complications. Obesity is also linked to polycystic ovary syndrome (PCOS), which involves abnormal hormone levels, irregular or absent menstrual cycles, and impairment of ovulation. Also, PCOS results in lower fertility rates. Often, overweight or obese women are also insulin resistant. If they do become pregnant, PCOS causes a three to four times higher risk for pregnancy-related forms of hypertension and diabetes than in healthy women. There is also twice the risk for preterm birth. In women with PCOS that are overweight or obese, weight loss is often the initial step of treatment.

A good diet before conception reduces risks for nutrition-related concerns during pregnancy. These concerns later affect the health of both mother and baby. Also, the father's nutrition and health before his partner becomes pregnant play a role. Poor paternal hygiene increases infection risk. An obese father may also have sperm abnormalities, impaired fertility, and altered gene expression. There is also an increased risk of loss of pregnancy and chronic disease in the baby. A father that drinks alcoholic beverages or uses some prescription or illegal drugs may have reduced sperm counts or reduced sperm motility. Paternal reproductive health requires a diet that has adequate levels of calcium, zinc, folic acid, vitamin D, and dietary antioxidants such as vitamin C.

PREGNANCY

During pregnancy, nutrients required in order for DNA synthesis to occur are provided by the mother. If she was insufficiently nourished before she became pregnant, there may be a lack of stored nutrients needed for this synthesis. The most important insufficiency is folacin, which is essential for DNA synthesis and cell replication, division, and specialization. Insufficient folacin increases the risks for abnormalities of the fetal brain and spinal cord, especially during first trimester of pregnancy.

For fetal bone formation, calcium, magnesium, and vitamin D are very important. When the mother's diet is lacking in these nutrients, the fetus will "pull" them from the mother's supply. Maternal bone turnover is greater during pregnancy. When the fetus pulls these nutrients from the mother, she experiences a loss of bone mineral. Supplementation of calcium and magnesium improves the health of the fetus and prevents bone loss seen in malnourished mothers. Deficiency of vitamin D during pregnancy is linked to low-birthweight infants, preeclampsia, and asthma. Racial differences exist, with African American and Hispanic women having more problems because of vitamin D deficiency than Caucasian mothers.

The brain and central nervous system (CNS) develop earlier than many other body systems. With brain development, the reproductive and cardiovascular systems also form. By week 8 of gestation, there is development of embryonic male genitalia and a release of testosterone, which will influence future male behavioral patterns. By the same time, female embryos develop uterine tubes and a uterus. The body systems develop from the influence of maternal hormones, including human chorionic gonadotrophin (hCG), estradiol, estriol, progesterone, relaxin, and prolactin. Hormones that influence growth and development are produced by the placenta, including beta-endorphin, dynorphin, and inhibin. Prorenin is produced by the embryo, which affects development and function of the kidneys. Formation of steroid hormones occurs from an interaction between the fetus and placenta, which affect growth and metabolic development.

Fetal growth is estimated but actual measurements are not fully understood. Measurements, in part, have been estimated from the sizes of infants that are born prematurely, though they may not actually represent a fetus that has a few additional weeks or months of gestation before being born. Between weeks 24 and 40 of gestation, a normal fetus gains 11–14 g/day of fat, 8–20 g/day of protein, and also gains mineral mater while losing water as a percentage of body mass. The growth of the fetus involves all body compartments. Normal growth is accomplished with coordinated increases in bone, fat, muscle, and organ mass. During the embryonal and fetal periods over the 37–42 weeks of gestation, weight will increase from almost zero to between 7 and 8.5 pounds. At birth, the newborn's length ranges between 18 and 21 inches (46 and 53 cm). The fetal weight and length are affected by the genetic background of both parents. Generally, if the parents are very small, the baby is as well, and the opposite is also true – taller parents generally have larger babies. For a mother with gestational diabetes, the infant is often excessively heavy (up to 16 pounds) at full-term birth, because of excessive fat gain during gestation. If the fetal weight gain appears to be excessive, the obstetrician often induces labor sooner. A cesarean section is required if the baby is too large to pass through the birth canal.

Test Your Knowledge

1. What should not be part of the diet before becoming pregnant?
2. What are the most important dietary nutrients during pregnancy?

NUTRIENT INTAKE RECOMMENDATIONS

In the first trimester, energy requirements increase slightly. The mother should consume about the same number of calories per day as she did before pregnancy. However, the nutrient density of the diet must be maximized. Examples include drinking low-fat milk instead of sodas, because this milk provides needed protein, minerals, and vitamins for the fetus. Sodas are nutritionally empty but high in calories. In the last two trimesters of pregnancy, caloric needs are higher, by 350–450 kcal/day. If a woman consumes 2,000 kcal daily, an extra 400 kcal means a 20% increase in caloric intake. The additional 400 kcal can be made up by one cup of low-fat yogurt and one g cracker with jam on top. However, some vitamin and mineral needs increase by up to 50%. Therefore, nutrient-dense foods are the way to go to have enough micronutrients without excessively high calories.

Intake of carbohydrates should be about 175 g/day, mostly from fruits, wholegrains, vegetables, and legumes. These sources are rich in vitamin B, other micronutrients, *phytochemicals*, and fiber. Foods rich in fiber make an individual feel full, helping to prevent excessive weight gain and lowering risks of constipation. Fat consumption during pregnancy is no different than before conception. However, **good fats** must be consumed, meaning that **saturated fats** and **trans fats** should be extremely limited. Some studies indicate that **docosahexaenoic acid** (DHA), an omega-3 polyunsaturated fatty acid, and **arachidonic acid** (ARA), an omega-6 fatty acid, are linked to enhance brain growth and eye development. The brain of the fetus grows quickly during the third trimester, making DHA very important in the mother's diet. Good sources include oily fish (anchovies, mackerel, salmon, and sardines). It is present in lower amounts in tuna and chicken, as well as eggs that are enhanced by feeding chickens a diet rich in DHA. The other fatty acid, ARA, is present in most types of meat, including fish and poultry.

Pregnant women that eat fish should be aware of possible mercury contamination, since even a small amount of mercury during pregnancy can impair development of the nervous system of the fetus. Large fish (king mackerel, shark, swordfish, and tile fish) should be avoided, but up to 12 ounces per week (properly cooked) of other types of fish are encouraged. Albacore tuna must be limited to only six ounces per week, since it is higher in mercury than other types of tuna.

The most important micronutrients during pregnancy begin with folate, because it is necessary for cell division. Sufficient folate is highly critical in the first 28 days after conception. It is needed for the formation and closure of the **neural tube**, which eventually becomes the CNS. Deficiency of folate is linked to neural tube defects such as **anencephaly** and **spina bifida** (see Figure 6.1). It is believed that 70% of all neural tube defects can be prevented if women of childbearing age consume enough folate or folic acid. Consuming at least 400 mcg/day before becoming pregnant and at least 600 mcg/day while pregnant is recommended. Other outcomes of insufficient folate include **macrocytic anemia**, low birthweight, preterm delivery, and failure of normal fetal growth. Folate sources include fortified cereals and grains, lentils, and spinach.

Iron is important during pregnancy because it is vital in the formation of red blood cells (RBCs), which transport oxygen. The expanded blood volume, increased uterine size, placenta, and fetus require more RBC and iron. During the last trimester, fetal needs for iron increase even more, as the fetus must store iron that will be used in the first few months of life. Insufficient iron intake by the mother can result in low birthweight, preterm birth, and even fetal death. However, the fetus "steals" iron from the

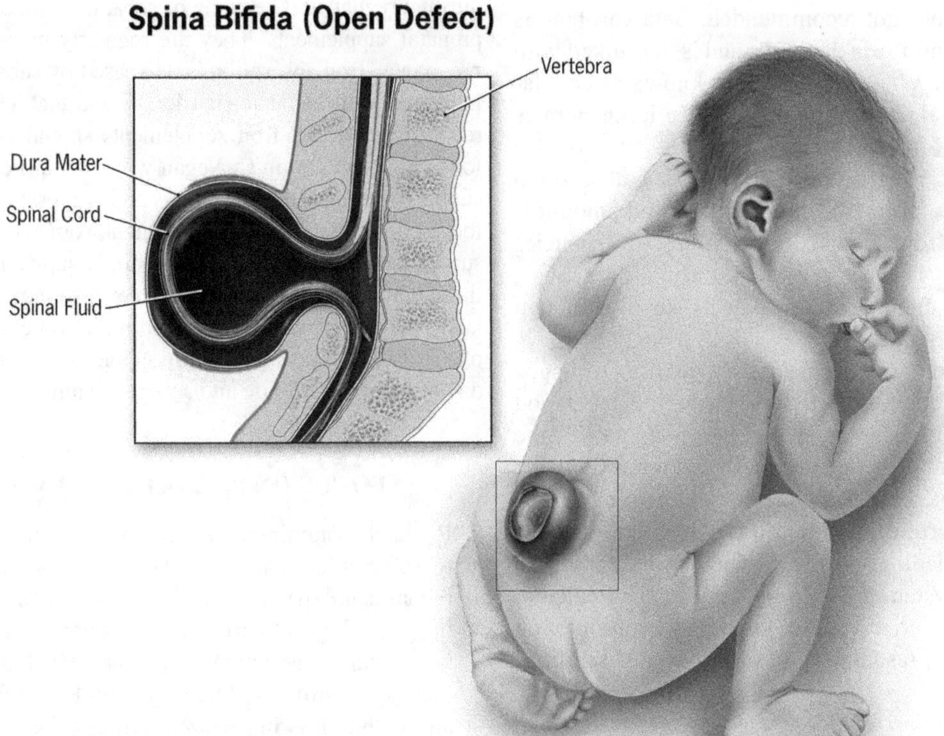

FIGURE 6.1 Spina bifida.

mother, which can result in her developing iron-deficiency anemia. She will become pale and exhausted. A significant point is that low iron at the time of delivery can danger the mother's life.

Calcium, in large amounts, contributes to the growth of the fetal skeleton. However, daily intake of calcium does not have to increase in comparison to non-pregnant women because pregnant women absorb more calcium from the diet. The extra demand for calcium is not proven to demineralize the bones of the mother or to increase risks for fractures. Sources of calcium include cheese, milk, yogurt, collard greens, kale, broccoli, and calcium-fortified cereals, juices, and soy milk.

Zinc is essential for synthesis of DNA, RNA, and protein. Insufficient intake can result in fetal malformations, and labor that is premature or extended. When food sources of zinc and iron are consumed together, the absorption of zinc is not affected. The heme form of iron is not believed to inhibit zinc absorption. Sodium, in excessive amounts, is related to bloating, fluid retention, and hypertension. However, since an increase in body fluids is normal (and required) during pregnancy, some amount of sodium is always necessary to maintain fluid and electrolyte balance. Iodine must increase greatly during pregnancy, but this can easily happen by using a small amount of iodized salt during cooking.

Vitamin A needs increase, but excess preformed vitamin A can result in fetal abnormalities – mostly heart defects and malformations of the face. A good diet supplies enough vitamin A, and supplements during pregnancy are therefore not recommended. Beta-carotene is converted to vitamin A in the body, and is not linked with any birth defects. Vitamin B12 is also known as cobalamin, and is crucial during pregnancy since it regenerates the active form of folate. Deficiencies of this vitamin also cause macrocytic anemia. During pregnancy, absorption of vitamin B12 is more efficient. The required amount is easily obtained from animal food sources. Deficiencies have been seen in vegan women during pregnancy, though fortified foods or supplements supply enough vitamin B12.

Vitamin C is required for collagen synthesis. Collagen is found in the connective tissues, including the blood vessels, skin, and tendons, and also makes up part of the organic matrix of bones. A deficiency of vitamin C during pregnancy will increase risks for preterm birth and other complications. Fortunately, vitamin C is abundant in many food source, including citrus fruits, other fruits, juices, and vegetables. Vitamin D is very important in calcium absorption. However, excessive vitamin D consumption can cause toxicity, resulting in developmental disabilities in newborns.

Table 6.1 summarizes the changes in nutrient intake required during pregnancy, for adult women.

Protein Intake

According to the *National Institutes of Health (NIH)*, the recommended dietary allowance (RDA) for protein in pregnant women is 0.88 g per kg of body weight per day. During the last trimester, the mother's protein needs increase to support the growth of the fetus. After delivery, the mother must increase protein intake to support lactation and the nutritional requirements of the baby. Studies of full-term babies indicate that a protein intake of 2–2.5 g per kg per day provide normal weight gain. Additional increases in protein intake do not significantly improve growth. Essential amino acids for growing infants include *histidine* and *methionine*. Insufficient intake will result in metabolic imbalances of *homocysteine*. **Hyperhomocysteinemia** during pregnancy is linked to neural tube defects, preeclampsia, miscarriage, and premature delivery. Low protein intake by the mother during pregnancy may have **epigenetic** effects upon the baby. Rich sources of protein include dairy products, eggs, meat, soy products, legumes, nuts, and seeds.

Supplements

Overall, prenatal multivitamin and mineral supplements are not extremely necessary during pregnancy, but they are still generally recommended. Prenatal supplements are very good for vegans, adolescent mothers, and others that may have a diet low in one or several micronutrients. Supplements are meant to be taken in addition to a nutrient-rich diet, not as a substitute for it. Folic acid and iron supplements are very important during pregnancy. They may be separate from or part of total prenatal supplements. They are regularly prescribed during pregnancy. Iron absorption is decreased by substances found in coffee, milk, oxalate-rich foods, and tea. Therefore, it is recommended that iron supplements should be taken with foods high in vitamin C. Vegan women require vitamin B12 supplements since this vitamin is highly present in the animal food sources that they avoid. Pregnant women that get enough sun exposure do not require vitamin D supplements, though those with dark skin or limited sun exposure that do not regularly consume vitamin D-fortified milk do benefit from supplements. Most prenatal vitamin supplements contain 10 mcg/day of vitamin D, a safe and acceptable amount.

FOCUS ON PRENATAL VITAMINS

Prenatal vitamins are available over-the-counter (OTC) in most pharmacies. Healthcare providers often recommend specific brands to women of childbearing age. They help promote development of teeth and bones during gestation. Other beneficial ingredients include vitamins A, C, and E, the B vitamins, zinc, and iodine. It is important to always take the correct amount of prenatal vitamins suggested by the provider.

TABLE 6.1
Changes in Nutrient Intake during Pregnancy (for Adult Women)

Micronutrient	Pre-pregnancy and Pregnancy Intake (per Day)	Percentage of Increase (%)
Folate	Pre-pregnancy: 400 mcg Pregnancy: 600 mcg	50
Iron	Pre-pregnancy: 18 mg Pregnancy: 27 mg	50
Calcium	Both: 1,000 mg	0
Zinc	Pre-pregnancy: 8 mg Pregnancy: 11 mg	38
Sodium	Both: 1,500 mg	0
Iodine	Pre-pregnancy: 150 mcg Pregnancy: 220 mcg	47
Vitamin A	Pre-pregnancy: 700 mcg Pregnancy: 770 mcg	10
Vitamin B12	Pre-pregnancy: 2.4 mcg Pregnancy: 2.6 mcg	8
Vitamin C	Pre-pregnancy: 75 mg Pregnancy: 85 mg	13
Vitamin D	Both: 600 International Units	0

Test Your Knowledge

1. What is the importance of zinc in the diet of a pregnant woman?
2. What are the outcomes of insufficient protein intake during pregnancy?

Food Choices

During the course of pregnancy more nutrients are needed. These include protein, iron, folic acid, iodine, and calcium. Smart food choices can ensure a healthy pregnancy and a healthy infant. A healthy eating pattern includes a variety of nutritious foods and drinks. Pregnant woman should eat a variety of vegetables, fruits, whole grains, fat-free or low-fat dairy products, and protein foods. Foods and drinks should have low levels of added sugars, sodium, and saturated fats. Refined grains and starches should be limited. These are found in foods such as cookies, snack foods, and white bread. For pregnancy-related **morning sickness**, whole-grain toast or crackers may be helpful. Healthy snacks include low-fat or fat-free yogurt with fruit and no added sugar, whole-grain crackers with fat-free or low-fat cheese, and carrots with hummus. Foods that may contain microorganisms and be harmful to the fetus include the following:

- Uncooked or undercooked fish or shellfish
- Soft, unpasteurized cheese (such as Brie, feta, or goat cheese)
- Raw or rare meats, poultry, or eggs
- Unpasteurized juices or milk
- Lunch or deli meats
- Smoked seafood
- Hot dogs (unless they are unheated until steaming hot)
- Prepared ham salad, chicken salad, or seafood salad
- Raw sprouts (alfalfa, clover, mung bean, or radish)
- Raw batter or dough (such as raw cookie dough)

Decaf coffee or tea is much better than the caffeinated forms, and sugar in them should be avoided if possible. Drinks that should be avoided include sodas, fruit drinks, and energy or sports drinks.

OBESITY AND WEIGHT GAIN

Obesity during pregnancy can increase obstetrical risks. Recent studies suggest that the heavier a woman is before she becomes pregnant, the greater her risk of pregnancy complications, including preeclampsia, stillbirth and cesarean delivery. Obesity during pregnancy is associated with increased use of health care and physician services, and longer hospital stays for delivery. Overweight and obese women who lose weight before pregnancy are likely to have healthier pregnancies.

An undernourished mother that does not gain enough weight during pregnancy has a greater chance of giving birth to a low-birthweight baby. A very-low-birthweight baby is one that is less than 3.3 pounds (1,500 g). Low-birthweight babies have an increased chance of developing infections, learning disabilities, and experiencing poor physical development. Some die within the first year of life. Many of these babies are born preterm, which is before 38 weeks of gestation. Others are born at full-term but are small for their gestational age, weighing less than expected.

Weight gain recommendations during pregnancy vary based on the mother's weight before becoming pregnant. For a woman of normal pre-pregnancy weight, the average weight gain should be 25–35 pounds. Underweight women must gain a little more than this, while overweight or obese women must gain less. For a teenage mother, the same recommendations exist. A woman of normal pre-pregnancy weight who is pregnant with twins should gain 37–54 pounds. These guidelines are also summarized as follows:

- Normal pre-pregnancy weight – body mass index (BMI) is 18.5–24.9, and recommended weight gain is 25–35 pounds
- Underweight before pregnancy – BMI is less than 18.5, and recommended weight gain is 28–40 pounds
- Overweight or obese before pregnancy – BMI is 25.0–29.9, and recommended weight gain is 15–25 pounds

An underweight woman that does not gain enough weight during pregnancy can have dangerous nutrient depletions because of the needs of the fetus.

A more common situation is an overweight or obese woman that becomes pregnant and gains too much weight. Children of these women have higher rates of childhood obesity and metabolic abnormalities. The more weight the mother gains during pregnancy, the harder it will be to return to the pre-pregnancy weight, and the more likely that the weight gain will be permanent. The pattern of weight gain is equally important. In the first trimester, a woman of normal weight should gain three to five pounds. In the second and third trimesters, one pound per week of weight gain is healthy. However, overweight woman should only gain six-tenths of a pound per week, and obese women should only gain five-tenths. Should weight gain be excessive within one week, month, or trimester, the woman should not try to lose weight, but instead, slow the rate of weight gain. The general rule is that weight gain during pregnancy must be slow and steady.

Pregnant woman often worry about weight gain because of societal pressures to be thin. It is important to focus on the quality of the food they eat, not the quantity. A physician-approved exercise program helps maintain a good body image and prevents excessive weight gain. Of the total weight gained during pregnancy, 10–12 pounds are for the fetus, amniotic fluid, and placenta. Blood volume will increase 40%–50%, which adds three to four additional pounds. After delivery, the mother will be 10–12 pounds lighter immediately. In about two weeks, fluid loss accounts for maternal weight to be five to eight pounds less. After that time, losing the rest of the pregnancy weight is based on more energy being expended than is taken in via the diet. Production of breast milk requires a lot of energy, but the effect of breastfeeding on weight loss is varied. Moderate weight loss is safe and does not interfere with the infant's weight gain.

FOCUS ON OBESITY DURING PREGNANCY

When obese women become pregnant, they are more at risk for serious health problems such as preeclampsia, gestational diabetes, and obstructive sleep apnea. Obesity increases the risk of harm to the fetus as well, including birth defects, problems with diagnostic tests.

HYPEREMESIS GRAVIDARUM

Hyperemesis gravidarum is a rare condition that occurs during pregnancy, in which there is severe, persistent nausea and vomiting that may require hospitalization. It is much more severe than common **morning sickness**, though in some cases this can progress into hyperemesis gravidarum, which results in dehydration, vitamin and mineral deficits, and loss of more than 5% of body weight. The cause of the condition is believed to be linked to the effects of the placenta hormone (progesterone). Hyperemesis gravidarum can develop quickly over a few weeks or slowly over a few months. This condition is severe before the 20th week of gestation that causes progressive weight loss. When a pregnant woman must be hospitalized because of the condition, management focuses on restoration of lost fluids and nutrients.

Other symptoms include increased pulse rate, excessive salivation, and tachycardia. Some women have a distinct **ketonic odor** of the breath. Symptoms can wax and wane, sometimes resulting in multiple hospitalizations. It may become difficult or impossible to work, perform normal tasks of daily living, care for children, or enjoy social activities and functions. Family relationships are often strained. Infants born to affected women are often of a lower birthweight, small for gestational age, or premature. Negative outcomes after delivery are linked to low maternal weight gain as well as chronic symptoms. Children of mothers with the condition in middle or late pregnancy often have attention and learning problems. About one of every ten women with weight loss during pregnancy of more than 15% of body weight have a child with a behavioral disorder. Exposure in utero to hyperemesis gravidarum increases risks for autism spectrum disorder, attention deficit disorder, learning problems or delays, depression, anxiety, and disorders of sensory integration or processing.

Many women with hyperemesis gravidarum cannot tolerate vitamins or normal nutrition. They may develop vitamin deficiencies, and metabolic disturbances. Most women (94%) have no psychiatric history, though they may have depression or anxiety because of being too nauseous to eat well or care for their families. Factors that may be related to the condition include family history of severe nausea and vomiting during pregnancy, younger maternal age, obesity, no previous completed pregnancies, having two or more fetuses in one pregnancy, first-time pregnancies, allergies, and restrictive diets.

Overall, hyperemesis gravidarum only occurs in 0.5%–2% of all pregnant woman, while generalized nausea and vomiting in pregnancy affects 50%–90%. Hyperemesis gravidarum is the second leading cause of hospitalization in early pregnancy. It is more common in Asian and other non-Caucasian populations. It appears to be increasing in incidence because of more emergency department visits than in previous decades. While most common in first-time pregnancies, it often recurs in subsequent pregnancies. Diagnosis is based on clinical evaluation, thorough patient history and the characteristic symptoms.

Test Your Knowledge

1. Which foods may contain microorganisms that may harm a fetus?
2. What amount of maternal weight gain is considered normal during the various periods of pregnancy?
3. What can hyperemesis gravidarum cause to occur in children born to women with the condition?

FOOD CRAVINGS AND AVERSIONS

Some women experience specific food cravings, but most actually crave a general type of food, not a particular food. In most cases, they ask for foods that are sweet or salty. There is no scientific proof that craving a specific type of food indicates that a pregnant woman is deficient in that type of food. More likely, cravings are caused by hormonal changes, physiologic changes, or they may be linked to family and culture. Most cravings are for various foods, though some women develop **pica** and crave non-foods such as clay from the ground or laundry starch.

Food aversions during pregnancy are linked to increasing hCG levels during the first 11 weeks. They affect about 60% of pregnant women. Food aversions are also associated with morning sickness. Some women unfortunately have them throughout the entire pregnancy, but mostly they continue through the first trimester. The most common aversions are toward foods with strong smells, such as meats, fatty foods, eggs, onions, garlic, tea, coffee, and spicy foods. Another common aversion is toward milk. Many women cannot stand the smell of any type of alcohol. Most women with food aversions during pregnancy prefer foods that are bland or sweet.

PREECLAMPSIA AND ECLAMPSIA

Preeclampsia involves a sudden increase in maternal blood pressure, edema, rapid weight gain that is not related to diet, and **proteinuria**. Untreated, it may progress to **eclampsia** which is a serious condition. Eclampsia may develop seizures, kidney failure, and possibly, death of the fetus, mother, or both. These disorders account for nearly 16% of pregnancy-related deaths in developed countries, including the United States. Their causes are not fully understood, though risks are increased by deficiencies of dietary protein, vitamins C and E, calcium, and magnesium. Risks are also higher in first-time pregnancies, maternal age over 40, the African American race, diabetes mellitus, obesity, multiple pregnancies, and family history of preeclampsia.

Diagnosis is made clinically, simply based on the symptoms. Treatment is focused on control of blood pressure, involving medications, close monitoring, and if required, hospitalization. For almost all women with no previous chronic hypertension, the blood pressure (BP) returns to normal within about one day after delivery.

ALCOHOL

During pregnancy, frequent drinking or occasional binge drinking increases the risk for **miscarriage**, delivery complications, preterm birth, and *sudden infant death syndrome (SIDS)*. Alcohol is a teratogen. Its consumption by a pregnant woman increases risks for birth defects of the heart, skeleton, kidneys, ears, and eyes. Other outcomes include developmental, behavioral, and mental problems throughout life. Examples include **attention deficit disorder** and hyperactivity. Heavy drinking, of more than three or four drinks per day, throughout pregnancy, may cause *fetal alcohol syndrome*. Even so about 10% of pregnant women report drinking alcohol at some time over the previous 30 days prior to being asked, and 3% binge drink. Some women have an occasional alcoholic drink with no obvious negative effects, yet no amount of alcohol during pregnancy is actually safe. Pregnant women are advised to abstain from alcohol prior to conception as much as possible, and definitely during pregnancy.

FETAL ALCOHOL SYNDROME

Fetal alcohol syndrome (FAS) is the most extreme outcome from maternal alcohol consumption. It causes malformations of the face, heart, limbs, and nervous system (see Figure 6.2). The facial features include a nose that is short and has a low and wide bridge. The eyes appear to "droop" and have an extra fold of skin. The upper lip is thin and flat. Most affected children also have behavioral problems and learning disorders. All of the effects of this syndrome are irreversible. Other outcomes include emotional, social, and development abnormalities. Also, the syndrome causes much higher rates of newborn and infant death. It is also one of the most common causes of mental retardation.

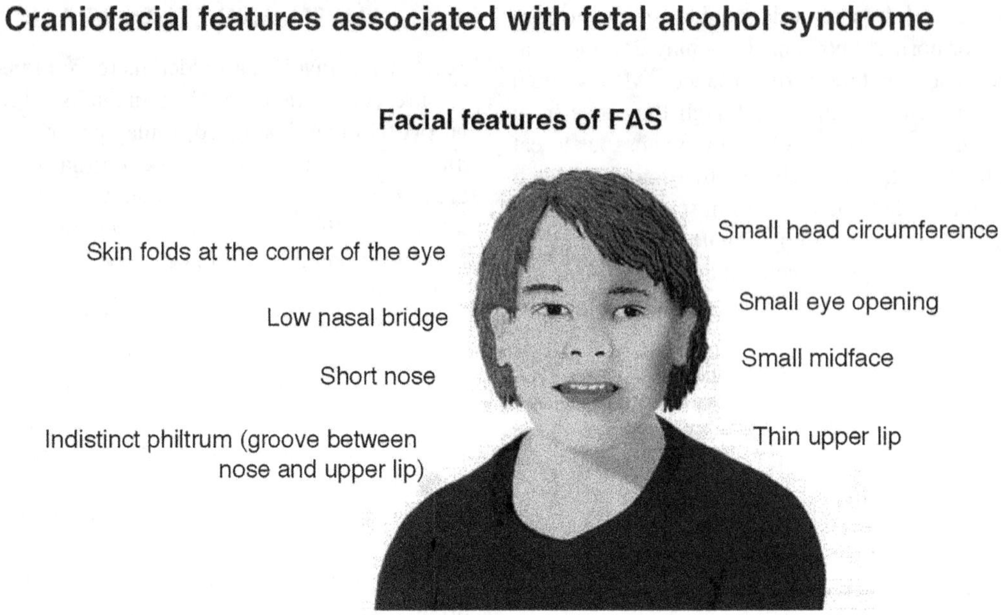

FIGURE 6.2 A child with fetal alcohol syndrome.

A less severe result of maternal alcohol use is referred to as **fetal alcohol effects** *(FAE)*, which is not usually diagnosed at birth. It is often first noticed as the child begins preschool or kindergarten, due to hyperactivity, attention deficit, or impaired learning ability. Incidence of FAE may be ten times more common than FAS. FAE can occur even with light to moderate alcohol consumption during pregnancy. Breastfeeding mothers should also abstain from alcohol. It passes into breast milk easily, at levels equivalent to the blood alcohol concentration. The infant may have slowed motor development and CNS depression as a result. Because of alcohol's diuretic effects, normal fluid losses of a breastfeeding women can be intensified by alcohol intake. The mother is at risk for dehydration, meaning a reduced ability to produce breast milk, and increased risk of malnutrition in the infant.

FOCUS ON FETAL ALCOHOL SPECTRUM DISORDERS

Fetal alcohol spectrum disorders are a group of conditions caused by exposure to alcohol before birth. Effects include physical, behavioral, and learning problems. Often, an individual with one of these disorders has a mixture of these problems.

Test Your Knowledge

1. What are the most common food aversions during pregnancy?
2. What are the risk factors for preeclampsia and eclampsia?
3. How much alcohol is safe during pregnancy?

GESTATIONAL DIABETES

Gestational diabetes is becoming more common and is diagnosed in up to 10% of pregnancies. It is usually temporary, with the pregnant woman being unable to produce enough insulin or becoming insulin resistant, with raised levels of blood glucose. Screening is regularly done as part of prenatal care. The symptoms include frequent urination, fatigue, and increased thirst and appetite. As long as blood glucose levels are strictly controlled with diet, exercise, medication, or all of these, the mother and fetus usually have good outcomes. Without control, gestational diabetes can cause **macrosomia**, due to excessive glucose crossing the placenta during gestation. A large infant is at risk for early delivery and trauma during vaginal birth, often requiring a cesarean section. Exposing a fetus to diabetes of the mother greatly increases risks for being overweight, obese, or having metabolic disorders (including type 2 diabetes) in later life. Diagnosis is made by taking blood samples every hour for 2–3 hours. High blood glucose over two or more times is indicative of the disease.

Gestational diabetes is more common in women that are obese, over age 35, or from the Native American, African American, or Hispanic racial or ethnic groups. A woman with gestational diabetes has a 40%–60% risk for type 2 diabetes developing in five to ten years, with risks increased for greater BMI. A healthy diet and regular physical activities will reduce risks for developing gestational diabetes. Treatment includes special meal plans, scheduled physical activity, and sometimes, daily blood glucose tests and insulin injections.

PREGNANCY AND HYPERTENSION

Hypertension prior to pregnancy is diagnosed by regular prenatal BP measurements. When severe hypertension occurs for the first time in a woman that is not having a multiple pregnancy or gestational **trophoblastic disease**, tests are usually done to rule out other causes such as **coarctation of the aorta**, renal artery stenosis, **Cushing's syndrome**, **pheochromocytoma**, or systemic lupus erythematosus. In gestational hypertension, increased BP usually occurs in third trimester. Treatments are based on severity of the hypertension. Decreasing the mother's BP with medications sometimes quickly decreases uteroplacental blood flow. Diuretics reduce the effective maternal circulating blood volume. If there is consistent reduction, risks for fetal growth restriction are increased. Hypertension with renal insufficiency, however, must be treated even if the hypertension is only mild to moderate.

Women taking methyldopa, a beta-blocker, or a calcium channel blocker before pregnancy can continue taking them. However, once pregnancy is confirmed, angiotensin-converting enzyme (ACE) inhibitors and angiotensin-receptor blockers (ARBs) must be stopped. Medications are required, however, for severe hypertension. Risks from this condition to the mother include preeclampsia and progression of end-organ dysfunction. Risks to the fetus include growth restriction, prematurity, and stillbirth. Several antihypertensive drugs may be needed.

When the BP is above 180/110 mm Hg, an immediate evaluation is needed, often with multiple drugs. Hospitalization is required during much of the final trimester of pregnancy. Sometimes, if the mother's condition gets worse, the pregnancy may have to be terminated. With chronic hypertension, all pregnant women are taught to monitor their BP and may need to be evaluated for target organ damage. Evaluation is done at baseline and periodically after that. It includes liver function tests, platelet count, serum creatinine, electrolyte levels, uric acid levels, urine protein assessment, and usually, funduscopy. If a woman has had hypertension for four or more years, echocardiography is considered. After the first ultrasound to assess the anatomy of the fetus, it is done monthly, beginning at 28 weeks or so to monitor fetal growth. **Antenatal testing** usually begins at 32 weeks. These techniques may start sooner if there are additional maternal complications such as kidney disorders, or if growth restriction occurs in the fetus. Delivery is induced earlier.

Medications for hypertension during pregnancy begin with methyldopa, beta-blockers, and calcium channel blockers. Methyldopa is increased as needed unless there is extreme somnolence, depression, or symptomatic orthostatic hypotension. The most often-used beta-blocker is labetalol, which can also be used with methyldopa. However, beta-blockers have adverse effects such as increased risk of fetal growth restriction, decreased energy in the mother, and maternal depression. Extended-release nifedipine, a calcium channel blocker is sometimes preferable due to its once-a-day dosing, though it can cause headaches and pretibial edema. Thiazide diuretics are used to treat chronic hypertension during pregnancy only if benefits appear to outweigh fetal risks. Doses are adjusted to minimize hypokalemia and other adverse effects. Aldosterone antagonists such as eplerenone and spironolactone are avoided during pregnancy because they can cause feminization of a male fetus.

HIV/AIDS

The human immunodeficiency virus (HIV) can be transmitted to a newborn during pregnancy, labor, delivery, or breastfeeding. The virus is not spread to infants by casual contact, touching items that were previously touched by the mother, and by saliva, sweat, or tears – unless they contain blood. If an infant is infected with HIV, there are often no symptoms for two to three months. Early symptoms include yeast infections in the mouth, failure to grow and gain weight, **lymphedema**, enlarged spleen or liver, ear and sinus infections, upper respiratory tract infections, diarrhea, and being slow to walk, crawl, or speak. Early treatment often prevents progression of the HIV infection. Without treatment, the child's immune system will weaken slowly and uncommon infections will appear. They are severe and may be caused by bacteria, viruses, fungi, or protozoa. At this point, the child is diagnosed with full-blown acquired immunodeficiency syndrome (AIDS).

Tests to diagnose HIV in a pregnant woman occur regularly with other prenatal tests. High-risk women must be screened again during the third trimester. Mothers that were not tested can receive a rapid HIV test during labor. When a woman was known to be HIV-positive during pregnancy, regular blood tests will include CD4 counts, a viral load test, and a resistance test to determine if the virus will respond to medications. Tests to diagnose HIV in infants determine how much of the virus is in their bodies. If the mother is HIV-positive, testing on the infant is done 14–21 days after birth, at one to two months, and at four to six months. If the result of two tests is negative, the infant is HIV-negative. If the results of any test are positive, the infant is HIV-positive. Infants at very high risk may be tested at birth.

HIV-positive women are instructed to feed their infants formula in place of breast milk, regardless of whether they are receiving treatment. Use of infant formula does not occur throughout all countries of the world because formula may be expensive and not sanitary, due to the pathogens in the water supply that is used to mix the formula.

HIV/AIDS is treated with antiretroviral therapy (ART), which stops the virus from multiplying. Treating a pregnant woman stops the fetus from becoming infected. Usually, there is a three-drug regimen. They have a low risk of harm to the fetus. If a woman goes into labor and has not received prenatal care, HIV may be discovered at the time of labor, and she will be treated with antiretroviral drugs immediately (sometimes IV). If the first HIV-positive test is during labor, immediate ART can reduce rates of infection in the infant to approximately 10%. For infants born to an infected mother, ART starts within 6–12 hours after birth. One or more antiretroviral drugs are continued for six or more weeks.

Test Your Knowledge

1. If gestational diabetes is not controlled, what may occur?
2. What are the risks to the fetus from hypertension during pregnancy?
3. How is HIV/AIDS in a pregnant woman and/or fetus treated?

VIRAL HEPATITIS

The management of *viral hepatitis* during pregnancy requires special efforts. The mother's liver health, influence of pregnancy upon the infection's clinical course, and effects of the virus or liver disease on the developing fetus must all be considered. The greatest risk to maternal and fetal health is seen with acute hepatitis A or E viruses during pregnancy. By contrast, the main risks for hepatitis B, C, and D virus are related to severity of the underlying liver disease in the mother, and the risk of mother-to-child transmission for HBV and HCV. The prevention of this transmission is the key to reducing the global cases of chronic viral hepatitis. Prevention strategies consider local health care and socioeconomic problems. The following additional information summarizes the impact of each subtype of viral hepatitis during pregnancy:

- Acute hepatitis A virus (HAV) infection during pregnancy may increase rates of adverse outcomes – there have been cases that led to fetal liver injury and some were via mother-to-child transmission
- Pregnant women with HBV infection may have an increased risk of preterm delivery and gestational diabetes – there is a risk of HBV transmission to the fetus, especially if the mother has high levels of HBV DNA; this risk is reduced with maternal antiviral therapy and prompt administration of immunoprophylaxis to the infant
- Pregnant women with chronic HCV infection have higher rates of adverse outcomes – mother-to-child transmission occurs in 5%; it is linked with invasive fetal monitoring and lengthy rupture of membranes
- Pregnant women with HDV infection have more risks related to underlying cirrhosis; mother-to-child transmission of HDV is rare; treatments are the same as for HBV monoinfections
- Acute HEV infection during pregnancy results in a higher risk of maternal and fetal mortality, along with higher rates of preterm delivery and stillbirth; mother-to-child transmission of HEV has occurred; however it is much more common in developing countries in Asia, the Middle East, Africa, and Central America, where water supplies may be inadequate and environmental sanitation may be poor; heavy rains that cause flooding have created favorable conditions for HEV to be transmitted

FOCUS ON HEPATITIS B

If a pregnant woman has hepatitis B, her newborn must receive hepatitis B immune globulin and an initial dose of the HBV vaccine within 24 hours of birth. The follow-up doses are given at one month of age and at six months of age. In the United States, the 3-dose series is sold under the trade names Engerix-B and Recombivax HB. Another option is the newer 4-dose vaccine series, which is administered within 24 hours of birth, at 6 weeks, 14 weeks, and at 24 weeks. The 4-dose series is sold under the trade names Vaxelis and Pediarix.

FOCUS ON HEPATITIS E

Hepatitis E causes high mortality in pregnant women due to fulminant hepatic failure. It also usually leads to spontaneous abortions, premature delivery, or still birth. About two billion people live in areas of the world endemic for HEV, and the World Health Organization estimates that over 20 million infections and 44,000 deaths occur every year, with pregnant women having the highest mortality rates.

IODINE DEFICIENCY

Iodine deficiency is signified by **goiter**, hypothyroidism, and **cretinism** in infants of mothers who are iodine deficient. It is rare in the United States and other countries that have added iodine to table salt for many decades. It is important to check package labels when buying table salt to make sure that it is iodized. Iodine deficiency impairs the synthesis of thyroid hormones. The thyroid enlarges to form a goiter as it attempts to correct the situation. Iodine deficiency is the main cause of goiter worldwide.

Symptoms of hypothyroidism include decreased body temperature, cold temperature intolerance, fatigue, sluggishness, and weight gain. During pregnancy, iodine deficiency greatly increases the risks of infant cretinism, which includes the features of deafness, muteness, stunted growth, mental retardation, bone growth retardation, and congenital heart disease (see Figure 6.3). Iodine deficiency is considered by the World Health Organization (WHO) to be the most significant cause of preventable brain damage and mental impairment, globally.

IRON-DEFICIENCY ANEMIA

Iron-deficiency anemia results in the RBCs being smaller than normal, with low hemoglobin. This makes them unable to transport enough oxygen, so the body produces less energy. The classic symptoms of this condition include reduced work performance, poor neurological function, generalized fatigue, pallor, and depressed immune function.

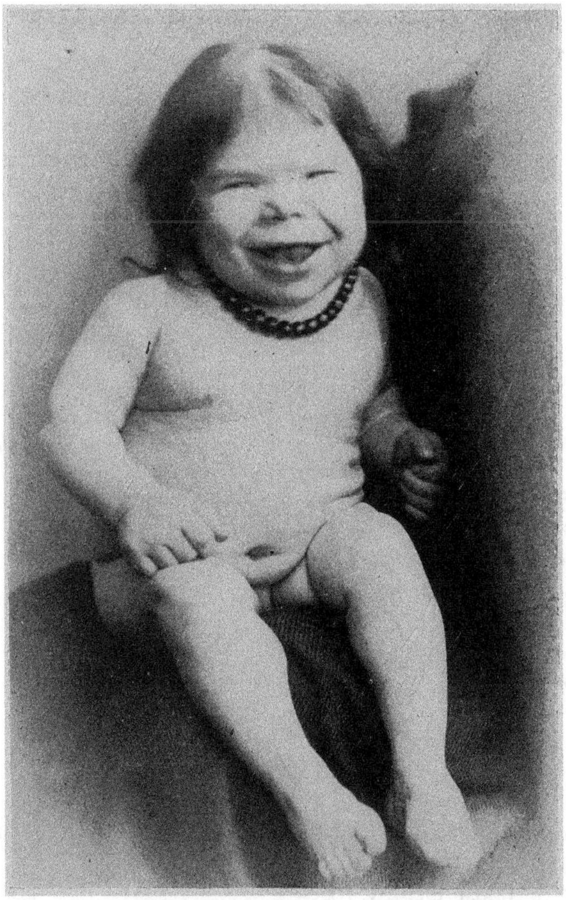

FIGURE 6.3 Cretinism.

When it is present in a pregnant woman, it increases the risks for low-birthweight infants, prematurity, infant mortality, and postpartum hemorrhage. Overall, iron-deficiency anemia is the most common micronutrient deficiency, on a global scale. It occurs in males and females of all ages, but is more prevalent in pregnant women and infants because of the demands of growth during the fetal and childhood periods. About 20% of maternal deaths involve iron-deficiency anemia.

Test Your Knowledge

1. What are the main risks during pregnancy for each type of viral hepatitis?
2. What does iodine deficiency during pregnancy increase risks for?

MENTAL HEALTH CONDITIONS

Pregnant women affected by various mental health conditions may have significant risks and outcomes. The primary maternal mental disorders that occur include depressive disorders, bipolar disorders, anxiety disorders, obsessive-compulsive disorder, and sleep disorders. Mental disorders during pregnancy are summarized as follows, along with their risks and outcomes:

- *Depressive disorders (major depression, persistent depressive disorder, minor depression)* – insufficient maternal weight gain, substance abuse, pre-eclampsia, preterm birth, low birthweight, fetal distress, increased risk of cesarean birth, increased risk of needed admission to a neonatal intensive care unit)
- *Bipolar disorders (bipolar I and II, bipolar not-otherwise-specified, cyclothymia)* – low birthweight, small size at birth, preterm birth, increased risk of cesarean birth, small head circumference, hypoglycemia, increased risk for long-term neurocognitive/behavioral/social deficits, high postpartum risk for bipolar episodes and hospitalization, substance use, poor prenatal care, maternal suicide
- *Anxiety disorders (generalized anxiety disorder, panic disorders, social anxiety disorder, specific phobias)* – increased risk for preterm birth, small for gestational age, spontaneous abortion, pre-eclampsia, decreased head circumference, low birthweight, excessive infant crying, long-term childhood behavioral disorders or anxiety, altered maternal/fetal cortisol levels
- *Obsessive-compulsive disorder* – low birthweight, preterm birth

- *Sleep disorders* – comorbid with mood/anxiety disorders, postpartum depression

Up to 20% of pregnant women suffer from mood or anxiety disorders. Those with histories of psychiatric illness that discontinue their psychotropic medications while pregnant are especially vulnerable. A recent study of women with histories of major depression showed that 26% continued to have depression that continued their medications through pregnancy, but 68% still had depression that stopped their medications. High relapse rates are also seen in women with bipolar disorder when they discontinue their medication during pregnancy.

The most frequently used antipsychotic medications during pregnancy are olanzapine, risperidone, and quetiapine. They do not appear to cause any consistent congenital harm to the fetus. There have been no specific patterns of fetal limb or organ malformations related to these drugs. There is some evidence that suggests use of antipsychotics during pregnancy may be linked to gestational diabetes. There is also a link between the medications and increased neonatal respiratory distress and withdrawal symptoms.

PRESCRIPTION MEDICATIONS

There are many prescription drugs that cause birth defects if taken during pregnancy. Examples include captopril, carbamazepine, codeine, enalapril, fluoxetine, hydrocodone, isotretinoin, morphine, oxycodone, paroxetine, thalidomide, tramadol, valproic acid, and warfarin. According to the Centers for Disease Control and Prevention (CDC), about one of every four pregnant women between ages 15 and 44 take prescription medications. About 90% of pregnant women take an OTC medication, and 70% take at least one prescription medication. The most common prescription medications during the first trimester include amoxicillin, progesterone, albuterol (for asthma), and promethazine (for allergies or nausea). Opioids such as oxycodone, hydrocodone, and morphine taken during pregnancy can be dangerous. They may cause **neonatal abstinence syndrome**. Drugs that are safe to take during pregnancy include bacitracin, diphenhydramine, docusate, hydrocortisone, loperamide, loratadine, miconazole, cetirizine, dextromethorphan, famotidine, guaifenesin, mentholated or non-mentholated cough drops, neomycin, phenylephrine, pseudoephedrine, ranitidine, and acetaminophen. Pregnant women can use saline nasal drops or sprays, and can gargle with warm saltwater.

Since many prescription medications can pass into breast milk, it is always important that breastfeeding women discuss all of them with their physician. If a safe, effective form of a required medication cannot be found, breastfeeding will have to stop while the woman is taking it. During this time, it is advised that she pump and discard her breast milk so that her milk supply will be enough when breastfeeding resumes.

Test Your Knowledge

1. Which type of mental health conditions during pregnancy increase risks for spontaneous abortion of the fetus?
2. Which drugs taken during pregnancy are the most common cause of neonatal abstinence syndrome?

KEY TERMS

Anencephaly

Antenatal testing

Attention deficit disorder

Coarctation of the aorta

Cretinism

Cushing's syndrome

Dynorphin

Eclampsia

Epigenetic

Fetal alcohol effects

Fetal alcohol syndrome

Folacin

Food aversions

Gestational diabetes

Goiter

Human chorionic gonadotrophin

Hyperhomocysteinemia

Inhibin

Ketonic odor

Lymphedema

Macrocytic anemia

Macrosomia

Miscarriage

Morning sickness

Neonatal abstinence syndrome

Neural tube

Nutrient density

Pheochromocytoma

Pica

Polycystic ovary syndrome

Preeclampsia

Proteinuria

Relaxin

Spina bifida

Systemic lupus erythematosus

Teratogens

Trophoblastic disease

CLINICAL CASE STUDIES

Clinical Case 1

A 25-year-old woman had recently become pregnant for the first time. She was extremely thin, with a BMI of only 14 kg/m2. As a child, she had surgery to correct a tracheo-esophageal fistula with esophageal atresia. Her menarche occurred later than normal, at age 16, and she had amenorrhea until the age of 20. Upon gaining sufficient weight around that time, regular menstrual cycles finally began. Her most recent visit to her physician was because she had developed dysphagia and started vomiting after meals. A CT scan revealed multiple redundant loops of her colon. A permanent gastrostomy was performed and the patient responded well. She began to be able to eat normally and slowly gained weight. It was planned that an early cesarean section would be performed to deliver the baby. This occurred at week 33 of gestation, and though he was underweight, he was healthy.

CRITICAL THINKING QUESTIONS

1. What does a pregnant woman that does not gain enough weight during pregnancy have a greater chance of?
2. What do low-birthweight babies have an increased chance of developing?
3. How much weight should be gained if a woman is underweight before becoming pregnant?

Clinical Case 2

A 34-year-old woman was diagnosed with gestational diabetes. She had experienced a loss of 22 pounds over the past 3 and ½ weeks, and had flu-like symptoms that included fatigue, nausea, polydipsia, and polyuria. The patient was hospitalized and started on an insulin drip. She developed gram-negative sepsis, adult respiratory distress syndrome, and Crohn's disease with a new rectovaginal fistula. She had to be intubated for further treatment. An emergency cesarean section was required at 31 weeks of gestation because of fetal distress. The patient's blood glucose levels improved postpartum and the insulin drip was gradually discontinued. Both mother and baby recovered well, though later, the new mother had a recurrence of raised blood glucose levels and required additional insulin therapy.

CRITICAL THINKING QUESTIONS

1. How often does gestational diabetes occur?
2. In which women is this condition more common?
3. How is gestational diabetes prevented and treated?

Clinical Case 3

A 36-year-old pregnant woman has had diabetes mellitus since the age of 17. She had not eaten a healthy diet for many years, but tried to reduce her caloric intake as she was planning to become pregnant with her husband. She complains of polyuria, polydipsia, and nocturia. A recent eye exam revealed moderate retinopathy. The patient's BMI is 31.2 kg/m2. She already has reductions in vibratory and touch sensations in her feet and lower legs. The patient is already on insulin therapy. She discusses her condition with her general physician and obstetrician, and asks how her health could impact the outcome of her pregnancy.

CRITICAL THINKING QUESTIONS

1. What is an obese woman who becomes pregnant more at risk for?
2. What do children of obese women have higher rates of?
3. If an obese woman develops polycystic ovary syndrome, which conditions are three to four times more likely to develop than in healthy women?

STUDY QUESTIONS

1. Which of the following nutrients is the most important during pregnancy for normal DNA synthesis?
   A. Vitamin C
   B. Folacin
   C. Zinc
   D. Iron

2. Which of the following hormones from the placenta does NOT influence growth and development of the fetus?
   A. Beta-endorphin
   B. Dynorphin
   C. Testosterone
   D. Inhibin

3. Which of the following types of fish contains the highest mercury, and should be limited to only six ounces per week during pregnancy?
   A. Tuna
   B. King mackerel
   C. Shark
   D. Swordfish

4. Insufficient iron intake by the mother may result in all of the following, EXCEPT:
   A. Low birthweight
   B. Preterm birth
   C. Spina bifida
   D. Fetal death

5. Hyperhomocysteinemia during pregnancy is linked to which of the following?
   A. Preeclampsia
   B. Hypertension
   C. Diabetes mellitus
   D. Pernicious anemia

6. Foods that are high in of the following should be consumed with iron supplements for better absorption?
   A. Folic acid
   B. Vitamin B12
   C. Vitamin C
   D. Sulfuric acid

7. Which of the following foods may be harmful to the fetus during pregnancy?
   A. Undercooked fish
   B. Chicken salad
   C. Pasteurized milk
   D. Undercooked broccoli

8. A woman who is pregnant with twins should gain how much weight?
   A. 18–25 lbs
   B. 25–30 lbs
   C. 37–54 lbs
   D. 45–62 lbs

9. Which of the following is the most common food aversion during pregnancy?
   A. Colorful foods
   B. Sweet foods
   C. Sour foods
   D. Strong food odors

10. Which of the following conditions during pregnancy may cause seizures?
    A. Eclampsia
    B. Hypertension
    C. Preeclampsia
    D. Alcoholism

11. Which of the following is NOT an affected by the malformations of fetal alcohol syndrome?
    A. Face
    B. Heart
    C. Liver
    D. Limbs

12. Without being controlled, gestational diabetes may cause which of the following?
    A. Lipidemia
    B. Azotemia
    C. Megaloblastic anemia
    D. Macrosomia

13. Which type of viral hepatitis during pregnancy results in a higher risk of maternal and fetal mortality?
    A. Type E
    B. Type C
    C. Type A
    D. Type B

14. Which of the following conditions in infants may be caused by an iodine deficiency during pregnancy?
    A. Endemic goiter
    B. Pheochromocytoma
    C. Macrosomia
    D. Cretinism

15. Which of the following medications may cause neonatal abstinence syndrome during pregnancy?
    A. Hydrocortisone
    B. Oxycodone
    C. Neomycin
    D. Acetaminophen

FURTHER READING

1. American College of Obstetricians and Gynecologists. (2021). *Your Pregnancy and Childbirth – Month to Month*, 7th Edition. American College of Obstetricians and Gynecologists.
2. Briggs, G.G., Towers, C.V., and Forinash, A.B. (2021). *Briggs Drugs in Pregnancy and Lactation, 12th Edition – A Reference Guide to Fetal and Neonatal Risk.* Wolters Kluwer.
3. Bright, E. (2022). *Female Phases – The Ultimate Pregnancy Nutrition and Safety Guide.* Bright.
4. Brown, J.E. (2019). *Nutrition Through the Life Cycle*, 7th Edition. Cengage Learning.
5. Davies, L., and Deery, R. (2014). *Nutrition in Pregnancy and Childbirth – Food for Thought.* Routledge.
6. Dean, C., and Shortman, A. (2014). *Hyperemesis Gravidarum – The Definitive Guide.* Spewing Mummy.
7. Fett, R. (2019). *Brain Health from Birth – Nurturing Brain Development During Pregnancy and the First Year (It Starts with the Egg).* Franklin Fox Publishing LLC.
8. Galbally, M., Snellen, M., and Lewis, A. (2014). *Psychopharmacology and Pregnancy: Treatment Efficacy, Risks, and Guidelines.* Springer.

9. Gonik, B. (2012). *Viral Diseases in Pregnancy (Clinical Perspectives in Obstetrics and Gynecology)*. Springer.
10. Heyden, E.L., (2014). *Preventing Birth Defects: Understanding the Iodine/Thyroid Hormone Connection.* Impact Health Publishing.
11. Lammi-Keefe, C.J., Couch, S.C., and Philipson, E. (2008). *Handbook of Nutrition and Pregnancy (Nutrition and Health).* Humana Press.
12. Lang, J. (2016). *The Whole 9 Months – A Week-by-Week Pregnancy Nutrition Guide with Recipes for a Healthy Start.* Sonoma Press.
13. Liamputtong, P. (2013). *Women, Motherhood and Living with HIV/AIDS: A Cross-Cultural Perspective.* Springer.
14. May, S. (2018). *Iron Deficiency in Pregnancy – Symptoms, Causes and Prevention of Iron Deficiency.* May.
15. Mente, S. (2020). *Pregnancy and Nutrition – Conscious Nutrition in Pregnancy – Stages and Tips Not to Be Missed*! Mente.
16. Moore, L.E. (2017). *Diabetes in Pregnancy: The Complete Guide to Management.* Springer.
17. Nelson, D. (2022). *Nutrition in Pregnancy – Healthy Childbirth.* Nelson.
18. Nichols, L. (2018). *Real Food for Pregnancy: The Science and Wisdom of Optimal Prenatal Nutrition.* Lily Nichols.
19. Olug, S. (2016). *Preeclampsia: HELLP Syndrome, Eclampsia and other Hypertensive Disorders of Pregnancy.* Olug.
20. Orteaga, M. (2022). *Obesity and Pregnancy.* American Medical Publishers.
21. Shawe, J., Steegers, E.A.P., and Verbiest, S. (2020). *Preconception Health and Care: A Life Course Approach.* Springer.
22. Simpson, A.C. (2017). *Boost Your Breast Milk – An All-in-One Guide for Nursing Mothers to Build a Healthy Milk Supply.* The Experiment.
23. Smith, N. (2022). *Nutrition in (the) First Trimester of Pregnancy – Taking Care of You and Your Baby.* Smith.
24. Somer, E. (2002). *Nutrition for a Healthy Pregnancy: The complete Guide to Eating Before, During, and After Your Pregnancy – Revised Edition.* Holt Paperbacks.
25. Spohr, H.L. (2018). *Fetal Alcohol Syndrome: A Lifelong Challenge.* De Gruyter.
26. Thompson, S. (2021). *Functional Maternity: Using Functional Medicine and Nutrition to Improve Pregnancy and Childbirth Outcomes.* Modern Wisdom Press.
27. Tiran, D., and Conrad, P. (2021). *Using Natural Remedies Safely in Pregnancy and Childbirth – A Reference Guide for Maternity and Healthcare Professionals.* Singing Dragon.
28. Willick, E. (2016). *Your Fit Pregnancy: Nutrition & Exercise Handbook.* Union Square & Company.

Part III

Nutritional Disorders

7 Undernutrition and Eating Disorders

OUTLINE

Protein-energy Undernutrition
Essential Fatty Acid Deficiency
Blindness
Carnitine Deficiency
Keratomalacia
Iodine Deficiency Disorders
Iron-deficiency Anemia
Fad Diets
Vegetarian Diet
Malnutrition in the United States
Malnutrition in Developing Countries
Eating Disorders
  Anorexia Nervosa
  Bulimia Nervosa
  Binge-Eating Disorder
  Night Eating Syndrome
  Female Athlete Triad
Key Terms
Clinical Case Studies
Study Questions
Further Reading

LEARNING OBJECTIVES

After study of the chapter, readers should be able to:

1. Explain protein-energy undernutrition.
2. Identify the features of essential fatty acid deficiency.
3. Discuss the cause of corneal xerosis.
4. Explain the symptoms of primary carnitine deficiency.
5. Describe fad diets and their potential negative outcomes.
6. Explain the causes of keratomalacia.
7. Describe vegan diets and their advantages.
8. Identify the positive and negative attributes of vegetarian diets.
9. Compare anorexia nervosa with bulimia nervosa.
10. Describe binge-eating disorder.

OVERVIEW

Undernutrition occurs because of nutrient intake not meeting nutritional needs, resulting in surplus stores in the body to be used. When nutrient stores are depleted and there are very low tissue concentrations of essential nutrients, metabolic processes start to slow down, and may stop in some cases. Early nutrient deficiency is called subclinical, since no obvious signs and symptoms are detectable for a diagnosis. Severe deficiency causes obvious features that include skin flaking, tiredness, or body aches. Eating disorders are changes in eating patterns, occurring in response to stress, illness, or a need to change the diet for health or personal appearance reasons. These disorders result in altered body weight and nutritional problems. Dieting, skipping meals, eating at incorrect times of day, and having hectic lives all contribute to eating disorders. Obesity is the most common eating disorder, but other significant conditions include anorexia nervosa, bulimia nervosa, and binge-eating disorder. All eating disorders result in some form of malnutrition, on a global scale.

PROTEIN-ENERGY UNDERNUTRITION

Protein deficiency usually occurs along with a deficiency of energy and nutrients, resulting in **protein-energy malnutrition** (PEM) or **protein-calorie malnutrition** (PCM). Many developing countries have diets that are low in protein and energy, so PEM is a serious matter. It can affect people of all ages, but is most severe in children. Insufficient protein and energy cause a failure of normal growth, diarrhea, infections, a variety diseases, and early life. With about 156 million children malnourished throughout the world, there are 50 million that experience wasting, and 3 million that die annually.

In most cases, PEM occurs as marasmus or kwashiorkor. Marasmus develops slowly because of a severe deficiency of energy, protein, and micronutrients. There is extreme loss of weight, muscle, and fat, and growth is impaired. Kwashiorkor develops more quickly because of severe protein deficits. There is usually underlying infections or diseases. Edema develops, with mild to moderate weight loss, impaired growth, and excess accumulation of hepatic fat, known as fatty **liver**. Marasmus literally means to *waste away*, with affected individuals having little to no subcutaneous fat. It is most common in infants that are not breastfed or have stopped breastfeeding early in life. Weaning formulas are often not prepared correctly because of unsafe water supplies and lack of money to buy sufficient infant formula. Parents may be forced to dilute the formula to provide more feedings, but this deprives the infant of nutrients, including essential calories and proteins. Large amounts of energy and protein are need to return an infant with marasmus to normal growth, development, and overall health. When the condition affects normal brain growth in the first months of life, the child may have poor cognitive and intellectual growth.

DOI: 10.1201/b22969-10

Kwashiorkor often develops in a child when a younger sibling is more within 12–18 months, resulting in the new infant receiving breast milk, and the older one being switched to starchy roots and **gruels** that have low protein densities compared to energy content. The older child becomes unable to consume enough of these foods for energy needs – especially protein needs. Prevalent infections and parasites can elevate these needs, precipitating development of kwashiorkor. The hallmark sign is edema, when there is still some remaining subcutaneous fat. Other primary symptoms include apathy, diarrhea, failure to grow and gain weight, listlessness, infections, and withdrawal. The symptoms complicate any other concurrent diseases, such as measles, which can become severely debilitating or fatal. If the affected child is treated for infections and the diet is corrected, the disease process often reverses and normal growth resumes. However, by the time these children get care, severe infections have usually already developed, and many still die. Survivors often have chronic infections and diseases.

Protein-energy malnutrition is more prevalent in areas of Africa (Ethiopia, Kenya, Somalia, South Sudan, Sudan, Uganda), Southeast Asia (India, China, Bangladesh, Indonesia, Philippines, North Korea), Central America (Guatemala, Honduras, Mexico, El Salvador, Nicaragua), and South America (Peru, Bolivia, Colombia, Paraguay, Venezuela) – see Figure 7.1. It also occurs in certain populations, within industrialized countries, including the United States. The greatest risks are among people living in poverty or isolation, substance abusers, and in those with anorexia nervosa, AIDS, or cancer. In hospitals, some patients are at a higher risk of PEM because of previous poor health histories, low dietary intakes, and more needs for protein to recover from disease, trauma, or surgery. If a person is malnourished, the risks for additional complications and death are higher. Therefore, hospitals now have nutrition support teams for at-risk patients.

FOCUS ON PROTEIN-ENERGY MALNUTRITION

Protein-energy malnutrition is an undesirable loss of body cell mass that is secondary to reduce intake or inadequate utilization of nutrients. Children (especially infants) are highly prone to developing the condition since they have less metabolic reserves on hand to combat illness. Calorie deprivation is often called starvation, wasting, or marasmus. Protein-energy malnutrition greatly contributes to morbidity and mortality on a global scale.

Test Your Knowledge

1. What does insufficient protein and energy cause?
2. What are the features of marasmus and kwashiorkor?
3. Which groups of people have the highest risks of developing protein-energy metabolism?

ESSENTIAL FATTY ACID DEFICIENCY

Essential fatty acid (EFA) deficiency is a rare condition. It mostly occurs in infants that receive insufficiency EFAs in their diets, resulting in **alopecia**, scaly dermatitis, and thrombocytopenia. In children with EFA deficiency,

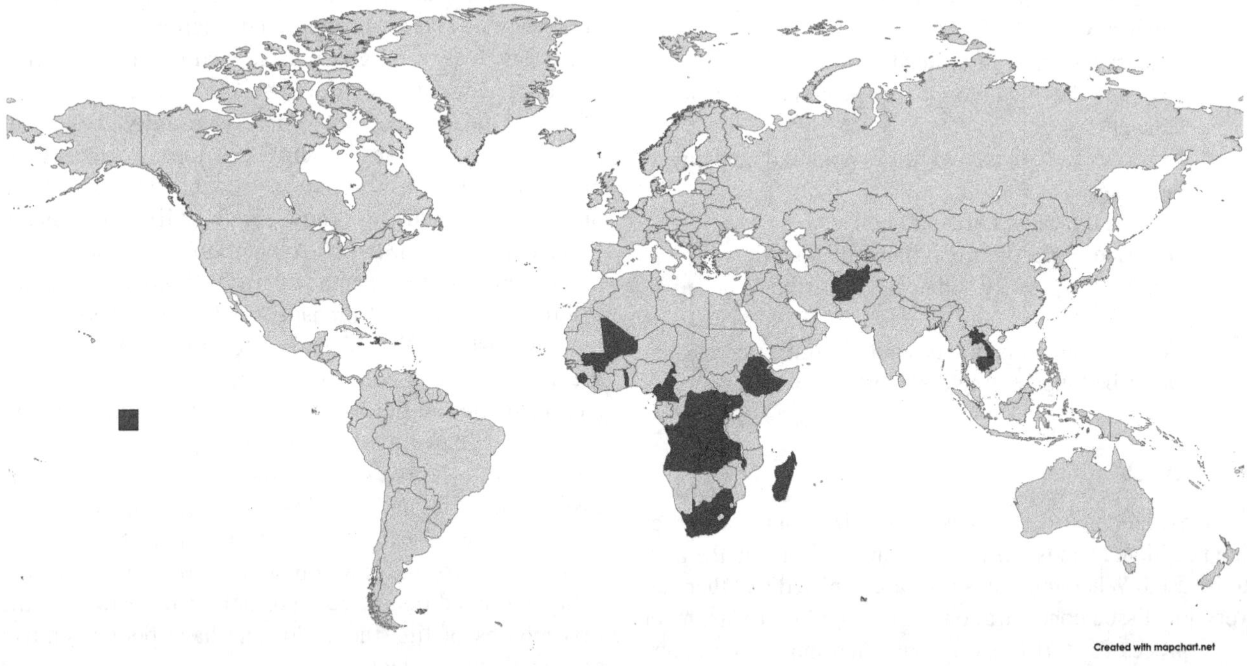

FIGURE 7.1 Countries with the highest rates of protein-energy malnutrition.

intellectual disability develops. The condition is easily reversed by dietary replenishment of EFAs. *Linoleic acid* and *linolenic acid* are substrates for endogenous synthesis of other fatty acids that are essential for a variety of physiologic processes. These include cell membrane and skin integrity maintenance, as well as the synthesis of **leukotrienes** and **prostaglandins**.

Dietary intake of EFAs must be extremely low in order for a deficiency to develop. Small amounts of EFAs are able to prevent deficiency. Though cow's milk has about 25% of the linoleic acid found in human breast milk, when it is ingested in recommended amounts, there is enough to prevent an EFA deficiency. The total fat intake in many countries that have high levels of food insecurity is often very low. However, the often vegetable-based fat is present in large amounts (linoleic acid and linolenic acid) to prevent any EFA deficiency.

Infants that are fed a formula that is low in linoleic acid, such as the skim-milk formulas, may develop an EFA deficiency. This condition, in previous times, resulted from long-term total parenteral nutrition (TPN) when fat was not included. Today, most TPN solutions contain fat emulsions, preventing EFA deficiency. A deficiency of EFA may be present, with no clinical manifestations, in patients that have fat malabsorption or increased metabolic needs such as those due to burns, multiple trauma, or surgery. The dermatitis caused by EFA deficiency is generalized and scaly.

BLINDNESS

Vitamin A deficiency causes serious consequences, including total blindness, night blindness, impaired growth, and higher rates of infections. The prevalence of vitamin A deficiency worldwide is significant, and it is the leading cause of preventable blindness in children, with 250,000–500,000 cases every year. About half of these children will die within one year from anemia, diarrhea, and severe infections.

Vitamin A deficiency-related blindness is common in developing countries but rarely seen in developed countries. It is a public health concern in over 50% of all countries, but mostly in those of Africa and Southeast Asia. The most severe effects are seen in young children as well as pregnant women in lower-income countries. Blindness results from conditions such as corneal xerosis and ulceration that may be caused by this deficiency. Vitamin A deficiency contributes to blindness by drying out the cornea and damaging it as well as the retina.

Test Your Knowledge

1. In which individuals is essential fatty acid deficiency most common?
2. In which patients can an EFA deficiency develop with no clinical manifestations?
3. How prevalent is vitamin A deficiency on a global scale?

CARNITINE DEFICIENCY

Carnitine is a carrier of fatty acids, moving them from cell **cytosol** into the inner portion of the mitochondria. It is also a popular nutritional supplement. When a person is healthy, the cells produce all the carnitine that is needed, and the supplements are not beneficial. However, in people that have acute illnesses, carnitine synthesis may be insufficient. These individuals may need supplemental carnitine added into total parenteral solutions if they are hospitalized for their acute conditions. Carnitine synthesis relies on sufficient amounts of vitamin C in the body. Once less than 10% of the required carnitine is not available to body cells, symptoms include muscle weakness and heart or liver conditions. Deficiency can occur in people of all ages, from all ethnic or racial backgrounds. Individuals who are at risk for carnitine deficiency include people with the abnormal gene, and those with liver or kidney disease.

The symptoms of primary carnitine deficiency are more severe than with the secondary form of the disease. Affected children usually have symptoms beginning in the first few years of life, though symptoms can also appear in adulthood. They range from mild to severe and may appear when meals are skipped, excessive exercise is done, or during other illnesses. The symptoms include decreased or **floppy muscle tone**, muscle weakness, delayed motor development, irritability, poor infant feeding, symptoms of hypoglycemia (if the liver is affected), shortness of breath or edema (if the heart is affected), and tiredness.

Diagnosis of carnitine deficiency requires a health history and physical examination, including family history. A neurological examination may be needed. Tests include blood tests for carnitine and **creatine kinase** (to assess muscle damage or liver disease), urine testing for **ketones**, exercise tests (to identify metabolic abnormalities), genetic tests (for primary carnitine deficiency), and heart tests such as echocardiography.

The main treatment for carnitine deficiency it with L-carnitine supplements (in pill form), which contain the usable form of carnitine. The amount of carnitine is increased in the bloodstream and cells, helping to prevent many of the symptoms of the disease. For primary carnitine deficiency, the supplements are often continued throughout life. For the secondary condition, they may only be needed for a short time. Repeated blood tests may be required. Heart or liver problems may require additional treatments. It is also important to not skip meals, be exposed to excessive cold temperatures, or engage in excessive exercise.

Complications of carnitine deficiency include heart and liver problems. A weak heart may not be able to pump blood as well, leading to inflammation and shortness of break, and possible early death. However, treatment with L-carnitine is able to correct many heart problems, though continual heart monitoring is needed. Heart problems are sometimes the first symptoms of carnitine deficiency. Liver problems often develop in children, early in live, causing hepatomegaly and physiological problems, resulting in poor feeding and irritability. Hypoglycemia may be triggered, often by infections. Severe hypoglycemia can lead to coma and death without treatment.

FOCUS ON CARNITINE DEFICIENCY

Carnitine was named from the Latin word *carnus*, meaning "flesh", since it was first isolated from various types of meat. In fact, the "redder" the meat, the higher the carnitine content. Primary carnitine deficiency usually develops in early childhood, signified by skeletal muscle weakness, hypoglycemia, and cardiomyopathy. Secondary carnitine deficiency is often caused by chronic renal failure or conditions that reduce its absorption or increase its excretion.

Test Your Knowledge

1. When do the signs of carnitine deficiency begin?
2. What are the symptoms of primary carnitine deficiency?
3. What are the potential complications of carnitine deficiency?

KERATOMALACIA

Keratomalacia is softening of the cornea. With vitamin A deficiency, eye abnormalities begin that lead to conjunctival xerosis, followed by **Bitot's spots**, which often progress to keratomalacia and scarring (see Figure 7.2). These sequential eye changes are collectively known as xerophthalmia, which causes irreversible blindness in millions of people throughout the world. Overall, keratomalacia is a rare disease. It usually affects both eyes, due to dietary or metabolic causes. Without sufficient treatment, there may be corneal infection, perforation, and degenerative tissue changes, which collective cause the person to become blind. In developing countries, vitamin A deficiency-related keratomalacia is a major cause of childhood blindness. It may also occur because of conditions related to impaired absorption, storage, or transport of vitamin A. These conditions include celiac disease, **ulcerative colitis**, liver disease, and **cystic fibrosis**.

Keratomalacia is caused by prolonged dietary deprivation of vitamin A. Primary vitamin A deficiency is common in areas where rice is a major dietary component, such as Southeast Asia. Rice lacks beta-carotene, which is converted into vitamin A. Keratomalacia is also common with malnutrition disorders caused by insufficient consumption of protein and energy. The deficiency can result from dietary deprivation as well as defective vitamin A storage and transport. Infants who are allergic to cow's milk or given diluted formula have a higher risk for vitamin A deficiency-related keratomalacia. Impaired vitamin A storage or absorption may be due to partial small intestine obstruction at birth, bile duct obstruction, or cirrhosis of the liver.

Diagnosis is via complete patient history, eye examination, blood studies, and trials with therapeutic doses of vitamin A. The condition is treated with vitamin A supplementation (avoiding excessively high doses), management of underlying conditions, administration of antibiotic drops or ointment for secondary infections, and symptomatic or supportive treatments as needed. Prevention of keratomalacia is with proper, balanced nutrition, prophylactic supplementation, and infant substitute formulas that contain adequate vitamin A within substrates.

IODINE DEFICIENCY DISORDERS

Iodine deficiency disorders are very common. Today, about 33% of the global population is at risk for iodine deficiency. The highest incidence occurs in Asia, Africa, the Middle East, and Europe. Because of the fortification of table salt with iodine, many countries have used iodized salt for decades, with great reductions in cases of iodine deficiency

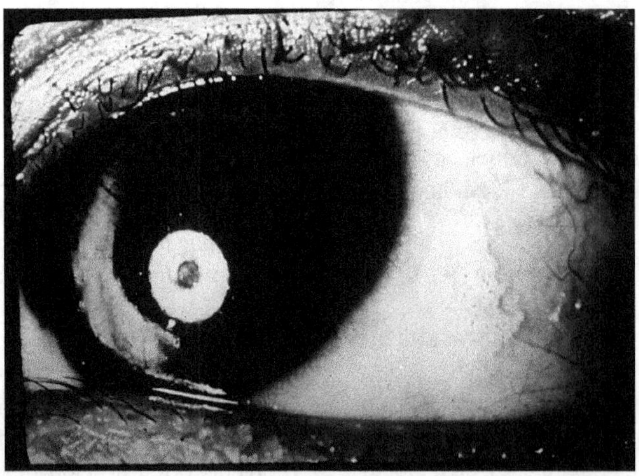

FIGURE 7.2 Bitot's spots.

and goiter. Still, about 30% of global households do not have access to iodized salt. Iodine deficiency disorders will be discussed in Chapters 11 and 15 in detail.

IRON-DEFICIENCY ANEMIA

Iron deficiency is the most common nutritional deficiency in the world. As iron deficiency progresses, body stores of iron are depleted. There is insufficient iron for synthesis of heme and hemoglobin, and iron-deficiency anemia develops. Then, there is impaired oxygen transport in the bloodstream, resulting in fatigue and a lowered ability to perform normal activities. This anemia compromises immune function, makes energy metabolism more difficult, and causes delayed cognitive development. Iron deficiency is serious in young children since there may be no way to reverse cognitive and developmental impairment.

In its early stages, the symptoms may be absent or very slight, since the body can use stored iron from the primary iron storage protein known as **ferritin**. As the deficiency progresses and the body's stores are depleted, a lack of iron needed for **heme** and hemoglobin synthesis causes *iron-deficiency anemia* to develop. Oxygen transport in the blood is impaired, resulting in fatigue and a lower ability to enjoy normal activities. Immune function, energy metabolism, and **cognitive** development are all affected. Iron-deficiency anemia is extremely dangerous in young children, since irreversible cognitive and developmental impairment may occur. Diagnosis of iron-deficiency anemia is partly achieved by viewing red blood cells under a microscope. They appear smaller than normal, known as *microcytic*, and paler in color, known as *hypochromic* (see Figure 7.3).

Another diagnostic method is to measure blood **hematocrit** and blood hemoglobin, since these are both decreased in iron-deficiency anemia. Even so, these are not excellent measures of iron status since they are unchanged in early stages of iron deficiency. They are also affected by inflammation, diseases, blood loss, and other nutrient deficiencies. At-risk individuals for iron-deficiency anemia include premature infants (born before week 37), since iron stores only accumulate during the last weeks of pregnancy. These infants have insufficient stores of iron that can be depleted quickly. Young children that are growing fast are also at risk, and often do not eat a lot of iron-rich meat, or drink iron-poor cow's milk. One of every four US children between 12 and 23 months of age does not have sufficient iron intake. However, iron-fortified formulas and cereals are provided to children from limited-resource families that are at nutritional risk. This has helped decrease rates of iron-deficiency anemia. Unfortunately, young children in poorer countries are iron deficient because supplementation programs often do not exist.

Because of menstrual blood losses and insufficient intake of iron-rich foods, teenage girls and women of childbearing age are also at risk. About 10% of US women aged 12–49 have iron-deficiency anemia. Pregnant women must consume enough iron because their blood volume and red blood cell (RBC) numbers are increasing during pregnancy along with those of the fetus. People that do not eat enough dietary iron, such as vegetarians, are also at increased risk of iron deficiency. Even with high intakes of plant-based iron foods, their diets include factors that may decrease iron bioavailability. They must add vitamin C-rich foods and consider iron-fortified foods, plus multivitamin-mineral supplements containing iron. Anyone that donates blood more than two to four times annually may have a higher risk for iron deficiency. Each donation of one pint of blood results in a loss of 200–250 mg of iron. It usually takes sometimes to replace the iron. Blood banks regularly test donor blood for anemia before allowing an individual to donate.

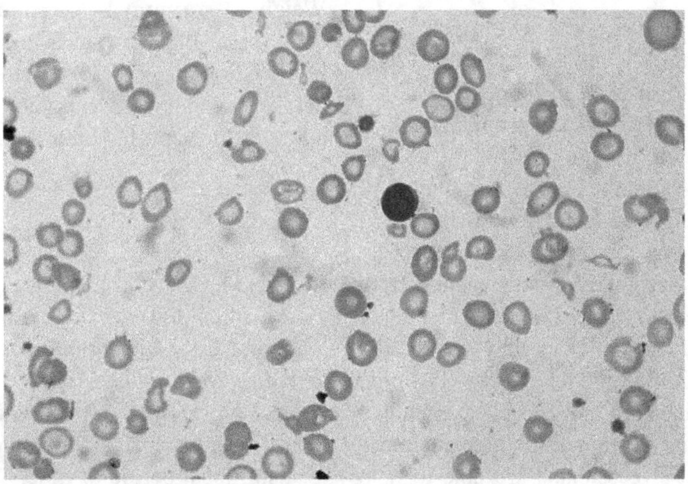

FIGURE 7.3 Red blood cells of normal size and color, and how these cells appear in iron-deficiency anemia, with the color loss due to decreased hemoglobin and a reduced capacity to carry oxygen.

FAD DIETS

Fad diets are named because they make outrageous claims for extreme weight loss or improved health. However, they often include unhealthy eating plans or promote eating only specific single foods. They sometimes encourage eating certain foods in excessively large amounts. Many are boring and cannot be followed for long. Though fad diets sometimes result in some amount of fast weight loss, this is simply because the individual on the diet is closely monitoring what they intake. Continued weight loss or changes in eating and exercise usually do not occur. Fad diets can also be extremely harmful. Negative outcomes of fad diets include multivitamin or mineral supplementation, **ketosis**, reduced exercise capacity, constipation, headaches, bad breath, muscle cramps, flatulence, poor mineral absorption, deprivation of nutrients, binging, relapses into previous poor diet, and malnutrition. Fad diets cost US civilians about $33 billion every year. It is much better to follow eating and exercise plans that can be maintained throughout life, which offer lifelong weight control but not immediate weight loss. There are 10 factors that indicate a diet is a "fad diet", as follows:

- The promise of a "quick fix" to improving weight
- Extreme warnings if one product or regimen is not followed
- Unrealistic-sounding claims
- Simplified ideas drawn out of complicated studies
- Recommendations base on only one study
- Dramatic claims that respected scientific organizations do not back up
- Lists of foods claimed to be good or bad
- Recommendations that influence sales, often with testimonials
- Recommendations based on published studies that were not peer-reviewed
- Recommendations based on studies that do not take into account differences between groups or individuals

Weight loss is often promised to occur very quickly, but fast weight loss does not mostly consist of fat since a high energy deficit is required to lose much adipose tissue. If 10–15 pounds of weight loss per week are promised, it will not be only from stores of fat. It is not possible to subtract enough energy from the daily intake to lose that amount of fat. When weight loss is more than a few pounds per week, it is lean tissue and water – instead of fat – that are mostly involved. Fad diets are not designed for permanent weight loss. Instead of fat, most dieters are unaware they are mostly losing muscle and other lean tissue. Once they start eating normally, the lost weight returns in a few weeks. The diet, not the dieter, has failed. This gain-and-loss cycle is known as *yo-yo dieting*. It causes significant guilt, blame, and poor health. Even though health professionals are able to help dieters succeed, trends suggest the more and more time and money is being spent on fad diets.

Examples of fad diets that do not usually work over the long term include restricted carbohydrate, low-fat, and novelty diets. Low carbohydrate diets result in less glycogen synthesis and reduced body water. If they are very low in carbohydrates, the liver must produce glucose through gluconeogenesis, with the source of needed carbons mostly being body proteins. While weight loss occurs, the extent of weight lost and possible health improvements are not greater than for those that follow a moderate fat, moderate protein, higher carbohydrate diet. Low carbohydrate diets are mostly effective in the short term since they limit total food intake. These diets may even increase low-density lipoprotein (LDL)-cholesterol. For each restricted carbohydrate diet, see if breads, cereals, fruits, and vegetables are very limited in the diet plan – this signifies a low carbohydrate diet.

Low-fat diets often include very high carbohydrate intakes. About 5%–10% of energy intake is as fat. These diets are not harmful in a healthy adult, but usually cannot be followed for long. Grains, fruits, and vegetables are the major components of low-fat diets. People usually get board since they cannot eat foods that are higher in fat or protein. These diets are extremely different from usually diets, making them difficult to follow.

Novelty diets consist of gimmicks, often emphasizing one food or food group, with most others being excluded. Examples include diets that include only eggs, grapefruit, or rice. The theory is that energy intake will be reduced because of simple boredom. However, most people abandon these diets before much weight can be lost. One extreme example of a novelty diet claims that food becomes stuck in the gastrointestinal tract and rots there, creating toxins. These diets suggest avoiding certain foods or eating them only at certain times. The claims are nonsensical because the GI tract efficiently digests foods and eliminates wastes.

Many fad diets require consumers to buy costly products or services, with no beneficial weight loss. People that try them and happen to lose some weight often become promoters of the diets even though the weight loss had little to nothing to do with the purchased products or services. Weight loss gimmicks come and go every year. Any new discoveries that appear in major peer-reviewed journals, however, should be looked at seriously. It is important to be skeptical about information that appears in diet books, advertisements, infomercials, and on websites.

FOCUS ON FAD DIETS

There are several major dangers of "fad diets". They are often too restrictive as to food choices, with severe limitations and sometimes, elimination of entire food groups. As a result, essential nutrients may be missing from the diet. Also, some fad diets are very expensive, and many are not sustainable for a sufficient period of time. Lastly, some fad diets can actually cause weight gain instead of weight loss.

Test Your Knowledge

1. Why is iron deficiency in young children serious?
2. How common is iron deficiency in American women?
3. What type of dietary regulation is preferred over fad diets?

VEGETARIAN DIET

A vegetarian diet requires people to have knowledge and creative planning so that high quality proteins and other important nutrients are obtained while not consuming some or any animal products. This requires *complimentary proteins*, in which essential amino acids that are deficient in one source of protein can be supplied by another that is consumed in the same meal or the next one. For example, while many legumes lack the essential amino acid *methionine*, many cereals are limited in their *lysine* content. Therefore, combining legumes such as beans with rice cereals, the body receives sufficient amounts of essential amino acids. For *vegans*, who do not eat any type of animal product (not even eggs), this type of dietary variety is extremely important. About 2.5% of adults in the United States and 4% of adults in Canada are vegetarians. There is an estimated 1.5 billion vegetarians globally, though vegetarians that choose this type of diet make up only 75 million people – the rest do not have the resources to be able to consume a diet that is rich in meat products. Up to one in four Americans consume at least four meals without any type of meat per week. Vegetarian diets are commonly chosen for religious, philosophical, ecological, or health-related reasons. Other people are concerned about the impact of meat-based diets upon the economy, and upon ecology. Meat is not an efficient way of obtaining protein, since about 40% of the global grain production is needed to raise animals for meat products.

Diets that are rich in fruits, vegetables, legumes, and grains often result in higher intakes of antioxidants, such as the carotenoids and vitamins C and E. There is also more intake of dietary fiber and healthy phytochemicals, with less intake of cholesterol and saturated fat. Vegetarians are less likely to be obese. Plant-based diets are encouraged for health promotion and to reduce risks of chronic disease by many associations, including the World Cancer Research Fund. The following list explains basic differences between various types of vegetarians:

- Lacto-ovo-vegetarians – exclude meat, poultry, and fish, but do include eggs
- Lacto-vegetarians – exclude meat, poultry, eggs, and fish from their diets, but do include dairy products
- Vegans – eat only plant foods without any type of animal foods – their diets may be low in valuable protein, riboflavin, vitamins B12 and D, calcium, and zinc

In North America, milk is a major source of riboflavin, vitamin D, and calcium – which vegans do not consume. However, riboflavin is obtainable from green leafy vegetables, whole-grain cereals and breads, yeast, and legumes – all of which vegans include in their diets. Other sources of vitamin D include soy milk and dietary supplements, plus regular sun exposure. For vegans, calcium-fortified foods are important, including fortified soy milk, orange juice, tofu, and some ready-to-eat cereals, breads, and snacks. Though green leafy vegetables contain calcium, absorption is not high. Dietary supplements provide another option for calcium. Supplement labels must be read carefully, since common multivitamin and mineral supplements supply 25%–45% of daily calcium. The only natural occurrence of vitamin B12 is in animal foods. Trace amounts are in plants that have soil or microbial contaminants, but these are vastly insufficient. Vegans must eat foods fortified with vitamin B12 or take supplements. For iron, whole-grain cereals and breads, dried fruits, nuts, and legumes can be consumed, but the iron is not as well-absorbed as from animal foods. However, eating a good source of vitamin C will enhance iron absorption. Zinc can also be obtained from whole-grain cereals and breads, nuts, and legumes, though phytic acid and other substances that are present limit its absorption. Grains have the most nutrition when eaten as breads, since **leavening** of the dough reduces the effects of **phytic acid**. Suggested food plans for lacto-vegetarians and vegans, based on MyPlate, are summarized in Table 7.1.

For infants and children, poorly planned vegetarian diets increase risks for undernutrition. Nutritional needs can be met by using complementary proteins and adequate sources of the "problem" nutrients. For infants and children, the most common deficiencies to be concerned with are of iron, calcium, zinc, and vitamins B12 and D.

Vegetarian and vegan diets are often high in fiber, with low calorie, bulky foods that make individuals feel full, which is an advantage for adults. However, the small stomach volume and high nutrient needs for children may result in a problem, if a child feels full before meeting energy needs. Therefore, the fiber content may need to be decreased by replacing high fiber sources with some refined grain products, fruit juices, and peeled fruit. Caloric and nutritional needs can be met by including concentrated sources of energy. These include fortified soy milk, dried fruits, avocados, and nuts. Though vegetarian and vegan diets can be good during infancy and childhood, it is important to ensure adequate nutrient intake to achieve normal growth. These diets should be guided by nutritionists and dieticians.

FOCUS ON VEGETARIAN DIETS

There are several positive and negative attributes of vegetarian diets. On the positive side, they provide many important vitamins, minerals, antioxidants, and fiber – lowering risks for heart disease, diabetes, certain cancers, and obesity. On the negative side, if a vegetarian diet includes a lot of highly processed foods, the risk for some chronic diseases actually increases.

TABLE 7.1
Food Plans for Vegetarians, Based on MyPlate

Food Group	Lacto-vegetarian Servings (75 g of protein in 1,650 kcal)	Vegan Servings (79 g of protein in 1,800 kcal)	Key Nutrients
Grains	5	6	Fiber, folate, iron, magnesium, niacin, protein, thiamin, vitamin E, zinc
Protein foods such as beans, nuts, and seeds	5	5	Fiber, magnesium, protein, vitamin B6, zinc
Vegetables	2 (including one dark green daily)	2½ (including one dark green daily)	Folate, magnesium, potassium, and vitamins A, C, and K
Fruits	1½	1½	Folate, and vitamins A and C
Milk	3	N/A	Calcium, protein, riboflavin, and vitamins B12 and D
Fortified soy milk	N/A	3	Calcium, protein, riboflavin, and vitamins B12 and D

Note: One serving of vitamin- and mineral-enriched ready-to-eat breakfast cereal is recommended, to fill any nutrient gaps, or a balanced multivitamin and mineral supplement can be taken.

Test Your Knowledge

1. What is the "vegan" form of vegetarian dieting?
2. What are the most common deficiencies, in infants and children, related to vegetarian diets?

MALNUTRITION IN THE UNITED STATES

Though many other countries have more significant problems with malnutrition, the condition is still prevalent in certain populations within the United States. It includes undernutrition, being overweight or obese, and micronutrient deficiency or excess. About 40 million Americans (and 12 million children) have food insecurity, often skipping meals or purchasing inexpensive and non-nutritious foods. Hunger and poverty are most prevalent in areas where fresh, unprocessed foods are not available or are too expensive. Americans from all income groups do not consume enough fruits, vegetables, whole grains, or low-fat dairy products. Lower-income families are most vulnerable to poor nutrition and obesity. Obesity affects children in lower socioeconomic levels in much higher proportions than other groups. In over 50% of all US households with malnourishment, malnutrition is often present along with non-communicable diseases.

According to the American Academy of Pediatrics, the nutrition that a child receives during the first 1,000 days of life greatly impacts future development. No compensation can totally repair the lost time for physical, mental, and cognitive growth. The most important nutrients that support neurodevelopment include protein, choline, zinc, folate, iodine, and vitamins A, D, B6, and B12. Brain malnourishment results in a lower intelligence quotient (IQ), increased risks for obesity, hypertension, and diabetes mellitus, and outcomes that negatively impact future success in job-related activities.

Over 50% of adult Americans are now overweight, which reduces productivity and lowers life expectancy. In young adults, obesity increases changes for diabetes, hypertension, gallbladder disease, heart disease, and cancer. Because of these conditions, about 71% of young Americans between ages 17 and 24 are ineligible to serve in the United States military – about 24 million individuals. Older people are also at risk of malnutrition due to aging-related physical changes, dementia, isolation-related depression, and limited income. Malnutrition causes more of them to require hospitalization, increased falls and fractures, weakened immunity, and higher risks for death.

Solutions for malnutrition in the United States include better public policies to provide adequate nutrients and healthy diets during life. These can reduce food insecurity, prevent poverty, support better economic stability, improve diets and health, protect against obesity, and increase learning and development. Federal nutrition programs help to educate, support, and improve public health. To reduce obesity, non-profit organizations are focusing on nutrient-dense foods being offered to low-income recipients instead of calorie-dense foods. The quality of food that is served is much more important than the quantity.

MALNUTRITION IN DEVELOPING COUNTRIES

Though malnutrition is still a significant problem in developing countries, undernutrition is decreasing. Underweight children today make up 16% of their population, but this percentage was 28% in 1990. Young children and women are disproportionately affected by undernutrition. About 2.6 million children under age five die annually in low- and middle-income countries because of undernutrition-related causes. This makes up 45% of all deaths of infants and preschool children. Approximately 95 million children throughout the world are underweight, and about 25% have stunted growth. These children are more likely to suffer from infectious diseases and to have problems in school. Women often have less access to food than men due to certain social customs. A poorly nourished woman may have a fetus or breastfed infant that is also malnourished. Hunger mostly affects people in rural areas of developing countries, or in those who operate **subsistence farms** – meaning they only grow enough food for their own families, and have little left over to sell in order to make money. Farming is difficult in various areas due to poor-quality land, droughts, floods, or lack of farming equipment, fertilizer, and seeds. Food crises and famine can be triggered by natural disasters, wars, and political instability.

By 2050, it is predicted that the global population will reach 9.5 billion. This growth and increases in economic growth and urbanization will mean that world food demand will explode. It is of supreme importance to reduce malnutrition and improve food security. Increasing agricultural productivity will allow people to grow more crops, eat more healthy meals, and earn a better income. This will be expensive and complicate, and require roads, electricity, irrigation, and banking. Also needed are agricultural research, education, and better overall health of the population. Elimination of micronutrient deficiencies will improve health, as will clean food and water, plus family-planning.

Test Your Knowledge

1. In the United States, where are hunger and poverty most prevalent?
2. What does early brain malnourishment result in?
3. Which global populations are disproportionately affected by undernutrition?

EATING DISORDERS

Eating disorders that result in varying degrees of global malnutrition include anorexia nervosa, bulimia nervosa, binge-eating disorder, night eating syndrome, and the female athlete triad. *Disordered eating* involves mild, short-term changes in eating patterns, related to stress, illness, or a desire to improve health or personal appearance. Eating patterns may be simply bad habits, learned from other people, or be implicated in preparations for athletic competition. It may lead to changes in weight and nutritional abnormalities. Dieting, skipping meals, eating at irregular times, or having hectic lives may press individuals with disordered eating to develop actual eating disorders. In the United States, about 20 million women and 10 million men have some type of eating disorder. About 500,000 adolescents have either disordered eating or an eating disorder. Eating disorders, overall, are six to ten times more common in women. As many as 5% of North Americans will develop some type of anorexia nervosa or bulimia nervosa. These disorders are increasing in prevalence.

Often, an eating disorder begins with a diet, but this may worsen because of insufficient coping mechanisms, dysfunctional families, or drug abuse. Stress may be due to puberty, an expected weight that must be maintained for employment, overall leanness for sports competitions, losing friends, or leaving for college. About 85% of eating disorders develop during adolescence or early adulthood. Disordered eating can evolve into chronic food restriction, binge eating, purging, and life-altering weight fluctuations. It involves emotional and cognitive changes affecting self-perception of body shape or weight. Eating disorders are common with depression, anxiety, and substance abuse. Eating disorders are treatable medical illnesses that require complicated professional interventions. They can cause serious physical health problems without treatment, including heart conditions, kidney failure, and even lead to death. Initial steps into treatment include self-help groups, and support from family members and friends. Self-help group meetings help people understand if an eating disorder is actually present.

Anorexia Nervosa

Anorexia nervosa involves extreme weight loss, distortions of body image, and an irrational fear of weight gain and obesity. The affected person often denies his or her appetite and hates looking in a mirror. Anorexics believe they are fat no matter what the truth is and what others tell them. Some people focus on body areas, such as the stomach, thighs, and buttocks, which they believe to be excessively fat. The severity of anorexia nervosa is determined by discrepancies between actual and perceived body shape. Prevalence of anorexia nervosa is uncertain because it is widely underreported. However, about 0.5% of adolescent girls will develop the condition in North America. In part, they blame themselves for the weight gain that occurs during puberty. This self-blame is less common in adult women or in African-American woman of all ages. Men make up only about 10% of all cases, since their ideal image is considered normal when they are larger and more muscular. Anorexia nervosa in males occurs more often in homosexuals and athletes participating in sports with weight classes – such as boxers, jockeys, and wrestlers. Eating disorders in men may be encouraged by activities such as cycling, dancing, modeling, and swimming.

Anorexia nervosa is more psychological than related to food. Family conflict is a common underlying factor. If a family's expectations are very high, including expectations about body weight, frustration results in arguments. Anorexic individuals often feel hopeless about human relationships and become socially isolated by family dysfunction. The two main forms of anorexia nervosa are as follows:

- Restricting – dieting, fasting, and/or excessive exercising
- Binge eating/purging – binge eating, and then purging in response to severe food restriction

Anorexics have very low body weights and fear gaining any amount of weight. They have a distorted view of their weight and their self-worth is nearly entirely based on it. There are continual thoughts about controlling food, eating, and weight, while human relationships are reduced. Health professionals can evaluate anorexics and make the correct diagnosis. It is important to seek help sooner rather than later because chances for recovery are much higher when treatment is received as early as possible.

Semistarvation causes the body to conserve as much energy as possible. There is a lowered body temperature and cold intolerance. The reduced synthesis of thyroid hormones causes a slower metabolic rate. The heart rate decreases, resulting in fatigue, fainting, and a greater need for sleep. Some people actually lose heart tissue to some degree or develop heart rhythm irregularities. If iron-deficiency anemia develops, the fatigue worsens. The skin becomes rough, dry, scaly, and cold. Bruising can occur because of less protective fat. Lower white blood cell counts increase risks for infection and even death. After eating anything, abnormal fullness or bloating may last for hours. Hair loss is common. **Lanugo hair** may appear, which helps trap air, and reduce heat loss caused by reduced fatty tissue. Semistarvation and laxative abuse may cause constipation. Low blood potassium increases risks for heart rhythm disturbances, which can lead to death. Loss of menstrual periods and related hormonal changes cause reduced bone mass and increased risks for **osteoporosis**. Neurotransmitter function in the brain is altered, and depression results. If frequent vomiting occurs, acid erosion will lead to eventual loss of teeth. Athletes experience muscle tears and stress fractures.

Treatment of anorexia nervosa requires experienced physicians, registered dietitians, psychologists, and additional health professionals. Eating disorder clinics are often preferred and treatment may require outpatient therapy, day hospitalization for up to 12 hours, or total hospitalization, which is required if the patient is below 75% of expected weight, has acute medical conditions, or has severe psychological problems (or is suicidal). Efforts sometimes fail regardless of the treatment team, so prevention of the disease is extremely important. Many anorexics try to hide their weight loss in various ways. It usually takes an anorexic about seven years to fully recover, but many insurers only cover a small amount of the costs of treatment.

Nutrition therapy begins by gaining the cooperation of the patient, as well as trust, to increase intake of foods. Weight gain is best if it is sufficient to increase the metabolic rate to normal and reverse many physical signs. An early goal is to minimize or stop additional weight loss. Appropriate food habits are slowly restored. Then, slow weight gain of two to three pounds per week is attempted. If immediate renourishment is needed, some patients require tube feeding, TPN, or both – but these efforts often cause the patient to distrust the treatment team. Calories are slowly increased and a multivitamin and mineral supplement is added. Enough calcium is added to increase intake to about 1,500 mg/day. Dietitians provide nutritional information, promote health food attitudes, and teach patients to eat when they are hungry and stop when they are feeling full. Reassurance is considerable because of uncomfortable bloating, and increases in body heat and fat. The medical team must assure the patient he or she will not be abandoned once gaining back normal weight.

After this, the underlying emotional problems are addressed. The patient learns to reject a feeling of accomplishment they previously associated with emaciation, and starts to accept the healthy body weight. Recovery is based on strong relationships with therapists and other support personnel. Patients are taught to regain control of their lives and how to cope with adverse situations. Once eating becomes normalized, the patient can return to activities they stopped enjoying while anorexic. Family therapy is important for younger patient still living at home. Medications are sometimes required for anorexic patients, but these are mostly focused at preventing relapses after treatment when psychiatric disorders are still present. These disorders include depression, anxiety, and obsessive-compulsive disorder.

FOCUS ON ANOREXIA NERVOSA

Weight loss caused by anorexia nervosa is generally to less than 85% of what is expected for the individual's age, or a body mass index of 17.5 or less. Many anorexics find security in rigid control of their weight. Even a small weight gain makes them panic. Strict discipline and self-denial provides feelings of purity, power, and superiority. However, they often feel helpless in the presence of food. Anorexic women often lack menstrual periods after the normal age of puberty.

Test Your Knowledge

1. In which age groups do eating disorders usually begin?
2. What are the two main forms of anorexia nervosa?
3. What are the effects of anorexia nervosa upon the heart and brain?

Bulimia Nervosa

Bulimia nervosa involves episodes of binge eating that are followed by attempts to purge via vomiting or excessive use of laxatives, diuretics, or enemas. Another way some bulimics try to burn off excess energy after binge eating is to exercise excessively. Bulimics use food to cope with extreme situations. They understand that their behaviors are abnormal, while anorexics do not. Often, there is very low self-esteem and depression underlying bulimia. Approximately 50% of patients have major depression. As many as 4% of adolescent and college-age women suffer from the condition. Overall, most patients are successful women who are of normal weight or only slightly above this, with only 10% of cases occurring in men. Many people are not diagnosed due to lack of obvious symptoms. Also, many of them hide their abnormal eating habits. Susceptible individuals often have genetic factors and lifestyle patterns that predispose them to being overweight. They often try weight reduction diets that fail.

Common characteristics of bulimia nervosa include secretive binging, eating while depressed or feeling stress, binging on large amounts of food and then purging, feelings of shame and embarrassment, fluctuating weight of ten pounds (more or less), fear of not being able to stop eating, being a perfectionist to try and please everyone, erosion of teeth due to excessive vomiting, and purchases of syrup of ipecac (which induces vomiting). Though this syrup is not used as much today as in previous years, it is still available in over 50% of US pharmacies. However, healthcare providers should advise against its use and encourage pharmacies to remove it from their inventories. Many affected individuals have elaborate rules about food, often avoiding all types of sweets. A single cookie can cause a feeling of severe guilt and trigger binging, and this usually leads to extreme overeating. Binges can be triggered by hunger from dieting, stress, loneliness, boredom, and depression. Binging is common after strict dieting and may be linked to extreme hunger. The individual eats quickly, loses control of eating, and may not be able to enjoy flavors. Binge-purge cycles may be daily, weekly, or with longer intervals. Binge eating is common at night when interruptions are less likely, and may continue from 30 minutes to 2 hours.

Bulimics often consume foods that are sweet and contain high levels of carbohydrates while binging. This is because these foods are more easily purged by vomiting. In one binge, the individual may consume 3,000 kilocalories or more. The purging is thought to prevent any weight gain. Even when vomiting is induced however, there is still an absorption of 33%–75% of the consumed food energy, causing some weight gain. Also, about 90% of the food energy is absorbed when laxatives or enemas are used, since these products affect the large intestine, which is past the point of where most nutrients are absorbed. Bulimics are under a severe misconception that purging soon after binging will prevent excess energy absorption and the gaining of weight. The other option – excessive exercise – is often done at odd times of day, or it continues even though injuries or medical complications occur. The exercise practice of *debting* is an attempt to undergo physical activity that is enough to counteract the kilocalorie intake. Once binging and purging is complete, the individual usually feels guilty and depressed. They have low self-esteem and feelings of hopelessness. They become distant from other people, spending more time alone focusing on their bulimia.

The majority of negative health outcomes are caused by the repeated vomiting. The teeth become demineralized so they are painful and sensitive to temperatures and acids. Eventual severe tooth decay occurs, with erosion from fillings, and over time, the teeth fall out. Blood potassium may be very low because of vomiting or certain diuretics, which can disturb heart rhythm and lead to sudden death. Infections and irritation from vomiting may cause inflammation of the salivary glands. In some people, there are esophageal tears and stomach ulcers. Frequent laxative use may lead to constipation. Ipecac syrup, if used to induce vomiting, is toxic to the heart, liver, and kidneys. Repeated doses may result in accidental poisoning. The final outcomes of bulimia nervosa include death (mostly from suicide), severe hypokalemia, and widespread infections.

Treatment of bulimia nervosa requires an experienced team. For severe weight loss, treatment begins with measures to gain back needed weight, followed by psychological therapy and nutritional counseling. For extreme laxative abuse, chronic vomiting, substance abuse, and depression, hospitalization is often required. The initial treatment goal is to reduce how much food is consumed during binging. The patient is instructed about his or her condition and its likely consequences. They are taught that the disorder is serious, with potentially deadly complications.

Psychological therapy is required due to high rates of depression and suicide. The patient learns self-acceptance and becomes less concerned about his or her weight. All-or-non thinking is reversed. Group therapy helps supply strong social support. The bulimic person is thought that some amount of depression and self-doubt is normal. Antidepressants can be used, but they must accompany other therapies. Therapy for bulimia nervosa is long term due to high relapse potential. Approximately 50% of patients recover complexly. Others battle the disorder in different amounts throughout life. Therefore, the need for prevention of bulimia nervosa is essential.

FOCUS ON BULIMIA NERVOSA

Bulimia nervosa is an eating disorder that is also classified as a mental disorder. It is among the most fatal mental conditions of all because of related long-term health problems, and even suicide. Many patients with bulimia also have depression. Affected individuals often feel shame and guilt about their inability to control the compulsive behaviors, worsening any preexisting depression.

Test Your Knowledge

1. What is the difference between anorexia nervosa and bulimia nervosa, related to how affected individuals perceive their conditions?

2. What often triggers binging?
3. What are the final outcomes of bulimia nervosa?

Binge-Eating Disorder

Binge-eating disorder is less severe than bulimia nervosa, yet large amounts of food are still frequently consumed. While binging, food is consumed much more quickly than normal and eating continues until the individual feels uncomfortable. Other behaviors in the disorder include eating large amounts of food even when not feeling hungry, eating alone due to embarrassment about the condition, and experiencing distress, depression, and guilt after overeating. Food is consumed with no thought about biological needs. It recurs in "ritualistic" behaviors. Some affected individuals eat food continually over long periods of time while others have episodes of normal eating broken up by periods of binging.

Obesity and binge eating are not always related since many obese people do not binge-eat. Even so, binge-eating disorder is most prevalent in the severely obese, and in those with chronic restrictive dieting, though many binge-eaters are not obese. About 30%–50% of people in weight-control programs have been diagnosed with binge-eating disorder, though only 1%–2% of people in North America are affected. There are less severe forms of the disease in the general population that lack the criteria for a diagnosis of binge-eating disorder. Cases of the disorder are much more numerous than cases of anorexia nervosa or bulimia nervosa. The condition may be preceded by frequent dieting, starting in childhood or adolescence. At times when little food is eaten, the individual becomes extremely hungry and feels a need to eat compulsively, without control. About 40% of binge-eaters are males, and feel hungry more often than is normal. Nearly half of severe binge-eaters have clinical depression and isolate themselves.

Triggers of binge eating include stress, depression, and anxiety. Self-permission to eat "forbidden" foods may trigger a binge. Additional triggers include loneliness, anxiety, anger, alienation, rage, and frustration. Binge eating helps some people feel better or become numb to their amotions, often to avoid emotional pain and anxiety. Some stressed-out or frustrated people eat continually until they go to bed, in an attempt to forget about their jobs or other stressors. Some simply binge-eat only when emotional setbacks happen. Often, affected individuals have dysfunctional families that poorly cope with emotions, so turning to substance use or abuse, or binge eating, becomes an option.

Binge-eating disorder is often overcome by the individual, without professional help. If nutrition therapy is needed, it is similar to what is used for bulimia nervosa. Psychological therapy focuses on identifying emotional needs and expressing emotions. Communication issues must be assessed. The individual often requires help to recognize hidden emotions in situations that produce anxiety. They learn simple, yet appropriate phrases that help remind them to stop binging when the desire to do so is strong. Overeaters Anonymous and other self-help groups assist with recovery. Treatment tries to create environments of encouragement and accountability. Antidepressants sometimes help to reduce binge eating since depressive triggers are reduced.

Night Eating Syndrome

Some individuals only eat or purge large amounts of food at night. This is known as **night eating syndrome**. Most people with eating disorders are in this category. It is classified as an Unspecified Feeding or Eating Disorder (UFED) because this disorder does not meet the criteria for anorexia nervosa, bulimia nervosa, or binge-eating disorder. In night eating disorder, food is consumed in larger quantities late in the evening, or eating occurs after being awakened during the night in an attempt to fall asleep again. Night eating contributes to weight gain, so treatment should be obtained.

Female Athlete Triad

The **female athlete triad** is a combination of disordered eating, amenorrhea, and osteoporosis. It is often not recognized, but bone mineral density loss can be severe for female athletes. Early osteoporotic fractures can occur, and the lost bone mineral density may never return. The triad requires early recognition by family physicians, via assessing risk factors and offering specific screening questions. The natural return of menstruation may be achieved by a good diet and controlled frequency of exercise. To prevent loss of bone density, hormone replacement therapy may be needed. Treatment may require interactive efforts between athletic trainers, coaches, parents, physicians, and the athletes themselves. Possibly life-threatening illnesses can be prevented by increased education of everyone involved.

Disordered eating may involve food restriction, binging, and purging, to lose weight and remain thin. **Amenorrhea** related to athletic training and weight fluctuations is due to changes in the hypothalamus, which decrease estrogen levels. The amenorrhea may be primary or secondary. With primary amenorrhea there is no spontaneous uterine bleeding by the age of 14 and no development of secondary sexual characteristics, or no spontaneous uterine bleeding by age 16 with otherwise normal development. Secondary amenorrhea is the six-month lack of menstrual bleeding in a female with primary regular menses, or a 12-month lack with previous **oligomenorrhea**.

Premature osteoporosis increases risks for stress fractures along with severe hip or vertebral column fractures. Morbidity is high, and lost bone density may be permanent. Exact prevalence of the female athlete triad is generally unknown. Disordered eating occurs in 15%–62% of female college athletes. Amenorrhea occurs in 3.4%–66% which is much higher than the rates of 2%–5% in the general female population. Pathogenic weight-control behaviors may be due to frequent **weigh-ins**, disciplinary actions because of weight gain, increased pressure to always win in competitions, excessive control by coaches or parents, and social isolation because of obsessive focus on athletic activities. The female athlete triad is of highest occurrence in females that engage in figure skating, gymnastics, ballet, diving, swimming, and long-distance running. Prevention requires education for all parties involved. Coaches must never overemphasize weight control. For example, 75% of female college gymnasts use pathogenic behaviors for weight control after being told by coaches they are overweight.

Screening for the female athlete triad is best done during physical examinations prior to competitions. Screening can also be done during acute visits for fractures, disordered eating, weight changes, amenorrhea, arrhythmia, bradycardia, depression, and during visits for routine Pap smears. A history of amenorrhea is an easy way to detect the triad in early stages. The condition is not normal in female athletes and must be reported when it develops. Past eating behaviors should be discussed, since this is less threatening to the female athlete than focusing on any current eating disorders. Histories of menstruation, diet, and exercise should be taken, as follows:

- *Menstruation* – age at menarche, menstrual cycle frequency and duration, longest period without any menstruation, last menstrual period, signs of ovulation, any previous or current hormonal therapy
- *Diet* – diet in the last 24 hours, lists of any "forbidden" foods, highest and lowest weight since menarche, happiness with current weight, the patient's "ideal weight", binging or purging, and use of laxatives, diuretics, or diet pills
- *Exercise* – patterns and training intensity of exercise (hours per day, and days per week), additional exercise that is outside of required training, histories of previous fractures or overuse injuries

Common signs and symptoms of disordered eating include anorexia nervosa, bradycardia, cachexia, hypotension, hypothermia, lanugo, cold intolerance, dry hair and skin, hypercarotenemia, alopecia, pruritus, bulimia nervosa, abdominal pain, fatigue, chest pain, sore throat or esophagitis, swollen parotid glands, erosion of tooth enamel, constipation, knuckle scars or calluses, and bloodshot eyes.

FOCUS ON FEMALE ATHLETE TRIAD

Some female athletes that focus on being thinner eat too little or exercise too much, causing long-term damage to health, and even death. Abnormal eating habits or excessive exercise prevents the body from getting sufficient nutrition. Often, hormonal changes result, leading to irregular menses or amenorrhea. This disrupts bone-building processes, weakening the skeleton and increasing the likelihood of fractures. In severe cases, young female athletes have even developed early-onset osteoporosis.

Test Your Knowledge

1. In which individuals is binge-eating disorder most prevalent?
2. What are the three features of the female athlete triad?
3. In which types of athletes is the female athlete triad most common?

KEY TERMS

Alopecia

Amenorrhea

Anorexia nervosa

Binge-eating disorder

Bitot's spots

Bulimia nervosa

Corneal xerosis

Creatine kinase

Cretinism

Cystic fibrosis

Cytosol

Fad diets

Fatty liver

Female athlete triad

Floppy muscle tone

Goiter

Gruels

Hematocrit

Keratomalacia

Ketones

Ketosis

Lanugo hair

Leavening

Leukotrienes

Mitochondria

Night eating syndrome

Oligomenorrhea

Osteoporosis

Phytic acid

Prostaglandins

Protein-energy malnutrition

Protein-calorie malnutrition

Ulcerative colitis

Weigh-ins

CLINICAL CASE STUDIES

Clinical Case 1

A baby girl was born at 34 weeks of gestation. Her mother had pregnancy-induced hypertension. The infant was admitted to the neonatal intensive care unit (ICU) with respiratory distress and was given antibiotics and oxygen. About two weeks later, she was discharged and her parents were glad to take her home. Within a few more weeks, the parents brought the infant back to the hospital because of apnea and vomiting. She was found to have hypothermia, hypotonia, and delayed capillary refill time, plus low blood sugar. Dextrose was injected as a bolus and electrolyte imbalances were corrected. Antibiotics and inotropes helped her recover though she was lethargic. Carnitine screening resulted in a diagnosis of primary carnitine deficiency, and the infant was prescribed L-carnitine syrup to be given three times per day.

CRITICAL THINKING QUESTIONS

1. What is primary carnitine deficiency?
2. Are the symptoms of primary carnitine deficiency more or less severe than with secondary carnitine deficiency?
3. What should be done if a carnitine deficiency is familial?

Clinical Case 2

An 87-year-old man complained of itching and burning in his eyes, with generalized visual decline. Slit lamp examination revealed frothy, dry-appearing patches on the temporal bulbar conjunctiva of both eyes. There was a Bitot's spot in the patient's right eye. Vitamin A deficiency was suspected, and the patient was asked about his diet. He replied that he could not tolerate many vegetables because of their textures and flavors. The patient described eating a lot of tuna fish and rice pudding. A serum vitamin A level test revealed a significant deficiency. The patient was started on 100,000 international units of oral vitamin A supplements for three days, followed by 50,000 of these units daily for two weeks. His symptoms quickly resolved and his vision improved.

CRITICAL THINKING QUESTIONS

1. With vitamin A deficiency, what are the progressive eye abnormalities?
2. Which conditions related to impaired absorption, storage, or transport of vitamin A may cause keratomalacia?
3. Why are areas where rice is a major dietary component implicated in keratomalacia?

Clinical Case 3

A 20-year-old woman, previously diagnosed with anorexia nervosa, was admitted to a mental health center. She weighed only 84 pounds (which was about 50 pounds underweight for her height), and tests revealed that she had kidney, liver, and pancreatic damage. The patient remained in the facility for eight weeks and underwent significant psychiatric and physical treatments. It was found that her anorexia nervosa was based on feelings of "needing to get revenge" on her parents because of feeling emotionally distanced from them. At discharge, the patient had gained 23 pounds, and she agreed to return to the facility if her weight ever dropped below 100 pounds. She continued to undergo regular weight management regimens and utilized support groups for her condition to prevent any recurrence of her negative behaviors.

CRITICAL THINKING QUESTIONS

1. How is anorexia nervosa described?
2. What is a common underlying factor of anorexia nervosa?
3. What do anorexics fear, and how do they perceive themselves?

STUDY QUESTIONS

1. Which of the following disorders may be caused by protein-energy malnutrition?
   A. Scaly dermatitis
   B. Corneal xerosis
   C. Marasmus
   D. Keratomalacia

2. Which of the following nutrient types includes linoleic acid as one example?
   A. Folic acids
   B. Fatty acids
   C. Amino acids
   D. Ascorbic acids

3. Which of the following nutrient deficiencies may cause corneal xerosis?
   A. Fatty acid
   B. Essential amino acid
   C. Vitamin D
   D. Vitamin A

4. Carnitine synthesis relies on sufficient amounts of which of the following vitamins?
   A. Vitamin C
   B. Vitamin B12
   C. Vitamin B6
   D. Vitamin A

5. Treatment with L-carnitine is able to correct disorders of which of the following organs?
   A. Brain
   B. Heart
   C. Prostate
   D. Bladder

6. Which of the following is NOT a symptom of primary carnitine deficiency?
   A. Decreased muscle tone
   B. Delayed motor development
   C. Hyperglycemia
   D. Irritability

7. Xerophthalmia may cause which of the following?
   A. Irreversible blindness
   B. Celiac disease
   C. Ulcerative colitis
   D. Cystic fibrosis

8. Microcytic and hypochromic red blood cells occur because of which of the following nutritional deficiencies?
   A. Iodine
   B. Vitamin A
   C. Vitamin D
   D. Iron

9. Which of the following is NOT a major component of a low-fat diet?
   A. Grains
   B. Whole milk
   C. Fruits
   D. Vegetables

10. Which of the following diets often emphasize one food or food group?
    A. Fat
    B. Carbohydrate
    C. Protein
    D. Novelty

11. People who do not eat *any type* of animal products are called:
    A. Lacto-ovo-vegetarians
    B. Fad dieters
    C. Vegans
    D. Lacto-vegetarians

12. Which of the following does NOT trigger binge eating?
    A. Depression
    B. Anxiety
    C. Happiness
    D. Stress

13. Bulimics often consume foods that contain high levels of which of the following?
    A. Carbohydrates
    B. Fats
    C. Vitamins
    D. Proteins

14. Which of the following disorders involves extreme weight loss, distortions of body image, and an irrational fear of weight gain?
    A. Binge eating
    B. Night eating
    C. Anorexia
    D. Bulimia

15. Premature osteoporosis may be seen in which of the following?
    A. Binge eating
    B. Anorexia
    C. Bulimia
    D. Female athlete triad

FURTHER READING

1. Agras, W.S., and Robinson, A. (2017). *The Oxford Handbook of Eating Disorders (Library of Psychology)*, 2nd Edition. Oxford University Press.
2. Anderson, L.K., Murray, S.B., and Kaye, W.H. (2017). *Clinical Handbook of Complex and Atypical Eating Disorders*. Oxford University Press.
3. Fries, J., and Sullivan, V. (2021). *Eating Disorders in Special Populations: Medical, Nutritional, and Psychological Treatments*. CRC Press / Taylor & Francis Group.
4. Gaudiani, J.L. (2018). *Sick Enough – A Guide to the Medical Complications of Eating Disorders*. Routledge.
5. Hickson, M., and Smith, S. (2018). *Advanced Nutrition and Dietetics in Nutrition Support (BDA)*. Wiley Blackwell.
6. Holmes, K. (2021). *Freed & Fierce – The 7 Untapped Essentials for Life-Long Eating Disorder Recovery*. Bowker Identifier Services.
7. Kalonji Ilunga, I. (2022). *Undernutrition and Nutritional Care in Hospitalized Adults – Need for the Creation of Food and Clinical Nutrition Services in Hospitals*. Our Knowledge Publishing.
8. Kerr, A., and Kerr, R. (2014). *The Bulimia Help Method – A Revolutionary New Approach That Works*. CreateSpace Independent Publishing Platform.
9. Leathers, H.D., and Foster, P. (2017). *The World Food Problem: Toward Understanding and Ending Undernutrition in the Developing World*, 5th Edition. Lynne Rienner Publishers, Inc.
10. Livingston, G. (2015). *Never Binge Again: How Thousands of People Have Stopped Overeating and Binge Eating – and Stuck To the Food Plan*. Psy Tech Inc.

11. Mehler, P.S., and Andersen, A.E. (2022). *Eating Disorders: A Comprehensive Guide to Medical Care and Complications*, 4th Edition. Johns Hopkins University Press.
12. Ramachandran, N. (2014). *Persisting Undernutrition in India – Causes, Consequences, and Possible Solutions*. Springer.
13. Selby, C.L.B. (2018). *The Psychology of Eating Disorders*. Springer.
14. Skolnik, R. (2019). *Global Health 101 (Essential Public Health)*, 4th Edition. Jones & Bartlett Learning.
15. Stein, N. (2014). *Public Health Nutrition: Principles and Practice in Community and Global Health*. Jones & Bartlett Learning.
16. Walraven, G. (2013). *Health and Poverty: Global Health Problems and Solutions*. Routledge.
17. Willis, A. (2019). *Nutritional Deficiencies – Diagnosis and Treatment*. Foster Academics.
18. World Bank, The. (2023). *Undernutrition in the Philippines – Scale, Scope, and Opportunities for Nutrition Policy and Programming*. The World Bank.

8 Obesity and Metabolic Syndrome

OUTLINE

LEARNING OBJECTIVES

After study of the chapter, readers should be able to:

1. Describe the causes of obesity and hyperplastic obesity.
2. Explain body mass index and a simple formula for its calculation.
3. Discuss the classifications of being overweight or obese.
4. Identify the risk factors for obesity.
5. Describe weight cycling.
6. Explain the prevention of obesity.
7. Discuss the outcome of bariatric surgery.
8. Describe the Mediterranean diet.
9. Compare the differences between the vegan diet and the paleo diet.
10. Explain metabolic syndrome and its relationship to chronic diseases.

OVERVIEW

Obesity, because of a poor diet and insufficient exercise, puts people at serious risks for many different health problems. Being overweight or obese constitutes one of the leading preventable causes of death. Complications of these conditions include coronary heart disease, type 2 diabetes mellitus, asthma, high cholesterol, osteoarthritis, hypertension, sleep apnea, certain cancers, and metabolic syndrome. An estimated one of every four adults has metabolic syndrome, and many of them are unaware of their condition. Obesity and lack of exercise are key components of metabolic syndrome. The syndrome is based on excessive abdominal obesity, high triglyceride levels, low HDL cholesterol, hypertension, and high fasting blood glucose. Most people with metabolic syndrome also have insulin resistance and diabetes.

DEFINITION AND MEASUREMENTS

Obesity is an abnormal increase in *adipocytes*, mainly within the viscera and subcutaneous tissues of the body. It is either exogenous or endogenous. **Hyperplastic obesity** is caused by an increase in the *number* of fat cells in the adipose tissue mass. **Hypertrophic obesity** results from an increase in the *size* of fat cells in the adipose tissue mass. The term *overweight* is determined by a *body mass index* (BMI) of 25–29.9 kg/m^2, and *obesity* is determined by a BMI of 30 kg/m^2 or higher. Body fat distribution can be assessed by waist-to-hip ratios. A ratio of greater than 1.0 for men and greater than 0.8 for women signals an increased risk of obesity. The Guideline for the Management of Overweight and Obesity in Adults gives recommendations on evaluation and management, based on scientific evidence. The use of BMI is the recommended approach for categorizing weight relative to height for adults (see Figure 8.1). The simple formula is as follows: weight in kilograms (kg) divided by height in square meters. The formula can also be calculated in pounds in inches, with the weight in pounds divided by the height in square inches, multiplied by 703. Table 8.1 summarizes classification of overweight and obesity by using BMI.

People classified as *overweight* may or may not appear to be excessively fat. Some adults are overweight because of

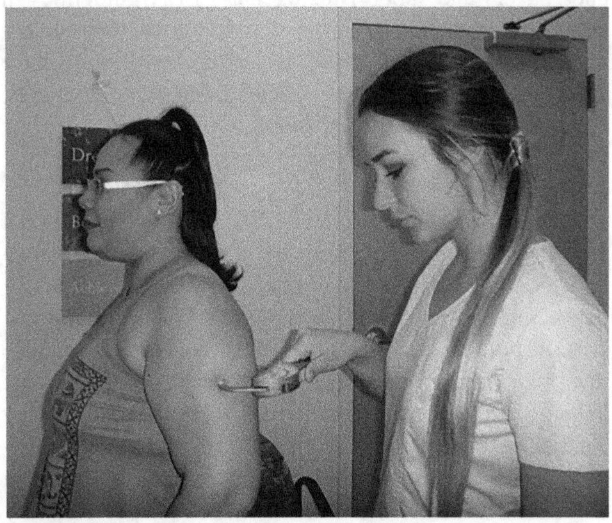

FIGURE 8.1 Measuring BMI.

DOI: 10.1201/b22969-11

TABLE 8.1
Classification of Overweight and Obesity by BMI

Classification	Obesity Class	BMI in kg/m²	BMI in lb/inches²
Underweight	None	Less than 18.5	Less than 1605.7
Normal	None	18.5–24.9	1605.7–2161.2
Overweight	None	25.0–29.9	2169.9–2595.2
Obesity	I	30.0–34.9	2603.8–3029.1
Obesity	II	35.0–39.9	3037.8–3463.1
Extreme Obesity	III	40 or higher	3471.8

increased muscle mass, which is easily observed clinically. Generally, risks for developing fat-related health problems continually increase as BMI exceeds 25. The use of waist circumference measurements is recommended in order to have a more accurate understanding of each patient's condition. For people in the overweight and *class I obese* categories, with a high-risk waist circumference, there must be discussion of lifestyle changes that will improve health and result in weight loss. Some patients with a BMI of 27.0–29.9 develop significant metabolic complications, which fortunately improve with weight loss. These patients are candidates for pharmacotherapy and other more aggressive treatments. Asians are at risk for typical metabolic complications of obesity at lower BMI and wait circumferences than Caucasians, Hispanics, African Americans, and Pacific Islanders. The guideline for at-risk BMI in Asians is 23–24.

Comorbidity is much higher incidence with a BMI higher than 30. The three classifications of obesity require different treatments. The US Food and Drug Administration (FDA) recommends that pharmacotherapy be used as adjunct treatment for all obesity classifications, even with no medical complications. Third-party insurance payers and supervising agencies FDA guidelines in determining patients who are eligible for treatment benefits. When a BMI is over 40 after medical treatments have failed, *bariatric surgery* is indicated. For class II obesity, bariatric surgery may be considered if medical treatments fail, and if there are severe, possibly life-threatening complications.

Previous waist circumference cutoff points of more than 40 inches for men and more than 35 inches for women indicate increased metabolic risks. However, relationships between waist circumference and disease risks are progressive and have no obvious cutoff points. Waist circumference must be measured in overweight and class I obese adults. When it exceeds the cutoff points, there must be further evaluation to detect other risk factors for cardiovascular disease. Class II or class III obese adults have a high enough risk so that waist circumference is not additionally important. The cutoff points for each overweight or obese classification apply to most people of European and African descent, but not to Asians.

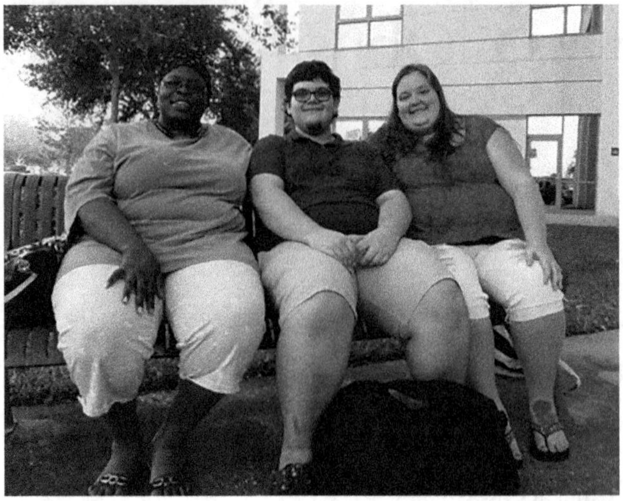

FIGURE 8.2 Obesity in young adults.

OBESITY AND TOTAL MORTALITY

Obesity causes increased *morbidity*, **mortality**, and a poorer quality of life. According to the World Health Organization (WHO), there are 2.8 million deaths every year from being overweight or obese. This puts these conditions in 5th place among the top ten leading causes of death globally. Obesity is associated with premature death. Men who are obese at age 20 are twice as likely to die prematurely compared to non-obese men at the same age. At all ages, obesity doubles the risk of early death up until 60 years of age. For each BMI unit that is above normal, the risk of early death is increased by 10% throughout life. Obese men die about eight years earlier than men that are not obese. About 60% of men and 51% of women are overweight or obese in the United States, though more women than men are actually obese. Large differences exist in prevalence of obesity by age, race, and socioeconomic level (see Figure 8.2).

In a study of women aged 30–55 who did not have cardiovascular disease or cancer at the start of the 16-year-long follow-up, obese women had a 90% higher total mortality. This was over four times higher for cardiovascular mortality, and more than twice as high for cancer mortality. About 53% of deaths among women with a BMI over 30 were because of their obesity. Gaining 10 kg or more of weight after age 18 and a BMI of more than 22 at age 18 predicted death from cardiovascular disease in middle adulthood. The lowest mortality rate was in thin women that maintained their weight since the age of 18. Obesity leads to most chronic diseases, via direct effects upon metabolic dysregulation.

RISK FACTORS FOR OBESITY

Obesity is a complicated condition. It is influenced by how we work, travel, and are affected by the presence of much more significant technology in daily life. Put most simply, obesity is caused by consuming more calories than the body can burn. Lifestyle changes that impact obesity include longer work hours, longer drive times, fewer meals prepared at home, eating in restaurants more often (due to larger portions of foods that are dense in calories), portion sizes of packaged foods, more time spent in sedentary activities (often with electronic technology), less physical types of labor, and less times spent in exercise-related activities.

Junk foods are more available today than ever before, sold in nearly every type of retail store and online. Television and other media regularly market foods products and restaurants. There are also plenty of shows related to desired types of foods that often are overloaded with calories, fats, and sugar. Many communities do not have safe routes for exercise, including walking, bicycling, or play areas for children. Many schools today have limited offering access to gymnasiums and recess periods. Fresh, healthy foods are often hard to obtain in poorer neighborhoods.

Stress also is a major risk factor for obesity. Overstressed people often make poor food choices and overeat. Hormone such as cortisol triggers release of triglycerides (fatty acids) from storage in the body, moving them to the deep abdominal fat cells. Cortisol additionally increases the appetite. Genetics result in many people being predisposed to being overweight or obese. This often becomes apparent only when lifestyle or environment changes significantly. Medical conditions that are linked to being overweight or obese include the following:

- Cushing's syndrome (from excessive cortisol production by the adrenal glands)
- Eating disorders (binge-eating and night eating disorders, and bulimia nervosa)
- Growth hormone deficiency
- Hypogonadism (low testosterone)
- Hypothyroidism (underactive thyroid)
- Insulinoma of the pancreas
- Polycystic ovarian syndrome

Sometimes, obesity can also cause another medical condition. Medications that can encourage weight gain, often by increasing appetite, include the following:

- Diabetes drugs – insulin, sulfonylureas, and thiazolidinediones
- Hypertension drugs – loop and thiazide diuretics, beta blockers, calcium channel blockers, and alpha-adrenergic blockers
- Antihistamines (especially cyproheptadine)
- Steroids (corticosteroids and birth control pills)
- Herbal remedies (chamomile, blessed thistle, gentian, dandelion root, chen pi, ginger, and custard apple)
- Antipsychotics (olanzapine and zotepine)
- Antidepressants (amitriptyline, mirtazapine, paroxetine, escitalopram, sertraline, duloxetine, and citalopram)
- Anticonvulsants (gabapentin, pregabalin, valproic acid, and vigabatrin)

FOCUS ON OBESITY AND ITS RISK FACTORS

The epidemic of obesity is tragic since it is highly preventable. The largest modifiable risk factors are diet, exercise, sleep, and stress.

Test Your Knowledge

1. What are the definitions of being overweight or being obese, according to BMI?
2. How is obesity implicated in global death rates?
3. Which foods are most highly implicated in becoming overweight or obese?

PREVENTION OF OBESITY

There are plenty of ways to prevent obesity for people of all ages. Obesity prevention begins early in life, and it is very important to help young people maintain a healthy weight. Breastfeeding compared to bottle feeding is associated with a reduced risk of childhood obesity. Once an infant becomes a toddler, from ages one to three, every inch of height should roughly equate to 40 calories of food intake. Older children should be encouraged to learn what correct food portion sizes look like. Children should be encouraged to try many different fruits, vegetables, and proteins as early as possible. As they grow, they may then be more likely to include these healthy foods into their diets. Eating habits should be improved on a family level, which allows children to experience healthy eating early in life. It makes the situation easier for them to continue to follow good eating habits throughout life. Children should be encouraged only to eat when they feel hungry, and to chew more slowly so that digestion will be improved. Unhealthy foods in the household must be limited. The refrigerator, freezer, and pantry should be stocked with healthy foods, and less-healthy snacks should only be considered as "rare" treats.

The role of good exercise can never be overstressed. Children and teenagers should have at least 60 minutes of physical activity every day, including games, sports, gym classes, and outdoor chores that involve a lot of movement, including gardening, raking leaves, pulling weeds, digging holes, or installing plants into the ground. Other good activities include painting the house, washing the car, power washing, vacuuming, cutting or trimming trees, mulching, cleaning out the garage, and removing or installing fences. Time spent watching television, using computers, or playing games on a cell phone must be minimized, with only a certain amount of time allowed for these activities every day. Other important considerations include getting adequate, high-quality sleep (using sleep schedules, bedtime rituals, and comfortable bedding), and keeping track of foods that are being consumed outside of the home, such as in school.

For adults, correct intake of healthy dietary fats such as polyunsaturated fats actually improves cholesterol levels and reduces obesity risks. Consumption of processed or ultra-processed foods is linked to a higher rate of obesity. Many processed foods are high in fat, salt, and sugar – encouraging overeating. Five to nine servings of fruits and vegetables is recommended per day. This helps keep dietary calories lower and reduces risks of overeating. Dietary fiber is also extremely important. Just taking fiber supplements on a regular basis can provide weight loss of up to 5% of overall body weight over 12 weeks.

It is important to engage in physical activities with family members as well as friends. Cooking or walking together help encourage a system of social support for a healthy lifestyle. Regular physical activity is vital for maintaining of losing weight and improving health. Adults should get 150 minutes of moderate aerobic activity or 75 minutes of vigorous aerobic activity per week. Weight training is equally important. Weight training involving all major muscles should occur at least twice per week.

Another important component in preventing obesity is to reduce daily stress, since stress can trigger brain responses that change eating patterns, leading to cravings for high-calorie foods. Many people learn that stress reduction helps them to follow healthy eating and exercise habits more easily. It is important to avoid *emotional eating*, which can be done by learning mindfulness-based stress and management and information about nutrition. Lower stress levels prevent emotional eating and lead to reduced abdominal fat over time. Keeping a food journal may be helpful in identifying excessive eating that occurred after anything stressful happened.

When shopping for foods, it is important to have a plan. Creating a food budget and shopping list helps avoid buying unhealthy foods that may seem tempting. Making multiple meals for the week helps to have healthy foods that are ready to eat. There are some basic healthy diets that have been widely studied and proven to be successful options for most people. They include the following:

- *The low-carbohydrate, whole-food diet* – high in vegetables, meat, fish, eggs, fruits, nuts, and fats; low in starches, sugars, and processed foods; perfect for losing weight, optimizing health, and lowering risks for disease; its flexibility allows people to fine-tune carbohydrate intake based on individual goals; foods that are highly encouraged include avocados, butter, dark chocolate, fat-dense meat and seafood, non-starchy vegetables
- *The Mediterranean diet* – emphasizes foods that were commonly consumed around the Mediterranean region in the 20th century and earlier, including many vegetables, fruits, fish, poultry, whole grains, legumes, dairy products, and extra virgin olive oil; it is especially effective in preventing heart disease; the ideal foods include tomatoes, broccoli, kale, spinach, onions, cauliflower, carrots, Brussels sprouts, cucumbers, sweet potatoes, turnips, apples, bananas, oranges, pears, strawberries, grapes, dates, figs, melons, peaches, almonds, walnuts, macadamia nuts, hazelnuts, cashews, sunflower seeds, pumpkin seeds, almond butter, peanut butter, beans, peas, lentils, peanuts, chickpeas, oats, brown rice, rye, barley, corn, buckwheat, whole wheat bread and pasta, salmon, sardines, trout, tuna, mackerel, shrimp, oysters, clams, crab, mussels, chicken, duck, turkey, eggs cheese, yogurt, milk, garlic, basil, mint, rosemary, sage, nutmeg, cinnamon, pepper, olives, avocados, and avocado oil
- *The paleo diet* – focuses on unprocessed foods that resemble food sources that were available to the paleolithic ancestors of humans. It is very effective for weight loss and general health improvement and has become the world's most popular diet. Foods that are encouraged for regular consumption include fruits, vegetables, nuts, seeds, lean meats (especially grass-fed animals), fish such as salmon, mackerel, and albacore tuna, and oils from fruits or nuts such as olive oil or walnut oil
- *The vegan diet* – based exclusively on plant foods, with all animal products eliminated; it results in weight loss, improved heart health, and better blood glucose control; there are several subtypes of the vegan diet, as follows:

    - *Whole-food vegan diet* – whole plant foods (fruits, vegetables, whole grains, legumes, nuts, and seeds)
    - *Raw food vegan diet* – raw fruits, vegetables, nuts, seeds, or plant foods cooked at temperatures below 118°F (48°C)
    - *80/10/10 diet* – raw foods that limit fat-rich plants such as nuts and avocados, mainly relying on raw fruits and soft greens (it is also called the low-fat, raw food vegan diet or the fruitarian diet)
    - *Starch solution* – low-fat, high-carb vegan diet, similar to the 80/10/10 diet, but focusing on cooked starches like potatoes, rice, and corn instead of fruit
    - *Raw till 4* – low-fat vegan diet in which raw foods are consumed until 4:00pm, and cooked plant-based meals for dinner may or may not be chosen
    - *Thrive diet* – a raw food vegan diet; plant-based whole foods are consumed raw or only minimally cooked at low temperatures

- *The gluten-free diet* – focuses on foods that are naturally **gluten-free**, though gluten-free "junk food" is still as unhealthy as junk food that contains glutens; it is essential for people that are intolerant to gluten

Preventing obesity helps to prevent many different chronic health conditions. A lot of the conditions in this list become more difficult to treat over time:

- Hypertension – since it increases risks for heart attack, stroke, heart failure, and kidney disease
- Diabetes mellitus (type 2) – since it eventually leads to circulatory, nervous, and immune system disorders
- Heart disease – signified by shortness of breath, problems exercising, fatigue, and swelling of the feet, ankles, and abdomen
- High triglycerides – contributing to arteriosclerosis and pancreatitis
- Low "good" (HDL) cholesterol – increasing risks for death from cardiovascular causes
- Sleep apnea – since it can lead to hypertension and heart disease
- Stroke – an initial stroke increases the likelihood of additional strokes
- Gallbladder disease – since it can cause the gallbladder to become scarred and stiff
- Sexual health problems – the complications of obesity often contribute to erectile dysfunction in men and poor sexual function in women
- Nonalcoholic fatty liver disease – can progress to nonalcoholic steatohepatitis (NASH), which involves liver inflammation that can worsen significantly
- Osteoarthritis – can cause chronic pain because of degeneration of joints
- Mental health conditions – excessive weight results in a 55% higher risk of depression

FOCUS ON THE GLYCEMIC INDEX

The **glycemic index** (GI) is a scale that is used to measure how quickly a food item increases blood glucose. Focusing on low-GI foods helps regulate blood glucose levels, which helps with weight management. Foods to avoid include corn chips, pretzels, soda, sweet tea, sports drinks, cheeseburgers, fried chicken, pizza, doughnuts, white bread, cereals that are not whole grain, mashed potatoes, and French fries.

WEIGHT CYCLING

Weight cycling is commonly referred to as *yo-yo dieting*. It involves losing and then regaining weight multiple times. In the United States, between 10% and 40% of adult females have a history of weight cycling. Individuals are able to successfully lose weight quickly, but then regain it. Over time, these weight changes affect health, body fat distribution, body composition, and the expenditure of energy. Weight cycling is linked to higher risks for developing metabolic syndrome and coronary heart disease. All causes of mortality are increased with weight cycling, and even when a person's BMI is in a healthy range, there is reduced quality of life. People who are obese but have extreme weight fluctuations have an increased taste preference for fat and sugar, making them likely to gain more weight in the future.

OBESITY THERAPY

The treatment of obesity is similar to treatment for other chronic conditions, requiring long-term changes in lifestyle. Diets should not be done temporarily, stopping once desired weight is lost. When diets are short-term, most people regain the lost weight, returning to being obese. The emphasis should be on healthy and active lifestyles, with lifelong dietary modifications. Weight loss must be slow and steady in order to promote lasting weight control. A goal of one to two pounds of weight loss per week is suggested. Weight maintenance occurs over a few months, with about 10% of body weight being lost. Then, there is an evaluation of a need for additional dieting before more weight loss should begin. Patients are encouraged to participate in normal activities, and the diet is adaptable to individual habits and tastes.

Dietary intake will meet nutrient needs, but not energy needs. A fortified ready-to-eat breakfast cereal is recommended, or a balanced multivitamin/mineral supplement is recommended, especially when less than 1,600 kcal are consumed per day. MyPlate.gov is used as a pattern for food choices. Behavior modification focuses on maintaining a lifelong healthy lifestyle and weight. Reasonable changes are encouraged since these are the ones that can best be maintained. Social support is important. A plan is made for any relapses, so that the patient does not quit after any setbacks. Changes that control problem eating behaviors are promoted. Existing health problems must be screened for. Screening is also required for men over 40 and women over 50 that plan to have substantial increases in physical activity, or those who plan to lose weight quickly. Regular physical activity, adequate sleep, and stress reduction are essential. Psychological weight issues such as depression or marital problems must be assessed and managed.

Surgical approaches to weight loss for obese patients are regularly successful in maintaining weight control. Bariatric surgery such as gastric bypass is performed when diet and exercise have not been effective, or when an individual has developed serious weight-related health problems. It is an option if the patient has a BMI of 40 or more, which indicates extreme obesity. It can also be done if the BMI is 35 to 39.9 (obesity) and there is concurrent type 2 diabetes, hypertension, or severe sleep apnea. Not every severely overweight person qualifies for bariatric surgery, and there is usually an extensive screening process. Patients must be willing to make permanent changes that will potentially lead to a healthier lifestyle. These may include long-term follow-up with nutrition monitoring, lifestyle and behavioral monitoring, and management of other medication conditions.

FOCUS ON BARIATRIC SURGERY

Bariatric surgery often improves hypertension, sleep apnea, joint pain, type 2 diabetes, fertility, and even depression. The surgery can even cure type 2 diabetes that is of recent onset. However, after bariatric surgery, there will be dietary restrictions. Recovering patients must eat more healthy than they did before, consume proteins first, follow their blood glucose tables, drink water, avoid snacking, and only consume small portions.

Test Your Knowledge

1. What are approved weight loss goals when dieting is used?
2. Which patients are candidates for bariatric surgery?

METABOLIC SYNDROME

Metabolic syndrome affects about 50 million adults in the United States alone. It is characterized by factors that increase risks for type 2 diabetes mellitus and cardiovascular disease. These include obesity (especially abdominal obesity), insulin resistance or glucose intolerance, which results in high blood glucose, high blood triglycerides and low-density lipoprotein (LDL) cholesterol, low HDL cholesterol, hypertension, increased *C-reactive protein* (CRP), and increased concentrations of oxidized LDL cholesterol. Metabolic syndrome is also related to physical inactivity, aging, and genetic predisposition. There are no established criteria for its diagnosis. According to the American Heart Association as well as the National Heart, Lung, and Blood Institute, three or more of the following criteria must be present for diagnosis:

- Waist circumference greater than 40 inches for men and 35 inches for women
- Fasting triglyceride levels above 150 mg/dL
- Blood HDL cholesterol below 40 mg/dL for men and below 50 mg/dL for women
- Elevated BP above 130/85 mm Hg
- Fasting blood glucose above 100 mg/dL

To decrease the health risks that are related to metabolic syndrome, lifestyle modifications focus on decreased dietary fat intake, increased physical activity, and regular, step-by-step weight loss.

People diagnosed with metabolic syndrome need to be completely aware that their health condition is serious. This knowledge may powerfully result in them making serious lifestyle changes. There are no quick results. The patient must change eating, exercise, and overall health habits for the rest of the lifespan. Slow and steady weight loss is essential, avoiding "fast" or "crash" diets, liquid diets, **fad diets**, and anything unsupervised such as fasting. There may be a need for regular monitoring and treatment for conditions that can accompany metabolic syndrome, including **polycystic ovarian syndrome**, gallstones, asthma, sleep disturbances, and fatty liver disease.

FOCUS ON METABOLIC SYNDROME

Metabolic syndrome is actually a cluster of conditions that increase risks for heart disease, stroke, and type 2 diabetes. The American Heart Association has estimated that metabolic syndrome will soon become the main risk factor for cardiovascular disease (instead of cigarette smoking).

Test Your Knowledge

1. What are the characteristic factors of metabolic syndrome?
2. Which criteria are required to diagnose metabolic syndrome?
3. Once diagnosed with metabolic syndrome, what essential changes must the patient make?

KEY TERMS

Comorbidity
Fad diets
Gluten-free
Hyperplastic obesity
Hypertrophic obesity
Mortality
Polycystic ovarian syndrome
Weight cycling

CLINICAL CASE STUDIES

Clinical Case Study 1

A 19-year-old man is evaluated because of his weight. Even though he has reached 5 feet 10 inches in height, his weight of 370 pounds classifies him as obese. He has completed his education in a home-schooled setting due to severe arthritis in his knees, obstructive sleep apnea causing extreme fatigue, and type 2 diabetes that requires him to inject insulin several times per day. Over time, the young man, his parents, and several physicians decide that gastric bypass surgery is needed. The surgery takes place, and immediately, the patient's insulin requirements decrease, along with his appetite. At six months of follow-up, the patient has lost 85 pounds and no longer needs insulin. His knee pain has been greatly reduced, and his sleep apnea is improving. By one year of follow-up, he no longer needs a continuous positive airway pressure (CPAP) machine. The patient continues to be monitored for long-term effects of the surgery and any potential complications.

CRITICAL THINKING QUESTIONS

1. What obesity classification is this patient classified as?
2. What can gastric bypass surgery improve or resolve?
3. How may gastric bypass affect insulin secretion and sensitivity?

Clinical Case Study 2

A 53-year-old obese woman has had type 2 diabetes mellitus for nine years. She complains of fatigue, difficulty losing weight, and depression. Since starting to take insulin, her weight has actually increased. Due to symptoms of hypoglycemia and severe sweating, she has not followed any specific diet and often eats extra snacks to prevent hypoglycemic attacks. Though exercise has been repeatedly suggested by her physicians, she complains that knee and ankle pain makes it too difficult to engage in. The patient receives education about the need to decrease her insulin doses along with her food intake to prevent hypoglycemia. She agreed to follow a restricted-calorie diet and slowly decrease her insulin. After three months, her depression was improving, she had lost seven pounds, but admitted to still sometimes snacking at night. Over two more months, with continual support, the patient has lost 21 pounds, has no depression, and feels much more energetic. She voluntarily begins a physician-moderated exercise program.

CRITICAL THINKING QUESTIONS

1. In relation to obesity, what does type 2 diabetes mellitus eventually lead to?
2. How should dieting be done as part of the treatment of obesity?
3. For women, how is obesity linked to mortality?

Clinical Case Study 3

A 39-year-old man presented with hypertension. He described his life as mostly centering around long, irregular work hours. He often went to fast food restaurants on his way home from work, smoked 15–20 cigarettes per day, and drank alcohol excessively a few times per week. The patient was obese (especially in the abdominal region), with high triglycerides, LDL cholesterol, and total cholesterol, as well as low HDL cholesterol. He was diagnosed with metabolic syndrome, and enrolled into an active, regular exercise program along with being started on the Mediterranean diet.

CRITICAL THINKING QUESTIONS

1. Which risk factors of metabolic syndrome increase risks for type 2 diabetes mellitus and cardiovascular disease?
2. What criteria must be present for diagnosis of metabolic syndrome?
3. What are the basics of the Mediterranean diet?

STUDY QUESTIONS

1. Which of the following terms describes an increase in the size of fat cells?
   A. Hyperplasia
   B. Hyperplastic
   C. Hypertrophic
   D. Hypoplastic

2. Which of the following waist-to-hip ratios for men signals an increased risk for obesity?
   A. Greater than one
   B. Greater than three
   C. Greater than five
   D. Less than one

3. Which of the following body mass indices indicates obesity class III?
   A. 18
   B. 30
   C. 35
   D. 40

4. What is the percentage of obesity for men in the United States?
   A. 10%
   B. 30%
   C. 50%
   D. 60%

5. Which of the following medical conditions is NOT linked to being overweight or obese?
   A. Hyperthyroidism
   B. Polycystic ovarian syndrome
   C. Hypogonadism
   D. Cushing's syndrome

6. All of the following medications may increase weight gain, EXCEPT:
   A. Steroids
   B. Antihypertensive drugs
   C. Antihistamines
   D. Antibiotics

7. Which of the following diets focuses on unprocessed foods?
   A. The vegan diet
   B. The paleo diet
   C. The gluten-free diet
   D. The low-protein diet

8. Which of the following diets is based exclusively on plant foods?
   A. The vegan diet
   B. The paleo diet
   C. The Mediterranean diet
   D. The gluten-free diet

9. All of the following chronic disorders may be prevented by weight loss, EXCEPT:
   A. Sleep apnea
   B. Stroke
   C. Diabetes insipidus
   D. Hypertension

10. Which of the following diets is referred to as "yo-yo dieting"?
    A. The paleo diet
    B. Weight cycling
    C. The vegan diet
    D. The thrive diet

11. Which of the following is a raw food vegan diet, in which plant-based whole foods are consumed raw or only minimally cooked at low temperatures?
    A. The thrive diet
    B. The Mediterranean diet
    C. The paleo diet
    D. The vegan diet

12. Which of the following is NOT a criterion for the diagnosis of metabolic syndrome?
    A. Hypertension
    B. Fasting blood glucose above 100 mg / dL
    C. Hyperthyroidism
    D. Fasting triglyceride levels above 150 mg / dL

13. How many adults in the United States are affected by metabolic syndrome?
    A. 5 million
    B. 24 million
    C. 50 million
    D. 110 million

14. Which of the following is linked to weight cycling?
    A. Pancreatitis
    B. Metabolic syndrome
    C. Hyperthyroidism
    D. Hypogonadism

15. Which of the following conditions may be caused by high triglycerides?
    A. Pancreatitis
    B. Hyperthyroidism
    C. Ovarian cancer
    D. Stomach cancer

FURTHER READING

1. Ahima, R.S. (2016). *Metabolic Syndrome: A Comprehensive Textbook*. Springer Reference.
2. Ali, N. (2015). *Living with Metabolic Syndrome – The Complete Guide to Risk Factors, Prevention, Symptoms, and Treatment Options*. Hatherleigh Press.
3. Aronne, L.J., and Kumar, R.B. (2019). *Obesity Management: A Clinical Casebook*. Springer.
4. Barnard, S.J. (2022). *The Metabolic Approach to Obesity 4.0 – Unlocking the Secrets of Weight Loss integrating Deep Nutrition, the Ketogenic Diet, Nontoxic Bio-Individualized Therapies, and Intermittent Fasting*. Barnard.
5. Beck-Nielsen, H. (2014). *The Metabolic Syndrome – Pharmacology and Clinical Aspects*. Springer.
6. Bray, G.A. (2014). *Contemporary Diagnosis and Management of Obesity and the Metabolic Syndrome*, 4th Edition. Handbooks in Health Care Company.
7. Bray, G.A., and Ryan, D.H. (2014). *Overweight and the Metabolic Syndrome – From Bench to Bedside*. Springer / Louisiana State University Pennington Biomedical Research Center.
8. Campbell, T. C. (2022). *Obesity and Metabolic Syndrome – Impact on Health Prevention and Treatment: Of Complicated Obesity, Weight Gain Patients after Successful Treatment (The Issue of Fat Diet Therapy)*. Campbell.
9. Chubenko, E.A. (2021). *Obesity and Metabolic Syndrome: The Role of Hyperleptinemia in the Development of Abdominal Obesity, Insulin Resistance, and Arterial Hypertension (and Approaches to Therapy)*. Our Knowledge Publishing.
10. Genazzani, A.R., Ibanex, L., Milewicz, A., Shah, D. (2021). *Impact of Polycystic Ovary, Metabolic Syndrome and Obesity on Women's Health – Volume 8: Frontiers in Gynecological Endocrinology*. Springer.
11. Jockers, D. (2020). *Keto Metabolic Breakthrough – A Radical Approach to Reversing Metabolic Dysfunction, Optimizing Nutrient Timing, and Balancing Hormones for Success on a Low-Carb Diet*. Victory Belt Publishing.
12. Kiess, W., Wabitsch, M., Maffeis, C., and Sharma, A.M. (2015). *Metabolic Syndrome and Obesity in Childhood and Adolescence* (Pediatric and Adolescent Medicine, Volume 19). S. Karger.
13. Kushner, R., Bessesen, D.H., and Gilden, A.H. (2020). *Primary Care – Evaluation and Management of Obesity*. Wolters Kluwer.
14. Lenzi, A., Migliaccio, S., and Donini, L.M. (2015). *Multidisciplinary Approach to Obesity – From Assessment to Treatment*. Springer.
15. Lipshultz, S.E., Messiah, S.E., and Miller, T.W. (2012). *Pediatric Metabolic Syndrome – Comprehensive Clinical Review and Related Health Issues*. Springer.

16. Migan, W. (2014). *Fatty Liver Disease – The Ultimate Guide for Understanding the Fatty Liver Diet and What You Need to Know*. Migan.
17. Mittal, S. (2014). *The Metabolic Syndrome in Clinical Practice*. Springer.
18. Noble, L.D.M., and James, R.H. (2020). *The Metabolic Syndrome Diet*. Noble and James.
19. Rippe, J.M., and Foreyt, J.P. (2021). *Obesity Prevention and Treatment – A Practical Guide (Lifestyle Medicine Series)*. CRC Press.
20. Stanhope, K.L. (2012). *Role of Fructose-Containing Sugars in the Epidemics of Obesity and Metabolic Syndrome (Review of Medicine, Book 63)*. Annual Reviews.

9 Complications of Obesity

OUTLINE

Cardiovascular Disorders
Diabetes and Metabolic Syndrome
Osteoarthritis
Gastroesophageal Reflux Disease
Skin Problems
  Candidiasis
  Cellulitis
Surgical Problems
Respiratory Problems
  Sleep Apnea
Gynecologic Problems
  Amenorrhea
  Dysfunctional Uterine Bleeding
  Dysmenorrhea
Infertility
Pregnancy Complications
  Impact of Obesity on Pregnancy
Social and Psychological Problems
Obesity and Cancer
  Breast Cancer
  Uterine Cancer
  Gallbladder Cancer
  Pancreatic Cancer
  Colon Cancer
Key Terms
Clinical Case Studies
Study Questions
Further Reading

LEARNING OBJECTIVES

After study of the chapter, readers should be able to:

1. Describe metabolic syndrome.
2. Explain degenerative joint disease and its causes.
3. Describe the prevention of gastroesophageal reflux disease.
4. List skin problems that affect obese individuals.
5. Describe the most common causes of cellulitis.
6. Identify the causes of obstructive sleep apnea.
7. Explain gynecologic problems in obese women.
8. Describe the impact of obesity during pregnancy.
9. Discuss social and psychological problems caused by obesity.
10. Explain the relationship between obesity and various cancers.

OVERVIEW

Global obesity rates have greatly increased in recent decades. People are becoming obese at younger ages, and morbid obesity is increasing, with the complete health implications only beginning to be seen. Usually, obesity results from inherited, physiological, and environmental factors, combined with diet, physical activity, and exercise choices. As obesity rates rise, there is a related increase in many diseases or conditions. These include type 2 diabetes mellitus, heart disease, stroke, dementia, certain cancers, digestive problems, sleep apnea, osteoarthritis, and even a worsening of COVID-19 symptoms. Other weight-related issues that affect quality of life include depression, disability, shame, guilt, social isolation, and lower work achievement. Therefore, obesity has the potential to shorten life expectancy.

CARDIOVASCULAR DISORDERS

Obesity is related to an increased risk of developing cardiovascular disorders. It changes the composition of the body, affecting *hemodynamics* and altering heart structure. Adipose tissue produces pro-inflammatory cytokines, which can cause cardiac dysfunction as well as promote the formation of atherosclerotic plaques. When obesity and heart failure or cardiovascular disease coexist, people with class I obesity have a better prognosis compared to those who are normal or underweight. This is known as the **obesity paradox**. The cardiovascular disorders that are complications of obesity include atherosclerosis, dyslipidemia, hypertension, stroke, and pulmonary embolism (see Chapter 14 for more detail).

DIABETES AND METABOLIC SYNDROME

Metabolic syndrome is increasing the risks for type 2 diabetes. These conditions include hypertension, high blood glucose, excess fat around the waist, and abnormal cholesterol or triglyceride levels. Metabolic syndrome is closely related to being overweight, obese, and inactive, plus the condition known as insulin resistance. In this condition, the cells do not respond normally to insulin, and glucose cannot enter them as easily. Therefore, blood glucose levels increase even as the body produces more and more insulin to try to compensate (see Chapter 8 for more detail).

OSTEOARTHRITIS

Long-term obesity also affects the musculoskeletal system, mostly the joints, bones, muscles, tendons, and ligaments.

DOI: 10.1201/b22969-12

Osteoarthritis, or *degenerative joint disease*, is a progressive loss of articular cartilage with related changes at joint margins. It is the most common form of arthritis, and usually develops later in life. In most cases, it affects weight-bearing joints, particularly knee joints. Osteoarthritis is the leading cause of disability in many countries, especially those in which the citizens have longer lifespans. Because humans are living longer, many more people will probably develop osteoarthritis than ever before in history. The condition often becomes symptomatic during a person's 40s or 50s.

Osteoarthritis affects about 80% of older adults. About 50% of patients with the pathologic changes of osteoarthritis have symptoms. Under age 40, most large-joint osteoarthritis occurs in men, often because of obesity, trauma, or conditions such as hip dysplasia. Women have the condition more than men between ages 40 and 70. After age 70, men and women are almost equally affected. In Europe, age-specific yearly prevalence rates of only osteoarthritis of the knees, after age 80, are approximately 32,000 of every 100,000 women, and about 20,000 of every 100,000 men. After 55 years of age, age-specific prevalence rates for women exceed rates for men by 50%–60%. Prevalence rates between women and men for hip osteoarthritis are only slightly higher in women, however. Globally, osteoarthritis in all of its forms makes up 3% of total cases of disability.

Age-specific annual incidence rates for osteoarthritis in the United States increase greatly from middle age, peaking after age 70. Surveys of knee and hip osteoarthritis between men and women are similar to those in Europe. According to the Third National Health and Nutrition Examination Survey (NHANES III), for adults 60 years or older, 42% of women had knee osteoarthritis but only 31% of men had the condition. Hip osteoarthritis affects 27% of women and 26% of men. The amount of US adults with osteoarthritis has increased by 30% over the last few decades, concurrent with the present obesity epidemic. There is a proven relationship between excessive weight and the likelihood of developing osteoarthritis. This is especially true for osteoarthritis of the knees. As of 2022, osteoarthritis affected 59 million people in the United States. By 2040, it is forecast that 78 million people will be affected, which is 26% of adults.

The global annual rate of years lost to disability (YLD) in women is 2.9 per 1,000 women, and about 1.8 per 1,000 men. Disability adjusted life years (DALY) equal years of life lost to premature death (YLL) plus the YLD. For osteoarthritis, the DALY mostly reflects years of life lost because of disability, not premature death. Countries with the highest rates include the Thailand, Japan, South Korea, Mexico, Sweden, Algeria, India, China, Canada, Spain, the United Kingdom, Italy, Iran, and the United States (see Figure 9.1). According to the 2019 Global Burden of Disease study, osteoarthritis cases increased from 247.51 million in 1990 to 527.81 million in 2019, an increase of 113%.

The cause of osteoarthritis is usually linked to normal wear and tear that occurs with aging. Major risk factors include the female gender (after age 55), being overweight or obese, and having had major joint trauma or sustained, repetitive joint trauma. Previous knee trauma, obesity, the presence

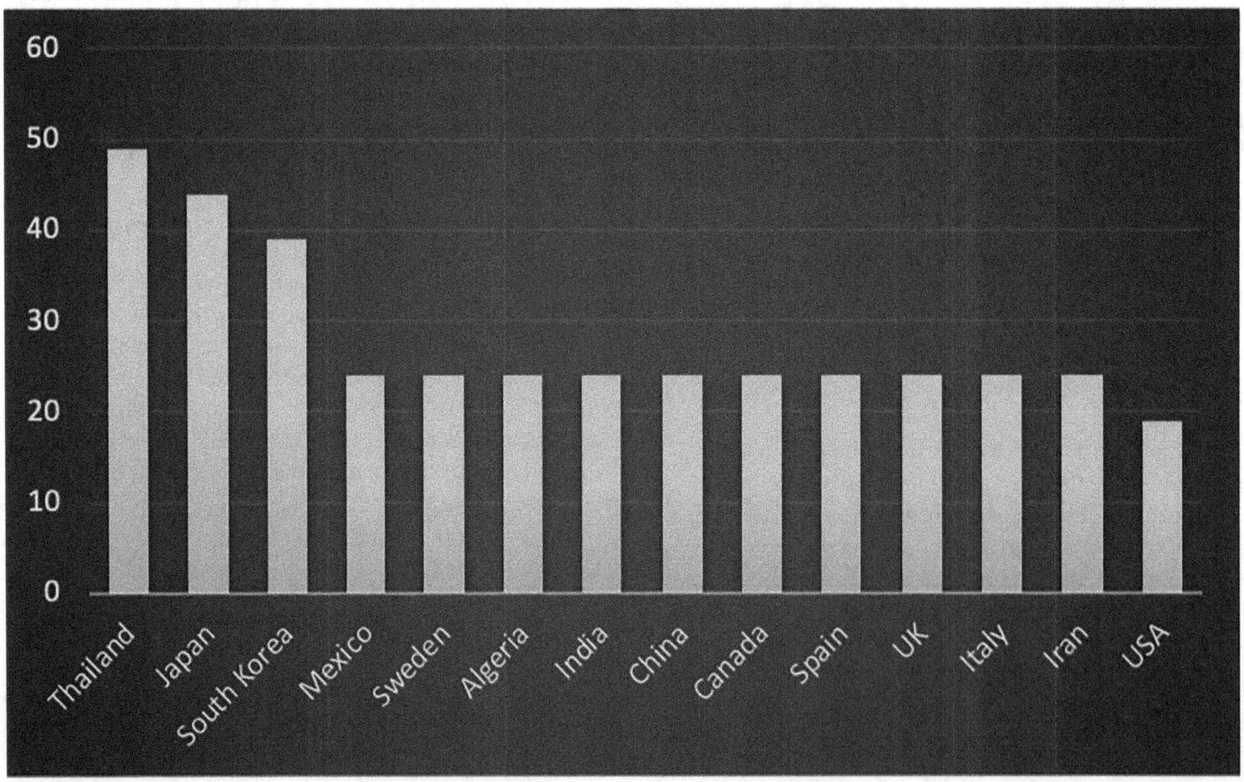

FIGURE 9.1 The countries with the highest percentages of citizens with osteoarthritis.

of Heberden nodes, and the female gender were the strongest risk factors for osteoarthritis. Additional risks are linked to regular strenuous exercise, a chronically high physical workload, repetitive kneeling and squatting, and higher bone mineral density. A positive family history also increases risks, and familial osteoarthritis may predispose patients to **Heberden nodes** (see Figure 9.2). In one study of twins, it was discovered that there was a concordance for nodal osteoarthritis in identical (monozygous) twins that was almost double that in fraternal (dizygous) twins. Afflicted twins (and other siblings) may have various genetic polymorphisms and point mutations related to defective collagen biosynthesis and repair, predisposing them to osteoarthritis. Hand osteoarthritis is most common in postmenopausal women.

The prevention of osteoarthritis includes maintaining a healthy weight, controlling blood glucose, being physically active on a regular basis, preventing joint injuries via warming up and stretching as well as avoiding carrying very heavy objects, using exercise equipment and protective devices. A physical therapist can help teach you the best exercises to protect the joints. A healthcare provider can provide education about the correct use of ice packs and pain medications before and after exercise.

The pathophysiology of osteoarthritis involves degradation of cartilage and remodeling of bone because of an active response of **chondrocytes** in articular cartilage, and in the inflammatory cells that surround tissues. Medications that help relieve osteoarthritis symptoms include acetaminophen, nonsteroidal anti-inflammatory drugs (NSAIDs), and duloxetine. Physical and occupational therapy may also be helpful, along with transcutaneous electrical nerve stimulation (TENS). Additional treatments include cortisone or lubricant injections, an osteotomy to realign bones, and joint replacement surgery.

Test Your Knowledge

1. What is the description of osteoarthritis?
2. How common is osteoarthritis?
3. What steps can help prevent the development of osteoarthritis?

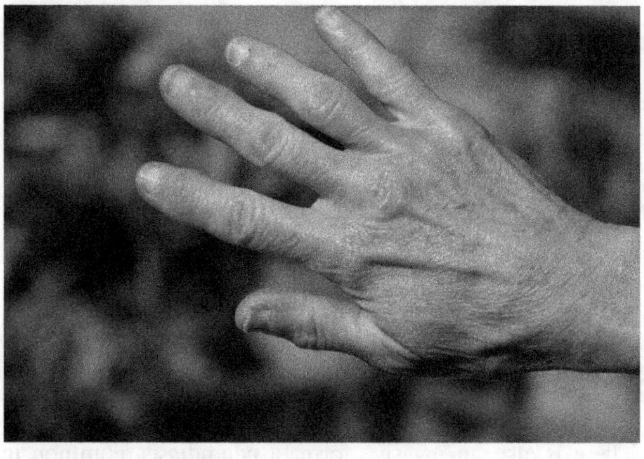

FIGURE 9.2 Heberden nodes.

GASTROESOPHAGEAL REFLUX DISEASE

Obesity causes many different gastrointestinal problems. The gastrointestinal system is very important concerning the pathogenesis of obesity and the facilitation of caloric imbalance. Gastroesophageal reflux disease (GERD) and fatty liver diseases such as non-alcoholic steatohepatitis are correlated to body weight and abdominal adiposity. Obesity can also trigger cirrhosis of the liver and gallstones. Obesity leads to gallstones because it alters the balance of cholesterol versus lecithin and bile acids within the gallbladder. Excessive body weight makes it more difficult for the gallbladder to empty, so cholesterol-rich bile accumulates and hardens into gallstones. When obesity is a risk factor for various gastrointestinal problems, it interacts with other mechanisms and results in earlier presentation or disease complications. Patients may require multidisciplinary management of obesity and the various disease states that result from it.

Gastroesophageal reflux disease is a chronic disorder caused by the retrograde flow of stomach contents back up into the esophagus. It is described as "heartburn" or "acid reflux". This causes a variety of symptoms and may or may not result in tissue damage. Incompetence of the lower esophageal sphincter allows gastric contents to reverse direction, and burning pain occurs. Overweight people have a 1.43 times higher risk for GERD, while obese people have a 1.94 times higher risk. Individuals with a waist circumference of over 90 centimeters have 7.2 times the risk of developing erosive esophagitis.

Though the epidemiology of GERD is hard to calculate, it is estimated that the condition 15.1%–30% of the global population. Every year about 0.4% of the population has symptoms for the first time. Prevalence rates of GERD in developed nations are linked to age, and adults between 60 and 70 are most commonly affected. About 20% of people have weekly symptoms, and about 7% have daily symptoms. There is no reported predominance between males and females. Lower esophageal sphincter incompetence may develop from a general loss of intrinsic sphincter tone, or from recurrent transient relaxations that are not related to swallowing. Transient lower esophageal sphincter relaxations are triggered by gastric distention, and can also be triggered by subthreshold stimulation of the pharynx.

Risk factors include the angle of the cardioesophageal junction, diaphragm activity, and position in comparison to gravity. Reflux may be induced by gaining weight, eating fatty foods, drinking caffeinated or carbonated beverages, alcohol use, tobacco smoking, and drugs. Drugs that lower pressure of the lower esophageal sphincter include anticholinergics, antihistamines, calcium channel blockers, tricyclic antidepressants, nitrates, and progesterone. Chronic GERD may contribute to esophagitis because of the caustic nature of the refluxate, an inability to clear refluxate out of the esophagus, gastric content volume, and local protective functions of the mucosa. Infants often aspirate reflux material, and patients of other ages may experience this as well.

Risk factors include alcohol or tobacco use, obesity, hiatal hernia, pregnancy, and scleroderma.

The prevention of GERD requires changing dietary habits to include small, frequent meals. Avoid trigger foods such as chocolate, citrus fruits and juices, peppermint, tomato products, foods that are fatty, fried, or spicy, and limiting garlic and onions. A food diary can help reveal patterns of foods that trigger the condition. Alcohol, tea, coffee, and carbonated drinks should be limited. It is important not to snack or eat a meal at least two to three hours before bedtime. While asleep, gravity pulls stomach contents toward the esophagus, initiating GERD symptoms. The head of the bed can be propped up six to ten inches, to reduce symptoms. Other preventive measures include losing weight, avoiding aspirin, ibuprofen, and naproxen, as well as prescription medications such as anticholinergics, beta-blockers, calcium channel blockers, dopamine-like drugs, progestin, sedatives, theophylline, and tricyclic antidepressants. Also, anything that helps relieve stress is indicated. Chewing gum after meals helps make more saliva, which neutralizes the acid that causes heartburn. Loose clothing also helps because tighter clothes around the stomach can push stomach acid upward.

GERD has a complex pathogenesis, with changes in reflux exposure, epithelial resistance, and visceral sensitivity. The gastric refluxate is noxious, and injures the esophagus. The refluxate is the main determinant of how serious the disease will be. Esophageal exposure arises from a compromised anti-reflux barrier and reduced ability to clear or buffer the refluxate. Complications and symptoms occur in relation to the normal reflux burden, with poor epithelial resistance or more visceral sensitivity. So, reflux develops due to alterations in the balance of the aggressive and protective forces.

Treatments for GERD include lifestyle and dietary changes, medications, endoscopic therapy, and surgery. Lifestyle changes include weight loss, quitting smoking, avoiding lying down immediately after a meal, and elevating the head of the bed. The affected individual must avoid foods that increase stomach acid such as caffeinated beverages, and foods that decrease lower esophageal pressure (alcohol, fatty foods, and peppermint). Other foods that should be avoided are those that affect peristalsis (acidic liquids, alcohol, and coffee) and those that slow gastric emptying (including fatty foods). Large meals should overall be avoided. Medications for GERD include antacids, histamine blockers, proton pump inhibitors, and prokinetic agents (which enhance activity of GI smooth muscle). Endoscopic therapies such as transoral incisionless fundoplication (TIF) are helpful, and TIF creates a passageway for an endoscope so that a surgeon can repair or recreate the valve that is a natural barrier to reflux. The surgical technique known as *Nissen fundoplication* involves wrapping the upper part of the stomach around the lower esophagus, which enhances the anti-reflux barrier, providing (potentially) permanent relief. This can be done laparoscopically, which is less invasive and requires a shorter recovery time.

Test Your Knowledge

1. What types of gastrointestinal problems are linked to obesity?
2. How can gastroesophageal reflux disease be prevented?
3. What foods must be avoided if GERD is present?

FOCUS ON GASTROESOPHAGEAL REFLUX DISEASE

Though heartburn and GERD start in the stomach, they are not necessarily caused by food. Being overweight or obese is a proven cause. Heartburn may cause hoarseness, sore throat, coughing, asthma, a feeling of a need to clear the throat, and overproduction of mucus. Chronic irritation from heartburn and GERD can damage the lining of the esophagus, leading to **Barrett's esophagus** and esophageal cancer.

SKIN PROBLEMS

Being overweight or obese may cause skin problems. Changes in hormones can cause acanthosis nigricans, resulting in darkened velvety areas, and stretching may result in stretch marks on the skin. Increased strain involving the leg veins may cause fluid retention, leg swelling, rupture of superficial capillaries, dermatitis, varicose veins, and ulcers. Retained moisture in body folds encourages growth of bacteria and fungi, causing skin rashes, potential skin breakdown, and infections such as intertrigo. Other obesity-related conditions include increased sweat and skin secretions, lymphedema, **cellulitis**, and hirsutism. Obesity can cause surgical problems because of difficulties accessing body sites requiring surgery, and the higher rates of infections, nerve injury, and even heart attack.

Candidiasis

Obese individuals often have fungal skin infections. Softening and moisture in intertriginous areas provide an excellent environment for yeasts such as *Candida* species to proliferate. This leads to redness and irritation, with satellite lesions under the breasts and abdominal folds, and in the inguinal area. Friction and softening play a role in the development of **candidiasis**. Candida folliculitis is less common, but is also seen in obese individuals. Topical antifungals such as ketoconazole or econazole creams, or oral agents such as fluconazole or itraconazole can treat the infection, but may not prevent recurrences. Candidiasis is a skin and mucous membrane infection, usually with *Candida albicans* (in 70%–80% of cases). Infections are most common in the skin folds, digital web spaces, genitals, cuticles, and oral mucosa. There is also an invasive form of candidiasis, common in immunosuppressed patients, and may be life threatening.

Community-acquired candidemia occurs in 22.4% of European populations, but is much more common in North America, with 63.5% of the population being affected. Infections of the mouth occur in 6% of infants less than one month old. About 20% of people receiving chemotherapy for cancer and 20% of AIDS patients will develop candidiasis. Approximately 20% of women may have asymptomatic colonization by vaginal yeasts. In the United States, *Candida* is the fifth most common pathogen causing nosocomial blood stream infections. *Candida* species cause 8%–10% of nosocomial bloodstream infections. Yearly incidence of *Candida* infections is 8 out of every 100,000 population. In 95% of *Candida* infections, the pathogens involved are *C. albicans*, *C. glabrata*, *C. parapsilosis*, *C. tropicalis*, and *C. krusei*. The pathogen *C. parapsilosis* causes 30% of candidemia in newborns, but only 10%–15% of candidemia cases in adults. *C. glabrata* is most common in older and neoplastic patients. *C. tropicalis* is more common in leukemia and neutropenic patients. Since *C. parapsilosis* colonizes the skin, it is common in catheter-related infections, and has caused outbreaks. *C. krusei* is more common in hematopoietic stem cell recipients or neutropenic **leukemia** patients that receive prophylactic fluconazole. In the United States, there are about 1.4 million cases of candidiasis documented by physicians. About 33% of women have at least one yeast infection at some time. Esophageal candidiasis is the most common esophageal infection in AIDS patients, accounting for 50% of all esophageal infections. It is often present with other esophageal disease. About 66% of patients with AIDS and esophageal candidiasis also have oral candidiasis.

Candida is a group of about 150 yeast species. The yeast is present on the skin and mucous membranes, activating when dampness, heat, and impaired local and systemic defenses encourage its growth. Risk factors include obesity, hot weather, poor hygiene, restrictive clothing, altered flora (from broad-spectrum antibiotics), corticosteroid use, infrequent undergarment changes, inflammatory skin fold diseases, endocrine alterations (diabetes mellitus, pregnancy, renal failure, and hypothyroidism), and immunosuppression. Candidal nail infections and **paronychia** can develop if the hands are continually exposed to water, or after an improper nail manicure. In obese patients, candidal infections are common beneath the abdominal fold. Oropharyngeal candidiasis may indicate local or systemic immunosuppression.

For those at high risk for developing invasive candidiasis, antifungal medications may be prescribed as part of antifungal **prophylaxis**. This is usually recommended for certain organ transplant patients, some people in intensive care units, those on certain types of chemotherapy or that have neutropenia, and patients with a stem cell or bone marrow transplant, plus **neutropenia**. Some physicians consider antifungal prophylaxis for very low birthweight infants in nurseries with high rates of invasive candidiasis. Preventive actions that can be taken include notifying your physician if the skin around a central venous catheter becomes red or painful, and regular adequate hand washing by the patient and all caregivers.

Candida species are usually transmitted through childbirth, sexual intercourse, in hospital settings between healthcare workers and immunocompromised patients, because of overuse of antibiotics, and uncontrolled diabetes mellitus. Pathogenesis involves yeast cells adhering to host cell surfaces via the expression of **adhesins**. Contact to host cells triggers a yeast to **hypha** transition, with growth directed through **thigmotropism**. The expression of **invasins** mediates uptake of the fungus by the host cell, via induced endocytosis.

The specific type and dose of antifungal medication used for invasive candidiasis is based on patient age, immune status, and the infection's location and severity. In most adults, the initial antifungal is usually an echinocandin such as anidulafungin, caspofungin, or micafungin, given IV. In some situations, amphotericin B, fluconazole, or other antifungals may be appropriate. Treatment should continue for two weeks after signs and symptoms have resolved and *Candida* yeasts are no long in the bloodstream. Treatments are usually longer for infections of the bones, central nervous system, heart, or joints.

Cellulitis

Bacterial skin infections are actually skin and soft tissue infections, and acute bacterial and skin structure infections. Cellulitis and **erythrasma** are influenced by obesity, and are considered to be complex bacterial infections. Other complex bacterial infections include erysipelas, wound infections, and major cutaneous abscesses. These are not directly linked to obesity. Cellulitis is an acute bacterial infection that involves the inner layers of the skin, mostly affecting the dermis and subcutaneous fat. It is most often affects the skin on the lower legs, but also the face, arms, and other areas (see Figure 9.3). Cellulitis is not usually considered to be a contagious disease. Periorbital cellulitis is a bacterial infection of the eyelids and surrounding tissues. Facial cellulitis may follow an upper respiratory infection or otitis media. Buccal cellulitis is an infection of the cheek, occurring in children, and associated with bacteremia. Abdominal wall cellulitis is most common in morbidly obese patients. **Necrotizing cellulitis** involves gas-producing bacteria in the lower extremities, more common in patients with diabetes.

Cellulitis is one of the most common bacterial infections occurring in primary care settings, occurring equally in males and females. Incidence is 200 of every 100,000 individuals per year. The exact prevalence is uncertain, since cellulitis is common but not reportable. All age groups and races are affected. In the United States, about 145 million annual cases of cellulitis occur, accounting for $3.7 billion in costs.

Most cases of cellulitis are caused by *Staphylococcus* or *Streptococcus* species. Cellulitis rarely occurs as a complication of strep throat. It usually starts with a minor scratch, cut, **abrasion**, insect bite, or another type of skin injury.

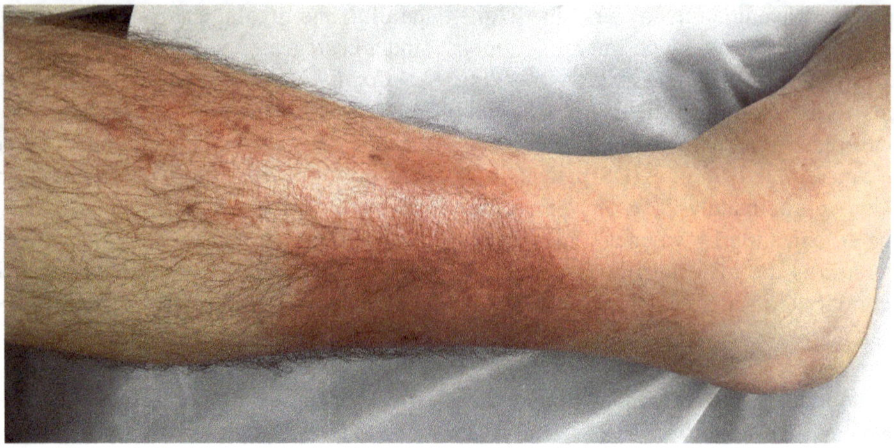

FIGURE 9.3 Cellulitis.

People with wounds should avoid exposures to fresh water or dirt. Wounds should be inspected daily to look for signs of infection such as redness, drainage, and swelling. Risk factors include immune compromise, a history of cellulitis, **psoriasis**, or **eczema**, being overweight or obese, **lymphedema**, and use of illicit injectable drugs. The prevention of cellulitis includes keeping the skin clean and well-moisturized, preventing cuts and scrapes with appropriate clothing and footwear, using gloves when needed, carefully trimming the nails, and promptly treating cuts or infections such as athlete's foot. As the causative organism of cellulitis invades a compromised area, it overwhelms defensive neutrophils, eosinophils, basophils, and mast cells. These cells normal contain and localize inflammation. Therefore, cellular debris accumulates. As cellulitis progresses, the organism invades tissues around the initial wound.

The treatment of cellulitis usually includes a prescribed oral antibiotic. Within three days, the infection should start responding. The antibiotic must be continued for its full course – usually seven to ten days – even if symptoms are improving. Some patients must be hospitalized so that they can be given IV antibiotics. This occurs if signs and symptoms do not respond to oral antibiotics, become extensive, or if a high fever develops.

Test Your Knowledge

1. Which fungal skin infections may affect people who are obese?
2. What are the risk factors for candidiasis?
3. What is the description of cellulitis?

SURGICAL PROBLEMS

Obesity is a risk factor for the development of postoperative complications. Obese patients experience more concomitant diseases, increased risks of wound infection, more intraoperative blood loss, and longer operation times. For some unknown reason, being obese is associated with improved long-term survival. This is described as the *obesity paradox*. Even so, obesity is definitely linked with longer operation times, an important predictor of postoperative wound infections. Impaired immunity, elevated blood glucose, and extensive tension upon the surgical incision also contribute to impaired wound healing.

According to John Hopkins University, obese patients are almost 12 times more likely to suffer a complication following a procedure such as elective plastic surgery than people of normal weight. Annual plastic surgeries increased between the years 1992 and 2005 by 725%. Any surgery on an obese person is more difficult than in patients of normal or near-normal weight. The procedures take longer, involve deeper operating fields, have spaces in which an infection can occur of larger size, and slower blood flow through fat tissue results in slower healing. The most common procedures include breast reduction/reconstruction/augmentation, and mastopexy. About 18.3% of obese patients experience at least once surgical complication, compared to only 2.2% of non-obese patients. The most common complications are inflammation, infection, and pain. After bariatric surgery, an obese person's body is usually left with excess skin and tissue that must be removed to complete the reshaping process. Procedures include **liposuction**, *body lift*, *plastic surgery*, and *tummy tuck* (see Figure 9.4).

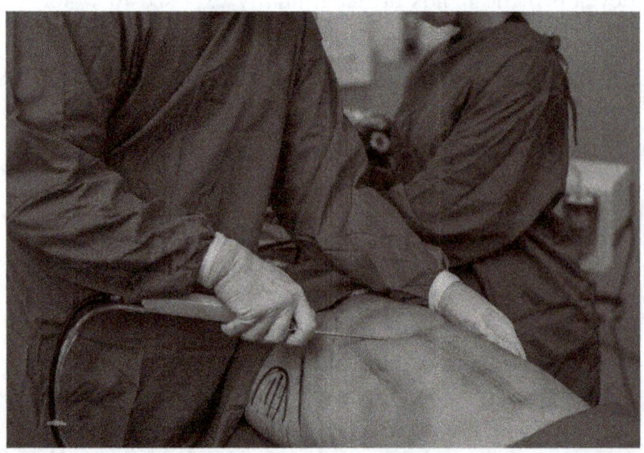

FIGURE 9.4 Liposuction.

RESPIRATORY PROBLEMS

Obesity significantly interferes with respiratory function by decreasing lung volume – especially the expiratory reserve volume and functional residual capacity. Due to ineffectiveness of the respiratory muscles, strength and resistance may be reduced. These factors lead to inspiratory overload, increasing respiratory effort, oxygen consumption, and respiratory energy expenditure. Patterns of body fat distribution greatly influence the function of the respiratory system, probably through the direct mechanical effect of chest and abdominal fat accumulation. The most common obesity-related respiratory condition is sleep apnea. Obesity also increases the risk of developing severe symptoms if individuals become infected with the virus that causes coronavirus disease 2019 (COVID-19). People who have severe cases of COVID-19 may require treatment in intensive care units or even need mechanical assistance to breathe. Mortality increases in obese people who are infected with the COVID-19.

Sleep Apnea

Sleep apnea involves episodes of partial or complete closure of the upper airway during sleep. Each episode results in breathing cessation. Being overweight or obese is a high risk factor for sleep apnea, along with other breathing problems during sleep. Alternately, a person who has a sleep-breathing disorder that is not treated can begin to gain weight as a result. In children, excess weight increases risks for developing lifelong obstructive sleep apnea. However, this can be preventable and even cured in children while they are still young, as long as weight management is undertaken along with continuous positive airway pressure (CPAP) or **tonsillectomy**. The impact of untreated sleep apnea on the developing brain and body will lead to changes in metabolism, due to systemic stress occurring nightly, during sleep. This results in abnormal food cravings, daytime fatigue, low energy levels, behavior problems, and other anomalies that may lead to unhealthy weight gain. The two forms of sleep apnea are *obstructive* and *central*.

Obstructive sleep apnea is the most common form, and is characterized by partial or complete obstructions of the upper airway. *Central sleep apnea* is usually associated with a reduction in blood oxygen saturation, and is less common. There is also an uncommon condition referred to as *obstructive sleep apnea syndrome* that occurs between the ages of 30 and 60. It is currently estimated that up to 4% of children, globally, suffer from sleep apnea. Many of these children are between the ages of two and eight years. Up to 25% of children with attention deficit problems may actually have undetected sleep apnea. Children are more likely to have other sleep disturbances, including restless leg syndrome, periodic limb movement disorder, narcolepsy, and insomnia. Up to 27% of children have loud snoring without sleep apnea. Insomnia affects 20%–30% of infants and toddlers, and as many as 5% of school-aged children.

Overall, sleep apnea affects about 5 in every 100 people. This is 3%–7% of adult men and 2%–5% of adult women. Prevalence estimates of obstructive sleep apnea from North America, Europe, Australia, and Asia are not very different – it is common everywhere. According to a four-year study, compared with participants of normal weight, those with just a 10% increase in body weight had an average of a 32% increase in their apnea-hypopnea index (AHI), and a six-times higher risk of developing moderate-to-severe obstructive sleep apnea. Conversely, a 10% decrease in body weight was associated with a 26% decrease in the AHI. Obstructive sleep apnea is increasing, affecting more than 25 million adults in the United States alone. It is estimated that 26% of adults between ages 30 and 70 have sleep apnea. In younger adults, sleep apnea is more common in men than in women by a larger margin, but this reduces with aging. In some elderly groups, obstructive sleep apnea is as high as 90% in men and 78% in women. Incidence averages 4.9% in women, but 11.1% in men. In both women and men, it is most common in middle age. Accurate statistics on YLD and DALYs related to sleep apnea are not available. Prevalence of obstructive sleep apnea is greater in obese and hypertensive patients. Undiagnosed obstructive sleep apnea is estimated to cost the United States more than $149 billion per year.

The causes of obstructive sleep apnea are a natural relaxation of throat muscles as sleeping begins. There may be additional complicating factors, such as being overweight or obese, a smaller than normal jaw, enlarged tonsils or adenoids that partially block breathing passages, or having a large tongue. In children, who often outgrow the condition, the primary cause is **adenotonsillar hypertrophy**. In adults, those who consume alcohol before sleep or take sleeping pills or tranquilizers experience further relaxation and narrowing of breathing passages. This makes the passages more likely to close. Though many people take sleeping pills or tranquilizers to get better and more continuous sleep, these agents often make things worse.

Endocrine disorders linked to sleep apnea include hypothyroidism, **acromegaly**, and **polycystic ovary syndrome** (since this is linked to being overweight or obese). Conditions that interfere with brain signals to the airway and chest muscles may be implicated in sleep apnea. These conditions include stroke, amyotrophic lateral sclerosis, Chiari malformations, **myotonic dystrophy**, post-polio syndrome, **dermatomyositis**, and **myasthenia gravis**. Sleep apnea is common with advanced heart or kidney failure, since there may be fluid build-up in the neck, obstructing the upper airway. Genetic syndromes may affect facial or skull structures. These syndromes include cleft lip or palate, **Down syndrome**, and congenital central hypoventilation syndrome. Babies born before 37 weeks of gestation have an increased risk for sleep apnea, but risks usually decrease as the brain matures.

Risk factors for sleep apnea include unhealthy lifestyle habits and environments, age, family history, genetics, race, ethnicity, and gender. Healthy lifestyle changes can decrease risks. With increased age, more fatty tissue builds up in the neck and tongue, raising risks. Studies of twins have revealed that sleep apnea is inheritable. Some genes are associated with obesity and inflammation. Race or ethnicity is a factor, with sleep apnea being more common in African-Americans, Hispanics, and Native Americans than in Caucasians.

There are preventive measures against the development or worsening of sleep apnea. It is important to stop drinking of alcohol or sleep medicines because they relax the muscles in the back of the throat, making it harder to breathe while asleep. Smokers must quit their habit. Weight loss is an essential method of preventing sleep apnea. Another suggestion is to try and sleep on one side instead of on the back for most of the night. The pathogenesis of sleep apnea involves upper airway anatomy, the ability of upper airway dilator muscles to respond to respiratory challenges while sleeping, the *arousal threshold, loop gain,* and the potential for state-related changes in lung volume to influence all of these factors. The arousal threshold is the propensity to wake from increased respiratory drive during sleep. The loop gain is the stability of the respiratory control system. The interaction between the patency of the pharynx and lung volume is important regarding obstructive sleep apnea. Deposition of fat around the pharyngeal airway increases its likelihood of collapse. Fat deposits around the abdomen reduce functional residual capacity. This may reduce lung volume effects upon the upper airway. Low lung volumes are related to reduced stores of oxygen, contributing to ventilatory control instability, known as *high loop gain.* Obesity is associated with functional impairment of the upper airway muscles.

Sleep quality problems usually manifest slowly, over years, especially with long-term weight increases. Most patients do not recognize the symptoms and rarely remember how many times they are awakened during the night. Often, patients attribute the effects of poor sleep to aging, medications, stress, or an uncomfortable bed. In children, sleep apnea may cause learning and behavioral problems. Apnea-related symptoms include bedwetting, sleepwalking, slow growth, hormone imbalances, worsening of **asthma**, hyperactivity, and failure to thrive. Brain function can be altered, with effects upon cognition, planning, self-monitoring, organization, and emotions. Signs and symptoms of sleep apnea in children include loud snoring, difficult or labored breathing, and chronic squeaking or gasping when breathing.

Snoring during sleep affects 10%–30% of adults, and loud snoring is a sign of sleep apnea. When the body does not get enough air, it signals the brain to breathe harder to force air inward, resulting in snoring. If the body cannot get any air in, breathing stops temporarily, and we awake so that the problem can be corrected. If this happens hundreds of times per night, it leads to chronic sleepiness, difficulty concentrating, and depression. If chronic, it can result in hypertension, heart attack, and stroke. *Obstructive sleep apnea syndrome (OSAS)* has two primary types: *hypopnea* and *apnea.* **Hypopnea** occurs if there is only slight narrowing of the breathing passages. The body can continue breathing, but only with increased effort, causing loud snoring or breathing. There are sleep disruptions and repeated sleep and wake cycles. These are often not remembered by the individual.

Apnea occurs when the breathing passages become so narrow that no air can pass, and breathing stops. The patient wakes up to breathe, and the cycle starts over. Some patients experience apnea along with hypopnea, as the throat muscles relax and the breathing passages narrow again. Apnea and hypopnea both drop the blood oxygen levels, causing many other symptoms. Additional signs and symptoms of sleep apnea include mood swings, difficulty concentrating, forgetfulness, irritability, anxiety, falling asleep at inappropriate times, morning headache, unexplained nausea, a frequent need to urinate at night, and chronic darkness of the skin below the eyes. Sleep apnea patients often complain of problems with motor skills and memory, dry mouth, sexual dysfunction, and decreased libido. Women more often report headache, fatigue, depression, anxiety, and insomnia than are reported by men.

Complications of sleep apnea include asthma, atrial fibrillation, cancers, chronic kidney disease, cognitive and behavioral disorders, heart disease and hypertension, eye disorders, metabolic disorders, and pregnancy abnormalities. The most common related cancers include pancreatic, renal, and skin cancers. Cognitive and behavioral disorders include decreased attention, vigilance, concentration, motor skills, and poor verbal or visuospatial memory. In older adults, dementia may be a result of sleep apnea. Diseases of the heart and blood vessels include atherosclerosis, heart attack or heart failure, hypertension that is difficult to control, and stroke. Eye disorders include dry eye, glaucoma, and keratoconus. Metabolic disorders include glucose intolerance and type 2 diabetes mellitus. Pregnancy complications include **gestational diabetes** or hypertension, along with having a baby of low birthweight. Sleep apnea can also cause inflammation, which may contribute to atherosclerosis and damage the pancreas.

The most common and reliable treatment method for obstructive sleep apnea is with a CPAP machine. This device pushes a steady stream of air through a mask to keep the airway open, helping the patient to snore less or not at all, and to sleep better. Another option is a bi-level positive airway pressure (BiPAP or BPAP) machine. It does not give the same, constant pressure all the time. Since it gives less air while the patient is breathing out, it makes the process of exhaling easier than with CPAP. The adaptive servo ventilation (ASV) machine adapts and adjusts airflow based on the patient's breathing. The variable positive airway pressure (VPAP) machine gives the patient different amounts of air while breathing. Oral appliances, also called mandibular advancement devices (MADs) are designed to either bring the jaw forward to open the airway, or to hold the tongue in place. Additional treatment options include weight loss, nasal decongestants, breathing strips, implantable upper airway stimulation (UAS) devices, uvulopalatopharyngoplasty (to surgically remove the tonsils and **uvula**).

FOCUS ON OBESITY AS A SURGICAL RISK FACTOR

Surgical operative time is lengthened when a patient's body mass index (BMI) category is high, for eight principal gastroenterological procedures. Mortality is also higher in patients with a BMI above 30. A high BMI can increase the risk of postoperative leakage, which is an important complication.

Test Your Knowledge

1. In relation to surgery, what problems affect obese patients more than non-obese patients?
2. How does obesity interfere with respiratory function?
3. How common is sleep apnea in relation to obesity?

GYNECOLOGIC PROBLEMS

Gynecologic problems increase significantly when obesity is an issue. These problems may be related to menstruation, including the absence of menstruation, light or infrequent periods, or abnormally heavy bleeding. There may be an increased risk for **infertility** and failure to ovulate, as well as poor responses to fertility drugs. Obesity increases risks for miscarriage, hypertension during pregnancy, gestational diabetes, increase the rate of cesarean section, and fetal abnormalities. Labor and delivery may cause harm to mother and baby. Polycystic ovary syndrome is associated with reproductive and metabolic abnormalities, many of which are exacerbated by obesity.

Women who are obese often have abnormal menstrual cycles, heaviness of menstruation, and pain. Obesity can cause unpredictable, irregular menses. This leads to frequent needs to urinate, leakage, and missing of work and recreational activities. Some obese women experience daily bleeding, continuing for weeks at a time, leading to vaginal irritation and problems with intimacy. Hormones at different levels can alter the menstrual cycle. While the ovaries normally produce estrogen, it is also produced in the adipose cells. More fat means more estrogen, thickening of the uterine lining, and heavy bleeding during menstruation. When excessive estrogen is produced, it can interrupt regular cycling of other menstrual hormones, causing irregular menses. There are various types of menstrual abnormalities, including amenorrhea, dysfunctional uterine bleeding, dysmenorrhea, and premenstrual syndrome. Excess estrogen causes conflicting signals to be sent to the brain and ovaries, resulting in irregular or absent ovulation, resulting in abnormal menses.

Those with irregular menses reported experiencing reduced flow or complete stoppage of flow for at least six months. Younger obese women have more menstrual problems later in life, as well as more ovulatory infertility. Women with a BMI of 32.5 at age 20 have about two times the chance for irregular menses and about 1.5 times the chance for ovulatory infertility. Irregular cycles are often treated with hormonal medications. However, treatment should always include a weight-loss program. Even just losing five to ten pounds may improve the menstrual cycle's regularity. Decreases in percentage of body fat can improve hormone balance between the brain and ovaries, causing more regular ovulation.

AMENORRHEA

Amenorrhea can be primary or secondary. *Primary amenorrhea* is the failure of menses to occur by the age of 13 years in girls with normal growth and secondary sexual characteristics. Even so, a patient who has had no menstrual period by age 15 and has no signs of puberty, such as any amount of breast development, must be evaluated for primary amenorrhea. *Secondary amenorrhea* is the absence of menses for six or more months, or the length of three cycles after regular menstrual cycles have been established. Patients with previously regular cycles are, however, evaluated for secondary amenorrhea if menses have not occurred for three or more months. Patients with previously irregular menstrual cycles are evaluated for secondary amenorrhea if menses have not occurred for six or more months.

Throughout the world, incidence of primary amenorrhea is less than 1% of the total population, and only about one of every 20 women of childbearing age has secondary amenorrhea. The prevalence of amenorrhea not due to pregnancy, lactation, or menopause is 3%–4% of the population. There is no evidence for race and ethnicity affecting prevalence. Most cases are linked to polycystic ovary syndrome, hypothalamic dysfunction, hyperprolactinemia, and ovarian failure. Amenorrhea is most often caused by pregnancy, delays in puberty, functional hypothalamic anovulation, use of various drugs (oral contraceptives, antidepressants, antipsychotics), and breastfeeding. Oral contraceptives cause thinning of the endometrium, but menses usually begin again after approximately three months. Antidepressants and antipsychotics can elevate **prolactin**, stimulating milk production, and resulting in amenorrhea. Congenital anatomic abnormalities cause only primary amenorrhea, but all disorders that cause secondary amenorrhea can also cause primary amenorrhea.

The most common causes of anovulatory amenorrhea include hypothalamic dysfunction such as functional hypothalamic anovulation, pituitary dysfunction, primary ovarian insufficiency (premature ovarian failure), and endocrine disorders that cause androgen excess such as especially polycystic ovary syndrome. Anovulatory amenorrhea is usually secondary, but can be primary if ovulation never begins, such as caused by a genetic disorder. If ovulation does not begin, puberty and development of secondary sexual characteristics will be abnormal. Genetic disorders that involve a Y-chromosome abnormality increase risks of ovarian germ cell cancer.

The most common causes of ovulatory amenorrhea include chromosomal abnormalities and congenital anatomic abnormalities that obstruct menstrual flow.

Obstructive abnormalities usually exist along with normal hormone function. Obstructions may result in hematocolpos or hematometra. **Hematocolpos** is accumulation of menstrual blood in the vagina, causing it to bulge. **Hematometra** is accumulation of blood in the uterus, causing uterine distortion, a mass, or cervical bulging. Since ovarian function is normal, the external genitals and other secondary sexual characteristics develop normally. Congenital disorders along with by vaginal aplasia or a vaginal septum also cause urinary tract and skeletal abnormalities. Acquired anatomic abnormalities such as endometrial scarring following instrumentation for postpartum hemorrhage or infection known as **Asherman syndrome** cause secondary ovulatory amenorrhea. Risk factors include obesity, the female athlete triad, stress, and anovulatory disorders.

The prevention of amenorrhea is based on maintaining a healthy weight, eating a well-balanced diet, exercising regularly, and learning to manage stress. The pathogenesis of amenorrhea is multifactorial, including hypothalamic, pituitary, thyroid, adrenal, ovarian, uterine, and vaginal factors. An immature *hypothalamic-pituitary-gonadal axis* may lead to anovulatory cycles, causing abnormal menstrual cycles. In hyperthyroidism, increased sex hormone binding globulins may lead to increased levels of androgens and estrogen. Any underlying condition that disrupts the **pulsatility** of gonadotropic-releasing hormone can lead to amenorrhea. Primary ovarian insufficiency can lead to ovarian failure, a decrease in estrogen, and amenorrhea.

The treatment of amenorrhea is based on the underlying cause. If obesity is related, a weight-loss program is highly recommended. Talk therapy, medications, and other treatments may be needed to manage any mental health issues. For thyroid issues, hormone replacements or surgery may be recommended. If ovarian cancer is underlying, a combination of medications, radiation therapy, and chemotherapy may be needed. Medication or surgery to treat other causative conditions are also options.

Test Your Knowledge

1. Which gynecologic problems are linked to obesity?
2. What are primary and secondary amenorrhea?
3. How can amenorrhea be prevented?

Dysfunctional Uterine Bleeding

Dysfunctional uterine bleeding is referred to also as *abnormal uterine bleeding.* It is caused by ovulatory dysfunction, and after examination and ultrasonography, cannot be attributed to common causes of cancer, structural gynecologic abnormalities, inflammation, pregnancy or its complications, systemic disorders, or use of oral contraceptives and other medications. Globally, about 90% of cases of dysfunctional uterine bleeding are anovulatory, while the other 10% are ovulatory. Abnormal bleeding due to ovulatory dysfunction occurs most often in women over age 45 (more than 50% of cases), and in adolescents (about 20% of cases). In premenopausal women, dysfunctional uterine bleeding has affects 10%–30% of the population. Up to 25% of women have at least one episode during their lifetimes. In adolescent girls, between 10% and 37% have dysfunctional uterine bleeding.

Anovulatory dysfunctional uterine bleeding results from any condition that causes anovulation. It is usually secondary to polycystic ovary syndrome, or idiopathic – sometimes occurring while gonadotropin levels are normal. This bleeding is linked to obesity, but anovulation may also result from hypothyroidism. In perimenopause, anovulatory uterine bleeding may be an early sign of ovarian insufficiency or failure. The follicles are still developing. Even with increased FSH levels, they do not produce enough estrogen to trigger ovulation. Approximately 20% of women who have endometriosis have anovulatory uterine bleeding from an unknown cause. Ovulatory dysfunctional uterine bleeding may occur in polycystic ovary syndrome since progesterone secretion is prolonged, or in endometriosis, which does not affect ovulation. Additional causes include a short follicular phase, plus luteal phase dysfunction from inadequate progesterone stimulation of the endometrium. A rapid estrogen decrease prior to ovulation can cause spotting. Risk factors for dysfunctional uterine bleeding include hormonal abnormalities, including thyroid problems and elevated prolactin; as well as medications, excessive exercise or weight loss, stress, illness, *menarche*, and menopause.

Dysfunctional uterine bleeding usually cannot be prevented, but being under or over the proper body weight can affect hormone production. This increases risks for the condition. Patients with this condition have lost cyclic endometrial stimulation arising from the ovulatory cycle. The patient has constant, noncycling estrogen levels that stimulate endometrial growth. Proliferation with no periodic shedding causes the endometrium to outgrow its blood supply. The tissue breaks down, sloughing off from the uterus. Healing is then irregular and not synchronized. Chronic stimulation by low levels of estrogen result in infrequent, light dysfunctional uterine bleeding. Chronic stimulation from higher estrogen levels lead to episodes of frequent, heavy bleeding.

Dysfunctional uterine bleeding can be treated medically or surgically. Medical treatments include anti-fibrinolytic tranexamic acid, nonsteroidal anti-inflammatory drugs, the combined contraception pill, progestogen, danazol, or analogs of gonadotrophin releasing hormone. The levonorgestrel-releasing intrauterine device is also effective for treatment. Surgical treatments include endometrial ablation and hysterectomy.

Dysmenorrhea

Dysmenorrhea is uterine pain occurring around the time of menses. The pain may occur before menses by one to three days, or occur during menses. The pain usually peaks 24 hours after onset of menses, and resolves after two to three days. It is usually sharp, but has been described as cramping, throbbing, or dull and constant aching, and may radiate to the legs. Estimates of the percentage of women of reproductive age affected by dysmenorrhea range widely (between 20% and 90% of the global population). It is the most common menstrual disorder of all. In the United States, about 25% of women are treated for dysmenorrhea. It mostly occurs in individuals in their late teens and 20s, declining with increased age. Primary onset is six to twelve months after menarche. Secondary dysmenorrhea is common between ages 20 and 30. Up to 42% of women lose school or work days due to dysmenorrhea. Up to 20% report impairment of daily activities or sleep.

Dysmenorrhea is caused when prostaglandin causes the uterus to contract. This can caused the uterus to press against blood vessels, cutting off the supply of oxygen to muscle tissues. When part of the muscle briefly loses its oxygen supply, it causes pain. Risk factors for dysmenorrhea include endometriosis, adenomyosis, pelvic inflammatory disease, cervical stenosis, fibroids, nulliparity, heavy menstrual flow, smoking, and depression. There is no way to prevent dysmenorrhea, but eating a balanced diet and getting regular exercise can help reduce the intensity of the condition. The pathogenesis of dysmenorrhea is based on the causative prostaglandins as well as the vasoconstrictive effects of vasopressin. Treatment options include nonsteroidal anti-inflammatory drugs, oral contraceptives, depo-medroxyprogesterone acetate, prolonged-cycle oral contraceptives, intravaginal contraceptives, topical heat, Japanese herbs, supplements (thiamine, vitamin E, and fish oil), a low-fat vegetarian diet, and acupressure. If these treatments are insufficient, additional options include transcutaneous electric nerve stimulation, acupuncture, nifedipine, and terbutaline. Otherwise, danazol or leuprolide may be considered. In rare cases, hysterectomy has been performed.

FOCUS ON MENSTRUAL ABNORMALITIES

Menstrual abnormalities include amenorrhea, dysmenorrhea, abnormal uterine bleeding, and premenstrual syndrome. Irregular or absent menses and non-menstrual vaginal bleeding have many causes. In women of reproductive age, pregnancy should be suspected. Abnormal vaginal bleeding in non-pregnant women is evaluated differently. Pelvic congestion syndrome is a common cause of chronic pelvic pain, and is sometimes accompanied by abnormal menstrual bleeding.

Test Your Knowledge

1. What are the causes of dysfunctional uterine bleeding?
2. How does excessive body weight affect dysfunctional uterine bleeding?
3. Does regular exercise have any impact upon dysmenorrhea?

INFERTILITY

Infertility is the lack of pregnancy despite regular, unprotected sexual intercourse after one year, or via therapeutic donor insemination in women below age 35 and after six months in women aged 35 or older. Infertility is one of the most common disorders of the reproductive system. The prevalence in obese women is very high in comparison to non-obese women, and is still being studied. Rates of miscarriage and pregnancy complications are higher in obese women. The risk of infertility is three times higher in obese women than in non-obese women. The probability of pregnancy is reduced by 5% per every unit of BMI that exceeds 29.

Obesity in early adulthood alters later reproductive functions. Obesity influences infertility to cause impaired **ovarian follicular** development, **oocyte** development, fertilization, embryo development, and implantation. Infertility is a common complication of polycystic ovary syndrome. This is related to chronic anovulation due to hyperandrogenism. Lack of ovulation also develops from the effects of hyperinsulinemia, insulin resistance, and hyperandrogenism upon steroidogenesis and the ovaries. Menstrual disturbances, anovulation, and infertility are more common in obese patients with polycystic ovary syndrome than in non-obese patients that have the syndrome. Risk factors for infertility include abnormal cervical mucus, decreased ovarian reserve, ovulatory dysfunction, tubal dysfunction, abnormal sperm, and pelvic lesions.

For some people, infertility can be prevented by maintaining a healthy weight, quitting smoking, avoiding alcohol, and reducing stress. The pathogenesis of infertility has different processes between males and females. In males, it involves a decrease in sperm count, blockages that prevent sperm from being released, sperm that have abnormal function, and genetic diseases (**Klinefelter syndrome**, **Noonan syndrome**, and chromosome Y deletions). In females, the pathogenesis of infertility involves more factors, which include the following:

- A fertilized egg or embryo does not survive once it adheres to the lining of the uterus
- The fertilized egg does not attach to the lining of the uterus
- The eggs cannot move from the ovaries to the uterus
- The ovaries cannot produce eggs normally
- There is a hormonal imbalance (hyperprolactinemia, hypothyroidism, diabetes mellitus, or polycystic ovary syndrome)

The treatment of infertility is based on the cause, the length of time being infertile, the age of the patients, and personal preferences. Some causes of infertility cannot be corrected. For men, treatments include changing lifestyle factors, medications, surgery, and sperm retrieval. Lifestyle factors include discontinuing certain medications, reducing or eliminating harmful substance intake, improving the frequency and timing of intercourse, regular exercise, and optimizing any factors that could impair fertility. Certain medications can improve sperm count and the likelihood for achieving a successful pregnancy. They may increase testicular function, including sperm production and quality. For some conditions, surgery can reverse sperm blockages and restore fertility. In others, surgically repairing a **varicocele** may improve chances for pregnancy. Sperm retrieval techniques obtain sperm when ejaculation is a problem, or when no sperm are present in the ejaculated fluid. They can also be used when assisted reproductive techniques are planned, and when sperm counts are low or abnormal.

For females, sometimes only a few therapies are needed to improve fertility, while other women may need several different types of treatment. The three basic techniques include stimulating ovulation with fertility drugs, **intrauterine insemination**, and surgery to restore fertility. Fertility drugs are the primary treatment for women who are infertile because of ovulation disorders. These medications regulate or induce ovulation. During intrauterine insemination, healthy sperm are placed directly in the uterus around the time the ovary releases the eggs to be fertilized. The timing of this procedure can be coordinated with the normal cycle, or with fertility medications. Uterine problems such as endometrial polyps, a uterine septum, intrauterine scar tissue, and some uterine fibroids can be treated with hysteroscopic surgery. **Endometriosis**, pelvic adhesions, and larger fibroids may require laparoscopic surgery.

Test Your Knowledge

1. How much more common is infertility in obese compared to non-obese women?
2. What is the pathogenesis of infertility in women?
3. What are the three basic therapeutic techniques for women dealing with infertility?

PREGNANCY COMPLICATIONS

Being obese during pregnancy results in many complications. It can cause loss of pregnancy, and obese women have a higher risk of miscarriage compared with women of normal weight. Obesity increases risks for birth defects. Babies born to obese women have an increased risk for heart defects and neural tube defects such as *spina bifida*. Also, excessive body fat during pregnancy can make it harder to visualize certain problems with the baby's anatomy in ultrasound exams. It may be harder to check the baby's heart rate during pregnancy and labor. Obesity complications include macrosomia, in which the baby is larger than normal. This increases risks for injury to the infant during birth. A shoulder can become stuck, causing structural and nerve damage. Macrosomia increases risks for cesarean delivery. Infants born with excessive body fat have a greater chance of future obesity as well. Pregnancy complications may lead to a medically indicated preterm birth, in delivery occurs earlier than normal for medical reasons. Since preterm babies are not as fully developed, there is an increased risk of short-term and long-term health problems. The higher a woman's body mass index, the greater the risk of stillbirth.

Impact of Obesity on Pregnancy

Obesity during pregnancy puts a woman at risk for serious health problems: gestational diabetes, **preeclampsia**, **eclampsia**, and sleep apnea. A woman who is short in height and has increased BMI is more likely to have a difficult labor. The World Health Organization has estimated that 60% of women between 20 and 40 are overweight or obese. More than 50% of pregnant women in the United States are overweight or obese, with 8% of woman in their reproductive years being *extremely* obese. According to the National Health and Nutrition Examination Survey (NHANES), this group is rapidly increasing in number. Obstetricians counsel patients about all factors related to obesity during pregnancy, including educating them about how obesity reduces the likelihood of actually becoming pregnant, and of maintaining a healthy and normal pregnancy. Preconception efforts must reduce or prevent fetal exposures to harmful *in utero* factors.

Between 25% and 35% of children from obese mothers are obese by age 11. They have a higher chance for metabolic syndrome, which involves obesity, dyslipidemia, hypertension, and glucose intolerance. Female children of obese mothers have an increased risk for many morbidities. Maternal obesity alters molecular structures of the oocytes. It also changes epigenetic reprogramming during conception, causing negative outcomes in embryonic and fetal development. In extremely obese women, 46.3% have chronic or gestational hypertensive diseases, or preeclampsia. About 31.8% have progestational or gestational diabetes.

In order to assess pregnancy in an obese patient, invasive, transvaginal evaluation is required, since early pregnancy (before 18 weeks) may be compromised. It is often difficult to completely survey the fetus, even with follow-up examinations. Some parts of the fetus are often not fully visualized throughout the entire pregnancy, and malformations or other defects may be unseen. Bariatric obstetrics is extremely challenging. Obese women nearing their third trimesters have a higher risk for intrauterine fetal death and altered fetal growth. Accurate serial fetal ultrasound procedures in late pregnancy are difficult in obese patients due to acoustic shadowing. Sometimes, the vaginal transducer is placed in the mother's navel, since the abdominal wall is thinner at this point. The patient may be required to change positions on the examination table in order to fully image the fetus, or may need to undergo transvaginal-trans-abdominal combination procedures.

In labor, obese women often have problems that are rare in non-obese women. There may be complications with anesthesia, or C-section delivery problems. The infant is at a higher risk for requiring resuscitation and intensive care unit treatment. Complications may continue into the postpartum period, with obese mothers experiencing hemorrhage, surgical site infections, and abnormal blood clotting. This makes recovery after delivery more prolonged, reducing the mother's ability to properly care for her infant. Chronic inflammation due to obesity may affect functioning of the placenta, which can affect development, growth, and maturity of the fetus. If uncorrected early in gestation, gene expression can be affected.

Obesity increases the risks for other complications, including miscarriage, stillbirth, recurrent miscarriage, and cardiac dysfunction. The baby may be much larger than normal, have excess body fat, and have a higher risk for birth defects. It is important that pregnant women understand how to avoid the impacts of obesity by gaining the appropriate amount of weight. For a single embryo, this means gaining 11–20 pounds. For multiple embryos, the recommended weight gain is 25–42 pounds. It is important not to gain or lose weight too quickly during pregnancy, since this increases risks for premature birth, and for the infant being less than the 10th percentile for gestational age.

Specialized care for obese mothers includes early testing for gestational diabetes, special accommodations for fetal ultrasound procedures, and screening for obstructive sleep apnea. A glucose challenge test is often recommended at the first prenatal visit for an obese woman, and is usually repeated between weeks 24 and 28 of pregnancy. If the results are abnormal, additional tests will be needed. The healthcare provider will advise about blood sugar monitoring and control. Since obesity during pregnancy can interfere with the effectiveness of fetal ultrasound, there may be a need for an experienced sonographer, repeated examinations, or more advanced equipment. If obstructive sleep apnea is suspected, the patient may be referred to a sleep medicine specialist.

FOCUS ON OBESITY DURING PREGNANCY

Despite excessive caloric intake, many obese women are deficient in the vitamins that are vital to a healthy pregnancy. For example, 40% are deficient in iron, 24% in folic acid, and 4% in vitamin B12. Respiratory disease due to obesity, including asthma and obstructive sleep apnea, increases risks for non-pulmonary pregnancy complications, such as cesarean delivery and preeclampsia.

Test Your Knowledge

1. What pregnancy complications are related to obesity?
2. What serious health problems can happen to an obese woman during pregnancy?
3. During labor, what problems can occur in relation to obesity?

SOCIAL AND PSYCHOLOGICAL PROBLEMS

Obesity is a physical, social, and psychological problem. The causative basis of obesity and eating disorders includes combinations of psychosocial, environmental, genetic, and biological attributes. Those with depression and anxiety may have more difficulty in controlling food consumption, and in exercising sufficiently. In many obese people, there is a continual cycle of mood disturbances, overeating, and weight gain. A continuous pattern of using food to cope with stress and emotions may appear. Society views obesity with extreme negativity. Obese people are regularly labeled as lacking willpower and being unmotivated to improve their health. They also experience workplace discrimination.

Adults with excess weight have a 55% higher risk of developing depression over their lifetimes compared to people that do not struggle with obesity. Obesity-related anxiety is up to 1.4 times more likely to occur than anxiety occurring in those who are not obese. Individuals are 1.5 times more likely to develop a mood disorder if they are obese. Global statistics on obesity-related depression ranges between 1.27 and 1.55 times more likely than depression in people that are not obese.

Losing weight can have a significant impact upon mental health and wellbeing, including greater self-esteem and being less self-conscious. One major mental block to weight loss is the desire to lose weight too much and too fast. Weight loss is simply "too slow" for most obese people. The prevention of social and psychological problems in the obese requires setting realistic goals, staying committed to weight loss, identifying inner motivations, monitoring signals from the body, being accountable, creating meal plans that fit lifestyles, reassessing exercise, and remembering to stay patient.

Obesity is associated with increased cases of anxiety, major depression, bipolar disorder, and panic disorder. Insulin resistance is an important contributor, linked not only to obesity, but also to most chronic diseases, including psychological problems. A diet that nourishes the gut microbiome reduces insulin resistance and optimizes mitochondrial function. Dietary sugar does the opposite. High-sugar diets actually encourage depression and anxiety. An individual consuming a high-sugar, processed food diet develops insulin resistance, paving the way for fat accumulation and type 2 diabetes. Sugar is extremely inflammatory, and chronic inflammation is a major factor for depression. Since the brain requires excessive energy for normal function, even a slight reduction in its fuel supply results in impairment, and therefore, a depressed mood.

OBESITY AND CANCER

Excessive body fat contributes to more than 100,500 yearly cases of cancer as well as 14%–20% of all cancer deaths in the United States. Excess body fat is estimated to be related to more than 33,000 postmenopausal breast cancers; 20,700 endometrial cancers; 13,900 kidney cancers; 13,200 colorectal cancers; 11,900 pancreatic cancers; 5,800 esophageal cancers; and 2,000 gallbladder cancers – annually in the United States. Not all subgroups are equally affected. For example, obese men have a higher risk for colon cancer than obese women. Obesity increases risks for breast cancer in postmenopausal women, but not in those who are not yet menopausal. This may be due to adipose tissue being the primary source of estrogen following menopause.

Breast Cancer

Breast cancer is the second most common cancer in women in the United States. The breast is mostly comprised of fat and glandular tissues. There are complicated networks of sac-like lobules, called *milk glands*, and ducts conveying the breast milk from the lobules to the nipple openings during breastfeeding. There are 15–20 distinctive clusters of lobules in each breast, called *breast lobes*. Each breast lobe has 20–40 *lobules*. Breast cancer usually involves the glandular cells of the ducts or lobules. Patients commonly present with an asymptomatic mass that is found during examination or mammography. Most breast lumps are benign, do not spread outside of the breast, and are not life threatening. However, some benign breast lumps increase risks of developing malignant breast cancer.

Worldwide, breast cancer is the most common invasive cancer in women. It makes up 22.9% of invasive cancers, and 16% of all female cancers. The average amount of deaths from breast cancer is over 450,000 annually. There is a one in eight chance of developing breast cancer. Incidence varies widely around the world. It is lowest in less-developed countries and highest in more-developed countries. Highest incidence is in North America (90 of every 100,000 women), followed by Western Europe (78 of every 100,000). Lowest incidence is in Eastern Asia (18 of every 100,000). Figure 9.5 illustrates the global incidence rates of breast cancer in 2018.

According to the American Cancer Society, in the United States, breast cancer is the second leading cause of cancer death, after lung cancer, in Caucasian, African-American, Asian/Pacific Islander, and American Indian/Alaska Native women. However, in Hispanic women, breast cancer is the leading cause of cancer death. Approximately 253,000 new cases of invasive breast cancer, with 41,000 deaths, occurred in 2017. Also, about 63,000 new cases of in situ breast cancer occurred. Though YLD and DALYs concerning breast cancer are inaccurate, the large range in total costs for treatment is significant. Overall costs are above $3 billion in the United States, over $143 million in Asia, and over $68 million in Africa. Per treated patient, costs begin at an average of $24,008.

The actual causes of breast cancer are unclear. The epidemic of obesity is linked to female breast cancer and benign tumors. It is highly important to maintain a healthy body mass index. In the United States, the cumulative risk of developing breast cancer is about 12%, with much of the risk focused on those over age 60. However, this data is misleading because it is based on risks *up to age 95*, and most people do not live that long. The cumulative risk of developing breast cancer in a 20-year period is much lower. The risk of dying from breast cancer is about 9% within five years after diagnosis. Risk factors for breast cancer include age, family history, gene mutations, personal and gynecologic history, breast changes, lobular carcinoma in situ (LCIS), use of oral contraceptives, hormone and radiation therapy, diet, and lifestyle factors.

The strongest risk factor is age, since most breast cancers occur in women older than 50. Having a first-degree

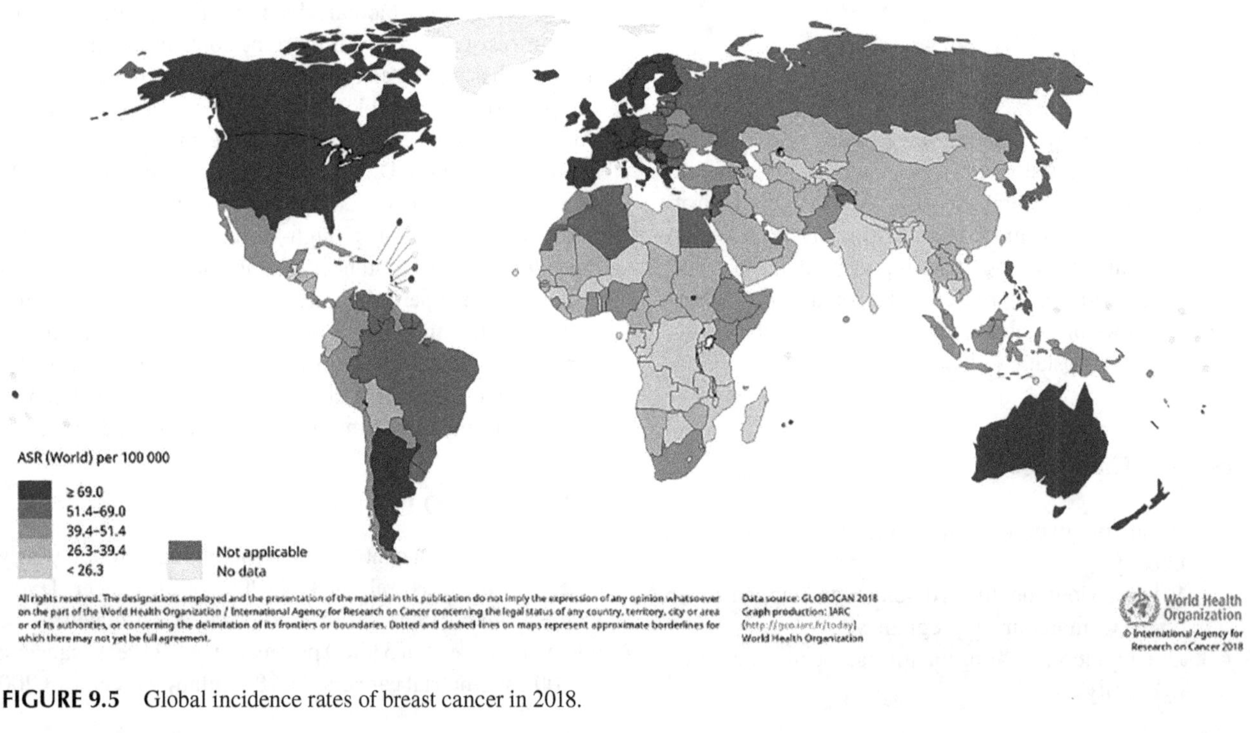

FIGURE 9.5 Global incidence rates of breast cancer in 2018.

relative (mother, sister, or daughter) with breast cancer doubles or triples the risks. However, breast cancer in more distant relatives only increases risk slightly. If two or more first-degree relatives have breast cancer, the risk may be five to six times higher. Between 5% and 10% of women with breast cancer have mutated genes. If a relative also carries one of these mutations, there is a 50%–85% lifetime risk of developing breast cancer. For gene mutations, there is also a 20%–40% lifetime risk of developing ovarian cancer. For those without a family history of breast cancer in two or more first-degree relatives, there is a low likelihood of carrying gene mutation.

A patient who has had in situ or invasive breast cancer also has an increased risk. The risk of cancer developing in the opposite breast after mastectomy is about 0.5%–1% per year of follow-up. Risks are increased by early menarche, late menopause, or a late first pregnancy. Women with their first pregnancy occurring after age 30 are at higher risk than those who have no children. Any history of a lesion requiring biopsy slightly increases risks. Women with multiple breast masses, but no histologic confirmation of high-risk patterns, are not considered to be high risk. Benign lesions that can slightly increase risks for invasive breast cancer include complex fibroadenoma, moderate or florid hyperplasia with or without atypia, papilloma, and sclerosing adenosis. Risks are about four to five times higher if the patient has atypical ductal or lobular hyperplasia. They are ten times higher if the patient also has family history of invasive breast cancer in a first-degree relative. Risks are also increased if increased breast density is seen during mammography.

LCIS increases risks for invasive carcinoma of either breast by approximately 25 times. Invasive carcinoma develops in 1%–2% of patients with LCIS annually. Use of oral contraceptives increases risks by about five cases per every 100,000 women. This is mostly during the years of contraceptive use, and tapers off during the ten years after stopping. Risks are highest in women who started using contraceptives before age 20, but absolute risks are still extremely low. Postmenopausal hormone therapy, with an estrogen plus a progestin, is believed to increase risk modestly, after three years of use. After five years of use, increased risk is about seven to eight cases per 10,000 women for each year of use, which is approximately a 24% increase in relative risk. Using estrogen alone does not appear to increase risk of breast cancer. Using raloxifene and other selective estrogen-receptor modulators reduces risks.

Risks for breast cancer are increased by exposure to radiation therapy before age 30. Mantle-field radiation therapy, for Hodgkin's lymphoma, nearly quadruples risks over the following 20–30 years. Diet can contribute to development or growth of breast cancer, though exactly which diet has not been proven. Obese postmenopausal women have a higher risk, but dietary modification has not been shown to reduce risk. Risks may be decreased in obese women who are menstruating later than is normal. Smoking and alcohol contribute to a higher risk of breast cancer, and women are instructed to stop smoking completely, and limit alcohol consumption. A woman's five-year and lifetime risk of developing breast cancer is calculated with the *Breast Cancer Risk Assessment Tool*, also known as the *Gail model*. This tool uses medical and reproductive history along with history among mother, sisters, or daughters to estimate absolute risks. It is accurate for Caucasian, African-American, Hispanic, and Asian/Pacific Islander women in the United States. However, it can underestimate risks in African-American women who have had previous biopsies, and in Hispanic women born outside the country. Data on American Indian/Alaska Native women are limited, so risk estimates are partly based on Caucasian women's data, and may not be highly accurate. The tool cannot accurately estimate risks for women with previous history of invasive or in situ breast cancer. Some higher-risk women do not develop breast cancer, while some lower-risk women do.

There is no sure way to prevent breast cancer, but there are ways to lower the risks for the disease. These include attaining and maintaining a healthy weight, being physically active, avoiding or limiting alcohol, choosing to breastfeed infants for at least several months after childbirth, and when possible, avoiding hormone therapy after menopause. For women at increased risk of breast cancer, options include genetic counseling and testing for breast cancer risks, medications that lower risks, prophylactic surgery, and close observations to monitor for early signs of breast cancer. Genetic counseling is indicated for women with a strong family history of breast cancer, or with a family member with a known breast cancer-related gene mutation.

Development of the disease involves breast pain or enlargement, or thickening. Paget's disease of the nipple causes erythema, crusting, scaling, and discharge that usually begin very benignly, and are often ignored. This can delay diagnosis for a year or even more. About half of patients have a palpable mass when first examined. Some patients with breast cancer show signs of metastatic disease, including pathologic fractures or pulmonary dysfunction. Often, physical examination reveals asymmetry or a mass that is very different from surrounding breast tissue. Benign disorders are usually signified by diffuse, fibrotic changes in a breast quadrant (most often the upper, outer quadrant). A slightly firmer thickening in one breast, but not in the other, may be an indicator of cancer.

Advanced breast cancers are characterized by one or more of the following: fixation of the mass to the chest wall or overlying skin, satellite nodules or ulcers of the skin, or exaggeration of common skin markings due to skin edema (via invasion of dermal lymphatic vessels). Inflammatory breast cancer is indicated by **peau d'orange**, erythema, and breast enlargement (often without a mass). Nipple discharge is common, and inflammatory breast cancer is exceedingly aggressive. The treatment of breast cancer is based on the type and the degree of the cancer spreading. Often, more than one type of treatment is used. Options include surgery, chemotherapy, hormonal therapy, biological therapy, and radiation therapy.

FOCUS ON OBESITY AND BREAST CANCER

The prevalence of obesity and metabolic syndrome among US women aged 60 years and older has increased. The rise of obesity is significantly associated with a higher postmenopausal breast cancer risk.

FOCUS ON OBESITY AND CANCER

Being obese is linked to a higher risk of getting 13 types of cancer, which make up 40% of all cancer diagnosed annually. These include meningioma, adenocarcinoma of the esophagus, multiple myeloma, kidney, uterine, ovarian, thyroid, breast, liver, gallbladder, upper stomach, pancreatic, and colon cancers.

Test Your Knowledge

1. How much more common are social and psychological problems in obese individuals?
2. What are the statistics between obesity and cancer?
3. What are advanced breast cancers signified by?

Uterine Cancer

Endometrial carcinoma is most often an **endometrioid adenocarcinoma**. It is usually signified by vaginal bleeding after menopause has occurred. This cancer is staged via surgical procedures. It begins in the endometrial lining of the uterus, and is often detected early since it frequently produces abnormal vaginal bleeding. If discovered early, removal of the uterus is quite often curative. The upper two-thirds of the uterus, above the internal orifice, is described as the *corpus*. Cancer of the corpus uteri is additionally referred to as endometrial cancer.

Worldwide, more than 287,000 women are diagnosed with endometrial carcinoma annually. As prevalence of metabolic syndrome increases, this cancer is anticipated to become more common. Incidence has been rising in most countries, which is believed to be linked to rising rates of obesity, having fewer children, and delaying childbirth until later in life. Endometrial carcinoma is more common in developed countries with diets that are high in fat. In the United States, endometrial carcinoma is the fourth most common female cancer. It accounts for 6% of all cancers in women, and is the most common gynecologic malignancy. About one in 40 women will develop endometrial cancer. Approximately 62,000 new cases are diagnosed each year, and over 12,250 cases are fatal. This type of cancer is most common in perimenopausal and postmenopausal women. The mean age at diagnosis is 63 years. The majority of cases are diagnosed between age 50 and 60, and 92% of cases occur in women older than age 50. It rarely develops before the age of 40 (in less than 5% of women). Caucasian women are affected more than any other racial or ethnic group. The YLD and DALYs regarding endometrial carcinoma are uncertain, and cost impacts are not well documented.

The major risk factors for endometrial cancer include age over 50, obesity, and diabetes mellitus. Additional risk factors include use of tamoxifen for five or more years, receiving previous pelvic radiation therapy, personal or family history of breast or ovarian cancer, family history of hereditary non-polyposis colorectal cancer, and hypertension. Unopposed estrogen involves high circulating levels of estrogen, with no progesterone or low levels of progesterone. This may be in relation to obesity, nulliparity, polycystic ovary syndrome, estrogen-producing tumors, late menopause, anovulation, and estrogen therapy without progesterone.

Over 90% of women with endometrial carcinoma have abnormal uterine bleeding, such as postmenopausal bleeding, or premenopausal recurrent metrorrhagia. About 33% of women with postmenopausal bleeding are found to endometrial carcinoma. Vaginal discharge may occur weeks or months prior to postmenopausal bleeding. Additional signs and symptoms include bleeding between periods and pelvic pain.

There are several methods of treatment for uterine cancer, including surgery, radiation, and/or chemotherapy. There is no way to prevent uterine cancer, but methods that can reduce risks include use of birth control pills, maintaining a healthy weight, being physically active, and if taking estrogen, adding progesterone.

Test Your Knowledge

1. Is the increased incidence of uterine cancer linked to the increasing rates of obesity?
2. What are the major risk factors for endometrial cancer?
3. What preventive measures may reduce these risks?

Gallbladder Cancer

Gallbladder tumors, plus bile duct tumors, can cause extrahepatic biliary obstruction. Nearly all are adenocarcinomas. Papillary adenocarcinoma is a rare type of adenocarcinoma that has cells with finger-like projections. Papillary cancers are generally less likely to spread to the liver or lymph nodes, and have a better prognosis than most other types of gallbladder adenocarcinomas. Gallbladder tumors may also be adenosquamous carcinomas, squamous cell carcinomas, and carcinosarcomas, but these are rarer. **Cholangiocarcinomas** form in bile ducts that connect the gallbladder to the liver. They may be described as *intrahepatic*, *hilar*, or *distal*.

Cholangiocarcinomas and other bile duct tumors occur in one to two of every 100,000 individuals, but are usually malignant. *Gallbladder carcinoma* occurs in 2.5 of every 100,000 individuals, mostly in American Indians, patients with gallstones larger than 3 centimeters, and those with significant gallbladder calcification due to chronic cholecystitis. Between 70% and 90% of patients also have gallstones. Most people who develop cholangiocarcinomas are over age 50, but these tumors can develop at any age. Compared to people of normal weight, individuals who are overweight have about a 20% higher chance for gallbladder cancer. However, obese people have a 60% increase in this risk, and the risk increase is greater in women than in men.

Gallbladder cancer is not fully understood, but chronic inflammation and irritation of the gallbladder are believed to influence the development of tumors. Risk factors for cholangiocarcinomas include obesity, old age, primary sclerosing cholangitis, choledochal cysts, and infestation with liver flukes. Other risks include chronic liver disease, bile duct abnormalities that have been present since birth, and smoking.

Gallbladder cancer is the result of persistent irritation of the gallbladder mucosa over a period of years. This predisposes an individual to malignant transformations or acts as an enhancer for carcinogenic exposure. The primary mechanism involves cholelithiasis, leading to cholecystitis, and appears to be the strongest pathogenic force, though gallbladder cancer is strongly related to gallstone disease, the female gender, and an age above 65 years.

Gallbladder cancer has various treatment options based on staging. If localized (stage 1), the cancer is in the wall of the gallbladder and can be completely removed by surgery. Stage 1 (unresectable) cancer cannot be removed completely by surgery. Unfortunately, most patients with gallbladder cancer have unresectable cancer. Recurrent (stage 3) gallbladder cancer may appear in the gallbladder or in other parts of the body. Metastatic (stage 4) gallbladder cancer may appear in surrounding tissues, organs, the abdominal cavity, or in distant areas of the body.

The treatment gallbladder cancers include cholecystectomy, radiation therapy, targeted therapy, and immunotherapy. There is no known way to prevent most gallbladder cancers since risk factors such as age, gender, ethnicity, and bile duct defects are beyond our control. Methods of reducing risk factors include attaining and maintaining a healthy weight, keeping physically active, limiting the time spend sitting or lying down, following a healthy diet with plenty of fruits, vegetables, and whole grains (limiting red and processed meats, sugary drinks, and highly processed foods), plus avoiding alcohol.

Test Your Knowledge

1. What is the most common type of gallbladder cancer?
2. Do overweight or obese people have a higher chance of developing gallbladder cancer?
3. What does gallbladder cancer result from?

Pancreatic Cancer

Most forms of pancreatic cancer involve exocrine tumors, developing from ductal and acinar cells. Adenocarcinomas of the exocrine pancreas develop from duct cells nine times more often than from the acinar cells. About 80% occur in the head of the pancreas. The disease is rare before age 40, and is most common in people older than 70. Approximately 12% of all pancreatic cancers are attributed to being overweight or obese. Obese women carrying most of their excess weight around their waist instead of their hips have a 70% higher chance or developing pancreatic cancer.

Globally, about 338,000 people have pancreatic cancer, making it the 11th most common cancer overall. Of these, about 331,000 cases are fatal. The American Cancer Society's estimates for pancreatic cancer in the United States, are nearly 57,000 cases and over 46,000 deaths. Prevalence is estimated to be one in 64 people. The highest incidence and mortality rates are in developed countries. Trends for incidence and mortality are varied widely on a global scale. The overall five-year survival rate is about 5% (ranging between 2% and 9% between developed and developing countries). The highest incidence is in North America and Western Europe, with the lowest rates in Middle Africa and South-Central Asia.

Adenocarcinomas appear at a mean age of 55 years. They occur 1.5–2 times as often in men compared to women. About 1.6% of the population will be diagnosed with pancreatic cancer at some point in life. Overall, pancreatic cancer ranks as the seventh leading cause of cancer death for both genders in the United States. While YLD and DALYs concerning pancreatic cancer are not accurate, mean total direct medical costs average $66,000 per patient, with mean total costs greater when there is resectable localized disease, at $135,000, than unresectable localized or distant disease (see Chapter 16).

Colon Cancer

Colon cancer is also commonly referred to as *colorectal cancer*. It is extremely common, with more than 50% of cases affecting the rectum and sigmoid colon. About 95% are adenocarcinomas. Insulin is the main biochemical mediator between obesity and colon cancer. Hyperinsulinemia is important in relation to the pathogenesis of colon cancer. Visceral abdominal fat is clearly linked to higher incidence of colon cancer. Obesity results in a higher risk of colon cancer for men of all ages, and for premenopausal women, but not for postmenopausal women. Direct radiographic evaluation of visceral abdominal fat may be the most accurate predictor for colon cancer, used in conjunction with measurement of BMI.

Colon cancers are a major cause of morbidity and mortality throughout the world, accounting for over 9% of all cancers. Colon cancer is the third most common cancer worldwide, and the fourth most common cause of death, affecting men and women almost equally. The American Cancer Society's estimate for colon cancer in the United States is approximately 135,000 new cases. Overall lifetime risk is about one in 22 men, and one in 24 women. There are more than one million people living with this type of cancer in the United States. Countries with the highest incidence include Australia and New Zealand, while countries with the lowest incidence include China and India. Worldwide statistics reveal that colon cancer represents about 9.4% of all cancers in men, and approximately 10.1% of all cancers in women.

Colon cancer accounts for more than 50,000 deaths in United States every year. Incidence increases sharply around ages 40–50. In 5% of patients, more than one other type of cancer occurs simultaneously. There are no accurate figures on YLD with colon cancer. However, colon cancer makes up about 0.38% of all DALYs, and 7.2% of DALYs due to malignant neoplasms. Costs of colon cancer interventions generally begin at around $14,000 and increase based on the severity of the malignancy. The global incidence rates of colorectal cancer for 2018 are depicted in Figure 9.6.

Colon cancer usually occurs as a transformation of adenomatous polyps. Most (80%) cases are sporadic, with the rest being inherited. Predisposing factors include chronic ulcerative colitis and Crohn's disease. The risk for developing colon cancer increases the longer that these disorders are present. In populations with a high incidence of colon cancer, the diets are usually high in animal protein, fat, and refined carbohydrates, but low in fiber. Though carcinogens can be ingested, they are usually produced by bacterial action upon dietary substances, or upon biliary or intestinal secretions.

Treatment for colon cancer usually involves surgical removal. If the cancer is very small, a minimally invasive approach can be used. This may involve removing polyps during a colonoscopy, endoscopic mucosal resection, and laparoscopic surgery. For more advanced colon cancer, options include partial **colectomy**, surgery to create a port so that feces can leave the body, and lymph node removal. If the cancer is extremely advanced or overall health is very poor, surgery can be done to relieve colon blockage or other conditions that cause bleeding or pain. Other treatment options include chemotherapy, radiation therapy, targeted therapy, immunotherapy, and palliative care.

There is no proven method of preventing colon cancer. However, regular screening is a powerful tool that may help catch the disease early. It allows for polyps to be found and removed before they have enough time to become cancerous. Screening can also find colon cancer when it is small and easier to treat. Screening should begin at age 45. People with a strong family history of colon polyps or cancer may benefit from genetic counseling to determine if there is a family cancer syndrome. Risks for colon cancer can be lowered by weight management, physical activity, and diet. Little or no alcohol consumption is beneficial, and smoking should be stopped.

FOCUS ON OBESITY AND COLON CANCER

Compared to people of normal weight, obese men have about a 50% higher risk of colon cancer. Obese women have about a 10% higher risk for the disease than non-obese women. Excess risk is also linked to higher abdominal fat, measured by waist circumference or the waist-to-hip ratio, and fat stored in the abdominal cavity.

Test Your Knowledge

1. What is the main biochemical mediator between obesity and colon cancer?
2. In populations with a high incidence of colon cancer, what do the diets consist of?
3. What is the most common treatment for colon cancer?

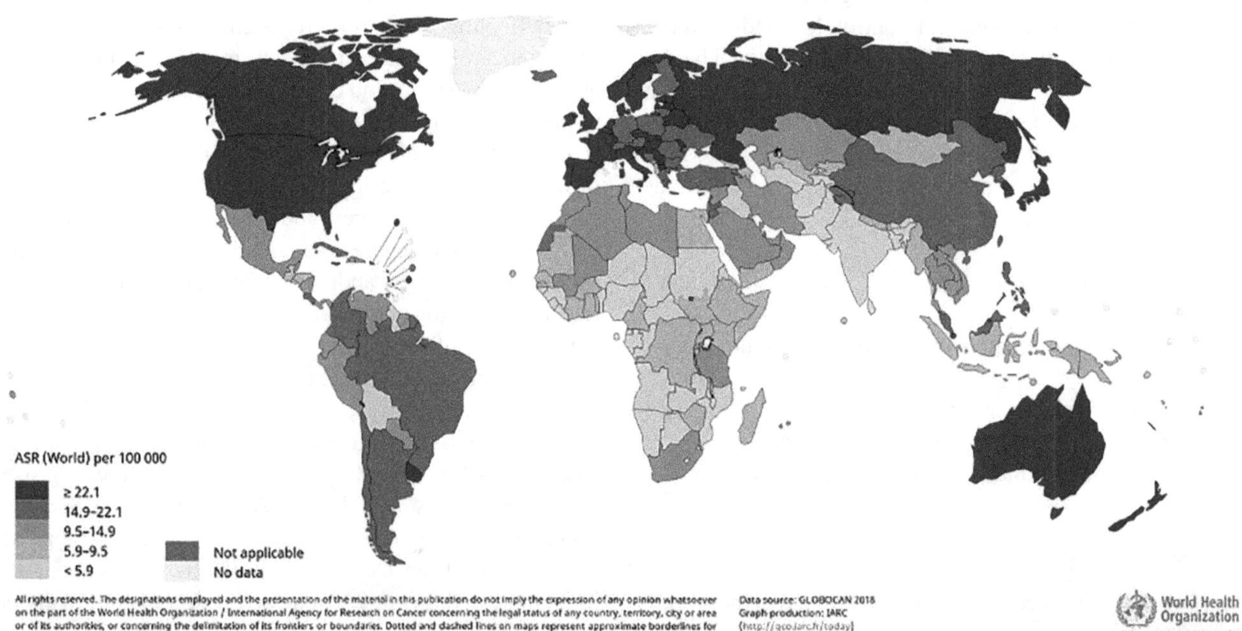

FIGURE 9.6 Estimated age-standardized incidence rates of colorectal cancer in women of all ages in 2018.

KEY TERMS

Abrasion
Acromegaly
Adenotonsillar hypertrophy
Adhesins
Amenorrhea
Apnea
Asherman syndrome
Asthma
Candida albicans
Candidiasis
Cellulitis
Cholangiocarcinomas
Chondrocytes
Colectomy
Dermatomyositis
Down syndrome
Dysmenorrhea
Eclampsia
Eczema
Endometrioid adenocarcinoma
Endometriosis
Erythrasma
Gestational diabetes
Heberden nodes
Hematocolpos
Hematometra
Hypha
Hypopnea
Infertility
Intrauterine insemination
Invasins
Klinefelter syndrome
Leukemia
Liposuction
Lymphedema
Myasthenia gravis
Myotonic dystrophy
Necrotizing cellulitis
Neutropenia
Noonan syndrome
Obesity paradox
Oocyte
Ovarian follicular
Paronychia
Polycystic ovary syndrome
Preeclampsia
Prolactin
Prophylaxis
Psoriasis
Pulsatility
Sleep apnea
Thigmotropism
Tonsillectomy
Uterine fibroids
Varicocele

CLINICAL CASE STUDIES

Clinical Case Study 1

An obese 64-year-old man was taken to the local hospital because of chest pain. He had previously experienced exertional chest tightness and mild shortness of breath after only minimal physical activity. These symptoms did not occur at rest. The patient has a history of type 2 diabetes and hypertension. He quit smoking 25 years ago. Tests reveal high LDL cholesterol and triglycerides as well as total cholesterol. An exercise test to evaluate his myocardial perfusion has to be stopped after 8 minutes due to chest pain and leg fatigue. The patient's signs and symptoms are highly indicative of peripheral arterial disease, and most patients with this condition have significant coronary artery disease as well. Treatment for his condition begins immediately.

CRITICAL THINKING QUESTIONS

1. How does obesity lead to cardiovascular disorders?
2. Which cardiovascular disorders are complications of obesity?
3. If this patient eventually requires surgery, how is his obesity potentially linked to postoperative complications?

Clinical Case Study 2

An obese 24-year-old man was assessed for symptoms of snoring, orthopnea, and restless sleep patterns. He complained of dyspnea, easy tiredness, extreme exercise intolerance, and poor self-esteem. The man's mother was morbidly obese. Obstructive sleep apnea was suspected for the man. He was prescribed a CPAP machine and discharged. Over one year of follow-up, the patient complained of headache, poor work performance, and progressive weight gain. He was determined to be a good candidate for bariatric surgery, and a laparoscopic sleeve gastrostomy operation was performed successfully. After one year, the patient's weight had dropped significantly, and the sleep apnea had completely resolved.

CRITICAL THINKING QUESTIONS

1. What is the most common form of sleep apnea, and what is it characterized by?
2. How much do weight increases and decreases affect sleep apnea?
3. What are the causes and complicating factors of obstructive sleep apnea?

Clinical Case Study 3

A 69-year-old obese woman found a lump in her left breast. She had a history of hypertension and a 25-year history of smoking one pack of cigarettes per day. Her sister recently had a lumpectomy with radiation therapy, and her mother and aunt died from breast cancer when they were in their 60s. The patient states she has too much stress in her life and cannot quit smoking. A bilateral mammogram and ultrasound are performed, revealing a 4 cm mass in her left breast. A core needle biopsy reveals it to be an infiltrating lobular carcinoma. A lumpectomy and axial lymph node dissection are performed, and six of the nodes are positive for cancer. Further treatment options are then discussed.

CRITICAL THINKING QUESTIONS

1. How common is breast cancer and what does it usually involve?
2. How fatal is breast cancer?
3. How does having a first-degree relative with breast cancer affect the risks of it developing?

STUDY QUESTIONS

1. The obesity paradox coexists with which of the following disorders?
   A. Renal failure
   B. Hepatic failure
   C. Heart failure
   D. Gastric cancer

2. Which of the following countries has the highest percentages of people with osteoarthritis?
   A. Thailand
   B. Iran
   C. Australia
   D. Israel

3. Which of the following gastrointestinal problems are linked to obesity?
   A. Hepatitis infection
   B. Esophagitis
   C. Mouth ulcers
   D. Gastroesophageal reflux disease

4. Which of the following describes paronychia?
   A. A bacterial infection of the eyelids
   B. A candidal nail infection
   C. An infection of the cheek
   D. An infection of the mucous membranes

5. Which of the following microorganisms is the most common cause of cellulitis?
   A. Coronavirus
   B. *Escherichia coli*
   C. Staphylococci
   D. *Pseudomonas*

6. Which of the following is associated with central sleep apnea?
   A. Blood oxygen saturation is reduced
   B. Complete obstruction of the upper airway
   C. It occurs only in elderly people
   D. Blood oxygen saturation is increased

7. In obese people, sleep apnea may be linked to all of the following endocrine disorders, EXCEPT:
   A. Polycystic ovary syndrome
   B. Acromegaly
   C. Hyperthyroidism
   D. Hypothyroidism

8. Obesity may increase risks for all of the following conditions or disorders, EXCEPT:
   A. Miscarriage
   B. Gestational diabetes
   C. Hypotension
   D. Fetal abnormalities

9. Which of the following hormones stimulates milk production?
   A. Prolactin
   B. Growth hormone
   C. Insulin
   D. Gastrin

10. Which of the following is NOT a complication of obesity in pregnant women?
    A. Macrosomia
    B. Miscarriage
    C. Birth defects
    D. Liver disease

11. Which of the following mental disorders is NOT associated with obesity?
    A. Depression
    B. Schizophrenia
    C. Anxiety
    D. Panic disorder

12. Which of the following is NOT a major risk factor for endometrial cancer?
    A. Obesity
    B. Diabetes mellitus
    C. Hyperthyroidism
    D. Family history

13. Which of the following hormones is the main biochemical mediator between obesity and colon cancer?
    A. Insulin
    B. Glucagon
    C. Growth hormone
    D. Gastrin

14. Which of the following is the cause of gallbladder cancer?
    A. Irritable bowel syndrome
    B. Gastritis
    C. Viral hepatitis C
    D. The actual cause is unknown

15. Which of the following increases the risk of breast cancer in obese women?
    A. History of eclampsia
    B. History of dysmenorrhea
    C. History of late pregnancy
    D. Being postmenopausal

FURTHER READING

1. Angrisani, L., De luca, M., Formisano, G., and Santonicola, A. (2017). *Bariatric and Metabolic Surgery – Indications, Complications, and Revisional Procedures (Updates in Surgery).* Springer.
2. Banks, D. (2017). *Quadruple Threat: Obesity, Sleep Apnea, Diabetes, and Heart Disease.* Timely Publishing.
3. Crum, C.P., Nucci, M.R., Howitt, B.E., Granter, S.R., Parast, M.M., Boyd, T., Haefner, K.R., and Peters, W.A. (2017). *Diagnostic Gynecologic and Obstetric Pathology*, 3rd Edition. Elsevier.
4. Dannenberg, A.J., and Berger, N.A. (2013). *Obesity, Inflammation and Cancer (Energy Balance and Cancer – 7).* Springer.
5. Ettinger, S. (2016). *Nutritional Pathophysiology of Obesity and Its Comorbidities – A Case-Study Approach.* Academic Press.
6. Faintuch, J., and Faintuch, S. (2020). *Obesity and Diabetes – Scientific Advances and Best Practice*, 2nd Edition. Springer.
7. Freemark, M.S. (2018). *Pediatric Obesity – Etiology, Pathogenesis, and Treatment (Contemporary Endocrinology).* Humana Press.
8. Genazzani, A.R., Ibanez, L., Milewicz, A., and Shah, D. (2021). *Impact of Polycystic Ovary, Metabolic Syndrome and Obesity on Women Health – Volume 8: Frontiers in Gynecological Endocrinology (ISGE Series).* Springer.
9. Govil Bhasker, A., Kantharia, N., Baig, S., Priya, P., Lakdawala, M., and Shah Sancheti, M. (2021). *Management of Nutritional and Metabolic Complications of Bariatric Surgery.* Springer.
10. Hamouda, A., and El Dien about El Noaman, S. (2016). *Obesity and Male Infertility: Diet Program on Human Semen.* Scholars' Press.
11. Kumar, S., and Gupta, S. (2021). *Obesity and Cancer.* Springer.
12. Marini, I., and Stebnicki, M.A. (2017). *The Psychological and Social Impact of Illness and Disability*, 7th Edition. Springer.
13. Martirosyan, D.M. (2009). *Functional Foods for Chronic Diseases, Volume 4 – Obesity, Diabetes, Cardiovascular Disorders, and AIDS (Functional Food Science).* D & A Incorporated.
14. Michaelson, J.A. (2014). *Obesity and Pregnancy: The Dangers and Risks – What You Should Know.* Michaelson.
15. Moini, J., Ahangari, R., Miller, C., and Samsam, M. (2020). *Global Health Complications of Obesity.* Elsevier.
16. Pischon, T., and Niptsch, K. (2016). *Obesity and Cancer (Recent Results in Cancer Research).* Springer.
17. Ramonde, P.R., and Fochas, E.H. (2009). *Obesity and Cancer Research.* Nova Biomedical.
18. Tappia, P.S., Ramjiawan, B., and Dhalla, N.S. (2020). *Pathophysiology of Obesity-Induced Health Complications (Advances in Biochemistry in Health and Disease).* Springer.
19. Tulasi Latha, A. (2022). *Obesity – Causes, Complications, and Strategies for Weight Loss.* Lap Lambert Academic Publishing.
20. Woodward, B.G. (2006). *A Complete Guide to Obesity Surgery – Everything You Need to Know about Weight Loss Surgery and How to Succeed.* Trafford Publishing.
21. Youness, E.R., and El Toukhy, S.E. (2020). *Obesity – (the) Most Common Metabolic Complication in Prader-Willi Syndrome.* Scholars' Press.

10 Vitamin Deficiency, Dependency, and Toxicity

OUTLINE

LEARNING OBJECTIVES

After study of the chapter, readers should be able to:

1. Explain the classifications of fat-soluble vitamins.
2. Describe the effects of retinoids in the human body.
3. Discuss the effects of vitamin D deficiency in children.
4. Identify good sources of vitamin E.
5. Discuss the outcomes of thiamin deficiency.
6. Describe the benefits of taking folic acid.
7. Discuss the consequences of vitamin B12 deficiency.
8. Identify foods with the highest levels of ascorbic acid.
9. Describe the signs and symptoms of vitamin B6 deficiency.
10. Identify the people that have the highest risks for vitamin B9 deficiency.

OVERVIEW

Vitamins are essential organic substances that do not provide energy, but are required in small dietary amounts. They aid in energy metabolism, tissue growth, development, and maintenance. Vitamins A, D, E, and K dissolve in organic solvents, so they are termed "fat-soluble vitamins". The B vitamins, along with vitamin C, dissolve in water and are termed "water-soluble vitamins". Vitamins either cannot be synthesized by the body or only in insufficient quantities. When vitamin intake is not sufficient to meet the body's needs, a deficiency develops, with a significant decline in health. Initially, a deficiency and its signs and symptoms can be reversed by increasing intake of the particular vitamin. Megadoses of certain vitamins have been used to prevent deficiencies and treat some non-deficiency conditions. Dietary vitamins are supplied by plant and animal foods, along with supplements. Vitamin dependency may result from a genetic defect concerning vitamin metabolism. Sometimes, doses that are one thousand times higher than the daily recommended intake improve the function of the affected metabolic pathway. Vitamin toxicity is also called hypervitaminosis, and usually occurs because of consumption of megadoses of vitamin A or D.

FAT-SOLUBLE VITAMINS

Fat-soluble vitamins are absorbed with dietary fat, so sufficient absorption of these vitamins is based on normal use of bile and pancreatic lipase in the small intestine in order to digest dietary fat, plus good absorption in the intestines. Normally, 40%–90% of fat-soluble vitamins are absorbed when consumed in the recommended amounts. Fat malabsorption, usually due to gastrointestinal (GI) tract and pancreatic diseases, may result in poor absorption of fat-soluble vitamins. After absorption, fat-soluble vitamins are readied to be transported through the lymphatic system and then into the bloodstream to reach target cells, via the **chylomicrons** and other blood **lipoproteins**. After body cells remove many triglycerides from the chylomicrons, the remainder is taken up by the liver, including dietary fat-soluble vitamins. The liver reorganizes the vitamins with new proteins for transport in the bloodstream, or stores them in the adipose tissue or the liver itself. Except for vitamin K, fat-soluble vitamins are not greatly excreted from the body.

Vitamin A

Vitamin A has been known about for over 3,500 years, including its effects that prevent night blindness. It is a reference to preformed **retinoids** and provitamin A carotenoids, which can be converted to active vitamin A. Retinoids are the biologically active forms of this vitamin. They are *preformed* because they do not have to be converted within

DOI: 10.1201/b22969-13

the body to be biologically active. There are three forms of retinoids, as follows:

- **Retinol** – an alcohol, sometimes referred to as *vitamin A1*
- **Retinal** – an aldehyde, sometimes referred to as *retinaldehyde*
- **Retinoic acid** – derived from retinal, it is important for cell growth, differentiation, and organogenesis

Carotenoids in fruits and vegetables are yellow to orange in color. Some of them are **provitamins** that can be converted into vitamin A. There are more than 600 known carotenoids, but the only ones that can be converted to biologically active forms of vitamin A are *alpha-carotene, beta-carotene,* and *beta-cryptoxanthin.* Provitamin A carotenoids are mostly found in vegetables of a dark green or yellow-orange color and in fruits. Good sources include carrots, spinach, sweet potatoes, winter squash, broccoli, cantaloupe, mangoes, apricots, and peaches. Beta-carotene has the largest amount of provitamin A activity and makes up some of the orange color of carrots and other foods rich in carotenoids. In dark green vegetables, the dark green pigment known as **chlorophyll** masks the yellow-orange color, but plenty of provitamin A is still present. This is why a diet rich in dark green and yellow-orange vegetables provides good amounts of vitamin A.

Retinoids are present in liver, fish and fish oil, fortified milk, and eggs. Foods that are fortified with vitamin A include fat-free, low-fat, and reduced-fat milks as well as margarine. Approximately 70% of the vitamin A in most North American diets come from animal sources. Adult men have a recommended daily allowance (RDA) of vitamin of 900 mcg while for adult women, the RDA is 700 mcg. Table 10.1 summarizes foods with the highest levels of vitamin A.

Preformed vitamin A is present in animal-based foods as retinol and **retinyl ester** compounds. These esters have no activity until retinol is separated in the intestinal tract from its attached fatty acid. This requires bile and pancreatic lipase enzymes. Up to 90% of retinol is absorbed by the small intestine cells, using carrier proteins. Once absorbed, a fatty acid is attached to retinol, forming a new retinyl ester, which is packaged into chylomicrons prior to entering the lymphatic circulation.

TABLE 10.1
Foods with the Highest Levels of Vitamin A

Food	Quantity	Percentage (%) of Daily Vitamin A
Beef liver	3 ounces (oz)	600
Sweet potato	½ cup	225
Carrots	½ cup	Over 200
Kale	½ cup	Just under 200
Broccoli	½ cup	About 175
Apricot	½ cup	About 40
Spinach	½ cup	About 30
Romaine lettuce	½ cup	About 28
Margarine	2 tablespoons (tbsp)	About 25
Acorn squash	½ cup	About 25

Carotenoids in the diet are often attached to proteins, from which they are split off by digestive enzymes before absorption. The free carotenoids are mostly absorbed by **passive diffusion**, with rates between 5% and 60% of intake. Provitamin A carotenoids are cleaved in intestinal cells to form retinal, and retinoic acid. Retinal is then converted into retinol, which may attach to a fatty acid, becoming a retinyl ester, entering the lymphatic system as a component of a chylomicron. Vitamin A is delivered to tissues by chylomicrons, for storage or use by cells. Retinoic acid can enter the bloodstream for direct transport to the liver. Carotenoids enter the bloodstream directly as well, but in small amounts. More than 90% of the vitamin A stores are in the liver. Smaller amounts are in the adipose tissue, bone marrow, kidneys, eyes, and testicles. The liver normally stores sufficient vitamin A as retinyl esters to last for months, protecting against deficiency.

Vitamin A as a retinoid is released by the liver into the bloodstream and binds to a retinol-binding protein. The synthesis of these proteins requires sufficient retinol, protein, and zinc. When carotenoids are released by the liver, lipoproteins carry them. They are taken up into cells by **apoprotein** receptors. In the cells, retinoids bind to retinol-binding proteins that direct them to function cell sites. Almost all cells have one or more of these binding proteins. Distribution of cellular proteins is different in various tissues, which may indicate different functional requirements for the vitamin. Most vitamin A is excreted in the urine, while carotenoids are excreted in the bile eliminated with the feces.

Retinoids mostly promote growth, development, cell differentiation, vision, and immune function. They are important in embryonic development. Vitamin A is part of the development of the eyes, limbs, cardiovascular system, and nervous system. A lack of the vitamin in early gestation results in birth defects and death of the fetus. Retinoic acid is required for production, structure, and function of epithelial cells of the lungs, trachea, skin, and GI tract. It is needed so that these organs can form and maintain mucous-forming cells. In cell nuclei, retinoids bind to two primary families of retinoid receptors. Vitamin A is highly important for maintaining normal differentiation of cells of the structural eye components, including the cornea and retina.

As retinal, vitamin A is required in the retinas to turn visual light into nerve signals within the brain. The sensory elements in the retina are the rods and cones. **Rods** handle visual processes in dim light and translate objects into black-and-white images while detecting motion. **Cones** handle visual processes in bright light and translate objects into color images. Thousands of rod cells contain millions of **rhodopsin** molecules. In bright light, the rhodopsin is totally activated and is unable to respond to any more light.

In each cycle, some retinal is stored in the eye, maintaining pools of vitamin A. As the pools become depleted, dark adaptation is impaired. It becomes difficult to adjust to seeing in dim light, which is known as *night blindness*. A similar experience occurs when walking into a dark room from outside during the day, or if driving at night when another vehicle shines its bright lights into your eyes. This short period of difficult vision is not due to a vitamin A deficiency, since the vision quickly normalizes once the eyes have adjusted to the light changes. Increased incidence of infections is an early symptom of vitamin A deficiency. Vitamin-deficient individuals also are more susceptible to other illnesses because vitamin A assists in maintaining the epithelium that protects against pathogens entering the skin. Globally, where vitamin A deficiency is common.

Diets rich in carotenoids may decrease risks for eye diseases, cancers, and cardiovascular disease. Beta-carotene has the most vitamin A activity and may act as an antioxidant in tissues, protecting them from damage from **free radicals**. People with high blood levels of antioxidant nutrients have a decreased risk of **cataracts**. However, long-term supplementation with beta-carotene plus vitamin E, with or without adding vitamin C, has not prevented or reduced cataract incidence. Though the effects of beta-carotene upon lung cancer are controversial, it has been shown, along with alpha-carotene, to reduce risks for breast cancer. The carotenoids called lutein and zeaxanthin may protect against age-related **macular degeneration** of the eyes in certain people, but more studies are continuing.

Vitamin A deficiency diseases are not common in developed countries because of the abundance of the vitamin in the food supply. However, this is not the case in underdeveloped or developing countries. Globally, vitamin A deficiency is the primary cause of non-accidental blindness. Children in Africa, Asia, and South America, in poorer regions, are very susceptible because of insufficient dietary intake and low stores. The countries with the highest rates of vitamin A deficiency include Zambia, India, Pakistan, Bangladesh, Sri Lanka, Afghanistan, Bhutan, Nepal, Mexico, Haiti, Peru, Honduras, Argentina, Ecuador, and Brazil (see Figure 10.1). The World Health Organization estimates that about 250 million preschool children are vitamin A deficient. Vitamin A deficiency in pregnant women increases the likelihood of transmission of human immunodeficiency virus (HIV) to developing fetuses, and increases maternal mortality rates. Vitamin A deficiency is the leading cause of preventable blindness in children (250,000–500,000 annual cases). In the poorest countries, about 500,000 children become blind annually (a global map).

In North America, poor people, older adults, alcoholics, people with liver disease, and those with the following conditions may develop vitamin A deficiency:

- Severe fat malabsorption **(celiac disease)**
- Chronic diarrhea
- Pancreatic insufficiency
- Crohn's disease
- Cystic fibrosis
- Acquired immunodeficiency syndrome (AIDS)

Eye changes are common with vitamin A deficiency. If blood retinol is lacking, the retinal lost in the visual cycle cannot be replaced, so the rods regenerate rhodopsin slower than normal. Night blindness results. Without sufficient retinoic acid, mucous-forming cells deteriorate and mucus cannot be synthesized. The cornea and other parts of the eyes are affected since mucus helps keep them moist and washes away dirt particles. As a result, **conjunctival xerosis** develops. Often,

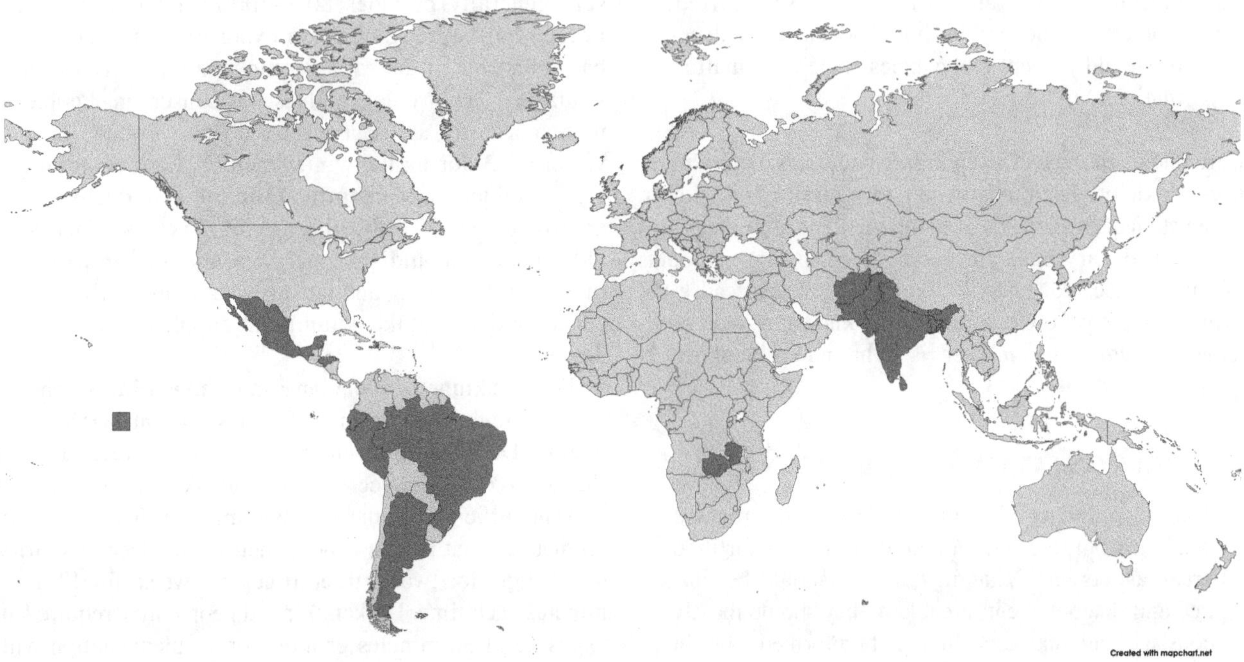

FIGURE 10.1 Map of countries with the highest rates of vitamin A deficiency.

keratomalacia and scarring occur. These changes are collectively known as **xerophthalmia**, resulting in irreversible blindness on a global scale, affecting millions of individuals.

Skin changes such as **follicular hyperkeratosis** may also occur. **Keratin** is the normal component of outer skin layers that protects inner layers and reduces water loss. When deficiency is severe, the keratinized cells replace normal mucous-forming epithelial cells in deeper skin layers. Hair follicles become plugged with keratin, and the skin texture becomes dry and rough, with a sandy feel. In infants and young children, deficiency of vitamin A impairs growth.

However, excessive vitamin A (*hypervitaminosis A*) from long-term use of supplements can occur if five to ten times the RDA is taken. The maximum amount of retinol per day is 3,000 mcg. There are three types of vitamin A toxicity as follows:

- *Acute* – caused by ingestion of a single extremely large dose of vitamin A or several large doses over a few days, which is about 100 times the RDA; effects include GI tract upset, blurred vision, headache, and poor muscle coordination; these disappear once dosing stops; extremely large doses (10 g in adults and 500 mg in children) can be fatal
- *Chronic* – caused by repeated ingestion of at least 10 times the RDA; effects include joint pain, loss of appetite, headache, skin disorders, liver damage, reduced bone minerals, double vision, hemorrhage, and coma; the supplement must be discontinued and symptoms will decrease over a few weeks; chronic ingestion of high amounts can cause permanent liver, bone, and eye damage
- *Teratogenic* – birth defects result from overuse of vitamin A and its analogs such as **Accutane** spontaneous abortions and birth defects have occurred; women of childbearing should not use these drugs or should prevent pregnancies since fetal malformations can be severe

Carotenoids in the diet, even in large amounts, nearly never cause toxicity. Their conversion to vitamin A is slower. Absorption of carotenoids from the small intestine decreases greatly as dietary intake increases. Even so, large amounts of carrots or carrot juice, or winter squash, can cause the skin to appear yellow-orange in color, known as *hypercarotenemia* or *carotenemia*. There is no harm to general health.

FOCUS ON VITAMIN A AND PREGNANCY

Too much dietary vitamin A can occur in pregnant women, from increased amounts of liver or fortified breakfast cereals. Vitamin A intake should be limited and if supplements are taken, they should mostly consist of beta-carotene. Intake of preformed vitamin A should not exceed 100% of the RDA.

Test Your Knowledge

1. What are three forms of retinoids?
2. What foods have the highest levels of vitamin A?
3. What conditions may develop because of vitamin A deficiency?
4. What are three types of vitamin A toxicity?

Vitamin D

Though vitamin D is generally classified as an actual vitamin, in sunlight, our skin cells can synthesize enough vitamin D from a cholesterol derivative. Therefore, vitamin D is better classified as a *conditional hormone* or **prohormone**. Without enough UV-light exposure, adequate dietary intake of vitamin D is required. The best food sources are fatty fish, cod liver oil, fortified milk, and fortified breakfast cereals. Fatty fish include mackerel, sardines, herring, and salmon. In North America, milk is usually fortified with 10 mcg of vitamin D in every quart. Products made from milk such as cheese and ice cream are usually not fortified. Eggs, butter, liver, and some types of margarine contain some amount of vitamin D, but large portions must be consumed to get enough of the vitamin. Most fortified foods and supplements that contain vitamin D have it in the form of **ergocalciferol** (vitamin D2). This is also the form found naturally in food sources.

Synthesis of vitamin D3 in the skin starts with *7-dehydrocholesterol*, which is a precursor of cholesterol synthesis. With sunlight exposure, a chemical transformation occurs and the more stable **cholecalciferol** (vitamin D3) is formed. This allows the new form to enter the bloodstream and be transported to the liver and kidneys, where it is converted to **calcitriol**, its bioactive form. Sun exposure generally provides 80%–100% of the vitamin D3 needed by the body. The sun exposure that is needed is based on time of day, geographic location, seasons, individual age, skin color, and use of sunscreen. People in more northerly areas generally do not produce enough vitamin D3 during the winter months. For people in any area, production of vitamin D3 in the skin decreases by approximately 70% by the age of 70 years. Therefore, older people should get small amounts of sun exposure in the early morning and late afternoon, minimizing skin cancer risks, or take vitamin D supplements to avoid deficiency.

Darker-skinned people have more **melanin**, which can block ultraviolet light and prevent sufficient synthesis of vitamin D3. Use of sunscreens with a sun protection factor (SPF) of 8 or higher decrease risks for skin cancer, but also prevent sufficient synthesis of vitamin D3. It is often recommended that people expose their hands, face, and arms to UV-light for two to three times per week, for 10 to 15 minutes each time. Darker-skinned people may require sun exposure of 30 minutes or more, or supplementation with vitamin D. Lengthy sun exposure usually does not cause synthesis of vitamin D any more than what is needed, or in toxic amounts. This is because excessive amounts of provitamin D3 in the skin are quickly degraded. Those with insufficient UV-light exposure should take steps to ensure correct amounts of vitamin D in the diet.

Adult men and women require 15 mcg of vitamin D per day, though the daily value listed on product labels is 20 mcg. This breaks down as follows: 15 mcg per day for people from age one to 70 years, but 20 mcg per day for those over 70. Full-term infants are born with a supply of vitamin D, but it is recommended that breastfed infants be given supplements to meet the current recommendation of 10 mcg for infants. Supplements continue until weaning off of breast milk onto infant foods fortified with or rich in vitamin D. Table 10.2 summarizes foods with the highest levels of vitamin D.

About 80% of vitamin D2 is incorporated, with dietary fats, into **micelles** of the small intestine. It is absorbed and transported to the liver by chylomicrons via the lymphatic system. Fat malabsorption syndromes increase risks of vitamin D2 malabsorption and deficiency.

Calcitriol is the most active form of vitamin D and primarily acts as a hormone to maintain concentrations of calcium and phosphorus. While this helps in maintaining the health of the bones, it can sometimes result in bone demineralization. Low blood calcium means that vitamin D promotes more intestinal absorption of calcium and phosphorus from foods. Calcium and phosphorus become available for the cells and incorporation into bones when at excessive levels. As blood calcium declines, vitamin D with parathyroid hormone (PTH) can take calcium from the bones to increase blood levels. Eventually, this weakens the bones over a long time, but temporarily provides enough calcium for basic life functions. Vitamin D also regulates immune function and secretion of insulin, PTH, and **renin**. It also involved in regulation of the cell cycle, decreases risks for certain infections and autoimmune diseases, and protects against diabetes mellitus, dementia, hypertension, and cancer.

Rickets is a childhood disease and caused by vitamin D deficiency. It characterized by imperfect calcification, softening, and distortion of bone and bowing of leg bones (see Figure 10.2). Other signs include an enlarged head, joints, ribs, and **pigeon chest**. The pelvis may also be deformed. Rickets in developed countries is usually due to fat malabsorption, such as with cystic fibrosis. In previous times, **cod liver oil** was used to cure rickets and became a daily childhood supplement until milk began to be fortified with vitamin D. There are more cases occurring in infants and children with darker skin, low milk intake, or reduced sun exposure.

TABLE 10.2
Foods with the Highest Levels of Vitamin D

Food	Quantity	Percentage (%) of Daily Vitamin D
Cod liver oil	2 tbsp	340
Eel	3 oz	100
Salmon	3 oz	About 38
Herring	3 oz	About 22
Tuna	3 oz	About 22
Fat-free milk	1 cup	About 15
Soy milk	1 cup	About 13
Rice/wheat/barley cereal	¾ cup	About 9
Bran cereal with raising	¾ cup	About 5
Egg	1 large	About 5

Osteomalacia occurs in adults because of insufficient calcium and phosphorus, resulting in the bones becoming soft and deformed. It is usually caused by low levels of vitamin D in the diet, not getting enough sunlight, or a problem with the way the body uses vitamin D. There is poor calcification of newly synthesized bone, so fractures of the hips or spine are common. Osteomalacia is most common with kidney or liver disease, which impair calcitriol synthesis, or intestinal diseases (see Chapter 18).

Excessive vitamin D supplementation, especially with cholecalciferol, can cause toxicity. This condition does not occur from too much sun exposure or natural dietary sources. The upper limit is 1,000–3,000 International Units per day for infants and children up to age eight. The limit is 4,000 International Units per day for people age nine and older. Once these levels are exceeded, vitamin D can cause overabsorption of calcium and hypercalcemia. Excessive blood calcium leads to calcium deposits in the kidneys, heart, and lungs. There is anorexia, nausea, vomiting, bone demineralization, joint pain, weakness, and kidney dysfunction. Early toxicity is often treatable if the vitamin D is stopped. If excess supplementation continues, the toxicity will be fatal.

Today, vitamin D deficiency has returned as a global health issue. It is now known that the vitamin is important for gene control and cell cycle regulation in most tissues, which can decrease risks for chronic illnesses such as diabetes, cardiovascular disease, autoimmune diseases, and cancers of the colon, prostate, and breast. It is sometimes estimated, therefore, that the body actually needs 75–100 mcg of daily vitamin D, but usually input from UV exposure often supply much of these requirements. Therefore, oral vitamin D between 1,000 and 4,000 International Units may be sufficient if sun exposure is limited. There is also link between vitamin D deficiency and dementia, which is discussed in detail in Chapter 13.

FOCUS ON VITAMIN D

There is some controversy as to whether vitamin D may have protective effects against infections such as that of the coronavirus (COVID-19). Some experts believe the vitamin can protect against the infection or decrease the severity of the illness, but studies are ongoing. So far, results have shown just a slightly better set of outcomes in patients with moderate to severe COVID-19 when vitamin D, specifically D3, was administered.

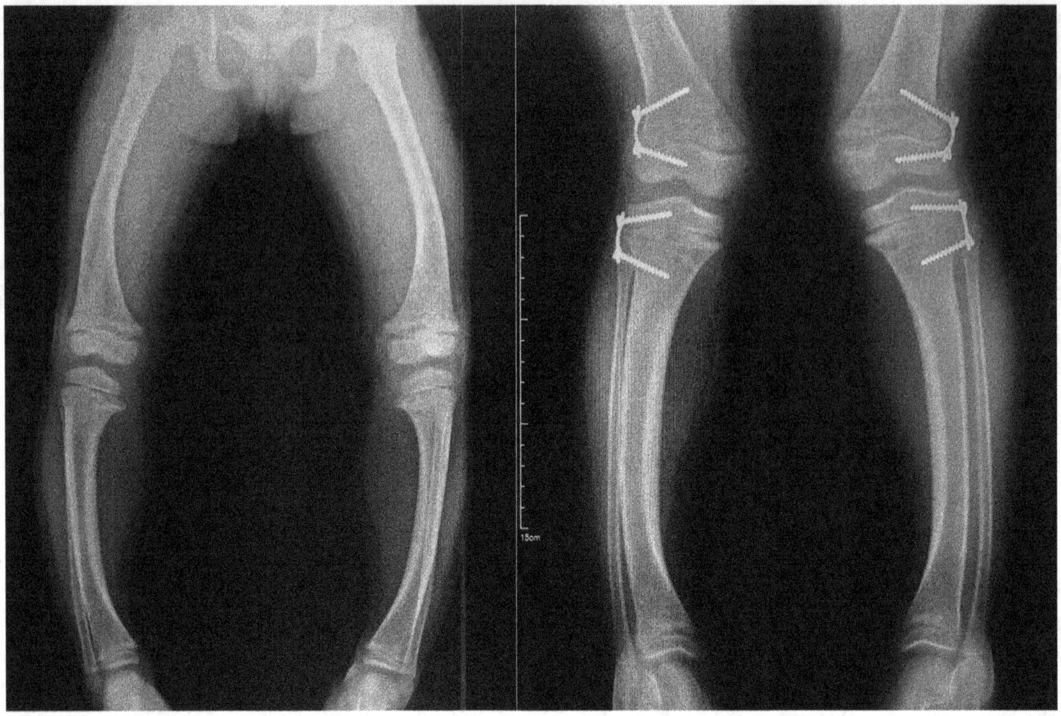

FIGURE 10.2 X-ray of a child, showing rickets.

Test Your Knowledge

1. What are the best food sources of vitamin D?
2. What type of vitamin D is the most active form?
3. What are the consequences of vitamin D deficiency?

Vitamin E

Vitamin E was discovered after vitamin D, hence its original name, though it is more commonly known as **tocopherol**. It was not recognized as an essential nutrient until the middle of the 1960s, when its deficiency was found in children that had fat malabsorption diseases. Vitamin E is actually a family of eight naturally occurring compounds, as follows:

- *Tocopherols* – alpha, beta, gamma, and delta
- *Tocotrienols* – also alpha, beta, gamma, and delta

Each of these eight compounds has its own amount of biological activity. The most active form is *alpha-tocopherol.* It is found in foods and vitamin supplements. *Gamma-tocopherol* does not have as much biological activity, but is a potentially beneficial form of vitamin E that is present in many vegetable oils. Good sources of vitamin E include canola, cottonseed, safflower, and sunflower oils, as well as avocado, wheat germ, almonds, peanuts, and sunflower seeds. Products manufactured from plant oils are also good sources, and include margarine, salad dressings, and shortenings. Very little vitamin E is contained in animal fats or dairy products. The content of vitamin E in food is based on the processes involved in harvesting, manufacturing, storage, and cooking of each source. Vitamin E is easily destroyed by oxygen, heat, light, and metals. Deep-fat frying easily destroys vitamin E.

The RDA for vitamin E is 15 mg per day for men and women. This is based on the amount needed to prevent **hemolysis** of red blood cell membranes. The 15 mg RDA is equivalent to about 22 International Units of a natural source and 33 International Units of a synthetic source. Adults usually consume only about 66% of RDA of vitamin E daily. Therefore, it is important to increase intake by eating breakfast cereals with the vitamin, or taking daily supplements. The daily value on food and supplement labels is also 15 mg. Table 10.3 summarizes foods with the highest levels of vitamin E.

Absorption of vitamin E is based on how much is consumed and the absorption of dietary fat. Absorption is via passive diffusion, at 20%–70% of dietary intake. The vitamin must be incorporated into the micelles of the small intestine, which depends on bile and pancreatic enzymes. After being taken up by intestinal cells, the vitamin is incorporated into chylomicrons and transported to the lymphatic system and bloodstream. Breakdown of chylomicrons results in most of the vitamin E reaching the liver as remnants of chylomicrons. A small amount directly moves to other tissues. In the liver, vitamin E is repackaged from the remnants with the very-low-density lipoprotein (VLDL), low-density lipoprotein (LDL), and high-density lipoprotein (HDL) lipoproteins, and delivered to the tissues. Vitamin E is unique in that it does not have a specific

TABLE 10.3
Foods with the Highest Levels of Vitamin E

Food	Quantity	Percentage (%) of Daily Vitamin E
Sunflower oil	1 tbsp	37
Sunflower seeds	½ oz	33
Safflower oil	1 tbsp	31
Almonds	½ oz	25
Mayonnaise	1 tbsp	20
Avocado	½ cup	18
Canola oil	1 tbsp	16
Peanut butter	2 tbsp	10
Wheat germ	1 tbsp	8
Margarine	2 tbsp	8

transport protein in the blood, requiring it to be carried by these lipoproteins. It also does not accumulate in the liver. Therefore, about 90% is localized in the adipose tissue. Vitamin E is excreted mostly via the bile within the feces, but also via the urine and skin.

Vitamin E helps maintain cell membrane integrity by preventing chain reactions caused by free radicals. Free radicals are unstable compounds with one or more unpaired electrons that act as strong oxidizing agents – meaning that they seek electrons. Free radicals can be highly destructive to cell membranes and DNA, which are electron-dense. However, free radicals also have some important roles. They aide the immune system in fighting pathogens, and they are generated by leukocytes to destroy infection-causing agents such as bacteria and viruses. For self-protection, the body must regulate free radical activity to avoid possible damage. Vitamin E is responsible for this along with other antioxidants. In areas where lipids are abundant, free radicals can start the chain reactions known as **peroxidation**.

Vitamin E is one of the most effective substances that stop lipid peroxidation. The peroxidation chain is stopped when vitamin E donates a hydrogen atom to lipid radicals. Since cell membranes are composed of a phospholipid bilayer, vitamin E protects integrity of the membrane by neutralizing lipid peroxyl radicals, preventing lipid peroxidation. Vitamin E reduces **oxidative stress**, which involves damage to DNA, lipids, and proteins from free radicals. One vitamin E molecule is used during the chain-breaking action. It must be regenerated by reducing agents. Along with other compounds, vitamin C aids in regenerating vitamin E so that it can resume functioning.

Vitamin E is a popular supplement along with other antioxidants, with the goal that they will help prevent cancer, cardiovascular disease, and other chronic diseases that are linked to free radical damage. However, studies have reported that vitamin E, selenium, or both do not decrease the risk of various cancers, though the effects of vitamin E may be varied based on the stage of prostate cancer and blood levels of the form of vitamin E known as alpha-tocopherol. Similar outcomes have been reported with use of vitamin E to decrease risks for *atherosclerosis*. There is also the possibility of vitamin E deficiency causing ataxia, but it is relatively rare. This condition is discussed in detail in Chapter 13.

Vitamin E deficiency is rare, and the highest risk is for people who have cystic fibrosis or Crohn's disease. Preterm infants are highly susceptible to vitamin E deficiency. Because, they are born with only limited amounts of stored vitamin E, and often have poor intestinal absorption of the vitamin. Smokers are also at risk since oxidative stress and lipid peroxidation from cigarette smoke makes their bodies require more vitamin E. Deficiency of the vitamin E is signified by early break down of red blood cells and **hemolytic anemia**. In preterm infants, this is very serious, so they are given supplemental vitamin E and specialized infant formula containing it. Deficiency of vitamin E can reduce immune function and cause spinal cord and peripheral nervous system neurological changes. These have occurred when the deficiency resulted from a genetic abnormality of lipoprotein synthesis that decreases vitamin E transport and distribution.

Vitamin E is relatively nontoxic, but large amounts can interfere with vitamin K, affecting blood clotting. Insufficient clotting results, and there is a risk of hemorrhaging. Risks are higher in people taking daily aspirin or anticoagulation medications such as warfarin to prevent blood clots. Therefore, vitamin E in megadoses can cause severe hemorrhaging. The upper limit for vitamin E is 1,000 mg (of alpha-tocopherol) from natural sources, and 1,100 International Units when it comes from synthetic sources. Large amounts may decrease antioxidant activities of gamma-tocopherol. Some experts recommend that vitamin E supplements should contain a mixture of natural tocopherols, but these are more expensive than natural or synthetic alpha-tocopherol.

FOCUS ON ANTIOXIDANTS

Antioxidants protect other compounds by becoming oxidized. Therefore, a better name for them is *redox agents* since they can undergo oxidation, the loss of an electron, and then reduction, regaining of the electron. *Antioxidant* is still the more common term, however.

Vitamin K

Vitamin K helps to make various proteins that are needed for blood clotting and the building of bones. Prothrombin is a vitamin K-dependent protein directly involved with blood clotting. Osteocalcin is another protein that requires vitamin K to produce healthy bone tissue. There are two main forms of vitamin K, also known as the *quinones*. They includes vitamin K1 (**phylloquinone**) found in plant foods like leafy greens, and vitamin K2 (**menaquinone**), which found in animal foods and fermented foods. The most biologically active form is phylloquinone, and is the primary dietary form.

Approximately 10% of vitamin K that body absorbs every day comes from bacterial synthesis within the colon, and the rest is provided by the diet. Content of vitamin K varies between food sources, with the best sources being kale, parsley, turnip greens, cabbage, salad greens, spinach, broccoli, green beans, and peas. Vegetable oils – especially canola and soy – are other good sources. The vitamin is highly stable to heat processing but can be destroyed by light exposure. Women need 90 mcg per day, while men need 120 mcg per day. These intakes are based on adequate dietary sources of the vitamin. It is not known whether increased dietary intake may be good for other body functions. The RDA for vitamin K is listed on labels as 120 mcg per day. Table 10.4 summarizes foods with the highest levels of vitamin K.

About 80% of dietary vitamin K, mostly phylloquinone, is taken up by the small intestine, then incorporated into chylomicrons. This requires bile and pancreatic enzymes. Menaquinones synthesized by colon bacteria are absorbed via passive diffusion. Vitamin K can be incorporated into VLDL in the liver to be stored, or carried by HDL and LDL to cells everywhere in the body. Most of the excretion of vitamin K occurs through the bile in the feces, but a small amount occurs in the urine.

Vitamin K is required for blood clotting factors to be synthesized by the liver, and for preprothrombin to be converted into prothrombin, an active blood clotting factor. Vitamin K is converted to an inactive form after activating clotting factors. Then, it must be reactivated in order for its biological actions to occur. Warfarin and similar drugs greatly inhibit this reactivation process, acting as powerful anticoagulants. People that take warfarin to reduce blood clotting must maintain a regular dietary intake of vitamin K, but avoid supplements with the vitamin K. Bone metabolism is also affected by vitamin K.

At birth, vitamin K stores are low, because the newborn intestinal tract does not have the bacteria needed to synthesize the vitamin. Therefore, there is a risk of bleeding from defective blood clotting, so newborns in North America are given vitamin K injections within 6 hours after birth. In older infants, children, teens, and adults, vitamin K deficiency is rare. However, it can occur because of extended use of antibiotics or impairment of fat absorption. Since deficiency causes poor clot formation and hemorrhaging, each patient's vitamin K status is checked before any surgical procedures. The actions of vitamin K are negatively affected by too much vitamin A and E intake. Vitamin A is believed to interfere with vitamin K absorption from the small intestine. Large doses of vitamin E lead to decreased vitamin K-dependent clotting factors, and a higher chance for bleeding. Megadose supplements of either of these vitamins increase risks for vitamin K deficiency and bleeding.

There is no upper level set for vitamin K, while it can be stored in the liver and bones. The vitamin is more highly excreted than the other fat-soluble vitamins. In its natural phylloquinone or menaquinone forms, increased amounts of vitamin K are not harmful. However, injections of synthetic menadione have caused hemolytic anemia, jaundice, and death in newborns. Therefore, menadione is no longer used to treat vitamin K deficiency. A summary of fat-soluble vitamin deficiency and toxicity symptoms is shown in Table 10.5.

TABLE 10.4
Foods with the Highest Levels of Vitamin K

Food	Quantity	Percentage (%) of Daily Vitamin K
Kale	½ cup	440
Spinach	½ cup	370
Turnip greens	½ cup	220
Brussels sprouts	½ cup	125
Broccoli	½ cup	90
Soybean oil	2 tbsp	45
Asparagus	½ cup	40
Cabbage	½ cup	35
Looseleaf lettuce	½ cup	25
Green peas	½ cup	15

Test Your Knowledge

1. What are the two main forms of vitamin K?
2. What foods have the highest levels of vitamin K?
3. Why is vitamin K storage low at birth?

WATER-SOLUBLE VITAMINS

Water-soluble vitamins are essential organic substances that, like fat-soluble vitamins, are also needed in small amounts. Thiamin, riboflavin, niacin, pantothenic acid, and biotin are very important for energy metabolism. Vitamins B6 and B12 as well as folate are important for amino acid metabolism and synthesis of red blood cells. Vitamin C helps to synthesize many compounds, including collagen. The essential nutrient called **choline**, while not a vitamin, is needed for nervous system function and also aids metabolism of amino acids and lipids. Only small amounts of water-soluble vitamins are stored in the body. Risk of toxicities is usually low since they are easily removed by the kidneys. Due to the limited storage of water-soluble vitamins, they should be consumed every day.

Water-soluble vitamins are more readily absorbed than fat-soluble vitamins, usually at rates between 90% and 100% in the small intestine, without any dependence upon dietary fat. Some B vitamins are malabsorbed because of alcohol abuse and intestinal diseases. Vitamin supplements are then usually needed to prevent deficiencies. Water-soluble vitamins are delivered directly to the bloodstream and then distributed everywhere in the body.

Water-soluble vitamins are more easily destroyed during cooking than the fat-soluble vitamins. Their vitamin content can be decreased by heat, light, air, or alkaline

TABLE 10.5
Fat-Soluble Vitamin Deficiency and Toxicity Symptoms

Vitamin	Deficiency Symptoms	Toxicity Symptoms
A – upper level: 3,000 mcg of preformed vitamin A	Dry skin, hyperkeratosis, impaired immune function, night blindness, poor growth, total blindness, xerophthalmia	Birth defects, bone and joint pain, double vision, dry mucous membranes, headache, hemorrhage, liver damage, spontaneous abortion, vomiting, coma
D – upper level: 100 mcg	Cell cycle regulation, maintenance of calcium and phosphorus concentrations, maintenance of immune function	Calcification of soft tissues, excess calcium in the blood, excretion in the urine, impaired growth
E – upper level: 1,000 mg	Antioxidant, prevention of free radical damage	Inhibition of vitamin K metabolism
K – upper level: none	Synthesis of blood clotting factors and bone proteins	Rare toxicity; can cause hemolytic anemia

TABLE 10.6
Coenzymes Formed from B Vitamins

B Vitamin	Example of Coenzyme(s)	Function
Thiamin (B1)	Thiamin pyrophosphate (TPP), also called thiamin diphosphate (TDP)	Decarboxylation
Riboflavin (B2)	Flavin adenine dinucleotide (FAD), flavin mononucleotide (FMN)	Electron (hydrogen) transfer
Niacin (B3)	Nicotinamide adenine dinucleotide (NAD), nicotinamide adenine dinucleotide phosphate (NADP)	Electron (hydrogen) transfer
Pantothenic acid (B5)	Coenzyme A (CoA)	Acyl (2-C groups) transfer
Pyridoxine (B6)	Pyridoxal phosphate (PLP)	Transamination, amino group transfer
Biotin (B7)	N-carboxylbiotinyl lysine	Carboxylation, carbon dioxide transfer
Folic acid (B9)	Tetrahydrofolic acid (THFA)	1-carbon unit transfer
Cobalamin (B12)	Methylcobalamin	1-carbon unit transfer

exposures. Water-soluble vitamins can enter cooking water. Retention of B vitamins and vitamin C is highest in foods that are steamed, stir-fried, and microwaved because these methods limit exposure to heat and water. All of the B vitamins act as **coenzymes**, which are nonprotein compounds needed for enzymes to function. Small organic molecules called **cofactors** are substances required for enzymes to be active. Examples include zinc and magnesium. These combine with inactive **apoenzymes**, forming active **holoenzymes**, which can catalyze reactions. The coenzymes that are formed from the B vitamins are summarized in Table 10.6.

The majority of the listed B vitamins are involved in energy metabolism, but some have other cellular roles. The need for these vitamins increases to some degree when a person has more physical activity. This is not a serious concern because greater food intake that usually occurs as more energy is expended adds more dietary B vitamins. For the water-soluble vitamins, Table 10.7 summarizes their roles in the body.

In food, the B vitamins are either vitamins or coenzymes, which can both be bound to protein. During digestion, the B vitamins are freed from proteins or coenzymes. These unbound vitamins are the primary form absorbed within the small intestine. Between 50% and 90% of dietary B vitamins are absorbed in most cases. In the cells, coenzyme forms of the vitamins are resynthesized. Any B vitamin supplements sold in the coenzyme forms have no specific benefits since the vitamins cannot be absorbed until they are released from the coenzyme.

Grains are rich sources of most B vitamins as well as minerals and fiber. Milling of grains often excludes the most nutrient-rich portions. As the seeds are crushed and the germ, bran, and husk layers are removed, only the

TABLE 10.7
Roles of the B Vitamins

B vitamin	Roles
Thiamin (B1)	Energy metabolism
Riboflavin (B2)	Energy metabolism, protein and amino acid metabolism, antioxidant defenses
Niacin (B3)	Energy metabolism
Pantothenic acid (B5)	Energy metabolism
Pyridoxine (B6)	Energy metabolism, blood production, protein and amino acid metabolism, immune function, one-carbon metabolism, normal nerve function
Biotin (B7)	Energy metabolism
Folic acid (B9)	Blood formation, protein and amino acid metabolism, one-carbon metabolism
Cobalamin (B12)	Energy metabolism, blood formation, protein and amino acid metabolism, one-carbon metabolism

TABLE 10.8
Foods with the Highest Levels of Thiamin (Vitamin B1)

Food	Quantity	Percentage (%) of Daily Vitamin B1 (Thiamin)
Sunflower seeds	2 oz	100
Whole-wheat cereal	¾ cup	100
Ham	3 oz	45
Bagel	4 inch	40
Egg noodles	1 cup	35
Pork chops	3 oz	35
Navy beans	1 cup	30
Tuna	3 oz	25
Flour tortilla	7 inch	20
Green peas	½ cup	15

starch-rich endosperm is left. This is the only part used to make white flour along with many bread and cereal products. As a result of milling, vitamins, minerals, and fiber are lost from many grains. Because of this fact, nearly all bread and cereal products, at least in the United States, are enriched with thiamin, riboflavin, niacin, folic acid, and iron. This program started in the 1940s and helps protect people from common deficiency diseases linked to lack of these nutrients. Only about 50% of the folate and thiamin, and 75% of the niacin and riboflavin that we consume actually occurs naturally in foods. At least half of the grains consumed every day should be whole grains. These include brown rice, oatmeal, popcorn, and bread or pasta made from whole-wheat.

Vitamin B1 (Thiamin)

In Asian countries where milled white rice was the primary food available, a disease called **beriberi** had serious health effects for centuries. People developed extreme weakness, fatigue, and paralysis – with death occurring in just a few months. It was discovered in the 1800s that simply adding fish, red meats, and barley to the diet could reverse the symptoms, but it was not until the early 1900s when it was actually discovered that the milling of rice removed a key ingredient for thiamin. The chemical bonds of thiamin molecules are easily broken by long heat exposure, such as during cooking. When this occurs, thiamin is no longer functional in the body. The vitamin can also be destroyed in alkaline conditions. This is why baking soda should never be added to the cooking water of green vegetables just to make them look greener.

Thiamin is present in many foods in small amounts, with the richest sources including sunflower seeds, whole-wheat cereals, and ham. Some foods contain *thiamin antagonists*, which reduce the *bioavailability* of thiamin. Some fresh fish and shellfish have *thiaminase enzymes* that destroy thiamin, but cooking inactivates these enzymes. Foods that have compounds that oxidize thiamin and inactivate it include coffee, tea, blueberries, Brussels sprouts, red cabbage, and beets. Even so, consuming these foods does not cause thiamin deficiency. The RDA for thiamin is 1.2mg for men and 1.1mg for women. The daily value on labels is 1.2mg in the United States and most developed countries at 1.4mg per day or higher. There is no adverse effect of excess thiamin intake because it is so easily excreted via the urine. There is no established upper level for thiamin. Table 10.8 summarizes the foods with the highest levels of thiamin.

Thiamin is easily absorbed in the small intestine via an active absorption process that relies on sodium. It is mostly transported by red blood cells (RBCs) in the coenzyme form of thiamin pyrophosphate. Very little thiamin is stores. There is a small amount of 25–30mg in the brain, muscles, kidneys, and liver.

The thiamin deficiency (beriberi) is much less common today but still persists in some Asian countries, mostly among refugees and poorer people of all ages. Beriberi is signified by peripheral neuropathy, muscle wasting, pain, tenderness, heart enlargement, difficulty breathing, anorexia, edema, poor memory and confusion, weight loss, and convulsions. The three subtypes are *dry, wet,* and *infantile* beriberi. Dry beriberi mostly affects the nervous and muscular systems. Wet beriberi has neurological and cardiovascular symptoms. The heart enlarges, breathing becomes difficult, and congestive heart failure may occur. **Infantile beriberi** develops if the mother's breast milk contains insufficient thiamin. It results in heart abnormalities, convulsions, and death without prompt treatment. Some signs of thiamin deficiency can appear after just two weeks on a thiamin-free diet.

Alcoholics may develop the thiamin deficiency disorder called *Wernicke encephalopathy.* These are discussed in greater detail in Chapter 13. Also called *cerebral beriberi,* the syndrome is related to decreased thiamin absorption due to alcohol consumption, increased thiamin excretion in the urine, and a poor-quality diet that lacks enough thiamin. The syndrome can develop quickly. There is damage to brain tissue, and symptoms include double vision, crossing of the eyes, rapid eye movements, apathy, **ataxia**, confusion, hallucinations, and **confabulation**. High doses of thiamin greatly improve the symptoms – especially those affecting the eyes. Some people that are elderly or have GI diseases, heart failure, critical illnesses, eating disorders, or obesity are at risk of thiamin deficiency to a moderate degree.

Vitamin B2 (Riboflavin)

Riboflavin has a distinct yellow-green fluorescence and was previously called the *yellow enzyme*. Nearly 25% of dietary riboflavin comes from milk products, though it is most prevalent in beef liver. Exposure to ultraviolet radiation in daylight causes riboflavin to quickly break down. Therefore, paper and plastic containers should be used for milk, milk products, and cereals. Glass containers should be avoided. The RDA for riboflavin is 1.3mg for men and 1.1mg for women. Daily values on labels are listed as

1.3 mg. Like thiamin, most daily intake for riboflavin is higher than the requirements. In the United States, this is 2.5 mg for men and 1.8 for women. No adverse effects are known from excessive dietary riboflavin due to its limited absorption and rapid excretion in the urine. No upper level for riboflavin has been set. Table 10.9 summaries the foods with the highest levels of vitamin B2 (riboflavin).

Between 60% and 65% of free riboflavin is absorbed, mostly through active transport or **facilitated diffusion** within the small intestine. Riboflavin is transported by protein carriers through the bloodstream. It is converted to its coenzymes in most tissues, mostly in the small intestine, liver, heart, and kidneys. A small amount is stored in the liver, kidneys, and heart. Excessive amounts are excreted in the urine. If excessive riboflavin supplements are taken, the urine becomes bright yellow and glows under a black light. Riboflavin is a component of the coenzymes needed for energy metabolism.

Ariboflavinosis is a deficiency of riboflavin and mostly affects the mouth, skin, and RBCs. Symptoms include inflammation that affects the throat, mouth, and tongue. There is cracking of skin around the corners of the mouth, and seborrheic dermatitis (see Figure 10.3). Some people have anemia, confusion, fatigue, headaches, and poor growth. Ariboflavinosis takes two months to develop if the diet is poor in riboflavin. Deficiency occurs in teenage girls, younger women, and in the elderly. Supplementation can correct moderate deficiency and improve the condition of the blood. Some diseases worsen riboflavin deficiency, such as cancer, diabetes mellitus, and some types of cardiovascular disease. Those at risk for riboflavin deficiency include alcoholics, and people with malabsorption disorders or very poor diets. Long-term use of phenobarbital also affects riboflavin levels since the drug increases its breakdown, along with other nutrients in the liver. Poor riboflavin intake occurs if milk or milk products are not consumed sufficiently.

TABLE 10.9
Foods with the Highest Levels of Riboflavin (Vitamin B2)

Food	Quantity	Percentage (%) of Daily Vitamin B2 (Riboflavin)
Beef liver	3 oz	223
Plain yogurt	8 oz	37.5
Cottage cheese	1 cup	26
Low-fat milk	1 cup	26
Whole-grain cereal	¾ cup	25
Pork chop	3 oz	22
Egg	1 large	21
Bagel	4 inch	20
Chili con carne	1 cup	20
Cheddar cheese	2 oz	18

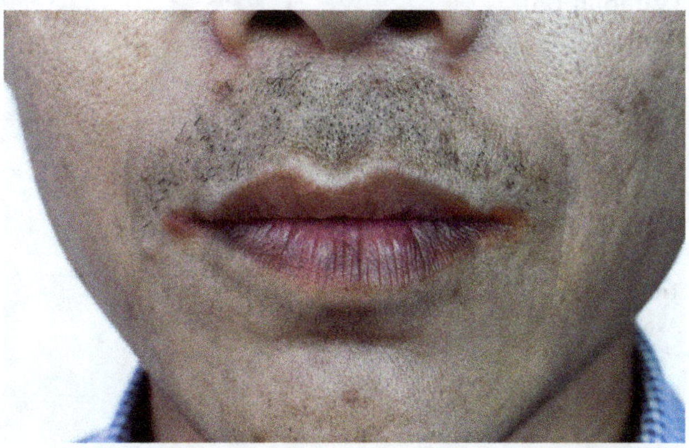

FIGURE 10.3 Ariboflavinosis, indicated by cracking of the skin around the corners of the mouth.

Test Your Knowledge

1. What are the classifications of water-soluble vitamins?
2. What are the three subtypes of beriberi?
3. What are the best sources of vitamin B2 (riboflavin)?

Vitamin B3 (Niacin)

Vitamin B3 (niacin) is the only vitamin of which there has been an epidemic of its deficiency in the United States. Niacin deficiency is called **pellagra**, which is discussed in greater detail in Chapter 17. About 27% of preformed niacin in North American diets comes from meats, including poultry and fish, with another 28% from enriched flour and grain products. Niacin is found in food sources such as liver, fish, red meat, legumes, and in cereals or breads that are whole grain or enriched. Insufficient dietary niacin can be compensated for by eating foods that are rich in tryptophan (such as dairy products), since dietary tryptophan is metabolized to niacin. Niacin is somewhat unique in that it is extremely stable in heat, so little is lost during cooking. About 60 mg of dietary tryptophan is required to make 1 milligram of niacin. Riboflavin and pyridoxine coenzymes are also needed for this. Since protein is about 1% tryptophan, 1 g of protein provides 10 mg of tryptophan. The adult recommended allowance is 14 mg per day for women and 16 mg per day for men. The daily value on labels is 16 mg. Fortunately, niacin intake, just in the United States, is much more. Preformed niacin from food averages 31.8 mg per day for men and 21.4 mg per day for women. The figures underestimate the niacin actually provided because they do not consider the niacin that is synthesized from tryptophan (which supplies about 50% of the niacin in the diet). The upper level for niacin is 35 mg per day, but this applies only to supplements and fortified foods. Table 10.10 summarizes foods with the highest levels of niacin.

Niacin (nicotinic acid), nicotinamide (niacinamide), and nicotinamide riboside are the three forms of vitamin B3 that are converted within the body to nicotinamide adenine dinucleotide (NAD). They are easily absorbed from the small intestine via active transport and passive diffusion. Nearly all niacin that is consumed is absorbed, but its

TABLE 10.10
Foods with the Highest Levels of Niacin (Vitamin B3)

Food	Quantity	Percentage (%) of Daily Vitamin B3 (Niacin)
Fortified cereal with corn, whole-grain oats, wheat flour, rice, and wheat germ	¾ cup	100
Chicken	3 oz	74
Wheat bran	2 oz	48
Tuna	3 oz	47
Halibut	3 oz	37.5
Salmon	3 oz	36
Peanut butter	2 tbsp	26
Steak	3 oz	24
Plain bagel	4 inch	23
Brown rice	1 cup	15

bioavailability is low in corn and other grains. Since niacin is tightly bound to protein, less than 30% is absorbed. Soaking corn in an alkaline solution of calcium hydroxide dissolved in water ("lime water") is done to prepare corn flour, releasing the skin from the corn kernels so that tortilla dough can be made. The soaking process also releases niacin from protein, protecting against deficiency. Once absorbed, niacin is carried through the portal vein to the liver, and stored or delivered to cells. Niacin is converted to coenzyme forms in every tissue and any excess niacin exits via the urine.

The coenzyme forms of niacin participate in oxidation-reduction reactions, and over 200 of them are in cellular metabolic pathways – primarily those that produce adenosine triphosphate (ATP). The metabolism of alcohol requires niacin coenzymes as well. Since nearly all metabolic pathways use the niacin coenzymes, deficiency of niacin causes extreme damage. High doses of niacin have been used for years to increase HDL-cholesterol and lower LDL-cholesterol and triglycerides, to reduce risks of stroke and heart attack. Even so, recent studies do not back this up. Large studies have revealed that niacin-containing medications did not reduce cardiovascular outcomes, but *did* cause GI bleeding, hyperglycemia, diarrhea, infections, and liver damage. Niacin-containing medications are no longer recommended for cardiovascular disease patients, except in a few cases.

FOCUS ON NIACIN

In general, niacin helps lower cholesterol, ease arthritis, and boost brain function, as long as it is taken in the correct doses. The top health benefits of niacin include increasing good (HDL) cholesterol while reducing bad (LDL) cholesterol and triglycerides, releasing prostaglandins to reduce blood pressure, lowering the risks for type 1 diabetes in at-risk children, boosting brain function, and protecting skin cells from sun damage.

Test Your Knowledge

1. What are the three forms of vitamin B3?
2. What are the best sources of vitamin B3?
3. What is the effect of high doses of niacin in lipids metabolism?

Vitamin B5 (Pantothenic Acid)

Vitamin B5 (pantothenic acid) is present in every body cell and also is supplied in most food sources. It is part of *acyl carrier protein (ACP)* used in biosynthetic reactions, and *coenzyme A (CoA)*, used for energy metabolism. The CoA forms as pantothenic acid combines with a substance derived from adenosine diphosphate (ADP) and a portion of the amino acid called *cysteine*, which provides the sulfur atom – the functional end of the coenzyme. Common sources of pantothenic acid include meat, milk, and vegetables. Unprocessed foods are generally higher in this vitamin than processed foods. This is because milling, freezing, heating, refining, and canning reduce the vitamin in food sources. The RDA is 5 mg per day (for men and women), but most adults consume more than this in the diet. The daily value on labels is also 5 mg. There is no known toxicity for this vitamin, so no upper level has been set. Table 10.11 summarizes foods with the highest levels of vitamin B5 (pantothenic acid).

The pantothenic acid portion of CoA in the diet is released during digestion, in the small intestine. It is absorbed and transported while being bound to RBCs. Storage is minimal, in the coenzyme form. Excretion of pantothenic acid is through the urine.

Coenzyme A is required for formation of acetyl-CoA, from breakdowns of alcohols, carbohydrates, fats, and proteins. The acetyl-CoA molecules enter the **citric acid cycle** with production of ATP. Acetyl-CoA is also important in building fatty acids, bile acids, cholesterol, and steroid hormones. Coenzyme A donates fatty acids to proteins that determine the location and function in cells. Pantothenic acid aids in fatty acid

TABLE 10.11
Foods with the Highest Levels of Pantothenic Acid (Vitamin B5)

Food	Quantity	Percentage (%) of Daily Vitamin B5 (Pantothenic Acid)
Cereal containing whole-grain wheat, raisins, and wheat bran	¾ cup	100
Sunflower seeds	2 oz	85
Pork sausage	3 oz	65
Trout	3 oz	40
Avocado	½ cup	38
Yogurt	1 cup	37
Blue cheese	2 oz	23
Milk	1 cup	22
Turkey	3 oz	21
Veal	3 oz	21

biosynthesis, with acyl carrier proteins attaching to fatty acids to move them through the metabolic pathway so that their chain length can be increased. Deficiency of pantothenic acid is very rare and only occurs if it is induced as part of a study. Symptoms include fatigue, headache, burning hands and feet, GI tract disturbances, and impaired muscle coordination.

Vitamin B6 (Pyridoxine)

All amino acid requires a vitamin B6 (pyridoxine) coenzyme for its metabolism. Vitamin B6 is actually a family of the compounds *pyridoxal, pyridoxine,* and *pyridoxamine.* They can be phosphorylated to become active coenzymes. Pyridoxal phosphate is the primary vitamin B6 coenzyme. Vitamin B6 is stored in animal muscle tissues, so rich sources include meats such as fish and poultry. The vitamin is better absorbed from animal foods than plant foods in most cases, but whole grains are also good sources. When grains are refined, the vitamin is lost and it is not added when the grains are enriched. The best fruit or vegetable sources are avocados, bananas, carrots, potatoes, and spinach. This vitamin can be lost from cooking or other processing. The RDA for vitamin B6 is 1.3 mg for men and woman under age 50. For those 50 or older, men need 1.7 mg per day and women need 1.5 mg per day. Daily value on labels is 1.7 g. Fortunately, average daily intake is usually higher, at 2.7 for adult men and 1.8 mg for adult woman. Vitamin B6 supplementation of 2–6 g per day has cause severe nerve damage and an inability to walk. Supplementation between 200 and 500 mg has caused tingling and numbness of the hands and feet. The upper level for adults is 100 mg per day to prevent nerve problems. Table 10.12 summarizes foods with the highest levels of vitamin B6 (pyridoxine).

Pyridoxine is absorbed by passive diffusion. The coenzyme form is generally converted to the free vitamin form for absorption, though a high concentrations some of the coenzyme is absorbed also. The vitamin is transported to the liver. The primary storage site is muscle tissue. Excess vitamin B6 is mostly excreted in the urine. Pyridoxine supports normal immune function and gene expression regulation. Low levels of pyridoxine have been seen in cardiovascular disease, diabetes mellitus, inflammatory bowel disease, and rheumatoid arthritis.

Deficiency of vitamin B6 is rare in most countries, but about 10% of the United States population have low concentrations. Signs and symptoms of deficiency include **microcytic hypochromic anemia**, convulsions, **seborrheic dermatitis**, depression, and confusion. Risk for deficiency is most prominent in women, older adults, African Americans, smokers, people taking oral contraceptives, alcoholics, underweight people, or those consuming a poor diet. Vitamin B6 supplements have long been used to treat carpal tunnel syndrome, premenstrual syndrome, and pregnancy-related nausea. Though evidence for its effectiveness is unproven, the Food and Drug Administration has approved a medication that contains vitamin B6 to treat mild to moderate pregnancy-related nausea. Another considered is the ingestion of megadoses of this vitamin, which can lead to peripheral neuropathy. This condition is discussed in detail in Chapter 13.

TABLE 10.12
Foods with the Highest Levels of Pyridoxine (Vitamin B6)

Food	Quantity	Percentage (%) of Daily Vitamin B6 (Pyridoxine)
Oatmeal	¾ cup	190
Pinto beans	1 cup	60
Pistachios	2 oz	49
Cereal containing milled corn	¾ cup	30
Banana	½ cup	28
Potato	½ cup	27
Turkey nuggets	3 oz	22
Beef	3 oz	22
Tuna	3 oz	21
Feta cheese	2 oz	16

Vitamin B7 (Biotin)

Vitamin B7 (biotin) is a coenzyme that participates in carboxylation reactions to add carbon dioxide to compounds. It was discovered in the 1920s when rats fed large amounts of raw egg whites developed rashes, lost fur, and became paralyzed. The feeding of yeast and liver to the test animals reversed the symptoms. Biotin is present in low amounts in foods, found as the free vitamin and **biocytin**, which is bound to lysine in proteins. Sources of biotin include chicken, salmon, peanuts, and eggs. Nutrient databases concerning biotin are not complete, and its content is only known for a small number of foods. Since humans excrete more biotin than is consumed, it is believed that large intestine bacteria synthesize this vitamin. Biotin is absorbed most efficiently from the small intestine. The recommended daily intake of biotin in men and women is 30 mcg per day, which is much less than for most other water-soluble vitamins. Most adults consume much more than this. The daily value on labels is also 30 mcg, and there is no upper level. Table 10.13 summarizes foods with the highest levels of vitamin B7 (biotin).

TABLE 10.13
Foods with the Highest Levels of Vitamin B7 (Biotin)

Food	Quantity	Percentage (%) of Daily Vitamin B7 (Biotin)
Chicken liver	3 oz	450
Chicken nuggets	3 oz	195
Salmon	3 oz	120
Peanuts	2 oz	115
Egg	1 large	52
Wheat germ	½ cup	49
Sunflower seeds	2 oz	25
Milk	1 cup	15
Mushrooms	½ cup	10
Swiss cheese	2 oz	9

The enzyme called *biotinidase* releases biotin in the small intestine from proteins and lysine. Free biotin is absorbed there through a sodium-dependent carrier, and stored in small amounts in the brain, liver, and muscles. Biotin is excreted mostly in the urine but also somewhat via the bile.

Biotin acts as a coenzyme for carboxylase enzymes, adding carbon dioxide to various compounds. The enzymes are needed for metabolism of carbohydrates, fats, and proteins. Biotin binds proteins that help DNA to fold in cell nuclei, which is believed to help maintain gene stability. Deficiencies are rare. About one of every 60,000 infants has a genetic defect, resulting in low amount so biotinidase, meaning they cannot break down biocytin in foods for absorption. Signs and symptoms of the resultant biotin deficiency include hair loss, skin rash, convulsions, impaired growth, and low muscle tone. These occur in a few weeks to months after birth. The infant is usually treated with regular biotin supplements, which have to continue throughout life in most cases. Deficiency of biotin has been caused by using anticonvulsants, because of malabsorption from severe intestinal diseases, and regularly eating 12 or more raw eggs per day. Raw eggs contain **avidin**, a protein that binds biotin and limits its absorption. When eggs are cooked, the avidin is denatured, so it cannot bind to the biotin.

Vitamin B9 (Folic Acid)

Vitamin B9, also known as folic acid or *folate*, was named because it is present in large amounts in leafy green vegetables, and *folium* is the Latin word meaning "leaf". Folate is actually the generic name of the vitamin and refers to various subtypes found in food sources. *Folic acid* refers to the synthetic form present in supplements and fortified foods. There are three parts of a folate molecule: *pteridine, para-aminobenzoic acid,* and one or more molecules of glutamate, an amino acid. When only one glutamate molecule is present, it is termed to be folic acid (*folate monoglutamate*). However, in foods, approximately 90% of folate molecules have three or more glutamates jointed to the carboxyl group, also known as *polyglutamates.*

Fortified cereals, lentils, and black beans are the top sources of vitamin B9, and both liver and leafy green vegetables provide the most bioavailability of the vitamin. In 1998, the United States made it mandatory to fortify enriched cereal grains with vitamin B9. This provided an extra 190 micrograms, on average, to the diets of adults. Leading sources are foods made with fortified flours, including rolls, yeast bread, cakes, cookies, pancakes, pasta, and ready-to-eat cereals and rice. Legumes, lentils, and vegetables actually contribute smaller amounts to U.S. diets. Biological availability of natural folate in mixed diets if 50%–80% of the amount found in fortified foods. Food processing and preparation is able to destroy up to 90% of the vitamin B9 in food sources, and it is easily destroyed by heat, oxidation, and ultraviolet light. However, dietary vitamin C helps protect vitamin B9 from oxidative destruction. It is advised that people regularly consume fresh or lightly cooked fruits and vegetables in order to benefit from the vitamin B9 they contain. Table 10.14 summarizes the foods with the highest levels of vitamin B9.

TABLE 10.14
Foods with the Highest Levels of Vitamin B9 (Folic Acid)

Food	Quantity	Percentage (%) of Daily Vitamin B9 (Folic Acid)
Fortified whole-grain cereals	¾ cup	110
Lentils	1 cup	85
Black beans	1 cup	65
Edamame	½ cup	60
Turnip greens	½ cup	54
Spinach	½ cup	35
Asparagus	½ cup	35
Bagel	4 inch	33
Avocado	½ cup	26
Orange juice	1 cup	25

Folate coenzymes are essential for synthesis and maintenance of new cells. Normal cell division requires folate, which has functions very similar to those of vitamin B-12. Deficiencies of both vitamins have similar symptoms. Folate coenzymes influence DNA function via **methylation** of certain parts of DNA molecules, and can affect risks for cancer. Hypomethylation and hypermethylation of DNA are linked to development of cancer and other diseases. Alterations in folate metabolism, due to reduced enzyme activities, can influence DNA methylation. Testing for the defect is available but not regularly done. Folate also helps form **serotonin**, norepinephrine, and **dopamine** in the brain. Therefore, supplemental folic acid may be a helpful addition in treating depression. Folate may help maintain normal BP and reduce stroke risks. Low blood folate is much more common in countries that do not have mandatory folic acid fortification measures in place, such as China, the Netherlands, Australia, New Zealand, Norway, Italy, Germany, the United Kingdom, France, Austria, Brazil, Algeria, Belgium, India, Moldova, Malaysia, Pakistan, the Philippines, Portugal, Georgia, Singapore, Sri Lanka, and Slovakia (see Figure 10.4).

Vitamin B9 deficiency used to be relatively common in the United States, but fortification of the food supply has greatly decreased its prevalence. Before fortification, 30% of Americans had low folate in RBCs. Today, less than 1% have folate deficiency. However, this condition can occur from low intake, malabsorption, and increased requirements for the vitamin. Highest risks are for poor people, alcoholics, those with chronic GI diseases, or those that use certain anticonvulsants and methotrexate. People with a vitamin B12 deficiency have abnormal utilization and metabolism of folate. A deficiency of folate can lead to cognitive dysfunction and encephalopathy, which is discussed in detail in Chapter 13.

Also, pregnancy increases needs for vitamin B9 greatly (the RDA is 600 mcg per day) due to increased rates of cell division and DNA synthesis. Prenatal multivitamin supplements are fortified with folate to compensate for these extra

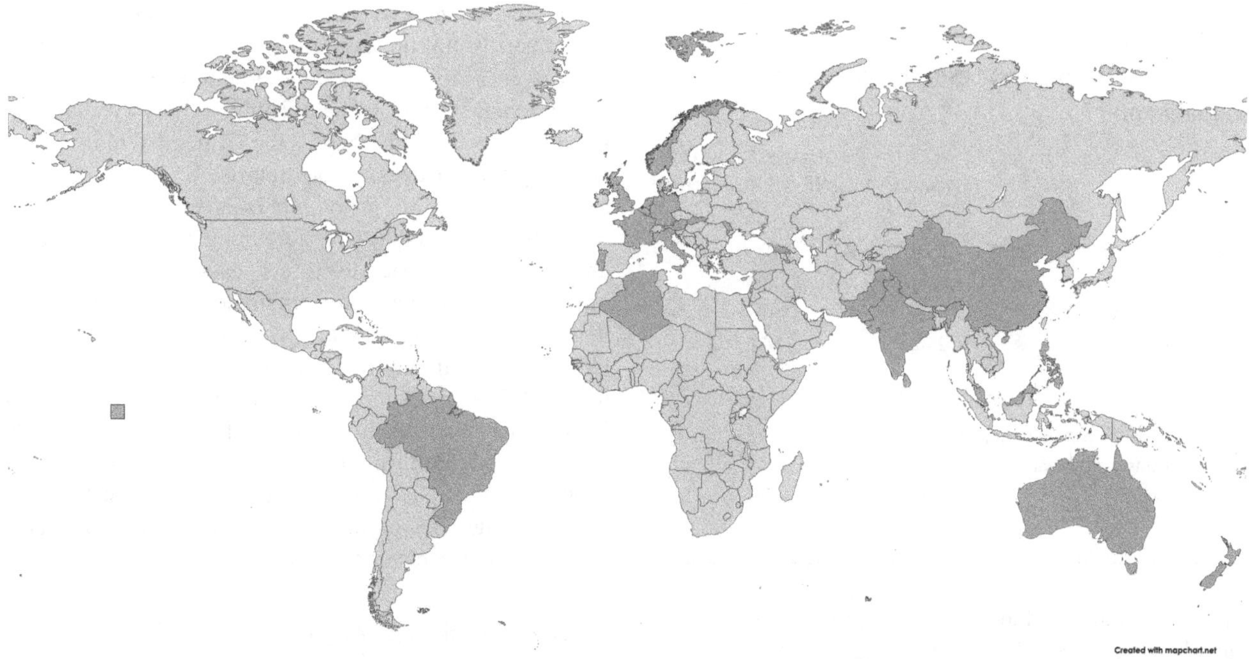

FIGURE 10.4 Countries with the highest rates of vitamin B9 deficiency.

needs during pregnancy. Deficiency of folate initially affects cells that actively synthesize DNA, since they have a short life span and rapid turnover RBCs. When a pregnant woman is deficient in folate, neural tube defects in the fetus are much more likely. The most common defects are spina bifida, and anencephaly, the lack of brain development. Spina bifida may cause incontinence, paralysis, and learning disabilities. Anencephaly is fatal. Therefore, ensuring good folate levels for all women of childbearing age is essential.

Precursor cells in bone marrow become unable to form new DNA and cannot divide normally to become mature RBCs. They grow larger due to continuous formation of RNA, resulting in more synthesis of components such as protein. Unlike normal mature RBCs, these **megaloblasts** keep their nuclei and remain large and immature. They mostly cannot exit the bone marrow. If they do enter the bloodstream, they are called macrocytes, resulting in **megaloblastic anemia**. Large and immature cells also appear in the GI tract if there is chronic deficiency of folate. This is because impaired DNA synthesis affects GI tract cell division. There is less absorptive capacity, and diarrhea becomes persistent. Other signs of deficiency are abnormal liver function and mouth sores. Synthesis of white blood cells (WBCs) is also disrupted by deficiency because they are made in short bursts during infections and other immune conditions. Folate deficiency, therefore, can reduce immune function.

Test Your Knowledge

1. What is polyglutamate?
2. Who has the highest risks for vitamin B9 deficiency?
3. What are the most common defects of vitamin B9 deficiency in newborns?

Vitamin B12 (Cobalamin)

Vitamin B12, or **cobalamin**, is quite different from other vitamins in that it almost only found in animal food products. It also is the only vitamin that incorporates the mineral called *cobalt* into its molecule. Between 1934 and 1965, researchers found out how the vitamin prevents deficiency-related *pernicious anemia*, resulting in multiple Nobel Prizes being awarded. No vitamin B12 is synthesized by plants, but nearly all related compounds are synthesized by bacteria and other microorganisms. Animals ingest vitamin B12 from soil as they eat and graze in fields, and some of them such as cows and sheep synthesize the vitamin from bacteria in their stomachs.

The best sources of vitamin B12 include liver, oysters, clams, and soy products. Vegans have difficulty getting enough dietary vitamin B12 because their food choices often are advertised as having good amounts, but actually contain analogs of the vitamin that do not function the same way in the body. Table 10.15 summarizes the foods with the highest levels of vitamin B12.

The RDA of vitamin B12 for adults is 2.4 mcg per day, and the daily value on labels is the same. Intake of the vitamin in the United States is usually higher than the RDA, with men averaging 6 mcg per day and women average 3.9 mcg per day. This means that the average American that consumes meat products has two to three years' worth of stored B12 in the liver. Excess vitamin B12 from food or supplements has never caused adverse effects, so there is no upper level.

About 50% of the vitamin B12 in food sources is absorbed, as long as an adult is healthy. In foods, vitamin B12 is bound to protein. Hydrochloric acid and pepsin in the gastric juice release the vitamin from these proteins. Free B12 combines with **intrinsic factor** from the **parietal cells** of the stomach and enhances absorption of the vitamin. The combination product travels to the ileum, where the vitamin is absorbed

TABLE 10.15
Foods with the Highest Levels of Vitamin B12 (Cobalamin)

Food	Quantity	Percentage (%) of Daily Vitamin B12 (Cobalamin)
Liver	3 oz	25,000
Oysters	3 oz	1,025
Clam chowder	1 cup	425
Soy milk	1 cup	125
Swiss cheese	2 oz	76
Roast beef	3 oz	52
Milk	1 cup	51
Fortified cereal with whole-grain wheat, raisins, and wheat bran	¾ cup	35
Turkey sausage	3 oz	34
Ham	3 oz	23

and transferred to a blood transport protein. Though continually secreted into the bile, most B12 is reabsorbed by the enterohepatic circulation and efficiently recycled. Very little B12 is excreted in the urine.

Vitamin B12 is needed for two enzyme reactions. Methionine, formed from homocysteine, is catalyzed by methionine synthase, which must have the B12 coenzyme called Methylcobalamin. Methylation reactions are important for DNA and RNA regulation, the regulation of **myelin**, and synthesis of biochemical compounds. The close link between vitamin B12 and folate is further emphasized in that methionine synthesis requires both vitamins

Pernicious anemia has been known of since the middle 19th century. It can be caused from insufficient production of intrinsic factor. Vitamin B12 deficiency also occurs because of malabsorption of intestinal conditions or certain medications. Very low intake of animal food products also causes B12 deficiency. Severe deficiency causes megaloblastic anemia. Some individuals have nerve degeneration that can lead to death. There are sensory disturbances in the legs, including burning, prickling, tingling, and numbness. Walking and balance become affected. Mental problems include loss of concentration and memory, disorientation, and **dementia**. Bowel and bladder control is eventually lost and visual disturbances are common. Gastrointestinal problems include tongue soreness and constipation. Neurological problems often precede anemia. Vitamin B12 deficiency-related large fiber peripheral neuropathy and encephalopathy are discussed in detail in Chapter 13.

The effects of low levels of B12, folate, and even B6 can cause high blood levels of **homocysteine**, increasing risks for heart attack and stroke. Homocysteine can damage the endothelial cells of the arterial linings. High levels are also linked to cognitive dysfunction and bone fractures. Good intake of B12 is essential for normal physiological function and health. Approximately 20% of older adults have insufficient vitamin B12 in their bodies, mostly due to atrophic gastritis. Taking crystalline B12 as a dietary supplement or in fortified foods can be helpful. When a person has an impairment of B12 absorption, he or she can receive monthly injections that bypass the GI tract. While vegetarians may become deficient in vitamin B12, vegans are much more likely to do so. When a person decides to become a vegetarian as an adult, B12 stores in the liver can hold off any signs of deficiency for a few years. Infants born to or breastfed by a vegetarian or vegan mother can develop B12 deficiency, with anemia and chronic neurological problems. Affected infants may have reduced brain growth, spinal cord degeneration, and poor intellectual development. Vegetarians can consume dairy products and eggs in order to get enough B12, or eat fortified food products or take supplements. Vegans *must* eat fortified foods at least two or three times per day, or take sufficient supplements as guided by a physician or dietitian.

Vitamin C (Ascorbic Acid)

Since human beings are unable to synthesize vitamin C, dietary sources are essential. Vitamin C (ascorbic acid) is involved in multiple body processes, mostly as a donor of electrons. Though present in most fruits and vegetables, the three best sources are guava, red peppers, and kiwi. Much vitamin C is taken in when an individual consumes five servings per day of fruits and vegetables. Vitamin C is the least stable of all the vitamins and is lost during storage, processing, and cooking. Juices are often fortified with vitamin C because the vitamin degrades less quickly due to their level of acidity. Table 10.16 summarizes the foods with the highest levels of vitamin C.

The RDA for vitamin C is 90 mg per day in men and 75 mg per day in women. The daily value on labels is 90 mg. For most adults in the United States, average intakes are close, at 83.3 mg per day for men and 75.1 mg per day for

TABLE 10.16
Foods with the Highest Levels of Vitamin C (Ascorbic Acid)

Food	Quantity	Percentage (%) of Daily Vitamin C (Ascorbic Acid)
Guava	½ cup	206
Red pepper	½ cup	106
Kiwi	½ cup	90
Strawberries	½ cup	60
Brussels sprouts	½ cup	53
Fortified cereal with milled corn, whole-grain out flour, wheat flour, and rice	¾ cup	51
Papaya	½ cup	47
Broccoli	½ cup	45
Orange juice	½ cup	45
Cranberry apple juice	½ cup	44

women. However, about 40% of adults do not get enough per day. Past studies have revealed that 10%–12% of people aged six years or older were low in vitamin C, and 6% were deficient. Vitamin C deficiency is more common in the poor, and in young or middle-aged adults.

People that smoke need more vitamin C, by about 35 mg per day, because smoking creates oxidative stress, increasing turnover of the vitamin. Women taking oral contraceptives may need more vitamin C as well. Obese people often have low serum vitamin C, in part due to a poor diet and a faster use of the vitamin by the body to try and reduce inflammation. Burn and trauma patients also need more vitamin C because it is linked to **collagen** synthesis, which greatly increases as tissues are rebuilt. An extra 500–1,000 mg of daily vitamin C may be needed.

The upper level for vitamin C is 2 g per day, based on adverse GI effects that include bloating, stomach inflammation, and diarrhea. High doses may increase risks for kidney stones and excessive iron absorption. High doses also give false medical test results for blood in the stool. Absorption of vitamin C happens in the small intestine, via active transport for ascorbic acid. As intake increases, absorption becomes less efficient. Approximately 70%–90% of vitamin C is absorbed at intakes between 30 and 200 mg per day. Excretion via the kidneys increases with higher levels of vitamin C in the diet. Stored vitamin C differs between body tissues. It is higher in the pituitary and adrenal glands, eyes, and brain. The lowest concentrations are in the blood and saliva.

Vitamin C has many important cell functions, based on donating electrons during oxidation-reduction reactions. It acts as a cofactor for **metalloenzymes** and has antioxidant defense properties. Metalloenzymes contain iron, copper, or zinc, usually as an ion. Ascorbic acid keeps iron in its reduced *ferrous* form and allows enzymatic actions to occur, and it is essential for wound healing. It also helps convert cholesterol to bile acids and aids in biosynthesis of corticosteroids and **aldosterone**. It inactivates free radicals, protecting DNA, proteins, and lipids from damage. In **neutrophils**, it protects against free radicals produced during immune functions. Vitamin C also regenerates active vitamin E to improve its functions.

Vitamin C is also believed to have additional roles in immune function. The vitamin C deficiency disease is known as **scurvy**, initially indicated after 20–40 days by fatigue and pinpoint hemorrhages around the hair follicles. The gums and joints bleed, indicating connective tissue failure. Other effects include slow wound healing, bone pain, fractures, and diarrhea. Advanced scurvy causes psychological problems such as depression. Untreated, scurvy is eventually fatal. Globally, scurvy is linked to poverty. It is highly common in infants fed boiled milk. Though rare in North America, scurvy still occurs in Canada, Afghanistan, and in countries with high rates of malnutrition. People at the greatest risk include the poor, alcoholics, smokers, and anyone with a diet that is poor.

Vitamin C is under continued study concerning its possibly preventive effects against cancer of the mouth, esophagus, stomach, and lungs. Some studies also suggest that good vitamin C status offers some protection against heart disease and stroke. Some evidence exists that high vitamin C intake may sometimes prevent or treat the common cold. A summary of water-soluble vitamin deficiency and toxicity symptoms is shown in Table 10.17.

KEY TERMS

Aldosterone

Apoenzymes

Apoprotein

Ariboflavinosis

Ataxia

Avidin

Biocytin

Calcitriol

TABLE 10.17
Water-Soluble Vitamin Deficiency and Toxicity Symptoms

Vitamin	Deficiency Symptoms	Toxicity Symptoms
B1 (Thiamin)	Beriberi (anorexia, peripheral neuropathy, weakness, weight loss), Wernicke-Korsakoff syndrome	None recognized
B2 (Riboflavin)	Ariboflavinosis (cracks at the corner of the mouth, inflammation of the mouth and tongue)	None recognized
B3 (Niacin)	Pellagra (dementia, dermatitis, diarrhea, and eventually, death)	Skin flushing
B5 (Pantothenic acid)	Fatigue, GI tract disturbances, impaired muscle function, weakness	None recognized
B6 (Pyridoxine)	Anemia, confusion, convulsions, depression, dermatitis	None from food; excessive supplementation can cause neuropathy, skin lesions
B7 (Biotin)	Conjunctivitis, dermatitis, hair loss, nervous system abnormalities	None recognized
B9 (Folic acid)	Birth defects, megaloblastic (macrocytic) anemia	None recognized
B12 (Cobalamin)	Megaloblastic (macrocytic) anemia, paresthesia, pernicious anemia	None recognized
C (Ascorbic acid)	Scurvy (bleeding gums, pinpoint hemorrhages, poor wound healing)	GI tract problems, including diarrhea

Carotenoids
Cataracts
Cholecalciferol
Choline
Chylomicrons
Citric acid cycle
Coenzymes
Cofactors
Cones
Confabulation
Conjunctival xerosis
Dementia
Dopamine
Ergocalciferol
Facilitated diffusion
Follicular hyperkeratosis
Free radicals
Homocysteine
Hemolysis
Hemolytic anemia
Holoenzymes
Infantile beriberi
Keratin
Keratomalacia
Lipoproteins
Macular degeneration
Megaloblastic anemia
Megaloblasts
Melanin
Menaquinone
Metalloenzymes
Methylation
Micelles
Microcytic hypochromic anemia
Myelin
Neutrophils
Osteomalacia
Oxidative stress
Parietal cells
Passive diffusion
Pellagra
Peroxidation
Phylloquinone
Pigeon chest
Prohormone
Provitamin D3
Renin
Retinal
Retinoic acid
Retinoids
Retinol
Rhodopsin
Rods
Scurvy
Seborrheic dermatitis
Serotonin
Tocopherol

CLINICAL CASE STUDIES

Clinical Case 1

A four-year-old boy who lived in Zambia on the African continent was assessed by a physician because of his symptoms, which included chronic diarrhea and recurring infections. His mother also told the physician that he would not go into his bedroom at night unless someone turned the light on for him, because he said he "couldn't see in there". A blood test revealed that is serum retinol was low, and the boy was diagnosed with vitamin A deficiency. A thorough review of his diet was conducted, and the physician suggested that the entire family follow his suggested changes, and seek help from United National International Children's Emergency Fund (UNICEF) to obtain other types of food. The boy was started on oral vitamin A supplementation.

CRITICAL THINKING QUESTIONS

1. What are the top three food sources that contain the most vitamin A?
2. Where is vitamin A stored in the body?
3. How does vitamin A deficiency lead to vision problems, including blindness?

Clinical Case 2

Vitamin D deficiency is endemic in Saudi Arabia, especially in younger males and those with diabetes or hypercholesterolemia. A 29-year-old man with diabetes mellitus went to see his physician because of severe fatigue, bone pain, and muscle cramps. He had suffered with these symptoms for a few months and admitted to feeling rather depressed about his health situation. The physician discussed the patient's diet and the patient stated that he never ate fish because he couldn't stand the taste, and was allergic to cow's milk. Tests revealed that his vitamin D levels were much lower than normal. The patient was given oral vitamin D2 (ergocalciferol) supplements for eight weeks. His levels normalized, and he was then started on maintenance doses of vitamin D3 (cholecalciferol).

CRITICAL THINKING QUESTIONS

1. How does melanin affect the skin's synthesis of vitamin D3 and what can be done to make sure enough vitamin D is being obtained?
2. Which food sources supply more than 20% of the daily percentage of vitamin D that is required?
3. Which adult disease occurs because of insufficient calcium and phosphorus but is usually caused by low levels of vitamin D in the diet.

Clinical Case 3

An Algerian woman, aged 32 years, had previously given birth to a baby boy with spina bifida. Vitamin B9 deficiency is a real problem in Algeria, and this vitamin is essential in the prevention of neural tube defects. The woman was planning on becoming pregnant again, and her physician counseled her on the importance of folic acid or folate supplementation in order to reduce the chance of having a second baby with the same type of condition. He also discussed her diet and gave her a list of foods that supply a good amount of folate. The physician additionally educated his patient on the other pregnancy-supporting results of having good levels of folate in the bloodstream.

CRITICAL THINKING QUESTIONS

1. What is the difference between the terms "folate" and "folic acid"?
2. What impact does pregnancy have upon vitamin B9 requirements?
3. Why is ensuring good folate levels for all women of childbearing age essential?

STUDY QUESTIONS

1. Which of the following forms of retinoids is an alcohol and may be referred to as vitamin A1?
   A. Retinal
   B. Retinoic acid
   C. Retinol
   D. Retinyl ester

2. Which of the following promotes growth, development, cell differentiation, vision, and immune function?
   A. Calcitriol
   B. Retinoids
   C. Tocopherol
   D. Phylloquinone

3. Which of the following vitamins primarily acts as a hormone?
   A. Vitamin K
   B. Vitamin A
   C. Vitamin D
   D. Vitamin E

4. Which of the following substances can be synthesized by bacteria in the colon?
   A. Menaquinones
   B. Tocopherol
   C. Retinoids
   D. Calcitriol

5. Which of the following substances may protect against macular degeneration?
   A. Ergocalciferol
   B. Carotenoids
   C. Phylloquinone
   D. Tocopherol

6. Which of the following is referred to as vitamin B1?
   A. Riboflavin
   B. Pyridoxine
   C. Niacin
   D. Thiamin

7. Which of the following vitamin deficiencies can cause pernicious anemia?
   A. Cobalamin
   B. Pyridoxine
   C. Riboflavin
   D. Biotin

8. Which of the following vitamins is also known as biotin?
   A. Vitamin B12
   B. Vitamin B7

C. Vitamin B3
D. Vitamin B1

9. Which of the following vitamins helps to form serotonin, norepinephrine, and dopamine in the brain?
 A. Cobalamin
 B. Niacin
 C. Folate
 D. Riboflavin

10. Which of the following vitamin deficiencies may cause rickets in children?
 A. Retinoid
 B. Calcitriol
 C. Phylloquinone
 D. Tocopherol

11. Which of the following vitamins can interfere with vitamin K, affecting blood clotting?
 A. Vitamin E
 B. Vitamin B1
 C. Vitamin A
 D. Vitamin B3

12. Which of the following vitamin deficiencies can cause beriberi?
 A. Biotin
 B. Retinoid
 C. Thiamin
 D. Tocopherol

13. Which of the following substances is required for the absorption of vitamin B12 in the small intestine?
 A. Dopamine
 B. Intrinsic factor
 C. Homocysteine
 D. Coenzyme A

14. Metalloenzyme is a cofactor that has antioxidant defense properties. It contains all of the following minerals, EXCEPT:
 A. Calcium
 B. Copper
 C. Iron
 D. Zinc

15. Which of the following vitamin deficiencies may cause scurvy?
 A. Folic acid
 B. Pantothenic acid
 C. Retinoic acid
 D. Ascorbic acid

FURTHER READING

1. Adefemi, O.E. (2023). Benefit, *Deficiency, and Sources of Vitamins*. Adefemi.
2. Allison-Francis, E. (2011). *Correcting the Vitamin D Deficiency Epidemic – Strategies to Fight Diseases and Prolong Life for Black People*. Dare Books.
3. Anderson, D.C., and Grimes, D.S. (2020). *Vitamin D Deficiency and COVID-19 – Its Central Role in the World Pandemic – Stay Safe & Take Vitamin D*. Tennison Publishing.
4. Berdanier, C.D., and Berdanier, L.A. (2021). *Advanced Nutrition: Macronutrients, Micronutrients, and Metabolism*, 3rd Edition. CRC Press.
5. Bever, M. (2015). *Vitamins, Minerals, & More! – Food Sources, Functions of the Body, and Deficiencies (Symptoms)*. CreateSpace Independent Publishing Platform.
6. Chandy Kayyalackakom, J., and Minney, H. (2019). *Vitamin B12 Deficiency in Clinical Practice – Doctor, You Gave Me My Life Back*! Kayyalackakom and Minney.
7. Crow, M. (2015). *Vitamin D Miracle – Health Benefits and Cure for Depression, Infertility, and Diabetes*. Transcendence Publishing.
8. Davis, M. (2020). *Eat Your Vitamins – Your Guide to Using Natural Foods to Get the Vitamins, Minerals, and Nutrients Your Body Needs – Reduce the Need for Costly Supplements*! Adams Media.
9. Ghazanfar, A., and Elya, R. (2014). *The B12 Deficiency Survival Handbook – Fix Your Vitamin B12 Deficiency Before Any Permanent Nerve and Brain Damage*. CreateSpace Independent Publishing Platform.
10. Guidi, L., De Bellis, L., and Pardossi, A. (2022). *Nutritional and Antioxidant Value of Horticulturae Products*. Mdpi AG.
11. Gupta, R.C., Lall, R., and Srivastava, A. (2021). *Neutraceuticals: Efficacy, Safety, and Toxicity*, 2nd Edition. Academic Press.
12. Kreisler Horwitt, M., Liebert, E., and Wittman, P. (2013). *Investigations of Human Requirements for B-Complex Vitamins: Bulletin of the National Research Council, Number 116*. Literary Licensing, LLC.
13. Leigh, I. (2022). *A Guidebook to Nutrition – A Comprehensive Guide to Essential Vitamins, Minerals & Omega Oils*. Leigh.
14. Lonsdale, D., and Marrs, C. (2017). *Thiamine Deficiency Disease, Dysautonomia, and High Calorie Malnutrition*. Academic Press.
15. Luciya, F. (2021). *Vitamin B6 Deficiency Symptoms – Cracks and Sores on the Lips, Tingling Sensations, Weakened Immunity, Skin Rashes, Etc*. Luciya.
16. Luyase, N. (2021). *Vitamin A Deficiency Symptoms – Dry Skin, Night Blindness, Acne, Dry Eyes, Dry Hair, Infertility, Miscarriage, Thick Skin, Itchiness, Frequent Respiratory Tract Infections*. Luyase.
17. Patel, V.B. (2019). *Molecular Nutrition: Vitamins*. Academic Press.
18. Purser, D., and Larkin, J. (2019). *Vitamin Deficiency Symptoms & Cures – Using Intracellular Micronutrient Results (Modern Deficiency Illness)*. Purser.
19. Somerville, J. (2018). *The Optimal Dose: Restore Your Health with the Power of Vitamin D3*. Big Bend Press.

20. Stone, I. (2017). *The Healing Factor – Vitamin C Against Disease: How to Live Longer and Better.* Books on Demand.
21. Wartian Smith, P. (2019). *What You Must Know About Vitamins, Minerals, Herbs and So Much More – Choosing the Nutrients That Are Right for You*, 2nd Edition. Square One.
22. World Health Organization. (2005). *Vitamin and Mineral Requirements in Human Nutrition*, 2nd Edition. World Health Organization.

11 Mineral Deficiency and Toxicity

OUTLINE

Food Sources of Minerals
Absorption and Bioavailability
Transport, Storage, Functions, and Excretion
Mineral Deficiency and Toxicity
Major Minerals
- Sodium
- Potassium
- Chloride
- Calcium
- Phosphorus
- Magnesium
- Sulfur

Trace Minerals
- Iron
- Iodine
- Copper
- Manganese
- Fluoride
- Zinc
- Selenium
- Chromium

Key Terms
Clinical Case Studies
Study Questions
Further Reading

LEARNING OBJECTIVES

After study of the chapter, readers should be able to:

1. Explain the essential minerals in the human body.
2. Describe the factors that decrease the bioavailability of minerals.
3. Discuss the effects of hyponatremia in the body.
4. Identify the signs and symptoms of hyperkalemia.
5. Discuss calcium deficiency.
6. Describe the signs and symptoms of Mg deficiency.
7. List the microminerals and their requirements.
8. Explain the outcome of iron overload in the body.
9. Describe the outcome of copper deficiency and Wilson's disease.
10. Discuss the signs and symptoms of selenium toxicity.

OVERVIEW

Minerals occur naturally and are solid, inorganic substances that the human body cannot synthesize. While about 4,000 minerals are known of, only 16 of them plus a few *ultratrace elements* such as cobalt, molybdenum, and nickel have nutritional value. They are required in small amounts in the diet in order for the body to function normally, grow, and for tissues to be maintained. A substance is considered as a nutrient when biological function or overall health declines if it is not consumed sufficiently. Unless permanent damage has taken place, when the substance is consumed in the diet, health should improve. There are major minerals as well as trace minerals. A major mineral must be consumed in a quantity of 100mg or more daily. Examples of major minerals include calcium and phosphorus. A trace mineral is needed in amounts less than 100mg per day. Examples of minor minerals include iron and copper. Minerals serve many functions, and structurally, they provide rigidity and strength to the teeth and bones. Skeletal components also serve as a storage area of some minerals for other needs of the body. Minerals provide proper muscle contraction and nerve functions. Some minerals act as cofactors for enzymes and maintain proper acid–base balance in body fluids. Minerals are also required for blood clotting, as well as tissue repair and growth.

FOOD SOURCES OF MINERALS

Minerals in most diets come from plant and animal sources. Animal-based foods are the richest source of some minerals and also have the highest *bioavailability*. Dairy products, for example, are rich in bioavailable calcium, while meat is rich in bioavailable iron and zinc. Plant sources are rich in Mg, manganese (Mn), and potassium, but there are compounds in plants that can reduce the bioavailability of these minerals. Minerals in various foods are affected by genetic variations that alter the ability of animals and plants to absorb and store minerals. Other factors include mineral compositions of foods eaten by animals and medications given to them. Mineral content of water, soil, fertilizers, and pesticides also affects quantities of minerals that end up in food. Even food processing affects mineral content. Iron from pots and pans can actually move, in small amounts, into our food. Essential minerals in the human body are summarized in Table 11.1.

Various minerals, including calcium and phosphorus, are present in *additives* that enhance flavor, preserve foods, and maintain their texture. Solutions used to sanitize foods can leave behind residues that contain minerals such as *iodine*, which is absorbed by any food that is prepared in the sanitized equipment. Processing methods may also decrease the amount of minerals present. Usually, minerals are present in lower amounts in plant foods that have undergone more refining procedures. When grains are milled, minerals that are removed include copper, iron, selenium, and zinc. The boiling of potatoes can reduce, by 50%–70%, minerals

DOI: 10.1201/b22969-14

TABLE 11.1
Essential Minerals in the Human Body

Major Minerals	Trace Minerals
Sodium	Iron
Potassium	Iodine
Chloride	Copper
Calcium	Manganese
Phosphorus	Fluoride
Magnesium	Zinc
Sulfur	Selenium
	Chromium
	Molybdenum

such as Mg, Mn, potassium, sulfur, and zinc. They simply exit the potatoes and are left behind in the cooking water. Today, increased amounts of foods are mineral-fortified. Since the 1940s, iron has been added to milled grains, and in the United States, table salt that is iodine-fortified has been available for about nine decades. Breakfast cereals are often fortified with many minerals, and drink options such as orange juice may be contain added calcium.

ABSORPTION AND BIOAVAILABILITY

Though minerals are highly prevalent in many foods, the human body has varying ability to absorb and utilize them. Many different factors interact. One is a physiological requirement for a certain mineral when the food source is consumed. Usually, if the need for a mineral is extreme, absorption of the mineral is increased. One example is the requirement for iron during growth spurts in children. Absorption often declines when the body has enough of the mineral present.

Bioavailability is also important and can be affected by the amount of minerals consumed, since many have similar molecular weights and charges, known as **valences**. Calcium, copper, iron, and Mg each exist in the 2+ *valence state*, and compete with each other for absorption, affecting overall bioavailability of each. Excessive dietary zinc may decrease absorption and metabolism of copper. The competition is not important if minerals are supplied in a balanced diet, but serious imbalances can occur from individual mineral supplementation. The best mineral supplements have 100% of less of the recommended daily value. Mineral supplementation should only be done with medical supervision. Factors that increase the bioavailability of minerals include good vitamin D status, normal gastric acidity, and vitamin C intake. Factors that decrease bioavailability of minerals include high-dose supplements of individual minerals; **oxalic acid** present in leafy vegetables; **phytic acid** present in legumes and whole grains; **polyphenols** present in coffee, tea, and red wine; and reduced gastric acidity. Phytic acid is also known as *phytate* and affects mineral absorption by chemically binding to them, preventing their release as we digest.

Fiber intake above the daily adequate intake of 25–38 grams (g) can negatively affect mineral status. When grains are leavened with yeast, enzymes from the yeast can break chemical bonds between minerals and phytic acid, increasing mineral bioavailability. Zinc deficiencies in some Middle Eastern people are related in part to heavy use of **unleavened breads**. This results in low dietary zinc bioavailability. Oxalic acid is also known as *oxalate* and is found in green leafy plants. It can bind to minerals to make them less bioavailable. Though spinach contains a large amount of calcium, just 5% can be absorbed due to the high oxalic acid concentration that is present. From milk and milk products, about 32% of dietary calcium can be absorbed. Polyphenols contain two or more ring structures, each with one or more hydroxyl groups (OH) attached. These compounds can lower mineral bioavailability – primarily calcium and iron. Many polyphenols are present naturally in plants, including tea, cacao beans (used to make dark chocolate), and grapes (used to make wine). Flavonoids and **tannins** (tannic acid) are types of polyphenols that can help prevent cancer and heart disease.

Some vitamins enhance mineral bioavailability. When vitamin C is consumed in the same meal as iron, the absorption of the iron is better. Calcitriol is a vitamin D hormone that improves absorption of calcium, Mg, and phosphorus. Gastric acidity also affects mineral bioavailability. In the stomach, hydrochloric acid (HCl) increases their bioavailability by dissolving minerals and converting them into a more easily absorbable form. The HCl provides one **electron** to the ferric ion, yielding ferrous iron – a more absorbable form. Mineral bioavailability can be reduced in older people or excessive use of antacids, since stomach acid production is lower. Most mineral absorption occurs in the small intestine. It is usually proportional to dietary intake. The absorption of calcium and iron can be regulated according to the needs of the body. Calcium absorption is related to the amount of specific binding protein in the **enterocytes**. Iron absorption occurs in the duodenum and proximal jejunum.

TRANSPORT, STORAGE, FUNCTIONS, AND EXCRETION

After absorption, minerals are carried in a free form, or bound to proteins, through the bloodstream. Calcium ions, for example, may be free or bound to *albumin*, a blood protein. Trace minerals in the free form are usually extremely reactive, and toxic if they are not protein-bound. Therefore, a large amount of trace minerals have certain binding proteins, transporting them in the bloodstream. Many are bound by certain cellular proteins after being taken up by cells.

Storage of minerals allows for a source of the mineral when dietary intake is insufficient, and the body's mineral storage varies widely (see Figure 11.1). Calcium and phosphorus are stored in large quantities in the bones and teeth.

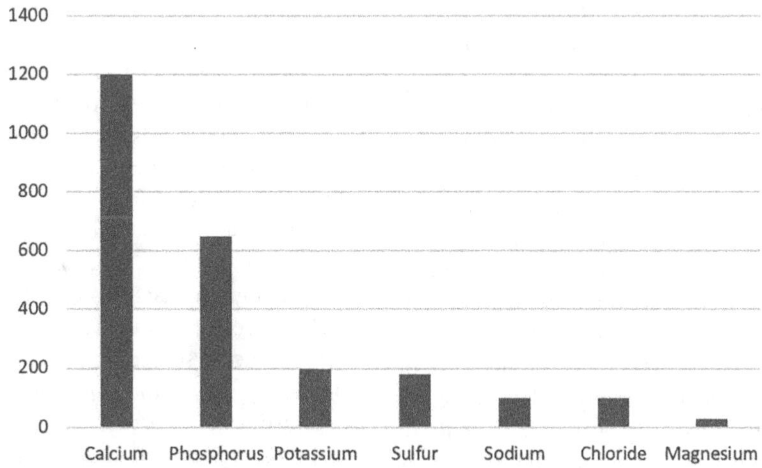

FIGURE 11.1 Storage of major minerals in the human body.

Iron is stored in smaller amounts in the **bone marrow** and liver. Also, there are tiny amounts of stored microminerals.

Minerals have widely different metabolic functions in the body. Chloride, phosphorus, potassium, and sodium are required for water balance. Nerve impulses are assisted by calcium, potassium, and sodium. Minerals that act as **cofactors** and allow enzymes to complete chemical reactions include copper, iron, Mg, and selenium. Many body compounds require minerals, such as hemoglobin in red blood cells, which needs iron in order to be synthesized. Minerals such as calcium and phosphorus are essential for body growth and development. Minerals play important parts in balancing body functions at the cellular, tissue, and organ levels, as well as the entire body.

Most major minerals are excreted via the urine. Some trace minerals, including copper, are secreted by the liver into the bile, so that they can be excreted via the feces. If kidney function should fail, it is very important to closely control mineral intake, in order to avoid mineral toxicity. This is especially true with phosphorus and potassium.

MINERAL DEFICIENCY AND TOXICITY

According to the latest Dietary Guidelines for Americans, the major minerals that are most likely to be insufficient, regarding daily recommended intake, include calcium, iron, Mg, and potassium. Serious public health problems in the United States include the following:

- Insufficient dietary calcium – poor bone health
- Insufficient dietary potassium – poor cardiovascular health
- Insufficient dietary iron – poor blood health, primarily during pregnancy, and in children

In other regions of the world, iodine and zinc deficiencies are common. Excessive amounts of minerals can also be toxic. This is true more often with the trace minerals, including iron and zinc. If the intake of mineral supplements will exceed the *upper level* that is recommended, a registered dietitian or physician should be consulted. Toxicity is just one reason to carefully evaluate use of mineral supplements. High intake of one mineral can reduce the absorption of other minerals. In past decades, some mineral supplements also became contaminated with lead or other toxic compounds. Therefore, it is important to use brands that are approved by the US Pharmacopoeia (USP). These brands are tested to make sure that no harmful amounts of contaminants are present, the listed ingredients are present, the ingredients will dissolve correctly, and safe/sanitary conditions were used in manufacturing.

MAJOR MINERALS

The major minerals **(macrominerals)** are inorganic substances that the human body cannot synthesize. Macrominerals include sodium, potassium, chloride, calcium, phosphorus, Mg, and sulfur. Major minerals are required in daily amounts of 100 mg or more.

SODIUM

Salt is a major mineral produced from the evaporation of seawater. It is the most important source of sodium (Na). The actual chemical name for salt is *sodium chloride* (NaCl), and it provides most dietary sodium. The actual makeup of salt is 60% chloride and 40% sodium. One teaspoon of salt is about 6 g, providing 2,300 mg of sodium. However, 75%–80% of sodium is not from table salt – instead, it is added during processing. It is important to understand that salt added during cooking or from a table salt shaker adds another 10%–15% of dietary sodium. Most unprocessed foods, however, do not contain much sodium, except for milk, which contains about 100 mg per cup. The dangers of sodium in the American diet are extreme. In general, men consume 4,094 mg per day, and women consume 2,997 per day. Processed foods are much higher in sodium than unprocessed foods. Foods that are highest in sodium content include table salt, pepperoni pizza, ham, chicken noodle soup, and chili with meat. Processing can greatly increase the sodium content of foods. For example, one cup of uncooked rice has no sodium, but one cup of fried rice, which is heavily processed, contains 705 mg of sodium.

Sodium deficiency is uncommon because there is so much of the mineral in the food supply, and the human body does not require very high amounts of it. However, sodium depletion may occur if losses exceed intake, which can happen via excess **perspiration**. Sodium losses are not significant unless weight loss from sweating is more than 2% of total body weight. For most people, simply adding some salt to foods is enough to restore sodium levels to normal. To avoid depletion of sodium and other electrolytes, athletes may need to consume sports drinks while they are competing. Sodium is not extremely concentrated in perspiration, despite sweat having a salty taste. Instead, water that evaporates from the skin leaves sodium on it. Sweat contains approximately 66% of the sodium concentration found in the blood. Sodium depletion may also occur due to diarrhea or vomiting – primarily in infants. In these cases, electrolyte drinks are used to replace sodium. *Hyponatremia* is a sign of sodium depletion. Symptoms include headache, nausea, vomiting, fatigue, and muscle cramps. If hyponatremia is severe, seizures, coma, and death may occur. The condition can also result from ingesting too much water.

Hypernatremia (excessive sodium) intake is well understood to be related to hypertension and cardiovascular disease. Blood pressure (BP) can often be reduced by decreasing sodium intake. Deaths from cardiovascular disease also are reduced. Though 2,300 mg per day is the upper level and daily value for adult sodium consumption, less than 33% of adults consume less than this. For most people, reducing sodium to less than the upper daily level will require that sodium levels – primarily in processed and restaurant foods – must be reduced. This is difficult to do, however. Many people enjoy salty foods in their diet. Reducing dietary sodium by 20% or more could prevent thousands of **strokes** and heart attacks per year. It is important for the public to look for food labels that include the terms *salt free, sodium free,* and *low sodium.*

FOCUS ON SODIUM AND HYPERTENSION

One of the key factors involved in development of hypertension is a poor diet with excessive sodium, insufficient potassium, and too many calories. Poor diets often lead to obesity, which is another primary risk factor for hypertension. The complications of hypertension include arterial damage, **aneurysm**, heart disease, brain damage, stroke, dementia, poor vision, kidney damage, sexual dysfunction, pregnancy abnormalities, and hypertensive crisis. Over 517,000 people die every year in the United States from hypertension as a primary cause of death.

POTASSIUM

Potassium (K) was first discovered in the 1800s as a silver-gray metal. Plant-based sources are rich sources of potassium. Even though it is widely abundant in foods, potassium intake is still low in many countries. Potassium occurs naturally in a variety of food sources, with unprocessed foods being the best sources – including kidney beans (73%), fruits and vegetables (20%), milk and milk drinks (11%), whole grains and grain-based dishes (10%), meats including poultry (10%), coffee and tea (7%), and fruit or vegetable juices (5%). Additional sources of potassium include salt substitutes (containing *potassium chloride*), and food additives such as the artificial sweetener *acesulfame-K*, and the preservative *potassium propionate*. Foods that provide potassium include apricots, artichokes, bananas, beef, broccoli, brussels sprouts, chicken, fish, kiwi fruit, milk, mushrooms, nuts, orange juice, pomegranate, spinach, tomatoes, and zucchini.

The adequate intake and daily value for adult dietary potassium is 4,700 mg, but average daily potassium intake is below this, at 3,016 mg in men and 2,320 in women. Men consume more potassium simply because they usually eat more food than women. Most adults need to increase potassium intake, which is best done by eating more fruits, vegetables, and whole-grain cereals and breads. Reducing milk and dairy products that are high in fat also helps. Low blood potassium is known as **hypokalemia** can be life-threatening. Symptoms include fatigue, weakness, muscle spasms, nausea, loss of appetite, constipation, and **arrhythmia**. Severe potassium deficiency can also cause muscle paralysis, and potentially fatal arrhythmias. Low potassium also raises risks for bone loss and kidney stones. Potassium depletion and low blood potassium are usually due to excessive losses of the mineral via the urine or gastrointestinal (GI) tract. Some diuretics used for hypertension deplete potassium by increasing the amount that is excreted in the urine. High-potassium foods should be added to the diet, or if recommended by a physician, potassium chloride supplements. *Potassium-sparing* diuretics do not increase potassium in the urine. In rare cases, extremely low dietary potassium results in low blood potassium. For example, eating disorder that involves low food intake plus induced vomiting and use of laxatives depletes potassium. Hypokalemia becomes a major concern. Also, alcoholics may have diets that are lacking in potassium. Heavy exercise causes excess loss of potassium via the sweat, but this can be replaced with a high-potassium, healthy diet.

Regarding potassium toxicity, hyperkalemia symptoms may include nausea, vomiting, weakness, tingling, or numbness. When hyperkalemia is severe symptoms such as difficulty breathing, heart palpitations, chest pain, arrhythmia, and sudden collapse may occur. It is extremely rare in healthy persons, since excess potassium is easily excreted in the urine. If kidney function is poor, potassium can quickly increase in the blood to cause arrhythmias or cardiac arrest. In these cases, dietary potassium must be carefully controlled.

FOCUS ON FOODS LOW IN POTASSIUM

Foods low in potassium include most refined fats and oils, grains (cornmeal, white rice, and pasta), cheeses (such as soft goat cheese), blueberries, eggs, leeks, Napa cabbage, and chia seeds. Boiling vegetables in water and discarding the water can help reduce their potassium and electrolyte content.

Test Your Knowledge

1. Why is sodium deficiency uncommon?
2. What could be a result of excessive sodium intake?
3. What are examples of foods that provide potassium?
4. What are the symptoms of hyperkalemia?

Chloride

Chloride (Cl) is the primary **anion** (Cl–) in the extracellular fluid, but the chloride ion is not the same as the element called *chlorine* (Cl2), a strong oxidant. Chlorine is used to disinfect swimming pools, purify water, bleach fabrics, and produce many paper and plastic products. Chlorine as well as chlorine gas is toxic. Nearly all dietary chloride comes from table salt. The same foods containing sodium also provide most of the dietary chloride. Other sources of chloride include olives, seaweed, lettuce, rye, and some fruits and vegetables. Potassium chloride is usually contained in salt substitutes. The adequate daily adult intake and daily value of chloride in foods and supplements is 2,300 mg. If the average daily consumption of salt is 9 gr, this yields 5,400 mg of chloride.

Chloride deficiency is uncommon because of the high intake of dietary salt. However, chloride deficiency may result from extended vomiting when an individual also has a diet that is poor in nutrients. This is related to a loss of HCl from the stomach. Symptoms of chloride deficiency include anorexia, **lethargy**, and weakness. Loss of HCl can cause an imbalance of acids and bases.

However, the upper level for daily chloride is 3,600 mg. Most adults consume much higher amounts, unfortunately. Dietary chloride may add to the effects of sodium chloride, increasing BP. As a person reduces sodium intake, such as during the treatment of hypertension, the chloride intake will also be reduced automatically.

Calcium

Calcium (Ca) is essential for normal development of the bones and teeth. It also plays an important role in blood clotting, helping muscles to contract, and regulating normal heart rhythms and nerve functions. A rich supply of bioavailable calcium is provided in dairy products, including milk and cheese. Nearly half of the US dietary calcium comes from these products. Other foods with good levels of calcium include crackers, rolls, yeast breads, and foods made with dairy products. Calcium also comes from collard greens, kale, broccoli, turnip greens, almonds, calcium-fortified juices and milk, breakfast cereals, canned fish, and **tofu** that is made by adding calcium carbonate. However, calcium levels are different between various food brands, so it is important to check labeling. In leafy greens and other plant foods, much calcium is poorly absorbed because it is bound to oxalic acid. As little as 5% of the calcium in one cup of spinach is bioavailable. However, about 33% of the calcium in a cup of milk is absorbable. For most adults, the recommended daily allowance of calcium is 1,000 mg per day, but in women over 50 and men over 70, this increases to 1,200 mg per day. During adolescence, 1,300 mg per day is needed to support increased bone mass during rapid growth. In pregnant women requirement for calcium is 2,400 mg. Calcium is essential for normal bone development in a fetus. The daily value of calcium on food and supplement labels is 1,300 mg. In the United States, average calcium intake is varied, as follows:

- Adolescent females – 842 mg per day
- Adult females – 852 mg per day
- Adolescent males – 1189 mg per day
- Adult males – 1086 mg per day

Females between 9 and 18 years, and those over age 71, have the lowest calcium intake. Just 15% of younger females and 39% of older females meet daily requirements even when dietary and supplemental sources are included. Nearly 70% of men over age 70 do not consume enough daily calcium.

Hypocalcemia is also known as *calcium deficiency disease*. It results in abnormal muscle function and increased likelihood of **osteoporosis** and **osteopenia**. Signs and symptoms of hypocalcemia include confusion, memory loss, muscle spasms and cramps, numbness, tingling, depression, **hallucinations**, nails that become brittle and weak, and easy bone fracturing. Tetany is a condition of intermittent muscle spasms related to calcium deficiency and malfunction of the parathyroid glands. When a child does not get enough calcium, their final height during adulthood may be shorter than average. In children, symptoms of *rickets* may occur due to poor bone mineralization. During menopause, women must increase calcium intake to reduce risks of bone abnormalities, especially since declines in the hormone *estrogen* also cause the bones to become thinner, more quickly. People with **hypoparathyroidism** do not produce enough *parathyroid hormone* (PTH) which controls calcium levels in the blood. Another factor is *vitamin D*, which in low levels, results in calcium absorption being compromised.

The upper level for daily calcium is 2,500 for adults between 19 and 50, and 2,000 per day for those over 50. The upper level is based on likelihood for increased risks of kidney stones and hypercalcemia. The small intestine usually prevents absorption of excess calcium. In some people, high amounts of calcium causes hypercalcemia. Excessive dietary calcium can cause headache, irritability, kidney stones or kidney failure, and decreased absorption of other minerals. Usually, dietary or supplemental calcium is not sufficient to cause hypercalcemia.

FOCUS ON OSTEOPOROSIS

Calcium is important in preventing osteoporosis because it helps build bone mass. Osteoporosis causes the body to break down more bone than it manufactures. The bones become weak, brittle, and more likely to fracture. However, calcium requires vitamin D and vitamin K2 in order to function correctly. Vitamin D helps the body absorb calcium that is consumed, while vitamin K2 activates proteins that help calcium move to the places where it is most needed. When dietary calcium is not keeping essential body processes functioning, it is taken from the bones, decreasing density and the likelihood of fractures. Osteoporosis is common in women after menopause and in men after age 70.

Test Your Knowledge

1. What is the requirement for calcium during pregnancy?
2. What are the complications of calcium deficiency disease in children and adults?
3. What are the signs and symptoms of hypercalcemia?

Phosphorus

Phosphorus (P) is needed by all cells in the body. Naturally, phosphorus occurs as a high amount of mineral that is extensively present in the bones. It is a major component of the teeth as well, and any excess is removed in the urine. Foods that provide large amounts of phosphorus include milk, cheese, bakery products, cereals, and meats. Other sources include bran, eggs, fish, and nuts. Up to 400 mg per day of dietary phosphorus is also supplied by food additives, which include the emulsifier *monosodium phosphate*, the jelling agent monocalcium phosphate, and fortifying nutrients such as *iron phosphate*. Phosphorus in food additives is often not included in nutrient databases or estimates of the daily intake of phosphorus. Adult men and women need about 700 mg per day of phosphorus. However, most adults consume much more. Men average 1,625 mg per day and women average 1,187 per day.

This means that phosphorus deficiency is extremely rare in healthy adults, primarily because the mineral is so well absorbed. The daily value for phosphorus on food and supplement labels is 1,250 mg. A chronic phosphorus deficiency can cause bone loss, reduced growth, and poor development of the teeth. Additional symptoms of phosphorus deficiency include anorexia, weakness, weight loss, irritability, bone pain, and stiff joints. Less than optimal phosphorus can be revealed in alcoholics, preterm infants, older adults that consume nutrient-poor diets, chronic diarrhea and weight loss, and excessive use of antacids that contain aluminum, since they may bind phosphorus in the small intestine.

Toxicity due to phosphorus is also rare. If there is hyperphosphatemia, calcium/phosphorus precipitates can form in the tissues. The most common cause of hyperphosphatemia is poor kidney function. Therefore, people with kidney failure must closely monitor their intake and blood concentrations of phosphorus. Most people in the United States have a low calcium intake combined with a high phosphorus intake. It is now believed that increased PTH and bone loss occurs because of insufficient calcium in the diet, and not from the calcium-to-phosphorus ratio, which was previously believed to be the cause. The upper level for adult dietary phosphorus is 3–4 gr per day, based on risks for hyperphosphatemia.

Magnesium

Magnesium (Mg) is naturally found as a silver-white metal in ocean water and soil. It is an essential nutrient for plants as well as human, and is present in many different foods. Mg is a component of **chlorophyll**, so rich sources include broccoli, green leafy vegetables, beans, squash, nuts, seeds, chocolate, and whole grains. Milk and meats supply some Mg, but in lower quantities. *Hard tap water* also contains a lot of Mg (as well as calcium). Coffee and tea also supply good amounts of dietary Mg. However, refined foods are usually low in this mineral. The type of Mg in mineral supplements (magnesium oxide) and multivitamins is poorly absorbed. The recommended daily allowance for Mg is 400 mg per day (for men 19–30) and 310 mg per day (for women of the same ages). Requirements increase by 10–20 mg per day past age 30. The daily value is 420 mg per day on food and supplement labels. In the United States, adults do not get quite enough Mg. Adult men average 345 mg per day, and adult women average 268 mg per day. Less than 25% of adults get enough daily Mg.

The signs and symptoms of Mg deficiency include arrhythmias that may be accompanied by muscle spasms, weakness, disorientation, nausea, vomiting, and seizures. There may be abnormal nerve cell function due to impaired Na/K pumping. Deficiency of Mg can also cause a decrease in PTH release that results in low blood calcium. The biologically active form of vitamin D (known as *1,25(OH)$_2$ vitamin D*) cannot be as effective during Mg deficiency. As a result, this condition contributes to increased risk of osteoporosis. However, since Mg is easily stored in the body, deficiency develops very slowly. A poor Mg status is also related to cardiovascular disease. Excessive loss of this mineral from the intestinal tract or urine causes the majority of Mg deficiencies. At-risk individuals include those with GI disorders involving chronic diarrhea and vomiting. More Mg is excreted in the urine of alcoholics, and those with poorly controlled diabetes mellitus.

The upper level of daily Mg is 350 mg, based on supplement and other non-food sources that include some antacids and laxatives. Intakes above this amount from non-food sources can cause diarrhea. With kidney failure, toxicity can occur since the kidneys are the main regulators of blood Mg. When there are high levels of blood Mg, symptoms include nausea, weakness, slowed breathing, and over time, malaise, coma, and death. Older people have a higher risk of Mg toxicity because of declining kidney function.

Sulfur

Sulfur (S) is mostly provided by the amino acids *cysteine* and *methionine*. It is a bright yellow mineral, and *inorganic sulfate* is also found in foods and water. Often, it is a preservative used to protect the color of white wines and dried fruits. Sulfur has no recommended daily allowance or adequate intake established, because it is highly present in foods containing protein. Sulfur helps stabilize protein structure such as in the collagen, hair, nails, and skin. It helps regulate acid–base balance. There is no established upper level for sulfur. As a result, there is no actual sulfur deficiency or toxicity. The requirements for major minerals are summarized in Table 11.2.

FOCUS ON MINERALS

Minerals are important for the health of the body. Minerals are needed to keep the bones, muscles, heart, and brain working properly. They are also important for manufacturing enzymes and hormones. Most people get the amount of minerals they need by eating a wide variety of foods. Those with certain health problems or if taking some medications may need to get lower quantities of a mineral. For example, patients with chronic kidney disease need to limit foods that are high in potassium.

TABLE 11.2
Major Minerals

Mineral and Intake	Functions	Sources	Deficiency	Toxicity
Sodium 1,500 mg (age 19–50) 1,300 mg (age 51–70) 1,200 mg (70+)	Amino acid absorption, glucose absorption, muscle contraction, nerve impulse transmission, water balance; it is the major positive ion of the extracellular fluid	Chips, condiments, processed foods, sauces, soups, table salt	Fatigue, headache, muscle cramps, nausea, vomiting	Contributes to hypertension (in susceptible people); increases calcium loss via the urine; upper level is 2300 mg
Potassium 4700 mg	Muscle contraction, nerve impulse transmission, water balance; it is the major positive ion of the intracellular fluid	Fruits, legumes, meats, milk and milk products, vegetables, whole grains	Increased risk of hypertension and stroke, irregular heartbeat, loss of appetite, muscle cramps	Slowed heartbeat (often with kidney failure)
Chloride 2,300 mg	Acid production in the stomach, nerve impulse transmission, water balance; it is the major negative ion of the extracellular fluid	Processed foods, some vegetables, table salt	Convulsions (in infants)	Hypertension when combined with sodium (in susceptible people); upper level is 3,600 mg
Calcium 1,300 mg (9–18 years) 1,000–1,200 mg (18+)	Blood clotting, bone structure, enzyme regulation, muscle contractions, nerve impulse transmission, tooth structure	Canned fish, fortified foods, leafy vegetables, milk and milk products, tofu	Higher risk of osteoporosis	Kidney stones (in susceptible people); the upper level is 2,500 mg
Phosphorus 1,250 mg (9–18 years) 700 mg (18+)	Acid–base balance, bone strength, part of adenosine triphosphate (ATP) and other metabolic compounds, tooth strength; it is the major ion of the intracellular fluid	Bakery products, fish, meats, milk and milk products, processed foods, soft drinks	Poor bone maintenance	Impaired bone health (in those with kidney failure); poor bone mineralization (when calcium intake is low); upper level is 3,000–4,000 mg
Magnesium 400–420 mg (men) 310–320 mg (women)	Bone formation, enzyme function, heart and nerve function	Chocolate, green vegetables, legumes, nuts, wheat bran	Muscle pain, poor heart function, seizures, weakness	Diarrhea, malaise, nausea, weakness (in those with kidney failure); upper level is 350 mg, but only to non-food sources such as supplements
Sulfur (none)	Acid–base balance, drug detoxification; is part of amino acids and vitamins	Protein foods	None seen	None likely

Test Your Knowledge

1. What are the differences between macrominerals and microminerals?
2. What are the signs and symptoms of potassium toxicity?
3. What are the effects of hypocalcemia?
4. What are the main sources of Mg?

TRACE MINERALS

The trace minerals (**microminerals**) include iron, iodine, copper, Mn, fluoride, zinc, selenium, chromium, and molybdenum. They are required in amounts of less than 100 mg per day. Trace minerals are inorganic but essential substances. They are found in tiny amounts in the human body, of less than 5 mg. All of the trace minerals combined make up less than 1% of body minerals. Even so, they are required for normal development, function, and good health. Iron helps to build red blood cells. Copper, Mn, selenium, and zinc help protect from harm caused by **free radicals**. Iodine is required for normal metabolism. Except for iodine and iron, the need for trace minerals was only discovered within about the last five decades. Due to their small amounts, it is quite difficult to assess changes in trace mineral concentrations and their effects upon the body. Recommended intake levels are also hard to determine.

Iron

The importance of iron in the diet has been known for centuries. Even so, about one in four people throughout the world has **anemia**, often due to iron deficiency. Younger children and pregnant women are most often affected. Iron deficiency is a leading global health risk, according to the World Health Organization, in many countries, though industrialized countries such as the United States have less overall cases based on population.

Most experts recommend using the *transferrin receptor number* to evaluate iron status. This is because it reveals the need for cellular iron, and it is unaffected by factors limiting use of other **biomarkers** of iron. Iron status may also be assessed by using laboratory data for transferrin receptors and ferritin. Individuals at highest risk of iron deficiency and its related anemia include the following:

- *Premature newborn before week 37* of gestation – since iron stores required for early life accumulate in the last weeks of gestation; these infants are born with low stores that may be quickly depleted by their high need for iron
- *Infants* – since they are growing fast and usually have low intake of meat and high intake of cow milk (which is low in iron)
- *Adolescent girls and women of childbearing age* – at risk, since monthly menstrual blood losses and low intake of iron-rich foods are common. In the United States, about 10% of women aged 12–49 have iron deficiency anemia
- *Pregnant women* – more iron is needed since the mother's blood volume and numbers of red blood cells is increasing along with those of the fetus
- *Blood donors* – those that donate blood more than two to four times per year are at increased risk of iron deficiency; for each pint of donated blood, there is a loss of 200–250 mg of iron; this usually requires several months to replace, but women may take longer; because of these factors, blood banks test donor blood for anemia before the donation can be done
- *Vegetarians* – even though they may have high intakes of plant-based foods with sufficient iron, the diet may have a variety of factors decreasing the bioavailability of the iron; therefore, these individuals must include vitamin C-rich foods and consider iron-fortified foods plus multivitamin–mineral supplements containing iron

Even though iron deficiency is a major concern, this mineral can also cause toxicity. Intakes above 45 mg per day, often from highly fortified foods and supplements, can cause nausea, vomiting, diarrhea, stomach irritation, and poor absorption of other trace minerals. In US children under age six, accidental iron overdose is the main cause of poisoning. Children are more vulnerable to this than adults since their ability to absorb iron is not as quick as in adults. Overconsumption of chewable supplements that contain iron is the primary cause of pediatric iron overload. Therefore, all iron supplements, according to the Food and Drug Administration (FDA), must carry a toxicity warning. Supplements containing 30 mg or more iron per tablet must be individually wrapped.

Iron overload in adults is usually from *hemochromatosis*, which is a genetic condition affects about one person of every 200–500 (see Figure 11.2). In this condition, the mucosal block that normally protects against excessive iron absorption does not function properly. Because of a **hepcidin** deficiency, higher amounts of iron are absorbed and transported across the enterocyte, to be bound to transferrin and distributed to tissues. Normally, hepcidin prevents degradation of the transport protein called *ferroportin*. Without an ability to eliminate the excess iron, it accumulates, causing iron overload and tissue damage. There is saturation of iron-binding proteins. Eventually, iron deposits collect in the heart, liver, and other organs. Without treatment, heart failure and liver disease develop.

Excess iron supplementation and regular blood transfusions can also cause iron overload in adults. Via blood transfusions, the increased iron in the blood overcomes the mucosal block, resulting in extremely high iron stores without close monitoring. Treatment of iron toxicity is based on the cause. Iron supplements, if used, should be stopped. With hemochromatosis, treatment requires periodic blood

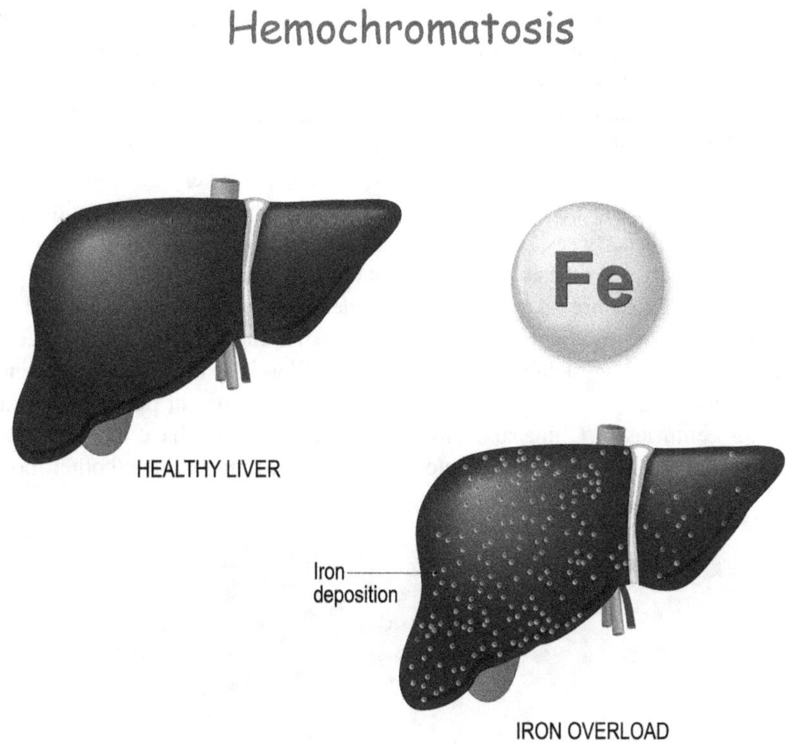

FIGURE 11.2 Hemochromatosis of the liver.

removal, or a chelator drug can be administered, which binds the iron and increases excretion. The problem with chelator drugs is that they also bind to other trace minerals, and can cause secondary deficiencies of them.

FOCUS ON IRON DEFICIENCY

Iron deficiency is one of most prevalent forms of malnutrition. Iron deficiency anemia accounts for several hundred millions of cases of anemia. Iron deficiency is an extreme risk factor for maternal and perinatal mortality. It has direct contributions to cognitive impairment, decreased work productivity, and death. Africa and parts of Asia make up 71% of the global mortality burden, while North America bears only 1.4% of the global burden. Therefore, an urgent need exists to develop effective, sustainable methods to control iron deficiency anemia.

Test Your Knowledge

1. What is the function of ferritin in the body?
2. Which individuals are at highest risk of iron deficiency?
3. What is hemochromatosis?

IODINE

Iodine is present in food as iodide and non-elemental forms. In many ways, it is distinct from the other trace minerals. Iodine is the heaviest element required for human health. In the body, it is only involved in the synthesis of thyroid hormones. Most foods contain low amounts of iodine. The best sources include saltwater seafood, iodized salt, seaweed, and dairy products. Though dairy products are not naturally good iodine sources, they usually provide good amounts because iodide is added to cattle feed and the sanitizing solutions used in dairy processing. Some breads and cereals also contribute dietary iodine. Plant-based foods may provide iodine but this is based on the type of soil in which they were grown. Iodine-rich soil is usually located close to oceans because seawater is naturally high in iodine. In the United States, iodized salt is regularly used during cooking or on the dinner table, so iodine intake is sufficient. There are about 76 micrograms (mcg) of iodine in every gram of iodized salt, so about one-half teaspoon (2 gr) is enough to supply daily requirements. It is important to understand that kosher salt and sea salts are not iodized. Bioavailability of iodine is decreased by **goitrogens** in raw vegetables that include cabbage, turnips, brussels sprouts, broccoli, cauliflower, potatoes, rutabagas, cassava, peanuts, peaches, soy, and strawberries. The goitrogens decrease absorption of iodine as well as inhibit the thyroid gland's use of it. Iodine deficiency is higher in part of the world where raw vegetable intake is high while iodine intake is low. Iodine is needed for adults in levels of 150 mcg per day. In the United States, iodine intake is between 190 and 300 mcg per day, without taking into account the amounts found in iodized salt added to meals. The daily value for iodine on food and supplement labels is 150 mcg per day.

Iodine deficiency disorders describe the conditions known as **endemic goiter**. They occur from insufficient iodine in the diet. When plasma levels of **thyroxine** (T4) drop, the pituitary gland secretes **thyroid-stimulating hormone** (TSH). The increased TSH levels cause the thyroid gland to enlarge so that it will become more efficient in trapping iodine. The enlargement of the thyroid gland is called a goiter (see Figure 11.3). This early response allows the gland to maintain thyroid hormone synthesis temporarily. A goiter is painless but can put pressure on the esophagus and trachea, impairing function. Without treatment, decreased T4 synthesis, abnormally slow metabolism, and serious complications can occur.

Goiter has been seen for centuries in China and other areas of the world. Before World War I, it was also common in areas of the United States in which soil or lake water was low in iodine. Today about 33% of the global population is at risk of iodine deficiency. A higher incidence occurs in parts of Asia, the Middle East, Africa, and Europe (see Figure 11.4). In the United States and Switzerland during the 1920s, discovery that iodine prevented goiter resulted in table salt becoming fortified with the mineral. Use of iodized salt has eradicated endemic iodine deficiency in areas where it has become common. Even so, about 30% of homes worldwide do not have access to iodized salt, so iodine deficiency is still an international public health problem. According to the World Health Organization, iodine deficiency is still the greatest cause of preventable brain damage and mental retardation. Goals have been established to increase use of iodized salt, milk, oil, and other food products.

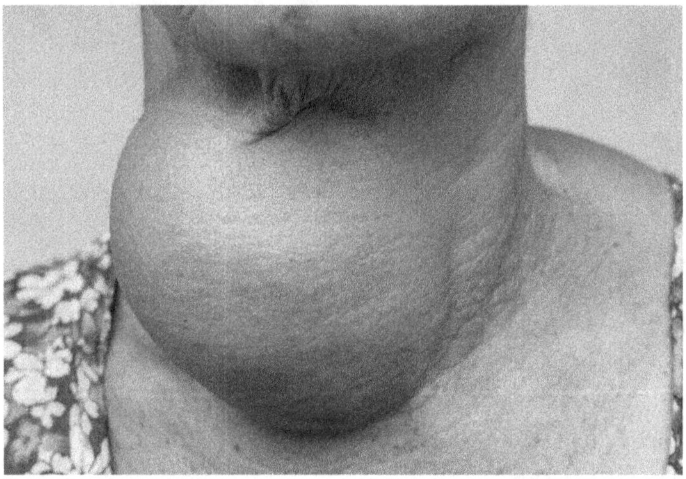

FIGURE 11.3 Goiter.

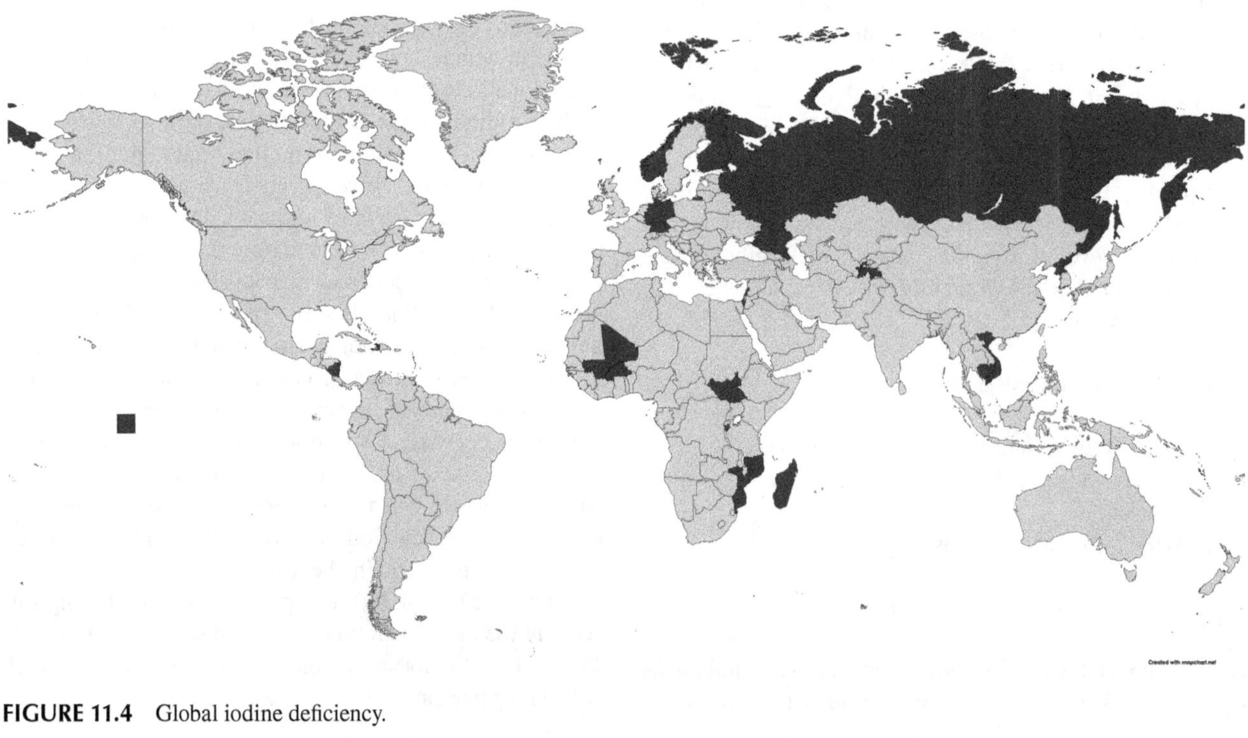

FIGURE 11.4 Global iodine deficiency.

For iodine, the upper level is 1,100 mcg per day for adults. Iodine toxicity can also cause an enlarged thyroid gland and reduced synthesis of thyroid hormone (TH). Toxicities have occurred in Japan because of high intake of seaweed, and in Chile due to high amounts of environmental iodine, over-fortification of salt, and increased use of iodine to purify water. In iodine-sufficient individuals, iodine excess causes elevated TSH levels, which inhibit thyroid hormone production. This leads to hypothyroidism and goiter. Excess iodine intake also can increase risks of autoimmune thyroid disease, hyperthyroidism, and thyroid cancer.

FOCUS ON IODINE

Iodine is a trace mineral that is mostly stored in the thyroid gland. It is essential for the body to convert food into energy. Deficiency of iodine leads to goiter or hypothyroidism. Iodine is most highly present in iodized salt and seafood, the type of seaweed known as "kelp", and in lower quantities, strawberries, yogurt, cow's milk, eggs, mozzarella, lima beans, soybeans, sesame seeds, and garlic.

Test Your Knowledge

1. What is a goiter?
2. How common is iodine deficiency, on a global scale?

Copper

Copper has been used to treat disease since 400 B.C., but it was not until 1964 when copper deficiencies in humans were found. Copper is vital in the function of many important enzymes and proteins. Fortunately, severe copper deficiency is relatively rare. It has occurred in premature infants being given milk-based formulas, during recovery from infantile malnutrition, in those receiving long-term total parenteral nutrition without copper being added. Severe copper deficiency is also seen in **Menkes disease**, which is an *X-linked recessive disorder* caused by mutations in genes coding for the copper-transport protein. Signs and symptoms of copper deficiency include anemia, **leukopenia**, osteopenia, cardiovascular changes, impaired immune function, and loss of pigmentation in the hair and skin.

Copper deficiency may increase risks for neurological disorders, including **Alzheimer's disease** and **amyotrophic lateral sclerosis** (Lou Gehrig's disease). Additional study is required to assess roles of copper **homeostasis** concerning these disorders. Mild copper deficiency may result from poor copper intake over time. There is a lack of reliable indicators to assess marginal copper deficiency. Like zinc, levels of copper in the blood and tissues may not be able to reflect copper status changes, and can be affected by different diseases. Symptoms of marginal copper intake include glucose intolerance, insufficient immune function, cardiac abnormalities, and increased serum cholesterol. Copper toxicity is not common, but has occurred in people that consumed food or water contaminated with copper. The genetic form of copper toxicity can cause **Wilson's disease** which will be discussed in greater detail in Chapter 13.

Test Your Knowledge

1. What are the best sources of iodine?
2. What are the consequences of iodine deficiency?
3. What are the risks for copper deficiency?

Manganese

Manganese (Mn) has long been known about, but its effects are less understood than other trace minerals. The best sources of Mn include legumes, leafy greens, nuts, tea, and whole-grain cereals. Specific food sources in these groups include walnuts, lima beans, pineapple, oatmeal, and peanuts. In the United States, the standard diet provides about 2–6 mg per day. The actual dietary requirements for Mn are not well understood. The adequate intake has been set at 2.3 mg per day for men and 1.8 mg per day for women. The daily value on food and supplement labels is 2.3 mg.

There is insufficient documentation of Mn deficiency in humans, with only a few reported cases. Symptoms of deficiency include nausea, vomiting, poor growth, abnormal reproductive function, impaired carbohydrate and lipid metabolism, and skeletal abnormalities.

Toxicities from Mn have been seen in children that were receiving long-term parenteral nutrition, as well as from the inhalation of automobile and industrial emissions in the air. Toxicity causes extreme neurological impairment and symptoms that resemble those of Parkinson's disease, including muscle stiffness and tremors. The upper level for Mn is set at 11 mg per day, in order to prevent nervous system damage.

Fluoride

Fluoride may not be an essential nutrient, since all basic functions in the body occur without it. In the 1930s, it was discovered that people in the southwestern United States, where water supplies had naturally higher concentrations of fluoride, had fewer cases of dental cavities (caries). However, excess fluoride in those areas of the country also caused **fluorosis**, a mottled discoloration of *tooth enamel*, even while lacking cavities (see Figure 11.5). This confirmed that fluorine had the ability to reduce cavities, so controlled water fluoridation was started in the United States. Even though no specific deficiency disorder or condition appears to be due to insufficient fluoride intake, increased incidence of dental caries is definitely seen.

Fluorine toxicity has been seen in young children after swallowing fluoride solutions or tablets. This rare but acute toxicity can develop quickly, and may be life-threatening.

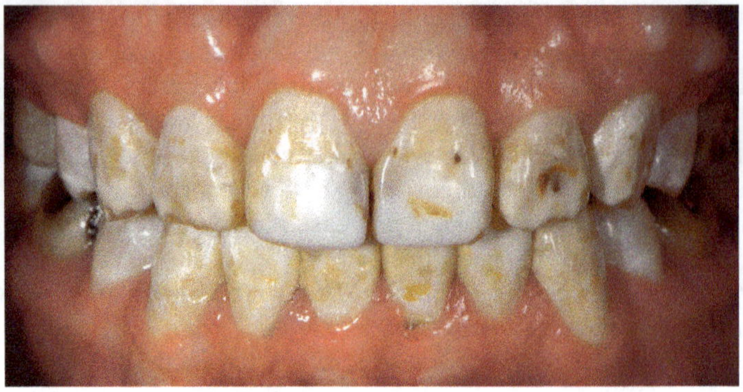

FIGURE 11.5 Fluorosis.

Therefore, it is very important to keep children away from fluoridated mouth rinses, supplements, and toothpaste. Toxicity from fluoride is signified by nausea, vomiting, diarrhea, spasms, sweating, convulsions, and coma. Chronic intake of excess fluoride during tooth development causes fluorosis. This is not related to any health risk, but the tooth enamel may become discolored or pitted. To reduce risks for fluorosis, the upper level for fluoride is set at 0.1 mg per kg of body weight per day, in a range of 0.7–2.2 mg per day, for infants and children up to age eight. The upper level for children over age eight and adults is 10 mg per day.

Zinc

Zinc has been known to be an essential component of nutrition since the 1930s. Only in the 1960s did it become known that zinc is also essential for normal growth and development. Nearly all body cells contain zinc and use it for a large variety of functions. However, zinc deficiency is a major problem in areas of the world in which the diet is affected by poverty. Symptoms of *zinc deficiency* include delayed growth and sexual maturation, loss of appetite, dermatitis, alopecia, impaired vitamin A function, decreased taste sensitivity, immune dysfunction, poor wound healing, birth defects, severe diarrhea, and higher occurrence of infant mortality. When the body's zinc status is compromised, the integrity of structural proteins that contain zinc is impaired in cell membranes, protein receptors, and **zinc finger proteins**. The proteins become unable to perform normal functions.

Severe zinc deficiencies were not seen in North American until the 1970s, after hospitalized patients received *total parenteral nutrition*. Zinc was not added to the first parenteral solutions since the protein source in them already contained zinc. Once the solutions' composition was altered to provide isolated amino acids (which did not contain zinc) as the primary protein source, cases of zinc deficiency developed quickly. Fortunately in North America, severe zinc deficiency is not common. There are mild zinc deficiencies seen in people with **Crohn's disease**, young children, patients undergoing kidney dialysis, *bariatric surgery* and in those that restrict intake of animal-based foods. Marginal zinc deficiencies are hard to detect since methods to assess changes in zinc status are insufficient. Studies are ongoing to find higher-sensitivity ways to measure mild zinc deficiencies. A rare genetic condition called **acrodermatitis enteropathica** can cause a severe zinc deficiency. It occurs after an infant is weaned off of maternal milk, and causes impaired intestinal zinc absorption. Treatment is with supplemental zinc. Also, about one in three patients that undergo bariatric surgery for obesity will eventually develop a zinc deficiency, which can be severe.

Zinc toxicity has been seen when supplements were taken at five or more times the recommended daily allowance. The upper level of zinc is 40 mg per day. Symptoms of toxicity include loss of appetite, nausea, vomiting, diarrhea, and intestinal cramps. Toxicities can impair immune function, while reducing absorption of copper and activity of enzymes that contain copper. To avoid toxicity and possible mineral to mineral interactions, people taking zinc supplements or lozenges to relive cold symptoms, should be very cautious and consult with a dietitian.

FOCUS ON ZINC AND COVID-19

Zinc is crucial for normal development and function of cells that mediate non-specific immunity, including neutrophils and natural killer cells. Therefore, zinc is currently being used in clinical trials against COVID-19 (coronavirus disease-2019). Some studies have shown that when administered at the onset of symptoms, zinc can reduce their duration.

Selenium

Selenium (Se) was not known to be essential for health until 1979, when it was found to prevent cardiac conditions. The presence of selenium in food sources is widely varied based on soil content. The best sources of selenium include cereals, grains, seafood, and other meats. Oysters (by far) have the highest content, followed by clams, sardines, egg noodles, and beef. The adult recommended daily allowance for selenium is 55 mcg per day, based on the amount needed to maximize *glutathione peroxidase* activity in the blood. In the United States, daily selenium intake is usually above the recommended amount. The daily value on food and supplement labels is also 55 mcg.

If selenium is insufficient in the diet, there is no known specific deficiency disease. Deficiency is linked to changes in thyroid hormone metabolism and a possibly higher risk of certain cancers. It is also related to development of **Keshan disease**, characterized by insufficient cardiac function. This was first seen in China in areas where the soil contained nearly no selenium. Other regions with a lack of soil selenium include Finland and New Zealand. Keshan disease can be prevented via selenium supplements, but the related cardiac abnormalities cannot be corrected by this once they have developed.

Excessive selenium supplementation can cause toxicity known as **selenosis**. This has occurred with only 1–3 mg per day taken over many months. Symptoms of selenium toxicity include diarrhea, nausea, fatigue, changes in nails, hair loss, and impaired protein and sulfur metabolism. The upper level for daily selenium is 400 mcg.

CHROMIUM

Chromium (Cr) has not been fully understood as an important trace mineral until relatively recently. It is widely distributed in many foods but information about the content of chromium is insufficient. Good sources of chromium include liver, red meat, fish, eggs, broccoli, whole-grain products, mushrooms, nuts, and dark chocolate. Since chromium is also used in steel manufacturing, small amounts may be transferred into foods via food processing equipment made of steel. For adults 19–50 years of age, adequate intake per day for chromium is 35 mcg for men and 25 mcg for women. Past age 50, adequate intake is lower, at 30 mcg for men and 20 mcg for women. Average intake in the United States usually is at these levels. The daily value for chromium is 35 mcg.

Chromium deficiency is hard to evaluate. This is because of a lack of sensitive measures of each person's chromium status. However, cases of chromium deficiency have been documented in people receiving **parenteral nutrition solutions** that did not include chromium. The symptoms of chromium deficiency include glucose intolerance, nerve damage, and weight loss.

Chromium toxicity has not been reported to cause many serious adverse effects. Therefore, no upper limit has yet been established. However, nutritionists have been expressing concern about just how safe high-dose chromium supplements – primarily *chromium picolinate* – may be. These are often used by athletes, so nutritionists recommend these supplements to be continually monitored concerning any possible toxicities.

The requirements for the trace minerals are summarized in Table 11.3.

FOCUS ON TRACE MINERALS

The human body cannot produce trace minerals, yet they are still essential nutrients. Some of them act as antioxidants, protecting the body from long-term damage. They help support the blood and hormones. Trace minerals also ensure proper development of neurological functions and enzymes.

TABLE 11.3
Trace Minerals

Mineral and Daily Intake	Functions	At Risk	Sources	Deficiency	Toxicity
Iron 8 mg (males) 18 mg (females)	Cognitive development, energy metabolism, immune function, respiration; is a functional component of hemoglobin	Infants, preschool children, women in childbearing years	Eggs, enriched breads, fortified cereals, meats, seafood	Anemia, fatigue upon exertion, poor immune function	GI upset; upper level is 45 mg per day
Iodine 150 micrograms (mcg)	Component of thyroid hormones regulating basal metabolism, growth, development	People living where soil iodine is low and fortified foods are not available	Dairy products, iodized salt, saltwater fish	Cretinism, goiter	Inhibited thyroid gland function; upper level is 1.1 mg per day
Copper 900 mcg	Aids iron metabolism, antioxidant enzymes, and those involved in connective tissue metabolism	People taking excessive zinc	Cocoa, legumes, liver, nuts, shellfish, whole grains	Anemia, low white blood cell counts, poor growth	Nausea, vomiting, diarrhea, liver and nervous system disorders; upper level is 10 mg per day

(*Continued*)

TABLE 11.3 (*Continued*)
Trace Minerals

Mineral and Daily Intake	Functions	At Risk	Sources	Deficiency	Toxicity
Manganese 2.3 mg (males) 1.8 mg (females)	Antioxidant protection, carbohydrate metabolism; is a cofactor of several enzymes	No significant risks	Legumes, nuts, tea, whole-grain cereals	Poor growth, skeletal abnormalities	Nervous system disorders; upper level is 11 mg per day
Fluoride 4 mg (males) 3 mg (females)	Increased resistance of tooth enamel to dental cavities; mineralization of bones and teeth	Areas with water that is not fluoridated	Dental treatments, fluoridated water, seaweed, tea, toothpaste	Dental cavities is a risk, but not a true deficiency symptom	Fluorosis or mottling of tooth enamel; acute toxicity can be fatal; upper level is 10 mg per day
Zinc 11 mg (males) 8 mg (females)	Growth, development, immune function, stabilization of body proteins and cell membranes; required for many enzymes	Alcoholics, elderly people, malnourished people, vegetarians	Meats, seafood, whole grains	Decreased appetite, decreased sense of taste, dermatitis, diarrhea, infections, poor growth and development	Cramps, decreased copper absorption, depressed immune function, diarrhea, nausea; upper level is 40 mg per day
Selenium 55 mcg	Activates thyroid hormones; is part of antioxidant system as glutathione peroxidase	Areas with low selenium soil content	Eggs, fish and other meats, nuts, seafood, whole grains	Keshan disease, reduced thyroid hormone	Changes in nails, diarrhea, hair loss, nausea, vomiting, upper level is 400 mg per day
Chromium 30–35 mcg (males) 20–25 mcg (females)	Enhances action of insulin	(Rare); in athletes, diabetics, pregnant women, and the elderly	Eggs, liver, mushrooms, nuts, processed meats, whole grains	Glucose tolerance	No report of dietary toxicity, no upper level set
Molybdenum 45 mcg	Acts as a coenzyme or cofactor so that the body can process proteins and genetic materials; also assists in breaking down drugs and toxic substances	None	Legumes, whole grains, rice, nuts, potatoes, bananas, leafy vegetables, dairy products, meat, eggs	(Rare); has caused increasing encephalopathy in newborns, over about one week, resulting in difficulty feeding and seizures	No reports of toxicity; upper level is 2,000 mcg per day

Test Your Knowledge

1. What is the role of iron in the human physiology?
2. What are the causes of endemic goiter?
3. What are the functions of copper?
4. What are the toxicities of fluoride?
5. What are the sources of selenium?

KEY TERMS

Acrodermatitis enteropathica
Alzheimer's disease
Amyotrophic lateral sclerosis
Anemia
Aneurysm
Anion
Arrhythmia
Biomarkers
Bone marrow
Chlorophyll
Cofactors
Cognitive
Crohn's disease
Electron
Endemic goiter
Enterocytes
Ferritin
Fluorosis
Free radicals

Goitrogens

Hallucinations

Heme

Hepcidin

Homeostasis

Hypokalemia

Hypoparathyroidism

Keshan disease

Lethargy

Leukopenia

Macrominerals

Menkes disease

Microminerals

Osteopenia

Osteoporosis

Oxalic acid

Parenteral nutrition solutions

Perspiration

Phytic acid

Polyphenols

Selenosis

Strokes

Tannins

Thyroid-stimulating hormone

Thyroxine

Tofu

Unleavened breads

Wilson's disease

Valences

Zinc fingers proteins

CLINICAL CASE STUDIES

Clinical Case Study 1

A 64-year-old man is hospitalized because he has symptoms of a gradually developing coma. He was diagnosed 10 years previously with type II diabetes and was also previously diagnosed with hypertension. Neurological examination reveals isolated left hemiplegia and a fever of 102.5 degrees Fahrenheit. Upon assessment, the patient has low blood pressure (90/60 mm Hg) but tachycardia at 133 beats per minute. The patient's skin is dry, along with the mucous membranes. A diagnosis of hypernatremia is made, along with metabolic acidosis. There is an inflammatory syndrome with leukocytosis, and blood glucose is high.

CRITICAL THINKING QUESTIONS

1. What is the description of hypernatremia?
2. What is the upper level and daily value for adult sodium consumption?
3. What are the possible complications of hypertension for this patient?

Clinical Case Study 2

A 58-year-old man had a previous history of coronary artery disease, hypertension, and gastrointestinal reflux, as well as type II diabetes mellitus. He was hospitalized due to carpal and calf spasms, leg pain, paresthesias, and malaise. Tests revealed the presence of hypomagnesemia, hypocalcemia, and hypokalemia. The patient reported having chronic diarrhea. His current medications were reviewed, and one of them was metformin, which is known to have diarrhea as an adverse effect. The medication was stopped, and the diarrhea resolved. The patient was given daily mineral supplements for his symptoms, which was successful. After discharge, a follow-up medical visit revealed high blood glucose. Sitagliptin was added to his medication regimen.

CRITICAL THINKING QUESTIONS

1. How serious is hypokalemia?
2. What does hypocalcemia result in?
3. What are the signs and symptoms of Mg deficiency?

Clinical Case Study 3

A 36-year-old pregnant woman has been fatigued for a few months. The pregnancy is her third within three years. She is not currently taking any prenatal vitamins and has developed cravings for ice. The woman has no other health conditions and does not smoke or drink. Physical examination by her physician reveals pale conjunctiva, spooning of her nails, and a systolic murmur of her heart. Stool testing is negative for occult blood. Blood testing leads to a diagnosis of iron deficiency anemia.

CRITICAL THINKING QUESTIONS

1. How does iron deficiency progress and worsen?
2. Why are pregnant women at high risk of iron deficiency?
3. How common is iron deficiency?

Clinical Case Study 4

A 73-year-old man was found unconscious on the floor of his home. Upon awakening, he complained of severe pain in his right hip. Arriving at the local emergency department, the man was confused and argumentative. The blood pressure was very low, and blood tests revealed high potassium. His past medical history indicates congestive heart failure, hypertension, type 2 diabetes mellitus, and osteoarthritis. His current medications include spironolactone, metoprolol and celecoxib. The diagnosis was of severe hyperkalemia.

CRITICAL THINKING QUESTIONS

1. What are the symptoms of severe hyperkalemia?
2. What are the food sources of potassium?
3. How common is hyperkalemia in healthy persons and how can it quickly increase in the blood?

Clinical Case Study 5

A 44-year-old woman underwent laparoscopic bariatric surgery because of obesity. In the years after the surgery, she developed health problems of unknown origin. After several misdiagnoses, it was found that she had a severe zinc deficiency. This occurs in about one of every three patients after having bariatric surgery. Treatment was started with zinc sulfate plus multivitamin supplements. The patient was educated about improving her diet as well.

CRITICAL THINKING QUESTIONS

1. What are the symptoms of zinc deficiency?
2. What happens to body proteins because of zinc deficiency?
3. Which people are most likely to develop zinc deficiency?

STUDY QUESTIONS

1. Which of the following is a trace mineral?
   A. Magnesium
   B. Sulfur
   C. Manganese
   D. Calcium

2. Excessive dietary zinc may decrease absorption and metabolism of all of the following, EXCEPT:
   A. Copper
   B. Fluoride
   C. Iron
   D. Magnesium

3. Which of the following parts of the digestive system can absorb iron?
   A. Mouth
   B. Stomach
   C. Duodenum
   D. Ileum

4. Which of the following mineral excesses in the diet causes hypertension?
   A. Sodium
   B. Copper
   C. Zinc
   D. Potassium

5. All of the following are examples of foods that provide adequate levels of potassium, EXCEPT:
   A. Kiwis
   B. Kidney beans
   C. Blueberries
   D. Bananas

6. Calcium is essential for all of the following body functions, EXCEPT:
   A. Blood clotting
   B. Secretion of insulin
   C. Normal heart rhythms
   D. Contraction of muscle

7. Which of the following is NOT a sign or symptom of magnesium deficiency?
   A. Blurred vision
   B. Disorientation
   C. Muscle spasm
   D. Arrhythmia

8. Which of the following mineral deficiencies may cause hemochromatosis?
   A. Iodine
   B. Copper
   C. Iron
   D. Manganese

9. Which of the following medical terms describes a mottled discoloration of tooth enamel?
   A. Selenosis
   B. Homeostasis
   C. Hemochromatosis
   D. Fluorosis

10. Which of the following mineral deficiencies decreases taste sensitivity?
    A. Zinc
    B. Iron
    C. Potassium
    D. Manganese

11. Which of the following mineral toxicities causes Wilson's disease?
    A. Selenium
    B. Manganese
    C. Zinc
    D. Copper

12. Which of the following is the outcome of iodine deficiency?
    A. Rickets
    B. Goiter
    C. Anemia
    D. Osteoporosis

13. All of the following are signs and symptoms of copper deficiency, EXCEPT:
    A. Leukopenia
    B. Osteopenia
    C. Hypercapnia
    D. Anemia

14. Which of the following disorders resembles the features of manganese toxicity?
    A. Parkinson's disease
    B. Alzheimer's disease
    C. Keshan disease
    D. Crohn's disease

15. Which of the following is NOT a result of iodine toxicity?
    A. Hyperthyroidism
    B. Autoimmune thyroid disease
    C. Osteopenia
    D. Thyroid cancer

FURTHER READING

1. Bagchi, D., and Swaroop, A. (2016). *Food Toxicology.* CRC Press.
2. Berdanier, C.D. (2021). *Advanced Nutrition – Macronutrients, Micronutrients, and Metabolism*, 3rd Edition. CRC Press.
3. Bever, M. (2015). *Vitamins, Minerals, & More! – Food Sources, Functions of the Body, and Deficiencies (Symptoms).* CreateSpace Independent Publishing Platform.
4. Davies, M. (2021). *Clinical Signs in Humans and Animals Associated with Minerals, Trace Elements,* and Rare Earth Elements. Academic Press.
5. DiNicolantonio, J., and Land, S. (2021). *The Mineral Fix: How to Optimize Your Mineral Intake for Energy, Longevity, Immunity, Sleep and More.* DiNicolantonio.
6. Gomes, C., and Rautureau, M. (2021). *Minerals latu sensu and Human Health – Benefits, Toxicity and Pathologies.* Springer.
7. Gualtieri, A.F. (2017). *Mineral Fibres: Crystal Chemistry, Chemical-Physical Properties, Biological Interaction, and Toxicity (EMU Notes in Mineralogy 18).* European Mineralogical Society.
8. Hommel, J. (2022). *The Copper Revolution: Healing with Minerals.* Hommel.
9. Lajusticia Bergasa, A.M. (2021). *Magnesium, Key to Health – The Importance of This Mineral and the Problems Caused by Its Deficiency.* Ennsthaler.
10. Liebermann, S., and Bruning, N. (2007). *The Real Vitamin and Mineral Book: The Definitive Guide to Designing Your Personal Supplement Program*, 4th Edition. Avery.
11. Malavolta, M., and Mocchegiani, E. (2018). *Trace Elements and Minerals in Health and Longevity (Healthy Aging and Longevity Book 8).* Springer.
12. Mozsik, G., and Diaz-Soto, G. (2021). *Mineral Deficiencies: Electrolyte Disturbances, Genes, Diet and Disease Interface.* Intechopen.
13. Ochsenham, P., and Vormann, J. (2015). *The Magnesium Deficiency Crisis: Is This the World's Number 1 Mineral Deficiency?* MadhouseMEDIA.
14. Rydon, R. (2017). *Profiles of the Nutrients: 2. Minerals and Trace Elements.* Rydon.
15. Tako, E. (2020). *Dietary Trace Minerals (Nutrients).* Mdpi AG.
16. Walters, C. (2013). *Minerals for the Genetic Code – An Exposition & Analysis of the Dr. Olree Standard Genetic Periodic Chart & The Physical, Chemical & Biological Connection.* Acres U.S.A.
17. Wartian Smith, P. (2019). *What You Must Know About Vitamins, Minerals, Herbs and So Much More – Choosing the Nutrients That Are Right For You*, 2nd Edition. Square One.

12 Electrolyte and Acid–Base Imbalance

OUTLINE

LEARNING OBJECTIVES

After study of the chapter, readers should be able to:

1. Explain the two primary fluid compartments.
2. Describe insensible and sensible water losses.
3. Discuss the regulation of water intake.
4. Identify the signs and symptoms of severe dehydr-ation.
5. Explain the signs and symptoms of hypotonic dehydration.
6. Describe the renin–angiotensin–aldosterone mechanism.
7. List the conditions caused by electrolyte imbalan-ces.
8. Explain acid–base imbalances.
9. Describe the medical conditions that can cause metabolic alkalosis.
10. Discuss chemical buffer systems.

OVERVIEW

In the human body, fluids are organized into functional compartments, which must be maintained in an orderly fashion for normal health. The composition and distribution of fluids in the internal environment and the roles of various body organs and functions are vital to understand the disorders related to body fluids. Electrolytes dissolved in the body fluids are essential for nearly every life process. As electrolytes move through cell membranes, electrical events occur, influencing nerve conduction, muscle contraction, and metabolic reactions. The body fluids' acidity or alkalinity is maintained within very narrow limits. Nearly all organ systems participate in fluid balance and can be affected by an imbalance. Many diseases alter fluid balance to damage organs or cause them to malfunction. The best treatment results are based on correctly evaluating fluid and electrolyte balances and then administering appropriate treatments. It is extremely crucial to understand the makeup of body fluids, pathologic changes to normal processes, and how to correct these changes.

CONTENT OF BODY WATER

Water content in human beings varies among individuals to some degree. Total body water is a function of age, body mass, gender, and the amount of body fat. During pregnancy, body fluid increases because of temporary hormonal changes. Infants have low body fat and bone mass, so their bodies are 75% made up of water. This large amount of hydration is why their skin is so soft and lustrous. As childhood progresses, total body water declines continually. By old age, the human body is made up of about 45% water. A healthy younger male has about 60% body water, while a healthy young female has about 50%. Differences between the genders are based on females having relatively more body fat and less skeletal muscle. The least hydrated body tissue, with less than 20% water, is adipose tissue. The bones contain more water than adipose tissue does. Skeletal muscles are about 75% body water, and individuals with more muscle mass have, in proportion, more body water.

FLUID COMPARTMENTS

Water is present into two primary **fluid compartments** (see Figure 12.1). Nearly 66% by volume is within the **intracellular fluid (ICF) compartment**. This is made up of trillions of individual cells, which act as tiny "compartments". An adult male of average build, about 154 pounds in weight (70 kg), has an ICF that makes up approximately 25 L of the 40 L of body water. The remaining 33% is outside the cells in the **extracellular fluid (ECF) compartment**. This compartment makes up the body's internal environment while remaining the external environment of the cells. The ECF compartment is divided into the following:

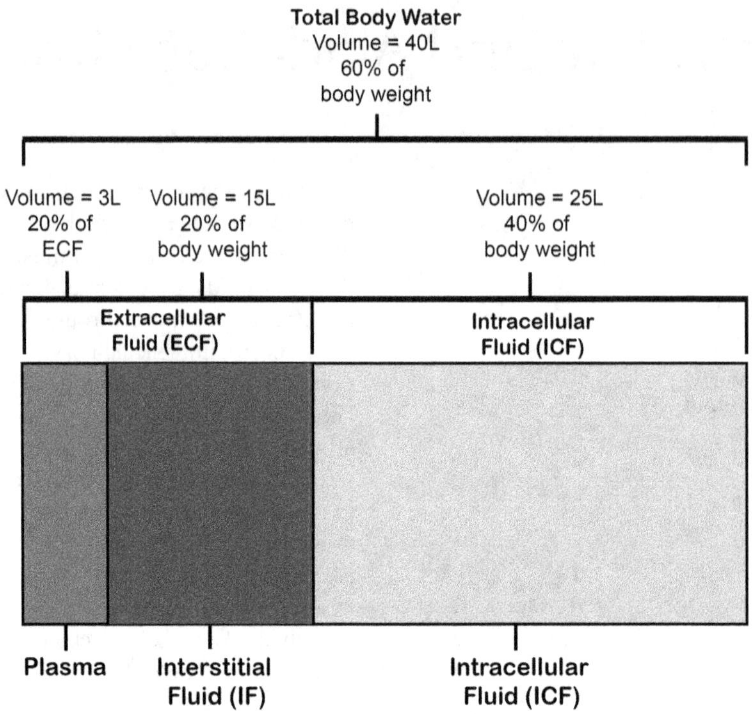

FIGURE 12.1 The intracellular fluid (ICF) and extracellular fluid (ECF) compartments.

- Plasma – in the blood vessels (20% out of 33% of fluid)
- **Interstitial fluid** – in the microscopic spaces between the tissue cells

Many other examples of ECF are different from the plasma and interstitial fluid. These examples include cerebrospinal fluid, lymph, the **vitreous humors** of the eyes, serous fluid, synovial fluid, and gastrointestinal secretions. Most are similar of the interstitial fluid, and usually considered to be part of it.

COMPOSITION OF BODY FLUIDS

The *universal solvent*, in which many solutes are dissolved, is water. Solutes are widely classified as *electrolytes* and *nonelectrolytes*. The **electrolytes** are chemical compounds, which dissociate in water into ions. The ions are charged particles that conduct an electrical current. Electrolytes consist of inorganic salts, inorganic acids and bases, organic acids and bases, and some proteins. The **nonelectrolytes** have **covalent bonds**, which stop them from dissociating in a solution. Therefore, no electrically charged species are formed as nonelectrolytes dissolve in water. The majority of nonelectrolytes are organic molecules, including *creatinine*, glucose, lipids, and urea.

All dissolved solutes contribute to a fluid's **osmotic** activity, but electrolytes have a much stronger osmotic power than nonelectrolytes, since every electrolyte molecule dissociated into two or more ions. A molecule of sodium chloride (NaCl), for example, contributes two times as many particles of solute as glucose, which remains undissociated. One molecule of magnesium chloride ($MgCl_2$) contributes three times as many. Water always moves according to osmotic gradients, from an area with less osmolality to an area with more osmolality. Therefore, electrolytes have the strongest ability to cause fluid shifts in the body.

Electrolyte concentrations of body fluids are primarily expressed in milliequivalents per liter (mEq/L). This is a measurement of the amount of electrical charges in one liter of solution. It is computed by dividing the ion concentration in mg/L by the atomic weight of the ion in mg/mmol, multiplied by the number of electrical charges on one ion. To calculate the mEq/L of sodium or calcium ions in solution within plasma, we first determine the normal concentration of these ions in plasma. Next, their atomic weight is looked up in the periodic table. The equations then look like this:

$$\text{Sodium ions}\left(\text{Na}^{+}\right) = \frac{3,300\ \text{mg/L}}{23\ \text{mg/mmol}} \times 1 = 143\ \text{mEq/L}$$

and

$$\text{Calcium ions}\left(\text{Ca}^{2+}\right) = \frac{100\ \text{mg/L}}{40\ \text{mg/mmol}} \times 2 = 5\ \text{mEq/L}$$

For ions with just one charge, 1 mEq is equal to 1 mmol. When this is dissolved in 1 kg of water, it produces 1 milliosmole (mOsm). However, 1 mEq of ions with a *double* charge, such as calcium, would be equal to ½ mOsm. Either way, 1 mEq provides the same amount of electrical charge.

Each fluid compartment has a unique pattern of electrolytes. Except for the fairly high-protein content in plasma, the extracellular fluids are very similar. Sodium is their primary **cation**, while chloride is their major **anion**. Plasma contains fewer chloride ions that interstitial fluid since the nonentering plasma proteins are usually anions, and plasma is electrically neutral. However, the ICF has only small amounts of sodium and chloride. The most abundant cation is potassium, while the primary anion is **hydrogen phosphate**. The cells also have large quantities of soluble proteins, which are about three times higher than the amount in plasma.

Sodium and potassium ion concentrations in the ECF and ICF are practically opposite. These distributions indicate the activity of cellular adenosine triphosphate (ATP)-dependent sodium–potassium pumps. These pumps keep the intracellular sodium ion concentrations low while potassium ion concentration remains high. The most abundant solutes in the body fluids determine most chemical and physical reactions, yet do not make up the majority of dissolves solutes in these fluids. The majority consists of large molecules, including proteins and nonelectrolytes, such as cholesterol, phospholipids, and triglycerides. These make up approximately 97% in the ICF, 90% of the mass of dissolved solutes in plasma, about 60% of dissolved solutes in the interstitial fluid.

Test Your Knowledge

1. What are the two primary fluid compartments in the human body?
2. What is the difference between electrolytes and nonelectrolytes?
3. What are the differences in electrolyte patterns between the two primary fluid compartments?

WATER BALANCE INTAKE AND OUTPUT

Water intake must equal output in order for the body to remain adequately hydrated. *Water intake* is different between individuals, greatly affected by our habits, but is usually about 2,500 mL per day in adults. The majority of water enters the body via ingested liquids, fruits, and vegetables. The body water produced by cellular metabolism is called the **metabolic water** or *water of oxidation. Water output* **includes insensible water** loss and **sensible water loss**. Insensible water loss is the water vaporizing out of the lungs in expired air, or via diffusion through the skin. Sensible water loss is any measurable water loss, including water lost via the urine (approximately 60%), visible sweat, and in the feces.

When healthy, humans maintain osmolality of body fluids in narrow limits of only 280–300 mOsm. An increase in plasma osmolality triggers two things: thirst and the release of **antidiuretic hormone (ADH)**. This hormone causes the kidneys to conserve water and excrete concentrated urine. Oppositely, a decline in osmolality inhibits thirst and ADH release, prompting the kidneys to excrete larger amounts of dilute urine. Water and sodium ions are closely tied together, with the sodium ions acting as strong *water magnets*. Even so, thirst and ADH that control osmolality regulate water independently of sodium.

Regulation of Water Intake

Water intake is regulated by thirst, which is triggered by receptors in the hypothalamus. These respond to as little as 2% increased plasma osmolality or decreased body fluid volume. In rare cases, hypothalamic dysfunction decreases thirst capacity. Water excretion by the kidneys is mostly regulated by ADH, which is also known as vasopressin, released by the posterior pituitary gland in the brain. ADH increases water reabsorption in the distal nephron. Release of vasopressin is stimulated by increased plasma osmolality, decreased blood volume, and blood pressure. The release of vasopressin can be impaired by substances such as ethanol or phenytoin, and posterior pituitary tumors. Water intake decreases plasma osmolality. If the plasma osmolality is low, secretion of vasopressin is inhibited. This allows the kidneys to produce dilute urine.

Regulation of Water Output

Certain amounts of water output cannot be prevented. These *obligatory water losses* show why humans cannot survive very long without drinking fluids. Zero water intake will eventually overcome all of the conservation efforts of the kidneys. Obligatory water loss includes insensible water losses, plus sensible water loss of 500 mL per day or more in the urine, plus water that is present in undigested food residues in the feces. Obligatory water loss in the urine indicates that the kidneys normally flush 600 mmol of urine solutes, per day, out of the body water. These solutes, in part, the end products of metabolism. The maximum concentration of the urine is approximately 1,200 mOsm. Therefore, at least 500 mL of water must be excreted.

Aside from obligatory water loss, the solute concentration and volume of urine that is excreted is based on fluid intake, diet, and other water loss. A person that sweats heavily on a hot day needs to excrete much less urine than usual in order to maintain water balance. In normal conditions, the kidneys start eliminating excess water about 30 minutes after it has been taken in. The delay indicates the time needed for the release of ADH to be inhibited. Diuresis peaks about 1 hour after drinking. It declines to its lowest level after 3 hours.

FOCUS ON DIABETES INSIPIDUS

Diabetes insipidus is a rare, treatable condition in which the body produces too much urine, resulting in polyuria, and polydipsia due to a deficiency of ADH. It is mostly caused by an abnormality in the creation and use of ADH. It can be temporary or chronic and mild or severe. Large volumes of urine must be voided every day, and the affected person drinks large amounts of water due to constant thirst.

Test Your Knowledge

1. What are sensible water loss and insensible water loss?
2. What regulates most water excretion by the kidneys?
3. What do obligatory water losses include?

PATHOLOGY OF WATER BALANCE

Most humans do not really understand how important water is for maintaining the peak functions of the body. The primary pathologies of water balance include dehydration, hypotonic dehydration, and edema. Fluid imbalance can be related to hypovolemia, normovolemia with maldistribution of fluid, and hypervolemia.

DEHYDRATION

Dehydration occurs when less fluid is consumed or more fluid is lost. The body then has insufficient fluids to function normally. Trauma is among the most common causes of hypovolemia, with its often extensive related blood loss. Another common cause is dehydration, which primarily involves a loss of plasma rather than whole blood. Dehydration can be caused by diarrhea, vomiting, sweating, urine abnormalities, fever, an inability to consume enough fluid (such as through unconsciousness), burns, poorly controlled diabetes mellitus, and diabetes insipidus, due to a deficiency of ADH. In healthy people, it can occur after heavy exercise, in hot or dry environments, at high altitudes – due to more rapid breathing – or by ignoring thirst. Normally, the thirst mechanism is controlled by the *hypothalamic thirst center*. This center is activated by **osmoreceptors** that detect extracellular fluid osmolality. The saliva glands then produce less saliva as the osmotic gradient that draws water from the blood into the salivary ducts is reduced. Dry mouth results. Next, there is a decrease in blood volume or pressure. If substantial, this also triggers the thirst mechanism. Changes in volume or pressure are signaled by **baroreceptors**, which directly activate the thirst center, and by **angiotensin II**. Baroreceptors in the heart and carotid arteries also affect kidney function to reduce blood pressure and volume. Table 12.1 summarizes the effects of dehydration, based on the extent of water weight lost. With extended physical activity, three to eight cups (750–2,000 mL) can be lost per hour. It is important to plan ahead, to have enough water available so that hydration is maintained.

Mild to moderate dehydration is signified by dry mouth and skin, fatigue, headache, dizziness, confusion, fatigue, dry mouth, chills, decreased urine output, and deep yellow urine. With progressive dehydration, tachycardia, hypotension, and constipation. If the loss of fluid continues, there can be kidney failure, seizures, **delirium**, and coma. Treatment is simply by replacing lost fluids. When dehydration is severe, fluid replacement requires medical supervision. Without replenishment, severe progression will lead to death. To avoid exercise-related dehydration, it is important to consume fluids adequately. This means before, during, and after exercise, as follows:

- Before exercise – drink water or sports drinks during the day before the exercise will begin, even if not very thirsty; drink two to three cups (500–750 mL) of fluid 2–3 hours before exercise, allowing for enough hydration and excretion of excess fluid; drink 250–375 mL of fluid 10–15 minutes before exercising or competing – especially if the event will last a long time
- During exercise – drink 1–1.5 cups of fluid every 10–15 minutes; fluid replacement is promoted by flavored fluids that are cooler than the temperature of the environment; drink sufficient fluid to maintain body weight during exercise; if the exercise lasts for 1 hour or more, fluid replacement beverages must contain 4%–8% carbohydrates in order to maintain blood glucose levels; sodium must be included in the beverage (0.5–0.7 g of sodium per liter) to replace the sodium that is lost in the sweat
- After exercise – drink three cups of fluid for each pound lost during exercise; restore body weight before the next period of exercise

FOCUS ON DEHYDRATION

A recent study revealed that about three of every four Americans suffer from constant dehydration due to poor drinking and eating habits. Though about 80% of our hydration comes from drinking water, a large amount of hydration comes from good food choice such as fruits and vegetables. Men need 3.7 L and women need 2.7 L per day. An easy way to judge adequate hydration is to check your urine – it should be pale yellow in color – not clear or very yellow. After consuming two bottles of water, it takes the body about 45 minutes to become perfectly hydrated.

FOCUS ON DEHYDRATION IN THE ELDERLY

Dehydration is the most common fluid and electrolyte problem in the elderly. The usual causes of water loss are often absent in dehydrated elderly patients. Age-related changes in total body water, thirst perception, renal concentrating ability, and the effectiveness of vasopressin (ADH) probably are involved. Dehydration related to infection, high-protein tube feedings, cerebral vascular accidents, and medication-related hypodipsia are especially relevant for elderly patients. Appropriate treatment depends on accurately assessing water deficits and slowly correcting them.

TABLE 12.1
The Effects of Dehydration, based on the Extent of Water Weight Lost

Percentage of Water Weight Lost	Effects
Up to 2%	Thirst
2%–3%	Stronger thirst, slight discomfort and a feeling of oppression, loss of appetite, increased hemoconcentration
4%–5%	Less movement, slow pace, flushed skin, impatience, weariness, sleepiness, apathy, nausea, emotional instability
6%–7%	Tingling, stumbling, headache, faintness, dizziness, fatigue, nausea, increased body temperature, increased pulse, increased respiratory rate, labored breathing, cyanosis
8%–9%	Indistinct speech, increased weakness, mental confusion
10%	Muscle cramps, inability to balance while the eyes are closed, general incapacity, delirium, wakefulness, tongue swelling, circulatory insufficiency, extreme hemoconcentration and decreased blood volume, failing kidney function
11% or higher	Increased risk of death, especially if dehydration is linked to an illness or extreme heat or exercise

FOCUS ON WATER IN INFANTS

When an infant is older than six months, small amounts of boiled tap water that have been cooled down can be offered. However, breastmilk or formula feeds should not be replaced with water. Breastmilk or formula should still be their primary fluid consumption up to 12 months of age. After 12 months, the main fluids should be water and cow's milk or breastmilk. Infants younger than six months should never be given water. Although water intoxication is rare, it can be brought about in infants whose kidneys are not yet fully developed. Without fully functioning kidneys, giving too much water to an infant can cause a removing sodium from the body, which is crucial for proper nerve function. Hyponatremia can be deadly to an infant.

Test Your Knowledge

1. What are the causes of dehydration?
2. What happens if more than 10% of body water is lost?
3. What should fluid consumption be while a person is exercising?

Hypotonic Dehydration

Hypotonic dehydration refers to a decrease of electrolyte concentration in the extracellular fluid. In hypotonic dehydration, the cells expand as water in the extracellular fluid moves toward the higher sodium concentration inside the cells. Reducing ECF osmolality inhibits ADH release. Less water is reabsorbed. Excess water is flushed quickly out of the body via the urine. If there is renal insufficiency, or if extremely large amounts of water are consumed quickly, hypotonic dehydration may occur. This is a type of cellular overhydration. Either way, the ECF is diluted. It has a normal sodium content, but the excess water results in the sodium concentration to be low. Therefore, the hallmark sign of hypotonic dehydration is hyponatremia. The low ECF sodium ion concentration promotes net osmosis into the tissue cells. Then, they swell due to being abnormally dehydrated. Various underlying conditions can cause hypotonic dehydration. Overall, these conditions result in a loss of body fluids, usually through the skin, gastrointestinal (GI) tract, or kidneys.

Hypotonic dehydration results in severe metabolic disturbances. Signs and symptoms include nausea, vomiting, dizziness, blurred vision, bradycardia, muscular cramping, **cerebral edema**, and unconsciousness. The neurons can be greatly damaged. If uncorrected, cerebral edema quickly causes disorientation, convulsions, coma, and death. People that have run in marathon races have died of overhydration after too much water was consumed too quickly. Sudden, severe hyponatremia is treated with IV hypertonic saline. This reverses the osmotic gradient, pulling water out of the cells. Treatment options include fluid replacement orally, if the child is conscious and able to drink. Water, fluids, and an oral rehydration solution can be used. In severe cases, intravenous fluids should be used.

Edema

Edema is an abnormal accumulation of fluid in the interstitial space. The tissues swell, but the cells do not. There is an increase in volume of the interstitial fluid alone. The extra fluid in the interstitial space can harm tissue function, since it increases the distance over which oxygen and nutrients must diffuse between the blood and the cells. Edema can be caused by events that increase the flow of fluid out of the blood, or that reduce the ability of fluid to return to the blood. There are different causes and types of edema. For example, *pulmonary edema* affects the lungs, while *pedal edema* causes swelling in the feet. Pulmonary edema occurs when excess fluid collects in the lungs, making breathing difficult. This can result from congestive heart failure or acute lung injury. It is a serious condition, can be a medical emergency, and it may lead to respiratory failure and death. Edema usually starts slowly, but onset can be sudden. It is a common condition, but it can also be a sign of a serious condition.

Cerebral edema occurs in the brain. It can happen for a range of reasons, many of which are potentially life-threatening. These causes include a sedentary lifestyle, too much dietary sodium, premenstrual signs and symptoms, pregnancy, because of certain medications (such as those for hypertension, nonsteroidal anti-inflammatory drugs, steroids, estrogens, and thiazolidinediones), and serious conditions such as congestive heart failure, cirrhosis, kidney disease, weakness or damage to leg veins, an inadequate lymphatic system, and a severe chronic protein deficiency. It most often occurs in the skin, especially in the hands, arms, ankles, legs, and feet. However, it can also affect the muscles, bowels, lungs, eyes, and brain (see Figure 12.2).

Symptoms depend on the underlying cause, but swelling, tightness, and pain are common. The skin may retain a "dimple" after a few seconds of pressure, with visible anomalies. There may be puffiness of the ankles, face, or eyes. Weight gain or weight loss, and decreased urine production also occur. Treatment depends on the cause of the edema. Diuretics help get rid of excess fluid by increasing the rate of urine production by the kidneys. There several types of edema, which include peripheral, pulmonary, cerebral, and **macular edema**. Complications of untreated edema can lead to the following:

- Painful swelling, with pain that gets worse
- Stiffness and difficulty walking
- Stretched, itchy skin
- Infection in the area of swelling
- Scarring between the layers of tissue
- Poor blood circulation
- Loss of elasticity in the arteries, veins, and joints
- Ulcerations on the skin

ELECTROLYTE BALANCE

The term electrolyte balance primarily refers to sodium balance in the body. Salts are important for controlling fluid movements. They provide minerals required for excitability, secretions, and membrane permeability. Though many electrolytes are needed for cellular activity, the regulation of sodium, potassium, calcium, and phosphate is most important. The flexibility of the kidney's mechanisms that regulate the blood's electrolyte balance is very important. The primary electrolytes, and their main functions, are as follows:

- Sodium – helps control body fluids and impacts blood pressure, and is necessary for muscle and nerve function
- Chloride – helps balance other electrolytes, balances acidity and alkalinity to maintain pH, and is essential to digestion
- Potassium – regulates the heart rhythm and blood pressure, helps balance other electrolytes, aids in nerve impulse transmission, contributes to bone health, and is essential for muscle contraction
- Calcium – is a key component of the bones and teeth, is important for movement of nerve impulses and muscle movements, and contributes to blood clotting
- Phosphate – strengthens the bones and teeth, and helps the cells produce needed energy for tissue growth and repair
- Magnesium – is important for DNA and RNA production, contributes to nerve and muscle function, helps to maintain heart rhythm, helps regulate blood glucose levels, and enhances the immune system

Renal regulation of sodium ions is based on the effects of **aldosterone**. It is a critical factor in the *renin–angiotensin–aldosterone mechanism*, which increases blood volume and pressure. When aldosterone concentrations are high,

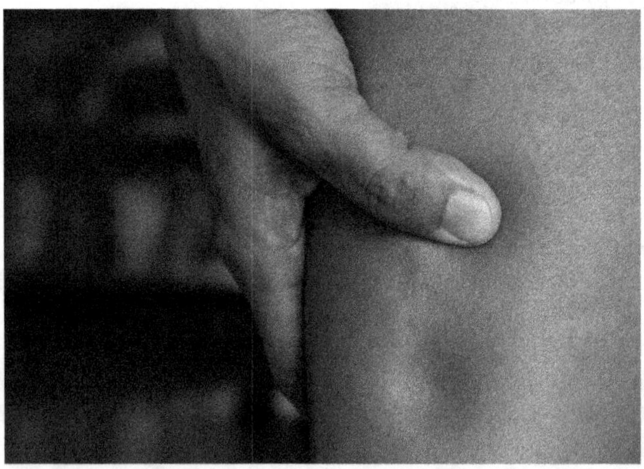

FIGURE 12.2 Edema.

nearly all remaining filtered sodium is actively reabsorbed in the distal convoluted tubules and collecting ducts. *Water always follows sodium.* This water comes from the intracellular fluid (ICF), or reabsorption from the collecting ducts by the presence of ADH. Either way, aldosterone increases the extracellular fluid volume. When aldosterone concentrations are low, nearly no sodium reabsorption occurs from the kidney. Urinary excretion of large amounts of sodium always means excretion of large amounts of water. The main trigger for aldosterone release from the adrenal cortex is the renin–angiotensin–aldosterone mechanism, regulated by the **juxtaglomerular complex** of nephrons (see Figure 12.3). Elevated potassium concentrations in the extracellular fluid can directly stimulate adrenal cortical cells to release aldosterone. This results in more reabsorption of sodium and more secretion of potassium. Aldosterone takes a few hours to exert its effects.

Any change in potassium concentrations in the extracellular fluid can have severe effects. Potassium also helps the body resist pH changes in body fluids. Potassium balance is mainly regulated by the kidneys. The distal convoluted tubule and collecting ducts achieve potassium balance mostly by changing how much potassium is secreted into the filtrate. If extracellular fluid potassium concentrations are too low, the renal principal cells conserve potassium by reducing its secretion and excretion to a minim. However, the main function of renal regulation of potassium is to excrete it. The most important factor related to potassium secretion is its concentration in the extracellular fluid. Another factor is aldosterone, which is released when potassium concentrations in the extracellular fluid increase to any degree, prompting increased potassium secretion.

Atrial natriuretic peptide (ANP) is a cardiac hormone which comes from the left atria. Its main function is to lower blood pressure and blood volume, by relaxation of smooth muscles in the walls of blood vessels. It also controls electrolyte **homeostasis**. This peptide accomplishes electrolyte homeostasis by inhibiting almost every event that promotes **vasoconstriction** and the retention of sodium ions, as well as water. It is a hormone secreted from the right atrium in response to atrial stretch from hypervolemia as well as when they are stretched because of hypertension, and has diuretic and sodium-excreting (natriuretic) effects. The hormone promotes excretion of sodium ions and water by the kidneys via inhibition of the ability of the collecting ducts to reabsorb sodium ions, plus by suppression of released ADH, renin, and aldosterone. Also, ANP has direct and indirect actions, such as by inhibition of renin-induced generation of angiotensin II, to relax vascular smooth muscle, causing **vasodilation**. All of these combined effects reduce sodium ion content and blood pressure.

Estrogens are sex hormones for maintaining the sexual and reproductive health. They are chemically similar hormones to aldosterone and enhance sodium chloride (NaCl) reabsorption by the rental tubules. Since water follows, many women retain fluid when their estrogen levels increase during the menstrual cycle. Estrogens are highly responsible for edema, as experienced by many women during pregnancy. Oppositely, **progesterone** has a slight diuretic effect, believed to be because it blocks aldosterone receptors. **Glucocorticoids**, including cortisol and hydrocortisol, enhance the tubular reabsorption of sodium ions, but also promote a higher glomerular filtration rate, which can obscure their effects upon the tubules. Another factor is

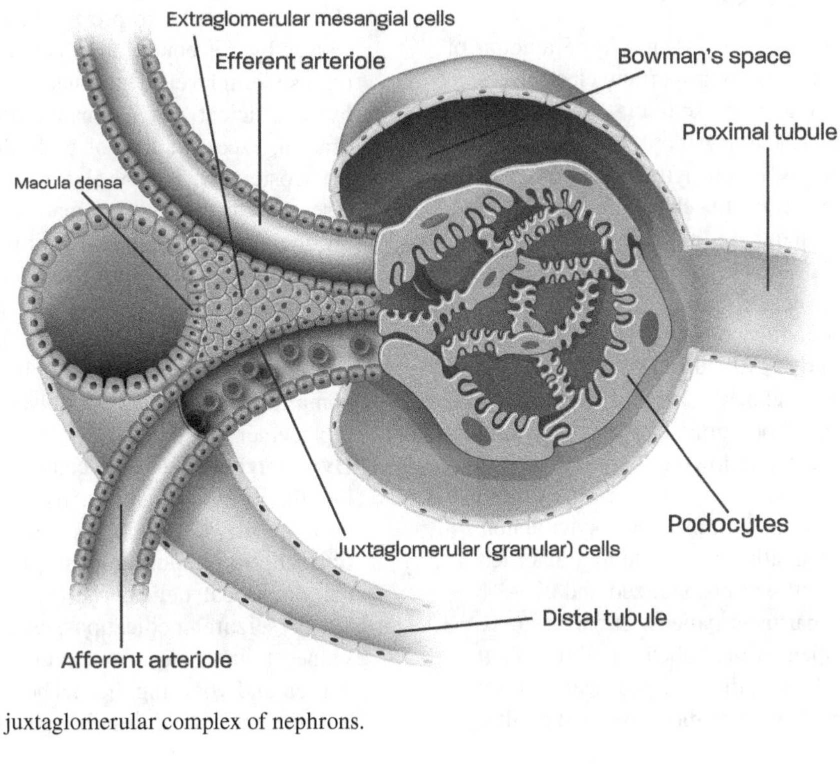

FIGURE 12.3 The juxtaglomerular complex of nephrons.

that when their plasma levels are high, glucocorticoids have strong aldosterone-like effects, promoting edema.

Parathyroid hormone (PTH) regulates calcium in the extracellular fluid. Reducing plasma levels of calcium stimulates the release of PTH, increasing calcium levels by targeting the bones, kidneys, and small intestine. It activates vitamin D in the distal tubules of the kidneys. Most calcium is passively reabsorbed in the proximal convoluted tubule through diffusion.

FOCUS ON ALDOSTERONE

Aldosterone is a steroid hormone secreted by adrenal glands. Its main role is to regulate salt (NaCl-) and water in the body. This influences the capillaries to increase reabsorption of sodium ions into the blood and to increase secretion of potassium ions into the urine. High aldosterone levels can cause hypertension and hypernatremia as well as hypokalemia (low potassium levels). Hypokalemia may cause weakness, tingling, muscle spasms, and periods of temporary paralysis.

Test Your Knowledge

1. What are the primary functions of chloride, sodium, and potassium?
2. What is the renin–angiotensin–aldosterone mechanism?
3. What can happen when potassium concentrations change in the extracellular fluid?

ELECTROLYTE IMBALANCE

An electrolyte imbalance occurs when a large amount of body fluids are lost. The most important electrolytes in body fluids include potassium, sodium, chloride, phosphate, magnesium, and calcium. All of these are important for normal body functions. Electrolyte imbalances may be caused by burns, medications for chronic kidney disease, insufficient food and fluids, chronic respiratory diseases, and use of laxatives or steroids. Symptoms of electrolyte imbalances commonly include cramps, dizziness, irregular heartbeat, and mental confusion. Other symptoms include tachycardia, fatigue, **lethargy**, nausea, vomiting, diarrhea, constipation, muscle weakness, irritability, headaches, numbness, and tingling. Conditions caused by electrolyte level imbalances include the following:

- **Hyperkalemia** – a common electrolyte abnormality and a potentially life-threatening disorder, occurring in 1%–10% of hospitalized and 2%–3% of emergency department patients. It occurs more commonly in patients with diabetes mellitus, renal failure, chronic kidney disease, and heart failure due to renal impairment or medications that alter potassium excretion. Hyperkalemia is caused by severe dehydration, kidney failure, severe acidosis, certain blood pressure medications or diuretics, and adrenal insufficiency **(Addison's disease)**. Signs and symptoms include fatigue, lethargy, muscle weakness, loss of appetite, increased thirst, craving for salty foods, depression, irritability, poor concentration, polyuria, and arrhythmia. People with Addison's disease may also have darkening of their skin. This darkening is most visible on scars, skin folds, and pressure points such as the elbows, knees, knuckles, and toes; the lips and mucous membranes such as those lining the cheeks (see Figure 12.4). Medications used in the acute setting are limited to shifting potassium, and there is insufficient safety and efficacy data available. The lack of guidelines has led to much variability in hyperkalemia treatment.
- **Hypokalemia** – caused by severe vomiting or diarrhea, dehydration, excessive sweating, dehydration, excessive alcohol use, chronic kidney disease, diabetic ketoacidosis, malnutrition, **Cushing's syndrome**, excessive aldosterone, hypomagnesemia, excessive laxatives, certain diuretics, and corticosteroids. Clinical manifestations include muscle cramps, severe muscle weakness (leading to paralysis), hypotension, faintness, arrhythmias, polyuria, and polydipsia. Hypokalemia is treated with oral or intravenous potassium. To prevent cardiac conduction disturbances, intravenous calcium is administered to patients with hyperkalemic changes discovered by electrocardiography.
- **Hypernatremia** – in many cases, hypernatremia is mild and doesn't cause serious problems. However, in order to prevent or reverse problems caused by this condition, it is important to correct high sodium levels. Hypernatremia may be caused by insufficient water consumption, severe dehydration, excessive loss of body fluids, and use of corticosteroids. It may also be caused by Conn's disease, which is a tumor made up of aldosterone-producing cells in the cortex of the adrenal gland. A major symptom is thirst. Other clinical manifestations are primarily neurologic (due to an osmotic shift of water out of brain cells), including confusion, neuromuscular excitability, seizures, and coma. Treatment usually involves controlled water replacement.
- **Hyponatremia** – usually caused by excessive fluid loss due to sweating or burns, vomiting, diarrhea, poor nutrition, alcohol use disorder, overhydration, chronic hypothyroidism, diabetes insipidus, adrenocortical deficiency, use of certain diuretics or seizure medications, and liver, heart, or kidney failure. Signs and symptoms may include nausea and vomiting, headache, confusion, irritability, muscle weakness or spasms, seizures, and

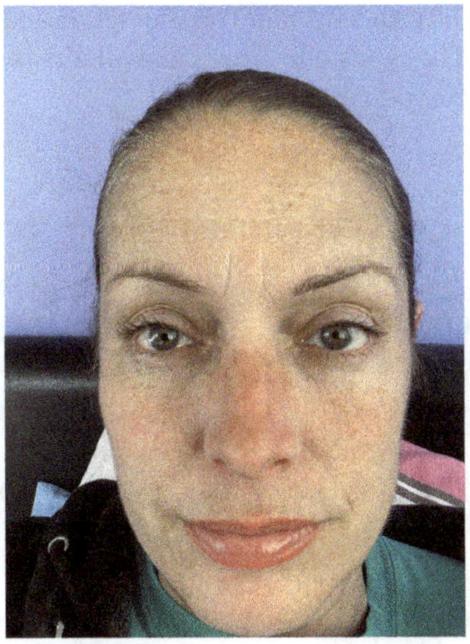

FIGURE 12.4 Darkening of the skin in Addison's disease.

coma. The mainstay of management is rehydration with sodium chloride (0.9% solution), and discontinuation of diuretic therapy where appropriate. Correction or maintenance of other serum electrolytes is vital. Correction of hypokalemia is particularly important because low potassium can impair correction of hyponatremia.

- **Hyperchloremia** – may be caused by severe dehydration, frequent diarrhea, ingestion of too much salt, renal acidosis, respiratory alkalosis, kidney failure, or dialysis. The signs and symptoms are fatigue, muscle weakness, excessive thirst, dry mouth, and hypertension. Complications of hyperchloremia include kidney stones, complete kidney failure, and heart and muscle problems. The exact treatment for hyperchloremia will depend on its cause.
- **Hypochloremia** – is usually caused by excessive use of loop diuretics, nasogastric suction, or vomiting. Metabolic alkalosis is usually present with hypochloremia. Vomiting causes a loss of hydrochloric acid. Also, certain medicines such as antacids can cause abnormal results. An intravenous (IV) saline solution to restore the electrolyte levels is an option for the treatment of hypochloremia.
- **Hyperphosphatemia** – usually caused by low calcium levels, chronic kidney disease, metabolic or respiratory acidosis, hypoparathyroidism, severe muscle injury, and excessive use of laxatives that contain phosphate. Clinical features may be due to accompanying hypocalcemia and include tetany, muscle cramps, and perioral numbness or tingling. Other symptoms include bone and joint pain, pruritus, and rash. The strategy for treatment of hyperphosphatemia in patients with normal kidney function is to enhance renal excretion. This can be accomplished effectively by volume repletion with saline, plus forced diuresis with a loop diuretic such as furosemide or bumetanide.
- **Hypophosphatemia** – usually caused by acute alcohol abuse, severe burns, starvation, vitamin D deficiency, hyperparathyroidism, medications such as intravenous iron, or use of niacin or certain antacids. Signs and symptoms of hypophosphatemia include bone pain and fractures, appetite loss, confusion, appetite loss, muscle weakness, tiredness, a general feeling of being upset, and tooth decay or late baby teeth eruption. Complications of hypophosphatemia include **rhabdomyolysis**, hemolytic anemia, arrhythmias, and respiratory failure. To treat mild to moderate cases of hypophosphatemia, oral phosphate replacement medications are usually used. If hypophosphatemia is severe, phosphate replacement through an IV is prescribed.
- **Hypermagnesemia** – occurs primarily in patients with acute or chronic kidney disease. malnourishment, and alcoholism. Hypothyroidism and especially cortico-adrenal insufficiency, are other recognized causes. The symptoms of hypermagnesemia include nausea, vomiting, headache, flushing, hypotension, and neurological impairment.
- Hypomagnesemia – usually caused by alcohol use disorder, malnutrition, malabsorption, chronic diarrhea, excessive sweating, heart failure, and use of certain diuretics or antibiotics. Symptoms of mild hypomagnesemia include tremors, tetany, nystagmus, fatigue, and weakness. Symptoms of severe hypomagnesemia include generalized tonic–clonic seizures, delirium, and arrhythmias. Treatment for hypomagnesemia depends on how mild or severe it is, and the underlying cause.
- **Hypercalcemia** – may be caused by primary hyperparathyroidism, lung and breast cancers, kidney stone, hyperthyroidism, excessive use of antacids, excessive use of calcium or vitamin D supplements, and use of lithium, theophylline, or certain diuretics. Calcium is one of the most important and common minerals in the body. Most of the body's calcium is stored in the bones. It is needed for blood coagulation. Two hormones called parathyroid hormone and calcitonin control the levels of calcium in the blood and bones. Vitamin D also plays an important role in maintaining calcium levels because the body needs it to absorb calcium from foods. Hypercalcemia can cause stomach upset, nausea, vomiting and constipation, bone pain, headaches, nausea, vomiting, constipation, loss of appetite, irritability, muscle pain, cramping, depression, and forgetfulness. Treatment of hypercalcemia depends on the cause and the severity of the condition. In mild cases of hypercalcemia, more water must be consumed, and any calcium-rich antacid tablets or calcium supplements must be stopped. If the hypercalcemia is due to an overactive parathyroid gland, surgery is done.

- **Hypocalcemia** – may be caused by kidney failure, hypoparathyroidism, vitamin D deficiency, pancreatitis, prostate cancer, malabsorption, and use of heparin, or antiepileptic drugs. Signs and symptoms of hypocalcemia most commonly include paresthesias, muscle spasms, cramps, tetany, circumoral numbness, and seizures. Oral calcium supplements are the most common treatment for hypocalcemia. Treating the cause is just as important as treating the hypocalcemia itself. Synthetic forms of parathyroid hormone, vitamin D supplements, and IV calcium gluconate are used.

FOCUS ON ELECTROLYTE IMBALANCES

Electrolyte imbalances can be life-threatening. If signs and symptoms such as confusion, sudden behavior changes, severe muscle weakness, rapid or irregular heartbeat, seizures, or chest pain are seen, 911 must be called immediately.

Test Your Knowledge

1. What are the symptoms of hyperkalemia?
2. What are the symptoms of hyponatremia?
3. What are the causes of hypophosphatemia?
4. What is caused by hypocalcemia?

ACID–BASE IMBALANCE

Acid–base imbalance results in disorders due to pathologic changes in carbon dioxide partial pressure (PCO_2) or serum bicarbonate (HCO_3^-). They usually produce abnormal arterial pH values. Acidemia exists if the serum pH is below 7.35. Alkalemia exists if it is above 7.45. **Acidosis** causes either accumulation of acid or loss of alkali. **Alkalosis** causes either accumulation of alkali or loss of acid. Actual pH changes are based on the amount of physiologic compensation, and if multiple processes are present. Primary acid–base disturbances are either metabolic or respiratory, based on whether the main change is in the serum PCO_2 or HCO_3^-.

The pH establishes whether acidosis or alkalosis is the primary process occurring, but it will move toward the normal range as compensatory efforts occur. Changes in the PCO_2 indicate the respiratory component, while changes in the HCO_3^- indicate the metabolic component. Metabolic and respiratory acidosis and alkalosis are further described here. The pH starts to be corrected by compensatory mechanisms, but these cannot totally return the pH to normal. A *simple acid–base disorder* is one acid–base disturbance with no accompanying compensatory response. A *complex acid–base disorder* consists of two or more primary disturbances. Compensated or mild acid–base disorders only cause a few signs or symptoms. Severe uncompensated acid–base disorders have many respiratory, cardiovascular, neurologic, and metabolic outcomes. The types of acidosis and alkalosis can be classified as metabolic or respiratory.

FOCUS ON SERUM BICARBONATE

Serum bicarbonate (HCO_3^-) helps the body maintain normal pH in the blood and regulates heart function. It mostly travels through the body as carbon dioxide, dissolved in the blood. This is why the amount of carbon dioxide in the blood is used to measure serum bicarbonate, a base, to check the acid–base balance.

Metabolic Acidosis

Metabolic acidosis develops when too much acid is produced in the body. It can also occur when the kidneys cannot remove enough acid from the body. There are several types of metabolic acidosis such as:

- Diabetic acidosis or diabetic ketoacidosis develops when ketone bodies build up during uncontrolled diabetes (usually type 1 diabetes)
- Hyperchloremic acidosis is caused by the loss of too much sodium bicarbonate from the body, which can happen with severe diarrhea
- Kidney disease (uremia, distal renal tubular acidosis, or proximal renal tubular acidosis)
- Lactic acidosis
- Poisoning by aspirin, ethylene glycol (antifreeze), or methanol
- Severe dehydration

Lactic acidosis results from a buildup of lactic acid. It is mainly produced in muscle cells and red blood cells. It forms when the body breaks down carbohydrates to use for energy when oxygen levels are low. Lactic acidosis can be caused by cancer, carbon monoxide poisoning, drinking too much alcohol, exercising vigorously for a very long time, liver failure, medicines such as salicylates and metformin, seizures, and prolonged lack of oxygen from severe anemia, shock, and heart failure.

Metabolic Alkalosis

Metabolic alkalosis develops from excessive bicarbonate in the body fluids, due to a variety of conditions. This condition is signified by a serum HCO3– higher than 28 mEq/L (28 mmol/L). It is caused by acid loss or retention of HCO_3^-. The blood pH increases. Symptoms include irritability, muscle twitching or cramping, muscle spasms, fatigue, confusion, tremor, tingling, numbness, arrhythmias, seizures, and coma. Healthcare assistance is required once arrhythmias, seizures, or confusion develop. Metabolic alkalosis is much less common than metabolic acidosis. Common causes include vomiting, gastric suctioning that removes too much of the normal stomach secretions, and intake of excess base, such as from too many antacids. Other causes include excessive use of baking soda, diuretics, certain laxatives, or steroids. Medical conditions that can cause metabolic alkalosis include **cystic fibrosis**, electrolyte imbalances, hyperaldosteronism, hypochloremia, and cyclic vomiting syndrome.

People at risk for metabolic alkalosis include those with severe, repeated vomiting, critical illnesses, dehydration, or if gastric suctioning is needed to rid the stomach of abnormal fluid or gas buildup, a poison, or a medication overdose. The condition is diagnosed via physical examination, blood tests (to measure blood gases, acid–base balance, and electrolyte levels, electrocardiogram, and urinalysis). Severe symptoms require immediate treatment. Options include infusion of saline, potassium and/or magnesium replacement, infusion of chloride, infusion of hydrochloric acid, and stopping any causative medications.

Respiratory Acidosis

Respiratory acidosis is a condition that occurs when the lungs cannot remove all of the carbon dioxide produced by the body, which results in the blood to become too acidic. This condition is signified by a PCO_2 higher than 40 mm Hg (**hypercapnia**). It is caused by hypoventilation. Physiologically, the lungs can eliminate carbon dioxide via **Kussmaul** breathing, a respiratory compensation for metabolic acidosis. Other causes include asthma, chronic obstructive pulmonary disease (COPD), **pulmonary fibrosis, scoliosis**, medications (such as opioids or benzodiazepines, often when combined with alcohol), severe obesity, and obstructive sleep apnea.

Chronic respiratory acidosis occurs over a long period of time. Some people with chronic respiratory acidosis develop the acute form when an acute illness disrupts the acid–base balance. Acute respiratory acidosis develops very quickly, before the kidneys can re-balance body fluids. Respiratory acidosis is a common cause of acid–base imbalances and may be related to pneumonia, cystic fibrosis, or **emphysema**, which all cause carbon dioxide to accumulate in the blood. The blood pH falls while the partial pressure of carbon dioxide rises (see Figure 12.5).

Respiratory Alkalosis

Respiratory alkalosis occurs when high levels of carbon dioxide disrupt the acid–base balance of the blood. This condition is signified by a PCO_2 less than 28 mm Hg (**hypocapnia**). It is caused by increased minute ventilation (hyperventilation). Respiratory alkalosis occurs when carbon dioxide is eliminated faster than it can be produced. The blood therefore becomes more alkaline. This condition is often related to stress or pain. Other causes of hyperventilation include anxiety, panic, fever, pregnancy, lung cancer, trauma, severe anemia, liver disease, overdose of salicylates or progesterone, pulmonary embolism, asthma, and stroke. People at risk for respiratory alkalosis are those experiencing intense stress, anxiety, panic, or anger. Patients receiving mechanical ventilation are also at risk. Symptoms include breathlessness, dizziness, numbness, tingling, irritability, nausea, muscle spasms or twitching, fatigue, lightheadedness, fainting, chest discomfort, shortness of breath, tremors, and confusion. Respiratory alkalosis and uncontrolled breathing often require immediate medical care in a hospital. Treatments are based on the underlying cause and focus on increasing blood carbon dioxide levels. The disorder may be prevented by learning methods of coping with stress, anxiety, pain, and anger. Preventive techniques include psychotherapy, relaxation techniques, lifestyle changes, and medications such as antidepressants. It is important to build a support system of others who can help the patient regain control of rapid breathing before it progresses to hyperventilation.

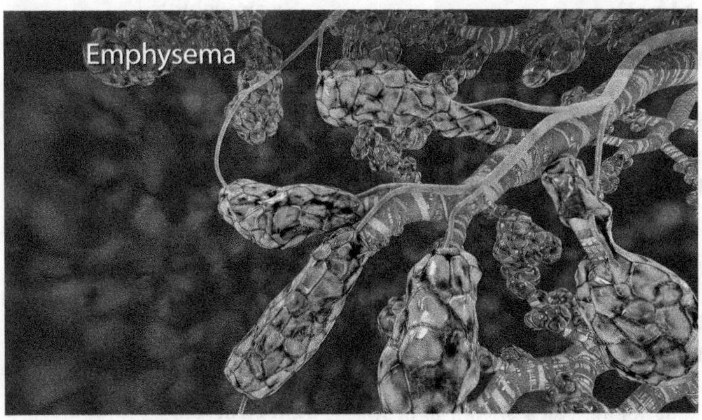

FIGURE 12.5 Damage to the walls of the lung alveoli in emphysema.

COMPLEX ACID–BASE IMBALANCES

Complex acid–base imbalances involve several primary processes. The values may appear close to normal – but this is not the case. Therefore, it is important to determine if changes in the PCO_2 and HCO_3^- indicate the expected compensation. If not, a second primary process is likely causing the abnormal compensation. Other clinical conditions such as chronic lung disease, drug overdose, and renal failure must also be considered. The **anion gap** is calculated, with elevations nearly always indicating metabolic acidosis. A normal anion gap has a low HCO_3^-, such as less than 24 mEq/L and high serum chloride (Cl^-). This indicates a nonanion gap or hyperchloremic metabolic acidosis. If there is metabolic acidosis present, a delta gap is calculated to identify any concurrent metabolic alkalosis. The **delta gap** is the difference between the anion gap of the patient and a normal anion gap. It is usually equivalent to the amount of HCO_3^-.

When the PCO_2 is higher than 40 mm Hg, respiratory acidosis is suggested. HCO_3^- should compensate, by increasing 3–4 mEq/L for every 10 mm Hg increase in PCO_2 that is sustained for 4–12 hours. There may be no increase or just an increase of 1–2 mEq/L that slowly increases to 3–4 mEq/L over a few days. A greater increase in HCO3– indicates a primary metabolic alkalosis. Metabolic alkalosis is indicated by HCO_3^- that is higher than 28 mEq/L. The PCO_2 should compensate by increasing 0.6–0.75 mm Hg for each 1 mEq/L increase in HCO_3^-, up to approximately 55 mm Hg. A greater increase indicates concurrent respiratory acidosis. A lesser increase indicates concurrent respiratory alkalosis.

Respiratory alkalosis is indicated by PCO_2 less than 38 mm Hg. The HCO_3^- should compensate over 4–12 hours by decreasing 4–5 mEq/L for each 10 mm Hg decrease in PCO_2. A lesser decrease means there was no time for compensation, or that there is a concurrent primary metabolic alkalosis. A greater decrease implies a primary metabolic acidosis. Another way to diagnose these mixed disorders is to use **nomograms**, which are acid–base maps that allow for plotting of pH, HCO_3^-, and PCO_2 at the same time.

CHEMICAL BUFFER SYSTEMS

There are a variety of **chemical buffer** systems in the human body. Acids are **proton** donors, while bases are proton acceptors. *Strong acids* dissociate completely and free all of the hydrogen ions in water, possibly changing a solution's pH dramatically. *Weak acids* dissociate only partially and have a smaller effect upon pH. Even so, weak acids can easily prevent pH changes, and therefore, they are important in chemical buffer systems. *Strong bases* dissociate easily in water and very quickly absorb hydrogen ions. *Weak acids* are not as likely to accept protons. A chemical buffer involves one or more compounds in a system that resists pH changes whenever a strong acid or base is added. The following are the three major chemical buffer systems:

- *Bicarbonate buffer system* – a mixture of carbonic acid and its salt, known as sodium bicarbonate; it is the only important extracellular fluid buffer; it also buffers the ICF
- *Phosphate buffer system* – very similar to the bicarbonate buffer system, this system's components are the salts of dihydrogen phosphate and monohydrogen phosphate; it is a very effective buffer in urine and the intercellular fluid, but not for the blood plasma to any great degree
- *Protein buffer system* – acts most effectively via proteins in the plasma and cells; hemoglobin is a good example of an intracellular protein buffer

Test Your Knowledge

1. What are the definitions of acidosis and alkalosis?
2. What are the neurologic outcomes of acidemia and alkalemia?
3. What are the differentiations between strong and weak acids and bases?

KEY TERMS

Acidosis

Addison's disease

Adipose

Aldosterone

Alkalosis

Angiotensin II

Anion

Anion gap

Antidiuretic hormone

Atrial natriuretic peptide

Baroreceptors

Cation

Cerebral edema

Chemical buffer systems

Covalent bonds

Cushing's syndrome

Delirium

Delta gap

Electrolytes

Emphysema

Estrogens

Extracellular fluid compartment

Fluid compartments

Glucocorticoids

Homeostasis

Hydrogen phosphate

Hydrostatic

Hypercapnia

Hypocapnia

Hypotonic hydration

Insensible water loss

Interstitial fluid

Intracellular fluid compartment

Juxtaglomerular complex

Lethargy

Macular edema

Metabolic acidosis

Metabolic alkalosis

Metabolic water

Nonelectrolytes

Nomograms

Osmolality

Osmolarity

Osmoreceptors

Osmotic

Parathyroid hormone

Plasma

Plasma proteins

Progesterone

Proton

Respiratory acidosis

Respiratory alkalosis

Rhabdomyolysis

Sensible water loss

Solutes

Tonicity

Universal solvent

Urea

Vasoconstriction

Vasodilation

Vitreous humors

Universal solvent

CLINICAL CASE STUDIES

Clinical Case Study 1

A 69-year-old man was brought to the local emergency department because his mental status had changed over the course of a single morning. His family reported he had not been eating or drinking as much as normal recently, and he had canceled his weekly social activities, which included playing golf and going to the theater. Past medical history included hypertension, hyperlipidemia, and osteoarthritis. He was also in the early stages of dementia. Upon examination, the patient had signs of wasting, dry mucous membranes, and confusion. He was relatively alert and could follow commands, but with some difficulty. Laboratory tests revealed that he had hypernatremia.

CRITICAL THINKING QUESTIONS

1. What are the common causes of hypernatremia?
2. What are the main functions of sodium in the body?
3. Is sodium the main extracellular or intracellular cation, and what are its concentrations in these fluids?

Clinical Case Study 2

A 29-year-old woman was brought to the emergency department by relatives after experiencing sudden stiffness and weakness in her arms and legs, plus lack of sensation and loss of mobility in her left leg. She also felt short of breath, anxious, and was perspiring heavily. Examination revealed signs of dehydration, and her heart rate was extremely fast. Laboratory tests revealed hypokalemia, hypochloremia, hypomagnesemia, and alkalemia. She also had a urinary tract infection. Immediate treatment was undertaken, and the patient's electrolytes were normalized within just over one day of hospitalization.

CRITICAL THINKING QUESTIONS

1. Why is hypokalemia potentially very dangerous?
2. What are the causes of hypomagnesemia?
3. What are the neurologic and respiratory outcomes of alkalemia?

Clinical Case Study 3

A 4-year-old boy was taken to the hospital by his parents due to a GI illness and severe dehydration. He had been having diarrhea for a few days, which started out as watery and yellow in color, but then turned to a red color, with visible clots. The boy also had severe abdominal cramping. Additional symptoms included vomiting and malaise. Examination revealed abdominal tenderness and altered mental status. Vital signs included hypertension and tachycardia. Blood tests showed significant leukocytosis and slight thrombocytopenia. Blood and stool specimens were collected for culture. The patient was started on fluids for rehydration therapy.

CRITICAL THINKING QUESTIONS

1. What can dehydration be caused by?
2. When dehydration is severe, what does fluid replacement require?
3. What is hypotonic dehydration?

Clinical Case Study 4

A 45-year-old man goes to an urgent care clinic with progressive pedal edema and shortness of breath. Both conditions got much worse over the previous two days. He has a history of chronic diarrhea with protein wasting, likely caused by a previous gastric bypass surgery. During physical examination, the patient's vital signs include a blood pressure of 133/83 mm Hg, a pulse of 143 beats per minute, and a respiratory rate of 24 breaths per minute. Heart sounds are tachycardiac and irregular. His legs have bilateral pitting edema. The patient has hypernatremia, metabolic acidosis, elevated blood urea nitrogen (BUN) and creatinine, and low magnesium.

CRITICAL THINKING QUESTIONS

1. What is the definition of pedal edema?
2. What are the common signs and symptoms of edema?
3. What are the complications of untreated edema?

Clinical Case Study 5

An 82-year-old man has had gastritis with severe vomiting for a few days. He also has a history of heart problems, and describes feeling dizzy and lethargic. His mouth is dry, his muscles are aching, and he cannot walk steadily. Though thirsty, any fluids or foods result in vomiting. His neighbor has brought him to the local emergency department. Examination reveals hypotension, but rapid pulse and respirations. Laboratory tests reveal combined fluid, electrolyte, and acid–base imbalances. The patient is diagnosed with alkalosis and hospitalized. Unable to resolve the patient's vomiting quickly, his serum sodium levels increase, and eventually, metabolic acidosis develops. He is started on fluid replacement therapy, and slowly, his imbalances begin to resolve.

CRITICAL THINKING QUESTIONS

1. What are the causes of metabolic and respiratory alkalosis?
2. How is pH used to assess acid–base imbalances?
3. What are the four steps used to interpret an acid–base imbalance?

STUDY QUESTIONS

1. What is the percentage of body fluid in infants?
   A. 20
   B. 45
   C. 65
   D. 74

2. All of the following are nonelectrolytes, EXCEPT:
   A. Creatinine
   B. Lipid
   C. Protein
   D. Glucose

3. Deficiency of ADH may cause which of the following disorders?
   A. Cushing's syndrome
   B. Diabetes insipidus
   C. Addison's disease
   D. Cystic fibrosis

4. How many milliliters of water are required per day in adults?
   A. 1,500 mL
   B. 2,000 mL
   C. 2,500 mL
   D. 5,000 mL

5. Which of the following hormones regulates water intake by the kidneys?
   A. Vasopressin
   B. Insulin
   C. Thyroid hormone
   D. Testosterone

6. Which of the following controls the thirst mechanism?
   A. Thalamus
   B. Internal capsule
   C. Hypothalamus
   D. Pineal gland

7. Which of the following is the hallmark sign of hypotonic hydration?
   A. Hyponatremia
   B. Hypercalcemia
   C. Hypocalcemia
   D. Hypernatremia

8. Which of the following may NOT cause edema?
   A. Cirrhosis of the liver
   B. Obesity
   C. Heart failure
   D. Chronic protein deficiency

9. Which of the following electrolytes may increase blood pressure?
   A. Sodium
   B. Potassium
   C. Magnesium
   D. Calcium

10. Which of the following electrolytes is a key component of blood clotting?
    A. Sodium
    B. Potassium
    C. Magnesium
    D. Calcium

11. Which of the following hormones increases the extracellular fluid volume?
    A. Parathyroid hormone
    B. Aldosterone
    C. Thyroid hormone
    D. Insulin

12. Which of the following hormones prompt increased potassium secretion?
    A. Thyroid hormone
    B. Growth hormone
    C. Aldosterone
    D. Estrogen

13. All of the following may be caused by hypercalcemia, EXCEPT:
    A. Hypoparathyroidism
    B. Hyperthyroidism
    C. Kidney stones
    D. Breast cancer

14. Which of the following disorders may cause metabolic acidosis?
    A. Stomach cancer
    B. Menopause
    C. Diabetic crisis
    D. Hyperthyroidism

15. Which of the following may cause hypercapnia?
    A. Respiratory acidosis
    B. Metabolic alkalosis
    C. Respiratory alkalosis
    D. Metabolic acidosis

FURTHER READING

1. Andersson, D., Mastenbjork, M.D., and Meloni, S. (2018). *Fluids and Electrolytes – A Thorough Guide covering Fluids, Electrolytes, and Acid-Base Balance of the Human Body.* Anderson / Mastenbjork / Meloni.
2. Connor, G.J. (2021). *Fluids and Electrolytes: A Fast and Easy Way to Understand Acid-Base Balance Without Memorization.* Connor.
3. Habibzadeh, F., Yadollahie, M., and Habibzadeh, P. (2021). *Pathophysiologic Basis of Acid-Base Disorders. Springer.*
4. Hale, A., and Hovey, M.J. (2013). *Fluid, Electrolyte, and Acid-Base Imbalances: Content Review Plus Practice Questions.* F.A. Davis.
5. Hassan Ketan, S. (2013). *A Guide for Management – Fluids and Electrolytes – Imbalances.* Scholars' Press.
6. Haws, J., and Haws, S. (2015). *A Nursing Guide to Fluids & Electrolytes and Acid-Base Balance.* CreateSpace Independent Publishing Platform.
7. Healy, Z. (2021). *Acid-Base Disturbance Cases (Critical Concept Mastery Series).* McGraw-Hill.
8. Hogan, M.A., Gingrich, M.M., Overby, P., and Ricci, M.J. (2006). *Fluids, Electrolytes, & Acid-Base Balance – Reviews & Rationales*, 2nd Edition. Prentice Hall.
9. Jameson, J.L., and Loscalzo, J. (2016). *Harrison's Nephrology and Acid-Base Disorders*, 3rd Edition. McGraw-Hill / Medical.
10. Johnson, J. (2018). *Fluids and Electrolytes Demystified*, 2nd Edition. McGraw Hill / Medical.
11. Kamel, K.S., and Halperin, M.L. (2016). *Fluid, Electrolyte, and Acid-Base Physiology*: A Problem-Based Approach, 5th Edition. Elsevier.
12. LeFever Kee, J., Paulanka, B.J., and Polek, C. (2009). *Handbook of Fluid, Electrolyte, and Acid-Base Imbalances*, 3rd Edition. Cengage Learning.
13. Mastenbjork, M., Meloni, S., and Andersson, D. (2018). *Fluids and Electrolytes: A Thorough Guide covering Fluids, Electrolytes, and Acid-Base Balance of the Human Body.* Medical Creations.
14. Nurse Academy. (2021). *Fluids and Electrolytes: A Quick and Easy Comprehensive Book to Understand the Acid-Base Balance of the Human Body – Clinical Assessment and Management.* Nurse Academy.
15. Preston, R.A. (2017). *Acid-Base, Fluids, and Electrolytes Made Ridiculously Simple*, 3rd Edition. MedMaster.
16. Reddi, A.S. (2014). *Fluid, Electrolyte and Acid-Base Disorders – Clinical Evaluation and Management.* Springer.
17. Rudiger Kulpmann, W., Stummvoll, H.K., and Lehmann, P. (2006). *Electrolytes, Acid-Base Balance and Blood Gases – Clinical Aspects and Laboratory*, 2nd Edition. Springer.
18. Schrier, R.W. (2017). *Renal and Electrolyte Disorders*, 8th Edition. Lippincott, Williams, and Wilkins.
19. Stephaniak, J. (2016). *The Acid-Alkaline Diet – Balancing the Body Naturally.* Live Healthy Now.
20. Tinawi, M. (2021). *Manual of Fluid, Electrolyte, and Acid-Base Disorders – A Pathophysiologic Approach to Common Clinical Problems.* Tinawi.

13 Nutritional Effects on the Nervous System

OUTLINE

LEARNING OBJECTIVES

After study of the chapter, readers should be able to:

1. Explain Wernicke encephalopathy and its causes.
2. Identify the risks of folic acid deficiency.
3. Describe reversible dementia and its outcome.
4. Discuss the combination of memory loss and Korsakoff psychosis.
5. Explain peripheral neuropathy and its prevention.
6. Describe large-fiber peripheral neuropathy.
7. Discuss Lewy body dementia.
8. Explain the causes of ataxia.
9. Identify the causes of slowly progressive encephalopathy.
10. Describe the effects of Wilson's disease in the body.

OVERVIEW

Proper nutrition is essential for the normal functioning of the nervous system. There are many deficiencies and toxicities from vitamins or minerals that cause diseases or conditions in the nervous system. Wernicke encephalopathy is a severe, life-threatening illness resulting from vitamin B1 deficiency. If not treated properly, a severe neurologic disorder called Korsakoff psychosis can occur, leading to death. Cognitive dysfunction refers to deficits in attention, verbal and nonverbal learning, short-term and working memory, visual and auditory processing, problem-solving, processing speed, and motor functioning. Cognitive disorders include dementia, amnesia, and delirium, with affected patients being no longer fully oriented to time and space. These disorders may be temporary or progressive, based on the cause. While delirium is temporary, dementias such as Alzheimer's disease are generally progressive. Inadequate nutrition can also lead to various types of peripheral neuropathies, which are among the most prevalent of all neurologic conditions. For example, a lack of vitamin B12 damages the protective myelin sheaths, resulting in nerves starting to function abnormally, leading to peripheral neuropathy.

NUTRITION AND THE BRAIN

Despite the limited effectiveness of current therapeutic approaches to reduce the consequences of brain injury, the brain has an incredible capability for plasticity. Much effort is being devoted to understanding how environmental conditions and lifestyle can influence the brain and body. Noninvasive approaches such as diet and exercise can have profound consequences for increasing resilience of the central nervous system to injuries and for maintaining cognitive abilities. Diet and exercise can influence the capability of the brain to fight disease and to react to challenges. Healthy diets, such as those high in omega-3 fatty acids (from salmon and other fish) and curcumin (from turmeric), can stimulate molecular systems that serve neuronal function and plasticity in the central nervous system (CNS). Oppositely, unhealthy "junk food" diets that consist of high amounts of saturated fats and sugars do the opposite. Exercise, augments the healing effects of the brain. It helps to reverse the mental decline associated with age, providing benefits underlying rehabilitative strategies after brain injuries, especially when implemented with a healthy diet.

Only recently, the actions of foods upon brain plasticity and function have been scrutinized. Selected dietary factors are important modifiers of brain plasticity and can have an impact on central nervous system health and disease. Dietary factors exert their effects by affecting molecular events related to the management of energy metabolism and synaptic plasticity. Select dietary factors have mechanisms similar to those of exercise and can complement the action of exercise. Nutrients can be taken in through whole foods and dietary supplements to reduce the consequences of neural damage. Therefore, exercise and dietary management appear to be a noninvasive and effective strategy to help counteract neurologic and cognitive disorders.

DOI: 10.1201/b22969-16

Green tea is rich in flavonoids, especially **catechins** such as epigallocatechin gallate, epigallocatechin, epicatechin, and epicatechin-3-gallate. Green tea is commonly consumed in China and throughout Asia, and is perceived as beneficial for general health. Green tea consumption is linked to reductions in cognitive deterioration in aging. Daily doses of the compound *Green Tea-catechin*, an antioxidant found in green tea, have been shown to help prevent memory loss and DNA oxidative damage. *Resveratrol* is most commonly found in berries, grapes, and red wine. It reduces oxidative stress in the spinal cord after an ischemia–reperfusion injury. Resveratrol has positive effects on body physiology, such as protecting cells in the heart, brain, and kidney; increasing apoptosis; and reducing tumor growth.

The amount of calories consumed per meal and the frequency of food consumption influence cognitive function and plasticity of the brain. Fasting every other day protects neurons in the hippocampus against excitotoxicity-induced death. Although certain foods contribute positively to neuronal health, diets high in saturated fats and sugar decrease levels of brain-derived neurotrophic factor in the brain, and lead to poorer neuronal performance.

It is necessary to control food intake to maintain optimal brain function and cognitive ability. Due to previous periods of food scarcity, we have adapted to eat whenever food becomes available. Brain circuits that control food intake are generally plastic and easily influenced by many stimuli, often leading to an exacerbation of their biological function. Eating disorders can follow similar mechanisms found in common types of addictive behaviors. This implies that the capacity of exercise to interact with the dietary signal can be used to control "food addictive behaviors".

FOCUS ON CURCUMIN

Curcumin is most commonly known for its traditional culinary and medicinal use in India. It comes from the rhizome (root) of the turmeric plant, and is used frequently in Indian dishes (producing the familiar yellow color of curry). Curcumin benefits the brain by providing protection, through multiple mechanisms, against neurologic disorders. As an antioxidant, anti-inflammatory, and antiamyloidal agent, curcumin can improve cognitive function in patients with Alzheimer disease.

WERNICKE ENCEPHALOPATHY

Encephalopathy is defined as a disease in which brain function is affected by an agent or a condition, resulting in an altered mental state, confusion, and actions that seem abnormal. **Wernicke encephalopathy** involves an acute onset of confusion, **nystagmus**, ataxia, and partial **ophthalmoplegia** that is linked to a thiamin deficiency. There may be insufficient intake or absorption of thiamin. Severe alcoholism is often an underlying this condition. When alcohol is consumed excessively, it interferes with the absorption of thiamin from the gastrointestinal (GI) tract. Poor nutrition that is related to alcoholism often prevents adequate intake of thiamin. Wernicke encephalopathy may also be caused by recurrent kidney dialysis, hyperemesis, **gastric plication**, starvation, cancer, and acquired immunodeficiency syndrome (AIDS). When a carbohydrate load is given to patients with a thiamin deficiency, such as refeeding following starvation or administration of intravenous (IV) dextrose-containing solutions to patients of high risk, Wernicke encephalopathy may develop.

People that abuse alcohol do not always develop Wernicke encephalopathy, so other factors may be implicated, such as genetic abnormalities causing a defective form of *transketolase*, an enzyme that processes thiamin. Usually, central nervous system lesions are distributed in symmetrical fashion around ventricles. Often, there are changes in the dorsomedial thalamus, **mammillary bodies**, ocular motor nuclei, **locus coeruleus**, and vestibular nuclei. The prevalence of Wernicke encephalopathy is based on autopsy studies, indicating that it affects 1% to 3% of the global population. Incidence is believed to be higher in developing countries because of vitamin deficiencies and malnutrition. The male to female ratio is 1.7 to 1, but there are no studies showing any particular racial predisposition to the disease.

As Wernicke encephalopathy develops, there are sudden clinical changes. Oculomotor abnormalities include horizontal and vertical nystagmus, along with partial ophthalmoplegia such as conjugate gaze palsies and lateral rectus palsy. The pupils are usually slow-moving or unequal in size. There is commonly vestibular dysfunction but no hearing loss, plus impairment of the oculovestibular reflex. Gait ataxia can be caused by cerebellar dysfunction, vestibular disturbances, and/or polyneuropathy. The gait is slow and wide-based, with short-spaced steps. Overall confusion is exemplified by indifference, extreme disorientation, drowsiness, inattention, or stupor. There are often elevations of peripheral nerve pain thresholds. Many patients have severe autonomic dysfunction with signs of sympathetic hyperactivity such as agitation and tremor. In some, hypoactivity may be present, signified by hypothermia, postural hypotension, and syncope. Without treatment, stupor may progress to coma and death.

The diagnosis of Wernicke encephalopathy is based on recognizing underlying vitamin B1(thiamin) deficiencies and poor nutrition. Outlook for Wernicke encephalopathy is based on an early diagnosis and early treatment, which can correct all of the abnormalities. Ocular symptoms usually start to resolve within one day after thiamin is administered. However, the ataxia and confusion can continue for days to months. Impairments of memory and learning may never totally return to normal. If not treated, the disorder progresses and death occurs in 10% to 20% of patients. Those that survive have an 80% rate of developing **Korsakoff psychosis**. The combination of the memory loss and Korsakoff psychosis is called *Wernicke-Korsakoff syndrome*.

The treatment of Wernicke encephalopathy requires immediate thiamin administration. Magnesium is a required as a cofactor for thiamin-dependent metabolism. Supportive treatment involves correction of electrolyte abnormalities, rehydration, and general nutritional therapy that includes multivitamins. When it is advanced, hospitalization is required. The patient must stop drinking alcoholic beverages. This is because the effects of alcohol can lead to permanent damage to the **Wernicke area** of the brain, which are irreversible. However, Wernicke encephalopathy is preventable, so undernourished patients must be given parenteral thiamin plus vitamin B12 and folate. Before any treatment of a patient that has reduced consciousness, thiamin is advised to be administered. Undernourished patients continue to take thiamin on an outpatient basis.

The prognosis of Wernicke encephalopathy is based on early diagnosis and treatment. Ocular symptoms usually start to resolve within 24 hours after early administration of thiamin. The ataxia and confusion can continue over days to months. Memory and learning impairment may not totally resolve. If untreated, the disorder will progress and mortality is 10%–20% of patients. Of those that survive, 80% develop Korsakoff psychosis as part of Wernicke-Korsakoff syndrome.

FOCUS ON WERNICKE ENCEPHALOPATHY

Wernicke encephalopathy is a degenerative brain disorder caused by the lack of vitamin B1. It can result from dietary deficiencies, alcohol abuse, prolonged vomiting, eating disorders, or chemotherapy. The thalamus and hypothalamus are primarily damaged.

Test Your Knowledge

1. What are the signs and symptoms of Wernicke encephalopathy?
2. What is Korsakoff psychosis?
3. What are the treatments of Wernicke encephalopathy?

COGNITIVE DYSFUNCTION

Folate deficiency may contribute to cognitive impairment of the brain with continued aging. This may lead to reversible *dementia*, and also increases risks for Alzheimer's disease (AD) and vascular dementia. Folate-deficient adults with impaired intellectual function that was confirmed by neuropsychological testing were greatly improved after 6–12 months of folic acid supplementation. Chronic folate deficiency is able to induce **cerebral atrophy**. The highest incidence of folate deficiency is in the elderly, and there is a close association with dementia and other cognitive dysfunction. Folate concentrations in the serum and cerebrospinal fluid (CSF) fall with age as plasma homocysteine levels rise, which may contribute to the aging process. In patients with AD, cognitive decline is significantly related to lower serum folate concentrations. Older people given folate supplements generally improve in their cognitive function to a large degree. Folate supplementation can improve **visuomotor** performance, **visuospatial** memory, associative memory, logical reasoning, and activities for daily living over four months.

Deficiency of folate may require months for encephalopathy to develop. Also, folate deficiency plays a role in developing acute and subacute encephalopathy, directly or indirectly, by reducing the absorption of thiamin. Encephalopathies include dementia, brain atrophy, reduced cerebral blood flow, and slowing of **brain waves**. A decrease of folate may be clinically diagnosed as frontal dementia, **Pick's disease**, and **amyotrophic lateral sclerosis** dementia. Approximately 70% of folate-deficient patients with a history of excessive alcohol intake have related encephalopathy. About 40% of patients with a history of **gastrectomy** also have encephalopathy. Primarily, encephalopathy involves mostly cognitive dysfunction with different features than those of AD. In almost 60% of cases, encephalopathy is accompanied by neuropathy in folate-deficient patients.

Though not always preventable, there are methods that help reduce the likelihood of developing cognitive dysfunction. These include regular, adequate exercise, a Mediterranean-style diet, minimal alcohol consumption, consistent good-quality sleep, staying mentally active as we age, and developing regular social interaction with as many people as possible. Frequent social engagement strengthens neural networks and slows normal age-related declines. It can help strengthen cognitive reserve and delay the onset of dementia.

Many cases of cognitive dysfunction can be reversed if a general health condition such as sleep deprivation is underlying. Addressing the underlying cause often greatly improves cognition. However, there is no single cure or treatment that can guarantee a cure. A worsened prognosis is given if there are significant amounts of abnormal plaque deposits, reductions in brain consumption of glucose in key areas, enlargement of brain ventricles, or shrinkage of the hippocampus. Better outlook is given if there is success with drugs that boost neurotransmitter levels, drugs that regulate the activity of glutamate, occupational therapy, and reducing environmental clutter and noise to allow for better focus and attention.

PERIPHERAL NEUROPATHY

Peripheral neuropathy is dysfunction of the peripheral nerves, which are the parts of nerves distal to the root and plexus. There are varying degrees of pain, sensory disturbances, diminished deep tendon reflexes, muscle weakness and atrophy, and vasomotor symptoms. All of these can occur singularly or in various combinations. Peripheral neuropathies can be *mononeuropathy* of a single nerve, *multiple mononeuropathy* of two or more discrete nerves

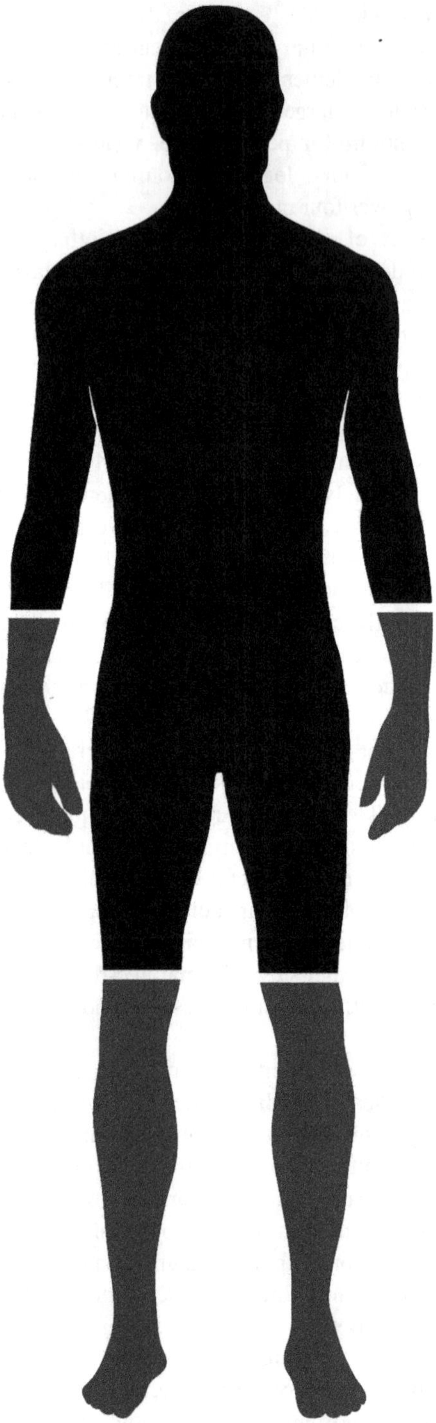

FIGURE 13.1 Stocking-glove distribution of peripheral neuropathy.

in separate areas, or *polyneuropathy*, with many nerves affected simultaneously, suggesting a diffuse disease process. The neuropathy due to thiamin deficiency is known as beriberi (see Chapter 10). Peripheral neuropathy may also be caused by ingesting megadoses (over 500 mg daily) of vitamin B6 (pyridoxine). Such doses are sometimes taken to treat **carpal tunnel syndrome** or **premenstrual syndrome**, even though the effectiveness of these doses has not been proven. Peripheral neuropathy may develop with deficits in a **stocking-glove distribution** (see Figure 13.1). These include progressive sensory ataxia, plus severely impaired position and vibration senses. The senses of pain, temperature, and touch are not affected as much, and the motor system and CNS are usually normal. The diagnosis of vitamin B6 toxicity is clinical, and treatment is simply to stop taking vitamin B6 supplements. Recovery, however, is slow, and some patients never fully recover.

There is distal sensory loss, burning pain, and in the toes and feet, paresthesias or muscle weakness. The lower legs often ache and cramp. Untreated, the peripheral neuropathy will cause ascending leg weakness, eventually evolving to sensorimotor neuropathy of the hands. The recurrent laryngeal nerve may be affected, causing hoarseness. Cranial nerve involvement is seen as weakness of the tongue and face. About 25% of patients with thiamin-deficient polyneuropathy also have Wernicke encephalopathy.

Electrodiagnostic testing will reveal an axonal sensorimotor polyneuropathy that is worse in the lower extremities. Nerve biopsies will show axonal degeneration. Once thiamin replacement is underway, cardiac problems can improve within hours to days. Neurological improvements may be required for three to six months. The motor manifestations respond better than the sensory manifestations. Improvement usually occurs slowly. In patients with severe neuropathy, there may be permanent deficits.

Prevention of peripheral neuropathy is based on a nutritious diet, regular exercise, limited alcohol use, avoiding injuries and toxic chemicals, and carefully managing underlying disorder such as diabetes mellitus. Also, correcting vitamin deficiencies and losing weight have some amount of preventive effects against peripheral neuropathy.

The prognosis of peripheral neuropathy varies, based on the underlying cause and which nerves have been damaged. Some cases improve over time with treatment of the underlying cause. Some patients experience permanent damage that cannot be reversed, or may gradually get worse over time. In most cases, the prognosis is intermediate since the neuropathy cannot be cured, but can be prevented from worsening.

Test Your Knowledge

1. What are the signs and symptoms of cognitive dysfunction?
2. What are the classifications of peripheral neuropathies?
3. What are the consequences of ingesting megadoses of pyridoxine?

LARGE-FIBER PERIPHERAL NEUROPATHY

Vitamin B12 deficiency may result in *demyelination* of axons, which is damage to the myelin sheath. Nerve conduction is slowed down. Demyelination mostly affects heavily myelinated fibers to cause **large-fiber sensory** dysfunction. These include buzzing and tingling sensations, diminished reflexes, and motor weakness. Acquired demyelinating polyneuropathy is usually signified by severe motor weakness with only slight atrophy. Nerve biopsy is sometimes done to differentiate demyelinating from vasculitic large-fiber neuropathies.

Dietary vitamin B12 deficiency usually occurs from inadequate absorption, but vegans that do not take vitamin supplements can also develop it. Deficiency of vitamin B12 causes damage to the white matter of the CNS, peripheral neuropathy, and megaloblastic anemia. Subacute combined degeneration of the nervous system may result in demyelinating or axonal peripheral neuropathies. In the early stages, the extremities have decreased position and vibratory sensation, with mild to moderate weakness and hyporeflexia. Later on, spasticity, extensor plantar responses, increased loss of position and vibratory sensation in the legs, and ataxia will appear. Though pain, temperature, and touch sensations usually remain normal, they may be hard to assess in elderly patients. Some patients develop irritability and slight depression. In advanced cases, delirium, **paranoia**, confusion, and postural hypotension may be seen. The patient's confusion may be very similar to that of age-related dementias. With vitamin B12 supplementation, resolution of neuropathy may take months. Neurologic symptoms that persist for months to years become irreversible. In most elderly people with a vitamin B12 deficiency plus dementia, their cognition does not improve with treatment. Vitamin B12 supplements must be continued throughout life unless the underlying mechanism that caused the deficiency is corrected.

Prevention of large-fiber peripheral neuropathy may occur if the underlying cause can be treated and cured, such as a vitamin deficiency. General preventive measures include managing diabetes mellitus, avoiding smoking, reviewing medications, addressing vitamin deficiencies, eating a healthy diet, exercising regularly, and avoiding repetitive motions, cramped positions, toxic chemicals, and excessive alcohol use.

Prognosis of large-fiber peripheral neuropathy is best when the condition is within the first three stages. Once stage 4 (constant numbness) develops, this is a sign that the nerves are dying and most nerve fibers have disintegrated. With irreversible damage of the large fibers, the prognosis is worsened. Much of the numbness will never be reversible and treatment must occur urgently. There is still a chance for improvement but it is usually slight. Prognosis is worst once stage 5 (a complete loss of feeling) has developed.

FOCUS ON LARGE-FIBER PERIPHERAL NEUROPATHY

Damage to the large sensory fibers disrupts the ability to feel vibrations and touch – primarily in the hands and feet. The damage can contribute to loss of reflexes. Vitamin B12 deficiency, high cholesterol, type 2 diabetes mellitus, chemotherapy, smoking, and HIV/AIDS are all potential causes. Large-fiber peripheral neuropathy manifests with loss of joint position and vibration sense, plus sensory ataxia.

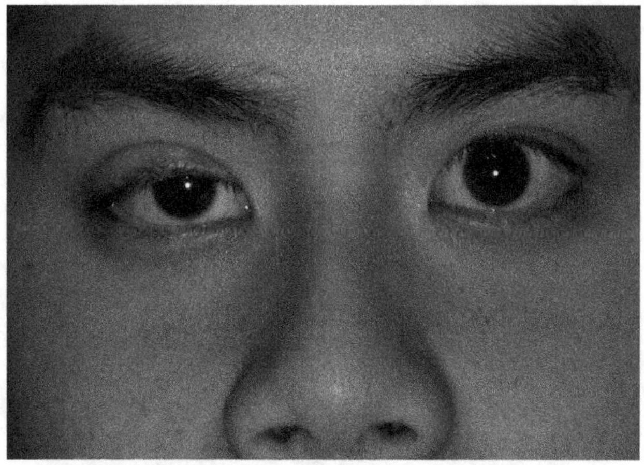

FIGURE 13.2 Ptosis.

ATAXIA

Ataxia is a lack of muscle coordination and control. Patients with ataxia have trouble with movement, fine motor tasks, and maintaining balance. It usually results from damage to the cerebellum that controls muscle coordination. Many conditions may cause ataxia, including alcohol misuse, brain degeneration, stroke, and vitamin E deficiency. In children, chronic **cholestatic hepatobiliary** disease or **cystic fibrosis** causes neurologic deficits. These include spinocerebellar ataxia, with a loss of deep tendon reflexes, truncal and limb ataxia, loss of sensation of vibration and position, muscle weakness, ophthalmoplegia, and **ptosis** (see Figure 13.2).

Ataxia with vitamin E deficiency is rare, an inherited neurodegenerative disorder that combines ataxia with peripheral neuropathy. The disorder is progressive and can affect many different body systems. Some patients have eye abnormalities, cardiomyopathy, and *scoliosis* (see Figure 13.3). Reflexes in the legs may become slow or be absent. The foot becomes highly arched, and there may be hyperextension of the big toe. If the throat muscles are involved, there can be impaired swallowing, choking, and difficulty eating. Some patients may develop tremor or shaking of the head. However, emotions and intellect are not usually affected. Fatty deposits known as **xanthomas** may affect the **Achilles tendon**. **Dystonia** may develop, with involuntary muscle contractions that force the body into abnormal, sometimes painful postures.

Ataxia with vitamin E deficiency results from mutations of a gene on chromosome 8. The gene regulates production of alpha-tocopherol transfer protein, which binds vitamin E into very low-density lipoprotein (VLDL) from the liver. There is an impaired ability to bind vitamin E into VLDL, resulting in vitamin E deficiency in certain tissues. Symptoms develop because of deficient vitamin E in the adipose tissue. Males and females are equally affected. The disorder occurs in less than one in every one million people. Onset may be in childhood or adulthood.

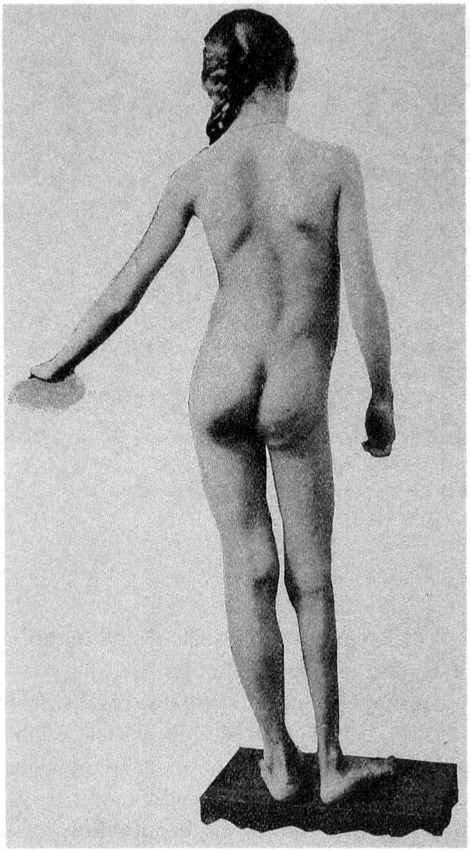

FIGURE 13.3 Scoliosis.

Diagnosis of ataxia with vitamin E deficiency is based on low levels of vitamin E, with normal levels of lipoproteins and lipids, and no evidence of fat malabsorption. Vitamin E supplements are given, which have often stopped progression of the disorder, and sometimes improved neurological symptoms.

Most forms of ataxia are not preventable since they may be inherited. Genetic counseling and screening are recommended to determine the chance of any offspring having the disease or carrying the gene without any symptoms. Prevention of ataxia in some cases requires only drinking alcohol in moderation or not at all, preventing concussions or traumatic brain injuries, avoiding recreational drugs, managing fatigue and stress, avoiding exposure to inhalants, preventing or treating infections, managing body weight, avoiding exposure to chemicals, metals, or toxic substances, and managing vitamin deficiencies or nutritional problems.

The prognosis for hereditary ataxia is varied since life expectancy is usually shorter than normal, though some people live well into their middle years or beyond. Severe cases have a poor prognosis since they can be fatal early in life. For acquired ataxia, prognosis depends on the underlying cause.

Test Your Knowledge

1. What area of the brain damage may cause ataxia?
2. What nutrient deficiency may cause ataxia?
3. What are xanthomas?

DEMENTIA

Dementia is a chronic disorder of mental processes, with loss of memory, language, and problem-solving. It is caused by brain disease or injury. The four common types of dementia including AD, Lewy body dementia, vascular dementia, and frontotemporal dementia. AD is the most common neurocognitive disorder. Between 60% and 80% of older adults with dementia have AD. There is progressive atrophy and death of brain cells, resulting in a continuous decline in cognition, behavior, and social skills. The affected individual becomes unable to function independently. *Vascular dementia* involves acute or chronic cognitive deterioration. It is usually due to diffuse or focal cerebral infarction from cerebrovascular disease. There are problems with reasoning, planning, judgment, memory, and other thought processes caused by brain damage from impaired brain blood flow. Vascular dementia is the second most common cause of dementia in older adults. It may be present concurrently with AD.

Lewy body dementia is chronic cognitive deterioration characterized by Lewy body inclusions in the cytoplasm of cortical neurons. Overall, it is the third most common type of dementia. Some patients also have neuritic plaques and neurofibrillary tangles, which also occur in patients with AD. *Frontotemporal dementia* (FTD) is actually a group of brain disorders, basically affecting the frontal and temporal lobes. These areas are associated with language, personality, and behavior. In FTD, areas of the lobes atrophy. This form is one of the less common types of dementia, and may be sporadic or hereditary. One example of FTD is called Pick disease, which includes severe atrophy, and loss of neurons.

Vitamin D deficiency may also cause dementia. Vitamin D is implicated in precognitive and neuroprotective functions. These include the reduction of AD factors such as **amyloid beta** and phosphorylated **tau**. Vitamin D concentrations are significantly lower in people with AD and cognitive impairment, compared to healthy control group subjects. Therefore, low vitamin D concentrations are linked to an increased risk of dementia and cognitive decline. In fact, deficiency of vitamin D is also implicated in vascular dementia and **Parkinson's disease**. Adults given vitamin D supplements have significant improvement in dementia and cognitive decline over three to six months periods compared to those that are not given supplements.

Dementia is difficult to prevent since its cause is often unknown. If caused by a stroke, future declines may be preventable by lower risk factors. Patients should avoid smoking, control body weight, exercise regularly, eat a healthy diet, manage diabetes, hypertension, or high cholesterol, remain mentally alert and active, engage in regular social activities, and if recommended by a physician, take aspirin.

The average prognosis for dementia is varied based on the type. Life expectancy for AD, for example, is about eight to ten years, but less if the person is diagnosed while in his or her 80s or 90s. Even so, a small amount of AD patients live for 15 or even 20 years. Some dementia patients require support soon after diagnosis while others are able to remain independent for several years. Early-stage dementia lasts about two to four years, while mid-stage dementia averages two to ten years. End-stage dementia lasts only one to three years.

SLOWLY PROGRESSIVE ENCEPHALOPATHY

Niacin (vitamin B3) deficiency may be linked to a variety of CNS symptoms. These include slowly progressive encephalopathy, which is primarily characterized by impaired consciousness. Other symptoms include psychosis and dementia. The psychosis caused by niacin deficiency is characterized by disorientation, memory impairment, confusion, and **confabulation**. The main symptoms may be depression, excitement, delirium, mania, or paranoia. Also, for undiagnosed encephalopathies in patients with alcoholism, treatment involves multiple vitamins that include niacin. There can also be *pellagrous encephalopathy*, which is delirium caused by pellagra (see Chapter 10). In industrialized countries such as the United States, niacin deficiency may present only with encephalopathy. Before the encephalopathy develops, cerebral manifestations include headache, irritability, confusion, fatigue, **apathy**, and insomnia. Mental changes include delirium, depression, and irritability. Additional symptoms include loss of appetite, nausea, tiredness, weight loss, a coated tongue, mouth sores, anemia, and forgetfulness. Without treatment, death may occur.

Niacin deficiency is associated with schizophreniform symptoms, bipolar symptoms, and anxiety. Alcoholic pellagra encephalopathy may result in neurological symptoms, confusion, decreased consciousness, oppositional hypertonia, and myoclonus. Treatment of niacin deficiency-related slowly progressive encephalopathy is with large doses of niacin given orally. Usually, improvements are dramatic, and continued use of niacin supplementation usually continues for at least three months, with regular follow-ups.

The prevention of slowly progressive encephalopathy is through niacin or multivitamin/mineral supplements that usually contain at least 20 mg of niacin. Supplements of niacin such as nicotinic acid are approved by the Food and Drug Administration (FDA) for treating and preventing niacin deficiency, and resultant slowly progressive encephalopathy. The prognosis of slowly progressive encephalopathy is generally good, since improvement is usually seen within several days of niacin supplementation. There is often a complete recovery.

WILSON'S DISEASE

The toxic accumulation of copper in the body is known as *hypercupremia*. It can be inherited or acquired. *Wilson's disease* is very rare that results in accumulation of copper in the brain and liver. It affects about one in every 30,000 people globally. Inherited Wilson's disease is more common in **homozygous** patients because of a mutant recessive gene located on chromosome 13. Hepatic fibrosis develops that eventually causes cirrhosis. Copper diffuses out of the liver into the bloodstream and accumulates in the brain. It seriously damages the brain, liver, and kidneys. In some cases, copper may deposit around the rim of the corneas and edge of the iris, **Kayser–Fleischer rings** appear.

Wilson's disease can occur at age two, but are most common between 5 and 35. In approximately 40% of patients – mostly young adults – initial signs and symptoms reflect CNS involvement. Motor deficits are common, with combinations being dystonia, tremors, dysarthria, dysphagia, **chorea**, incoordination, and **drooling**. The CNS symptoms may be cognitive or psychiatric problems. The clinical manifestations also include abdominal pain, fatigue, jaundice, ascites, and edema.

Wilson's disease is suspected in people under age 40 if they have an unexplained liver, neurologic, or psychiatric disorder; an unexplained chronic elevation of hepatic transaminases; **fulminant** hepatitis; or a parent, sibling, or cousin with Wilson's disease. Slit-lamp examination for Kayser–Fleischer rings is needed. Serum **ceruloplasmin** levels and 24-hour urinary copper excretion are assessed. The ceruloplasmin levels are usually sufficient, and the serum copper levels may be measured. Kayser–Fleischer rings plus motor neurologic abnormalities or decreased ceruloplasmin are highly diagnostic.

There is no way to prevent inherited Wilson's disease. Genetic counseling may be able to determine if current or future children are at risk for developing it. Genetic testing is important if there is a family or personal history of the condition. Prognosis is usually good unless the disease has advanced prior to treatment. If untreated, Wilson's disease is usually fatal by age 30. Treatment will be lifelong. A low-copper diet is needed, which avoids beef liver, black-eyed peas, cashews, shellfish, vegetable juice, cocoa, and mushrooms. Patients must not take the chelating drugs called penicillamine, trientine, and sometimes, oral zinc. Drinking water must be checked for its copper content. No vitamin or mineral supplements containing copper should be taken. For patients with Wilson's disease and fulminant hepatic failure or severe hepatic insufficiency that medications are not effective for, liver transplantation may be required.

FOCUS ON WILSON'S DISEASE

Wilson's disease is progressive and potentially fatal. It is a genetic disorder involving excess copper stored primarily in the liver, brain, and corneas. If untreated, Wilson's disease leads to liver disease, central nervous system dysfunction, and death. It mostly manifests between 12 and 23 years of age, and life expectancy without treatment is an average of 40 years. Early diagnosis and treatment can increase the life span.

Test Your Knowledge

1. Which organs are severely damage by accumulation of copper?
2. What are Kayser–Fleischer rings?
3. What foods are contained in copper diet?

KEY TERMS

Achilles tendon

Amyloid beta

Amyotrophic lateral sclerosis

Apathy

Brain waves

Carpal tunnel syndrome

Catechins

Cerebral atrophy

Ceruloplasmin

Cholestatic hepatobiliary

Confabulation

Cystic fibrosis

Drooling

Fulminant

Gastrectomy

Gastric plication

Homozygous

Kayser–Fleischer rings

Korsakoff psychosis

Large-fiber sensory

Lewy Body dementia

Locus coeruleus

Mammillary bodies

Nystagmus

Ophthalmoplegia

Paranoia

Parkinson's disease

Peripheral neuropathy

Pick's disease

Premenstrual syndrome

Ptosis

Stocking-glove distribution

Visuomotor

Visuospatial

Wernicke area

Wernicke encephalopathy

Xanthomas

CLINICAL CASE STUDIES

Clinical Case Study 1

A 54-year-old man was evaluated for possible Wernicke encephalopathy. He had a history of alcoholism and presented with extreme confusion, an upward gaze palsy of the left eye, and gait ataxia over the past week. A magnetic resonance imaging (MRI) of his brain revealed scattered nonenhanced low signal intensity lesions on T1-weighted imaging, and high signal intensity lesions on T2-weighted imaging. The bilateral basal ganglia, thalami, midbrain, pons, and periventricular regions were involved. There was evidence of atrophic changes and mammillary bodies. The patient was treated with IV thiamin, 100 mg per day. The left upward gaze palsy was resolved within one week, and the other symptoms gradually improved.

CRITICAL THINKING QUESTIONS

1. What does Wernicke encephalopathy involve?
2. When autonomic dysfunction is present as part of Wernicke encephalopathy, what signs and symptoms manifest?
3. With Wernicke encephalopathy, in regards to alcohol consumption, what *must* occur?

Clinical Case Study 2

A 46-year-old woman was evaluated because of weakness, irritability, loss of appetite, loose stools, dark-pigmented skin lesions, a burning sensation in the mouth, and disorientation. She had no history of significant medications and did not drink alcohol. The woman was a vegetarian, and was extremely thin, almost to the point of looking malnourished. She was dehydrated and pale. She also had cheilitis and glossitis. The skin lesions were on her face, neck, forearms, and feet. She was diagnosed with pellagra and a severe niacin deficiency. The patient was also anemic. Treatment was started with nicotinic acid at 375 mg, twice per day, and IV fluids were administered, with success.

CRITICAL THINKING QUESTIONS

1. How is the psychosis caused by niacin deficiency described?
2. What other manifestations may occur before encephalopathy develops?

Clinical Case Study 3

A 20-year-old woman presented to her physician with progressive burning sensations on her upper trunk, paresthesias, and numbness of the arms and legs. She also had mild weakness of her hands and feet, insomnia, irritability, and constipation. Extensive testing was undertaken, and eventually, the patient was diagnosed with vitamin B12 deficiency-related peripheral neuropathy. She was treated with sublingual vitamin B12 for three months, during which she experienced extreme improvements in her neurological symptoms.

CRITICAL THINKING QUESTIONS

1. What is peripheral neuropathy?
2. How does vitamin B12 deficiency lead to peripheral neuropathy?
3. How does dietary vitamin B12 deficiency usually occur, and what are the later manifestations?

Clinical Case Study 4

A 25-year-old woman had abdominal pain and a low grade fever, and also had vomited dark colored vomitus three times. She also had vaginal bleeding. The patient, upon examination, had pallor, puffiness around her eyes, and pedal edema. Her abdomen was distended and the spleen was palpable. Kayser–Fleischer rings were present in both eyes. The patient described having had similar symptoms twice before, and mentioned that her younger sister had died from the disease. Endoscopy revealed grade III esophageal varices. The patient was diagnosed with Wilson's disease, cirrhosis of the liver, portal hypertension, and chronic anemia. After repeated bouts of severe vomiting, the patient died on the fifth day of hospitalization.

CRITICAL THINKING QUESTIONS

1. What accumulates in the body as part of Wilson's disease?
2. When are the signs and the symptoms of Wilson's disease?
3. When is Wilson's disease suspected in people under age 40?

STUDY QUESTIONS

1. Which of the following is NOT a cause of Wernicke encephalopathy?
   A. Kidney dialysis
   B. Hyperemesis
   C. Niacin deficiency
   D. Thiamin deficiency

2. Which of the following mental disorders may be present with Wernicke encephalopathy?
   A. Dementia
   B. Korsakoff psychosis
   C. Paranoia
   D. Mania

3. Partial ophthalmoplegia and nystagmus may be seen in which of the following?
   A. Cognitive dysfunction
   B. Wilson's disease
   C. Slow progressive encephalopathy
   D. Wernicke encephalopathy

4. Which of the following may contribute to cognitive impairment of the brain?
   A. Folate deficiency
   B. Thiamin deficiency
   C. Niacin deficiency
   D. Biotin deficiency

5. A stocking-glove distribution of peripheral neuropathy may be caused by which of the following deficiencies?
   A. Thiamin
   B. Folate
   C. Pyridoxine
   D. Niacin

6. Which of the following may result from taking megadoses of vitamin B6?
   A. Cerebral atrophy
   B. Peripheral neuropathy
   C. Korsakoff psychosis
   D. Wilson's disease

7. Pellagrous encephalopathy may be caused by which of the following vitamin deficiencies?
   A. Riboflavin
   B. Cobalamin
   C. Ascorbic acid
   D. Niacin

8. Large-fiber sensory dysfunction may be caused by which of the following?
   A. Demyelination of axons
   B. Myelination of terminal axons
   C. Hardening of axons
   D. Kayser–Fleischer rings

9. Damage to which of the following may cause ataxia?
   A. Cerebrum
   B. Cerebellum
   C. Parietal
   D. Temporal

10. All of the following may cause ataxia, EXCEPT:
    A. Stroke
    B. Vitamin B6 deficiency
    C. Vitamin E deficiency
    D. Brain degeneration

11. Which of the following types of dementia affects language, personality, and behavior?
    A. Frontotemporal dementia
    B. Alzheimer's disease
    C. Lewy body dementia
    D. Wilson's disease

12. Which of the following is an example of frontotemporal dementia?
    A. Alzheimer's disease
    B. Wilson's disease
    C. Pick disease
    D. Pellagrous encephalopathy

13. Hypercupremia is also known as which of the following disorders?
    A. Pick disease
    B. Wilson's disease
    C. Parkinson's disease
    D. Alzheimer's disease

14. Kayser–Fleischer rings in the rim of the corneas and edge of the iris are seen in which of the following disorders?
    A. Parkinson's disease
    B. Pick disease
    C. Ophthalmoplegia
    D. Wilson's disease

15. In which of the following organs of the body is there the largest accumulation of copper?
    A. Liver
    B. Spleen
    C. Bone marrow
    D. Urinary bladder

FURTHER READING

1. Beller, J., and Beller Health Research Institute. (2022). *Dementia Overview – 49 Dementia Types, Symptoms, & Risk Factors.* Beller Health Research Institute.
2. Bowles, J.T. (2013). *Alzheimer's Treatment that Actually Worked in Small Studies That Will Never Be Tested; You Will Never Hear About.* CreateSpace Independent Publishing Platform.
3. Burgess, E.N., and Thornton, L.A. (2013). *Cognitive Dysfunctions: Biological Basis, Management of Symptoms and Long-Term Neurological Implications – Neuroscience Research Progress.* Nova Biomedical.
4. Burlison, L. (2016). *Understanding Alcoholism as a Brain Disease: Book 2 of the "A Prescription for Alcoholics – Medications for Alcoholism" Book Series (Rethinking Drinking).* Addiction Publishing.
5. Campbell, N. (2022). *Cognitive Dysfunction in Aging Adults: A Handbook on Techniques, Therapies, and Simple Hacks to Reversing Memory Loss in Your Old Age.* Campbell.
6. Campbell, W.W., and Barohn, R.J. (2019). *DeJong's The Neurologic Examination*, 8th Edition. Wolters Kluwer.
7. Colajuta, J., and Chapel, J. (2021). *The Gut-Brain Connection – How A Healthy Diet Improves Memory and Cognition Through the Relationship of the Immune System, Nervous System, and Hormones.* Nappi.
8. Dave, R. (2022). *Vitamin B12 – Truth Behind Deficiency.* Dave.
9. Gonzalez, N.J. (2017). *Nutrition and the Autonomic Nervous System: The Scientific Foundations of the Gonzalez Protocol.* New Spring Press.
10. Heinz Weiss, K., and Schilsky, M. (2019). *Wilson Disease – Pathogenesis, Molecular Mechanisms, Diagnosis, Treatment, and Monitoring.* Academic Press.
11. Icon Group International. (2010). *Tetany: Webster's Timeline History, 1880 to 2007.* Icon Group International, Inc.
12. Latrov, N. (2022). *Explaining Neuropathy – Symptoms, Diagnosis, and Treatment – When the Pain Won't Stop.* Latrov.
13. Mayor, J. (2021). *Peripheral Neuropathy Diet – Nerve Repair.* Mayor.
14. McCandless, D.W. (2009). *Metabolic Encephalopathy.* Springer.
15. Mein, C.L. (2023). *Nervous System Profile & Diet.* Mein.
16. Messaoudi, Y., Othmani, S., and Jeribi, B. (2022). *Postoperative Cognitive Dysfunction: Predictive Factors in Geriatrics.* Our Knowledge Publishing.
17. Miligui, J. (2013). *Nutrition During Hepatic Encephalopathy.* Books on Demand.
18. Mohajeri, H.M. (2020). *Nutrition and Central Nervous System.* Mdpi AG.
19. Naidoo, U. (2020). *This Is Your Brain on Food: An Indispensable Guide to the Surprising Foods that Fight Depression, Anxiety, PTSD, OCD, ADHD, and More.* Little, Brown Spark.
20. Pimentel, M., and Rezaie, A. (2022). *The Microbiome Connection – Your Guide to IBS, SIBO, and Low-Fermentation Eating.* Agate Surrey.
21. Quattina, C. (2021). *Wilson's Disease Symptoms – Increased Bleeding, Fatigue, Jaundice, Depression, Aggression, Anxiety, Abdomen Pain and Swelling, Difficulty Speaking and Swallowing, Difficulty Balancing, Tremors.* Quattina.
22. Schilsky, M.L. (2018). *Management of Wilson Disease – A Pocket Guide (Clinical Gastroenterology).* Humana Press.
23. Solanto, M.V. (2014). *Cognitive*-Behavioral *Therapy for Adult ADHD: Targeting Executive Dysfunction.* The Guilford Press.
24. Stephen, J. (2022). *Peripheral Neuropathy: A Patient's Guide to Self-Management.* Stephen.
25. Strupp, M., Brandt, T., and Dieterich, M. (2023). *Vertigo and Dizziness – Common Complaints*, 3rd Edition. Springer.

26. Veselak, M. (2017). *A Complete Guide to Understanding, Managing, & Improving Your Peripheral Neuropathy.* Veselak.
27. Vink, R., and Nechifor, M. (2011). *Magnesium in the Central Nervous System.* University of Adelaide Press.
28. Walsh, W.J. (2014). *Nutrient Power: Heal Your Biochemistry and Heal Your Brain.* Skyhorse.
29. Warren, S. (2019). *The Pain Relief Secret: How to Retrain Your Nervous System, Heal Your Body, and Overcome Chronic Pain.* TCK Publishing.
30. Weiss, K.H., and Schilsky, M. (2019). *Wilson Disease: Pathogenesis, Molecular Mechanisms, Diagnosis, Treatment and Monitoring.* Academic Press.
31. Wiesman, J.F. (2016). *Peripheral Neuropathy – What It Is and What You Can Do to Feel Better.* Johns Hopkins Press.

14 Nutritional Effects on the Cardiovascular System

OUTLINE

LEARNING OBJECTIVES

After study of the chapter, readers should be able to:

1. Describe the avoidable risk factors for atherosclerosis.
2. Discuss stable angina and unstable angina.
3. Explain the causes of primary dyslipidemias.
4. Describe the complications of dyslipidemias.
5. Explain coronary artery disease and its mortality rate.
6. Describe the categories of hypertension.
7. Identify the complications of uncontrolled hypertension.
8. Discuss the prevention of hypertension.
9. Explain the three different types of stroke.
10. Describe the most common signs and symptoms of stroke.

OVERVIEW

The term *cardiovascular disease* refers to any disorder of the heart and blood vessels, including hypertension, coronary artery disease, cardiac dysrhythmias, stroke, valvular heart disease, cardiomyopathies, peripheral vascular disease, and congenital cardiac abnormalities. Each disorder has incidence and prevalence rates that vary widely by country and culture. Hypertension, coronary artery disease, cardiac dysrhythmias, and stroke account for the majority of cardiovascular morbidity and mortality in developed countries. Evidence proves the effectiveness of health dietary patterns and lifestyles in order to prevent cardiovascular disease. Healthier dietary patterns reduce production of proinflammatory cytokines that are associated with the various cardiovascular diseases. A healthy dietary pattern has a greater range of beneficial effects than any one nutrient that is supplemented. Because of the prevalence of atherosclerosis, dyslipidemia, coronary artery disease, hypertension, and stroke, the identification and classification of nutrients, foods, and dietary patterns that can enhance their prevention has become a global priority. Sodium and potassium are two interrelated minerals that play major roles in regulating blood pressure and a healthy heart. Eating less salty foods and more potassium-rich foods may significantly lower the risk of cardiovascular disease.

NUTRITION AND CARDIOVASCULAR HEALTH

Cardiovascular disease (CVD) is the leading cause of death in Western countries, and represents almost 30% of all deaths worldwide. Evidence has proven the effectiveness of healthy dietary patterns and lifestyles for the prevention of CVD. The rising incidence of CVD over the last 25 years has become a public health priority, especially its prevention through lifestyle interventions. Current scientific evidence shows that Western dietary patterns lead to an excessive production of proinflammatory cytokines associated with a reduced synthesis of anti-inflammatory cytokines. Dietary intervention allows better combination of multiple foods and nutrients. A healthy dietary pattern shows a greater magnitude of beneficial effects than the potential effects of a single nutrient supplementation. Unhealthy dietary patterns, together with a lack of exercise, being overweight or obese, aging, gender, genetics, and smoking, often lead to the development of cardiovascular disease (see Figure 14.1).

ATHEROSCLEROSIS

Atherosclerosis is an inflammatory disease that contributes to the major incidence of CVD and its related mortality. Oxidative stress and systemic inflammation can be modified by good nutrition. Inflammatory processes involve the subendothelial area of the arterial wall, accumulating lipids, lipid-laden macrophages, and other cell types. Early stages of atherosclerosis involve the internalization of lipids in the intima. These are mainly low-density lipoproteins (LDL), which lead to endothelial dysfunction. The disruption of endothelial function promotes the inflammatory response, thrombus formation, and multiple pathological consequences such as calcifications, stenosis, rupture, or hemorrhage.

DOI: 10.1201/b22969-17

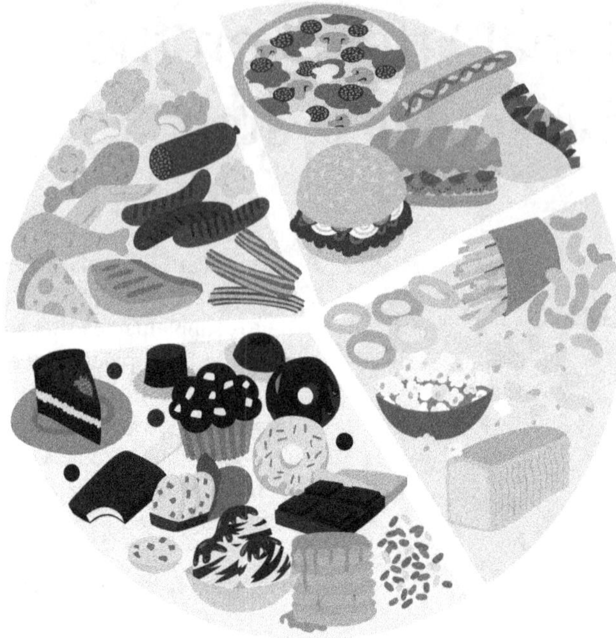

FIGURE 14.1 Unhealthy foods that lead to the development of cardiovascular disease.

Atherosclerosis is the buildup of waxy plaque inside blood vessels. It is part of the pathophysiology of coronary, cerebral, and peripheral vascular disease. Coronary artery disease is a significant manifestation. Many illnesses and deaths are also caused by aortic and carotid atherosclerotic disease and stroke. Atherosclerosis is the underlying cause of about 50% of all deaths in Western countries, which is more than any other disorder. According to the Surveillance, Epidemiology, and End Results Program (SEER), there is an average of 7.5 life years lost because of atherosclerosis. According to the World Health Organization (WHO), atherosclerosis is implicated in a disability-adjusted life year (DALY) calculation of over 5,100 per 100,000 population in Asia, South America, and Africa, and over 3,000 per 100,000 population in North America, Europe, and Australia.

Avoidable risk factors include obesity, high cholesterol, smoking, and hypertension. Inherited risk factors include LDL receptor gene mutations. **Atheromas**, also described as *atheromatous* or *atherosclerotic plaques*, are lesions that protrude into blood vessel lumens (see Figure 14.2). Being overweight or obese makes development of atherosclerosis more likely. Men with a waist size of more than 40 inches and women with a waist size of more than 35 inches are at higher risk. Excessive weight increases risks for blood clots, resulting in potentially severe cardiovascular complications.

The relationship between obesity and atherosclerosis involves abnormalities in lipid metabolism, insulin resistance, inflammation, endothelial dysfunction, **adipokine** imbalance, and **inflammasome** activation. By losing weight, getting more exercise, and eating healthier foods, there are many positive changes. These include better elasticity of blood vessels, lower blood pressure, higher High-density cholesterol (HDL) cholesterol, lower LDL cholesterol, and a reduced chance of developing type 2 diabetes.

The earliest visible lesion, a **fatty streak**, is an accumulation of lipid-laden **foam cells** in the intimal layer of an artery. Atherosclerotic plaques have three major components: lipids, inflammatory, and smooth muscle cells. Each plaque has a raised lesion with a soft core of lipid, made up of mostly cholesterol with a fibrous cap. The plaques mechanically obstruct blood flow and can rupture to cause severe obstructive vascular **thrombosis**. The plaques can result in ischemic injury and vessel wall weakening, and the formation of **aneurysms** (see Figure 14.3). *Stable plaques* sometimes grow slowly over decades until they cause stenosis or occlusion. *Unstable plaques* are more likely to spontaneously erode, develop fissures, or rupture. This causes acute thrombosis, occlusion, and infarction long before any thermodynamically significant stenosis.

Atherosclerosis is asymptomatic initially, and this may continue for decades. Once lesions block blood flow, transient ischemic symptoms include **stable angina**, transient ischemic attacks, and **intermittent claudication**. The arterial lumens may be reduced by over 70%. **Vasoconstriction** can alter lesions that do not limit blood flow into severe or complete stenosis. Symptoms of **unstable angina** or myocardial infarction, ischemic stroke, or resting limb pain may develop if unstable plaques rupture and block a major artery, with addition of thrombosis or **embolism**. Atherosclerosis can cause sudden death with no previous angina pectoris of any type. Atherosclerotic involvement of artery walls can lead to aneurysms and arterial dissection, with pain, a pulsing mass, lack of pulses, or death.

Ischemia is evaluated as to the location and amount of vascular occlusion. This involves history, physical

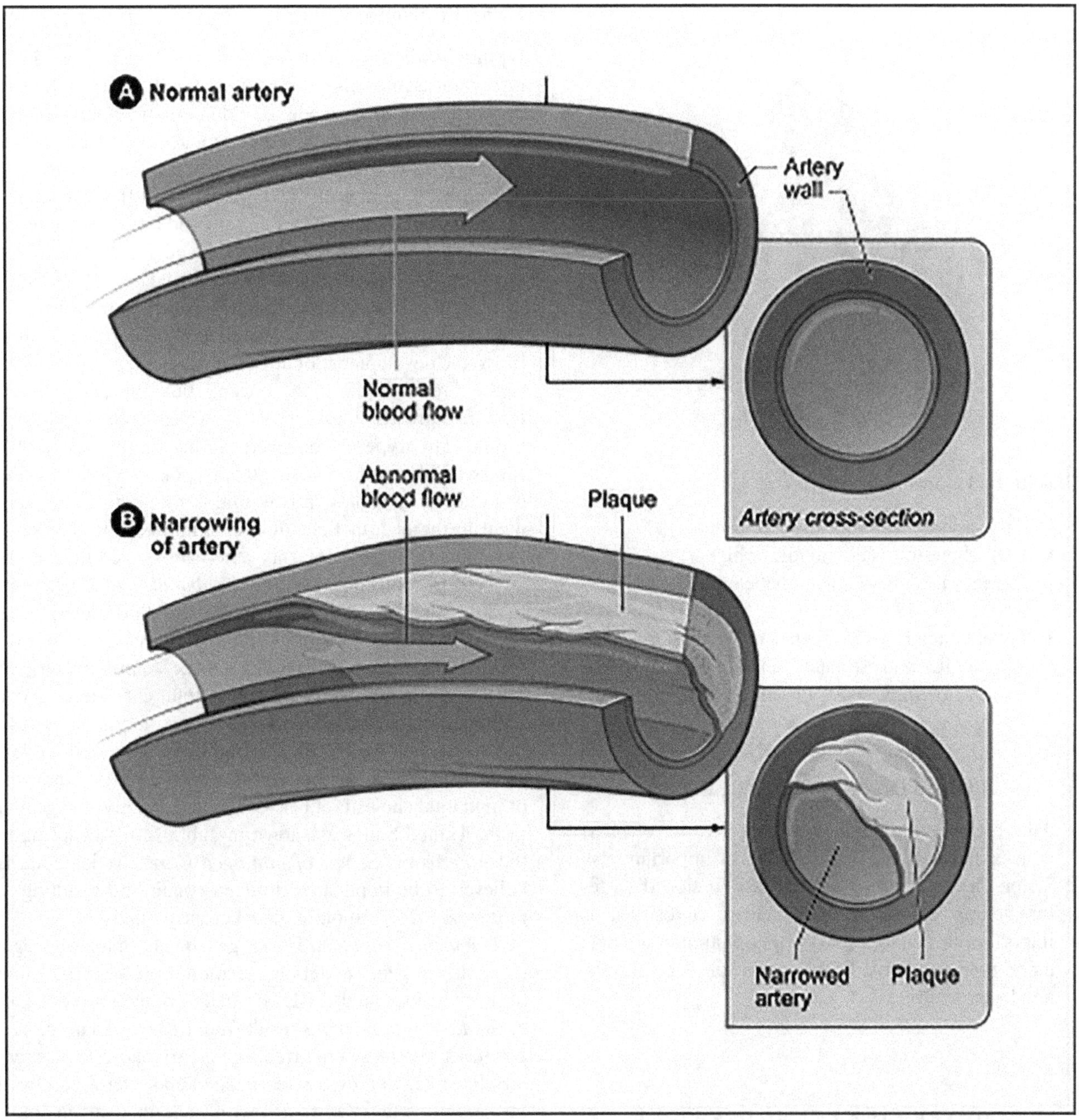

FIGURE 14.2 Atherosclerosis (showing atherosclerotic plaques).

examination, a fasting lipid profile, and plasma glucose levels. A significant marker for atherosclerosis is carotid artery intimal–medial thickness, which can be seen in imaging studies. Internal or external ultrasound is usually able to determine this measurement. High levels of C-reactive protein (CRP) in the blood may raise risks for atherosclerosis and myocardial infarction. This protein indicates inflammation in the body when it is present in high levels.

Treatment involves aggressive modification of risk factors to slow disease progression and aid in plaque regression. The lower that LDL levels become, the more the patient's condition will improve. Statins can decrease related morbidity and mortality, even if serum cholesterol is normal or slightly higher than normal. Antiplatelet drugs also help patients with atherosclerosis. Patients with coronary artery disease may receive additional benefit from angiotensin-converting enzyme (ACE) inhibitors and beta-blockers. Dietary changes include consuming less saturated fat, no trans fats, more fruits and vegetables, more fiber, and only moderate use of alcohol. Regular physical activity consists of 30–45 minutes of walking, running, swimming, or cycling, three to five times per week. Aerobic exercise is important in order to promote weight loss and prevent atherosclerosis. Antiplatelet drugs include aspirin and thienopyridines such as clopidogrel, prasugrel, and ticagrelor. Statins basically work by lowering LDL and enhance endothelial nitric oxide production. They stabilize and regress plaques while reducing lipid accumulation in artery walls. Statins are preventive therapy for:

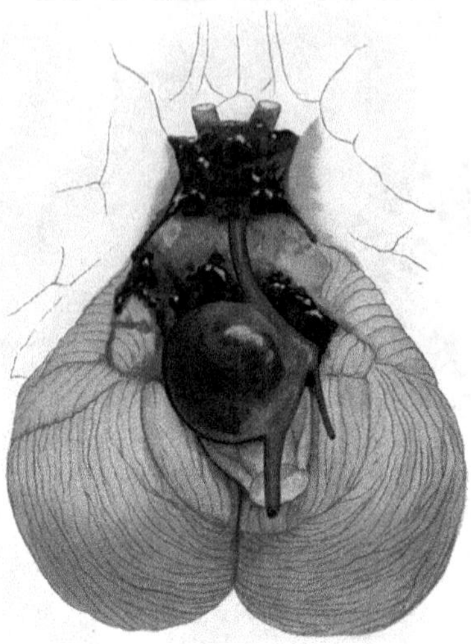

FIGURE 14.3 Aneurysm in the brain.

- Atherosclerotic cardiovascular disease
- LDL cholesterol (190 mg/dL or higher)
- Patients aged 40–75, with diabetes, and LDL cholesterol (70–189 mg/dL)
- Patients aged 40–75, with LDL cholesterol (70–189 mg/dL), and estimated ten-year risk of arteriosclerotic cardiovascular disease at 7.5% or higher

FOCUS ON ATHEROSCLEROSIS

Atherosclerosis is the most common cause of heart attacks and strokes. One of the most important risk factors is excessive abdominal fat. To stop the life-threatening complications of atherosclerosis, it is important to manage your weight, maintain a stable blood pressure, boost HDL (good cholesterol) levels, and lower triglycerides.

MEDITERRANEAN AND DASH DIETS

The Mediterranean and Dietary Approaches to Stop Hypertension (DASH) diets have been well-studied concerning their cardiovascular outcomes. Both diets may reduce the incidence CVD via the down-regulation of low-grade inflammation and better control of body weight. These factors also improve other risk factors and are correlated with lower numbers of clinical events.

Test Your Knowledge

1. How common is atherosclerosis?
2. What are the major components of atherosclerotic plaques?
3. What are the complications of atherosclerosis?

DYSLIPIDEMIA

Dyslipidemia has a close association with an increased risk of cardiovascular diseases, and especially, atherosclerosis. As efforts are being made to find alternative therapies and ways to prevent disease, there is a related increase in public interest in food or active food components that contribute to an improved lipid profile and better health. Besides supplying the basic nutrients required for good health, some foods add further physiologic benefits. In fact, specific foods and bioactive components could be beneficial. Dyslipidemia is signified by elevated plasma cholesterol, triglycerides, or both. It may also consist of low HDL cholesterol, contributing to the development of atherosclerosis.

Any reduction in the concentration of HDL cholesterol also greatly influences the prevalent atherogenic lipid profile. This type of cholesterol utilizes a pathway called reverse cholesterol transport. It is responsible for removing oxidized LDL cholesterol by inhibiting monocyte attachment to the endothelium. It also stimulates the release of nitric oxide, which prevents atherogenesis of the vascular beds. According to the *Dyslipidemia EpiCast Report*, in 2015, there were more than 580,000,000 global cases of dyslipidemia. This is estimated to increase to over 680,000,000 cases by the year 2025. Approximately 95 million US adults 20 or older have total cholesterol above 200 mg/dL, and nearly 29 million have levels above 240 mg/dL. About 7% of US children over age 6 and adolescents have high total cholesterol. There are different levels of high total cholesterol between race, ethnicity, and gender in the United States as shown in Table 14.1. According to the *American Journal of Managed Care*, dyslipidemia is believed to be implicated in many conditions, resulting in more than $200 billion in global costs annually.

Primary dyslipidemias are genetic, because of single or multiple gene mutations resulting in overproduction of triglycerides and LDL, or underproduction of HDL. *Secondary dyslipidemias* result from lifestyle. In developed countries, the most important secondary cause is a sedentary lifestyle, with excessive intake of cholesterol, saturated fat, and trans fats. Other factors include diabetes mellitus, overuse of alcohol, chronic kidney disease, hypothyroidism, cholestatic liver diseases such as primary **biliary cirrhosis**, and certain medications (antihypertensives, steroid hormones, immunosuppressants, antineoplastic agents, and more). Diabetes mellitus is a highly significant secondary

TABLE 14.1
High Total Cholesterol by Race, Ethnicity, and Gender

Racial/Ethnic Group	% of Men	% of Women
Hispanics	13.1	9.0
Non-Hispanic Asians	11.3	10.3
Non-Hispanic Whites	10.9	14.8
Non-Hispanic Blacks	10.6	10.3

cause, since patients usually have a combination of high triglycerides, high LDL, and low HDL. This is known as **diabetic dyslipidemia**. Patients with type 2 diabetes are at the highest risk. This may be related to obesity, poor diabetic control, or both, increasing circulating free fatty acids. It leads to increased production, in the liver, of very-low-density lipoprotein (VLDL). Diabetic dyslipidemia is often worsened by increased caloric intake and physical inactivity, which is regularly seen in patients with type 2 diabetes. As a result of this form of dyslipidemia, women with diabetes may have a specific risk of cardiac disease.

Dyslipidemia can be prevented by eating a diet lower in saturated fats, with no trans fats. The diet must include many fruits, vegetables, beans, nuts, whole grains, and fish, on a regular basis. Red and processed meats should be limited. These include bacon, sausage, and cold cuts. Another method of prevention for dyslipidemia is to maintain a healthy weight.

Dyslipidemia leads to symptomatic vascular disease, such as coronary artery disease, stroke, and peripheral arterial disease. High triglyceride levels can cause acute pancreatitis. If the levels of LDL become extremely high, they can cause confusion, **hepatosplenomegaly**, dyspnea, and **paresthesia**. High levels of LDL can cause **arcus senilis** of the corneas (see Figure 14.4) and **tendinous xanthomas** of the phalangeal joints, or near the elbow, knee, and Achilles tendons. Other findings with high LDL, such as familial hypercholesterolemia, include xanthelasma.

Dyslipidemia treatment focuses on preventing atherosclerotic cardiovascular disease, including acute coronary syndromes, stroke, transient ischemic attack, and peripheral arterial disease. Treatment is required for all patients with atherosclerotic cardiovascular disease and for some without it. Treatments include diet, exercise, dietary supplements, and medications. There must be reduced intake of saturated fats and cholesterol, increased dietary fiber and complex carbohydrates, and maintenance of ideal body weight. Dietitians are very helpful, especially for the elderly. Exercise lowers LDL cholesterol and helps maintain a healthy weight.

FOCUS ON DYSLIPIDEMIA

High cholesterol is the most common type of dyslipidemia. More than 71 million American adults have high LDL cholesterol. There are over 4 million deaths per year from dyslipidemia globally.

Test Your Knowledge

1. What is the difference between primary and secondary dyslipidemias?
2. How can dyslipidemia be prevented?
3. What do high or extremely high triglyceride levels cause?

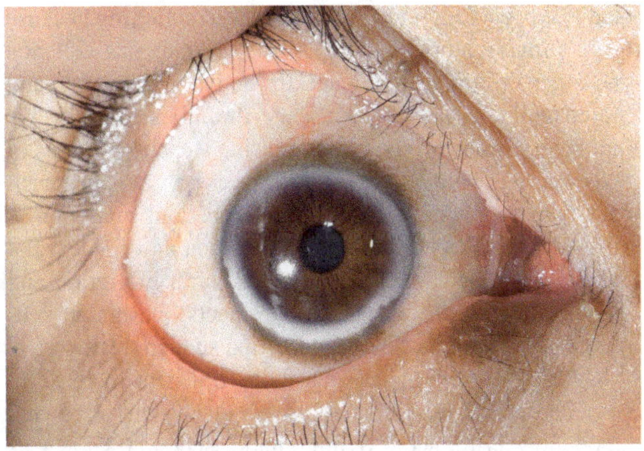

FIGURE 14.4 Arcus senilis.

CORONARY ARTERY DISEASE

Coronary artery disease (*CAD*) is a condition in which there is impaired blood flow due to a buildup, in the coronary arteries, of fatty substances like cholesterol, as well as the presence of atheromas. It is the most common heart disease in the United States. The disorder causes silent ischemia, acute coronary syndromes, and sudden cardiac death. Acute coronary syndromes are further described as unstable angina and myocardial infarction. In developed countries such as the United States, CAD is the primary cause of death for both men and women. About 33% of all deaths are from CAD. In Caucasian men, the mortality rate from CAD is one of every 10,000 people aged 25–34, and nearly 1 of every 100 at ages 55–64. The mortality rate in Caucasian men between 35 and 44 is 6.1 times higher than in Caucasian women of the same ages. It is not understood why other races, or patients with diabetes mellitus, do not have such as large difference between the genders. In women, mortality rates increase after menopause. By the age of 75, the mortality rate in women from CAD is equal to or higher than that of men.

CAD is usually caused by atherosclerosis of the coronary arteries, with subintimal deposition of atheromas in the large- and medium-sized arteries. Less often, CAD is caused by coronary artery spasm, as in **variant angina**. Vascular endothelial dysfunction can worsen atherosclerosis and contribute to coronary artery spasm. Endothelial dysfunction is now recognized as one cause of angina when there is no epicardial coronary artery stenosis or spasm. Rare causes of CAD include coronary artery embolism, aneurysm such as in **Kawasaki disease**, dissection, and vasculitis in **systemic lupus erythematosus** or *syphilis*.

There is often an irregular distribution of coronary atherosclerosis in different vessels. Even so, it usually occurs at **vessel bifurcations** and other points of turbulence. With growth of atheromatous plaques, there is progressive narrowing of the arterial lumen. Ischemia results, often causing **angina pectoris**. The amount of stenosis that causes ischemia is varied based on oxygen demand. An atheromatous plaque sometimes ruptures or splits. This is likely related to plaque morphology, calcium content, and softening because of an inflammatory process. A rupture exposes collagen and other thrombogenic materials, activating platelets and the coagulation cascade. An acute thrombus results. This interrupts coronary blood flow, causing various amounts of myocardial ischemia. Acute ischemia, as part of acute coronary syndrome (ACS), in relation to locations and degrees of obstruction, can cause unstable angina and myocardial infarction (MI). This can cause transmural infarction and complications such as conduction defects, malignant ventricular arrhythmias, heart failure, and sudden death.

Coronary artery spasm is a focal, transient increase in vascular tone. The lumen is progressively narrowed and blood flow is reduced. Symptomatic ischemia known as *variant angina* may occur. Extreme narrowing can trigger formation of a thrombus, then infarction or a life-threatening arrhythmia. Spasm may occur in arteries whether atheromas are present or not, as follows:

- *Arteries without atheromas* – basal coronary artery tone is likely increased; the response to vasoconstricting stimuli is usually exaggerated; the mechanism may involve endothelial cell problems in nitric oxide production, or imbalances between endothelium-derived factors of contraction and relaxation
- *Arteries with atheromas* – endothelial dysfunction occurs, which may cause local hypercontractility; there may be loss of sensitivity to acetylcholine or other intrinsic vasodilators, plus increased production of vasoconstrictors in the area of the atheroma (these include angiotensin II, endothelin, leukotrienes, serotonin, and thromboxane); recurring spasms may damage the intima and lead to formation of atheromas

Vasoconstricting drugs such as cocaine or nicotine, plus emotional stress, can trigger coronary spasms. A rare, non-traumatic tear in the coronary intima, with creation of a false lumen, is known as *coronary artery dissection.* As blood flows through the false lumen, it expands. This restricts blood flow through the true lumen, and coronary ischemia or infarction may result. Dissection can occur in coronary arteries with or without atherosclerosis. Non-atherosclerotic dissection is more common in pregnant or postpartum women, and if connective tissue disorder such as fibromuscular dysplasia are present. Risk factors for CAD and atherosclerosis are the same. They include the following:

- High blood levels of LDL cholesterol, lipoprotein(a), apoprotein B (apo B), and CRP
- Low blood levels of HDL cholesterol
- Diabetes mellitus (especially type 2)
- Smoking
- Obesity
- Physical inactivity

In women, especially under age 45, smoking may be a stronger predictor of MI. Genetic factors are implicated. Several systemic disorders contribute to risks. These include hypertension, hypothyroidism, and metabolic disorders such as hyperhomocysteinemia. High levels of apo B may indicate an increased risk if total cholesterol or LDL is normal.

High blood levels of CRP indicate instability of plaques and inflammation. They may be a stronger predictor for ischemic events than high LDL levels. High blood triglycerides and insulin may be risk factors, but this is not proven. The risk of CAD is increased by smoking tobacco, diets high in fat and calories, diets low in phytochemicals from fruits and vegetables, diets low in fiber and vitamins C, D, and E, diets low in omega-3 polyunsaturated fatty acids (in some people), and when there is poor stress management.

Treatment of CAD focuses on reducing cardiac workload, by decreasing oxygen demand and improving the coronary artery blood flow. Over time, treatment aims at stopping and reversing the atherosclerotic processes. Coronary artery blood flow may be improved via percutaneous coronary intervention (PCI) or coronary artery bypass grafting (CABG). Fibrinolytic drugs can be used to dissolve an acute coronary thrombosis. Medical treatments also include antiplatelet drugs to prevent clot formation, statins to lower LDL cholesterol levels, and beta-blockers to reduce angina symptoms. PCI is indicated for acute coronary syndrome or if a patient has stable ischemic heart disease yet still have angina even with medical treatments. CABG usually uses the internal mammary or radial arteries when possible. If necessary, CABG uses sections of the **saphenous veins** to bypass diseases segments of the coronary arteries. This procedure is better than PCI in patients with diabetes and those with multivessel disease that will respond well to grafting.

FOCUS ON CAUSES OF CORONARY ARTERY DISEASE

CAD is a multifactorial phenomenon. Etiologic factors can be categorized into non-modifiable and modifiable factors. Non-modifiable factors include gender, age, family history, and genetics. Modifiable risk factors include smoking, obesity, lipid levels, and psychosocial variables.

FOCUS ON CARDIAC CATHETERIZATION

Cardiac catheterization is the insertion of a catheter into a chamber or vessel of the heart, for both diagnostic and interventional purposes. It is the gold standard and most accurate modality to evaluate ischemic coronary heart disease. However, it is an invasive procedure with associated complications. Not everyone is a candidate for the procedure.

Test Your Knowledge

1. What are the mortality rates for coronary artery disease?
2. What are the risk factors for coronary artery disease?
3. What dietary choices may lead to development of coronary artery disease?

HYPERTENSION

Hypertension involves activation of the sympathetic nervous system and **renin–angiotensin system,** sodium retention, and various abnormalities. Obesity increases the risk for hypertension and is associated with increased blood flow, vasodilation, cardiac output, and glomerular filtration rate. As renal sodium retention increases, hypertension develops. Globally, hypertension is estimated to cause about 7.5 million deaths annually. Blood pressure (BP) levels are continuously related to risks of stroke and coronary heart disease. Global uncontrolled hypertension affects more than 1.13 billion people. Prevalence of hypertension was highest in Africa (46%) for both genders. Generally, prevalence is higher in low- and middle-income countries than in high-income countries. Countries with the highest prevalence of hypertension are shown in Figure 14.5.

In the United States, about 116 million people have hypertension. While 81% are aware of their condition, only about 75% receive treatment, and only 24% have adequate control of their BP. Adult hypertension is most common in African-Americans (56%) compared to Caucasians (48%) or Hispanics (39%) – see Figure 14.6. Morbidity and mortality are also greater in African-Americans. With age,

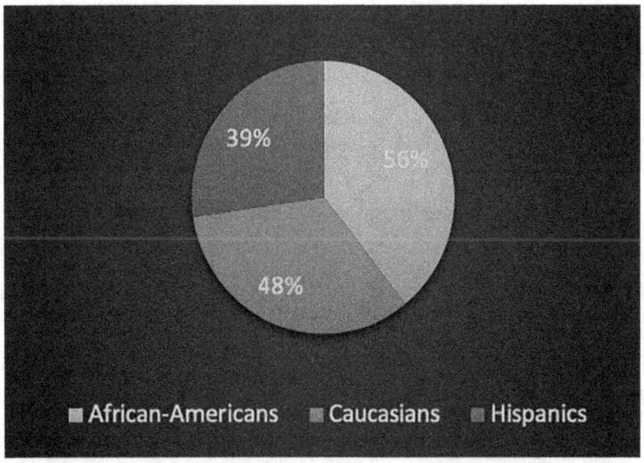

FIGURE 14.6 Percentages of adults with hypertension, in various racial or ethnic groups.

BP increases. About 70% of people over age 65 have hypertension. Higher BP increases morbidity and mortality risks. Globally, hypertension has an average incidence of 31.1% based on age, gender, and body type. The incidence of hypertension depends on age, gender, and body type. According to the WHO, hypertension is accounts for 57 million disability-adjusted life years, or 3.7% of total DALYs. The Centers for Disease Control and Prevention (CDC) report that total costs associated with hypertension in the United States exceed $131 billion annually.

Hypertension is classified as *primary* (essential) in over 90% of cases and as *secondary* in the remainder. In primary hypertension, there are multiple factors, and heredity is a predisposing factor. The exact causative mechanism is not clear. Environmental factors include

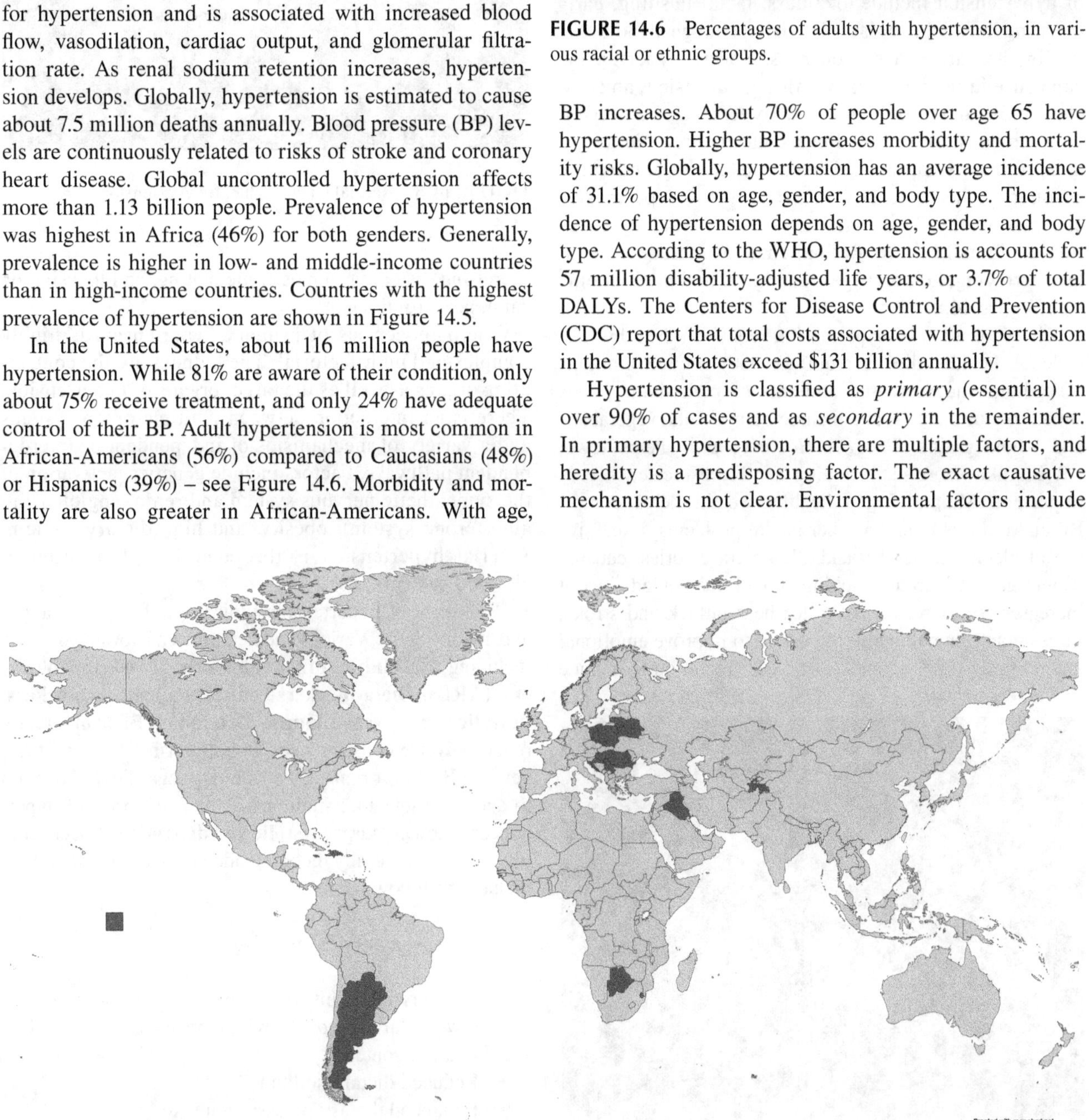

FIGURE 14.5 Countries with the highest prevalence of hypertension.

obesity, dietary sodium, and stress. These appear to affect only genetically susceptible individuals, at younger ages. In patients over age 65, high sodium intake is more likely to precede hypertension. Obesity, tobacco smoking, insulin resistance, and heavy alcohol consumption are additional risk factors. Common causes of secondary hypertension include primary aldosteronism, **parenchymal** diseases of the kidneys, renovascular disease, and sleep apnea. Renal parenchymal diseases include chronic **glomerulonephritis**, chronic **pyelonephritis**, and **polycystic renal disease** (see Figure 14.7). Other causes include Cushing syndrome, **pheochromocytoma**, hypothyroidism, hyperthyroidism, acromegaly, and coarctation of the aorta. Early signs and symptoms of hypertension include dizziness, facial flushing, early morning headache, **epistaxis**, vision changes, and buzzing in the ears and nervousness. Severe hypertension can cause fatigue, nausea, vomiting, confusion, anxiety, chest pain, and muscle tremors. Hypertensive emergencies can cause severe cardiovascular, neurologic, renal, and retinal symptoms. These include symptomatic coronary atherosclerosis, heart failure, hypertensive encephalopathy, heart attack, stroke, sexual dysfunction, and renal failure. Retinal changes include arteriolar narrowing, hemorrhages, exudates, and papilledema (see Figure 14.8).

The prevention of hypertension requires a healthy lifestyle. A healthy diet is required, with limited amounts of sodium and increased amounts of potassium. Foods should be lower in fat and include many fruits, vegetables, and whole grains. The *DASH eating plan* helps lower BP. Regular exercise, including aerobic exercise, is very important. Maintaining a healthy weight helps control BP and reduces risks for other health problems. Excessive use of alcohol raises BP and adds extra calories, causing weight gain. Cigarette smoking should be avoided since it increases BP as well as risks for heart attack and stroke. Stress management is also important to improve emotional and physical health, and lower BP. Techniques include exercising, listening to music, meditating, and focusing on calm, peaceful thoughts.

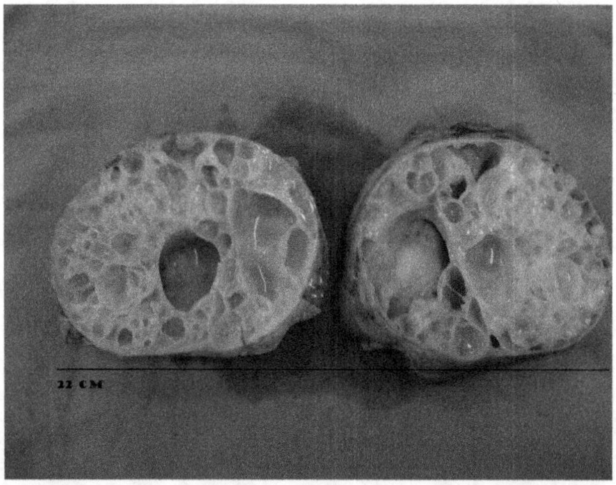

FIGURE 14.7 Polycystic renal disease.

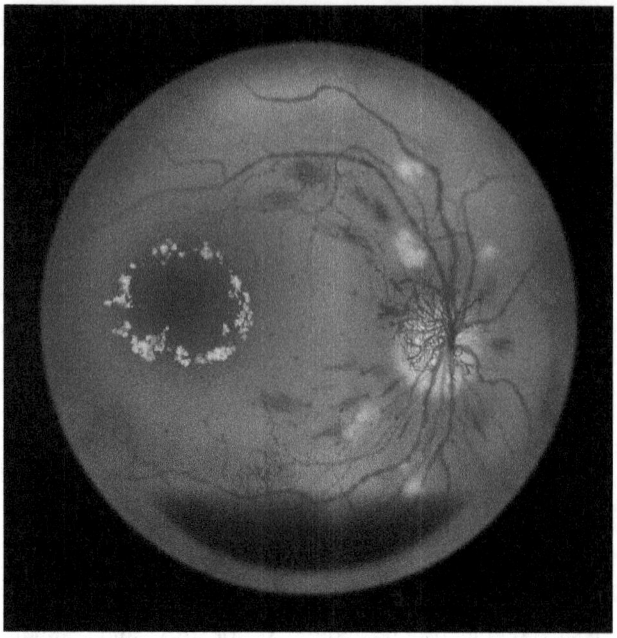

FIGURE 14.8 Retinal changes due to hypertension.

The pathogenesis of primary hypertension is highly complex and multifactorial. The kidneys are the contributing organs as well as the target organs of hypertension. There is an interaction between multiple organ systems and a variety of mechanisms of independent or interdependent pathways. Factors include genetics, activation of the sympathetic nervous system and renin–angiotensin–aldosterone system), obesity, and high dietary sodium. Arterial hypertension is the condition of persistently elevated systemic BP.

Treatment of hypertension typically is lifestyle changes and medications. Various medications can lower your BP, including **ACE inhibitors, angiotensin II receptor blockers (ARBs), beta-blockers, calcium channel blockers, diuretics, and vasodilators**. Control of BP can greatly reduce adverse consequences, in both forms. Treatment targets are BP lower than 120/80 mm Hg regardless of age, up to age 80. Table 14.2 summarizes the categories of hypertension, showing target **systolic** and **diastolic** BP, according to the CDC. Generally recommended lifestyle modifications include the following:

- Increased physical exercise
- Weight loss
- A diet rich in fruits, vegetables, whole grains, and low-fat dairy products, with reduced saturated and total fat content
- Reduced dietary sodium
- Enhanced dietary potassium intake
- Moderate or no use of alcohol
- Smoking cessation

TABLE 14.2
Categories of Hypertension

Blood Pressure Category	Systolic BP		Diastolic BP
NORMAL	Less than 120 mm Hg	and	Less than 80 mm Hg
ELEVATED	120–129 mm Hg	and	Less than 80 mm Hg
STAGE 1 HYPERTENSION	130–139 mm Hg	or	80–89 mm Hg
STAGE 2 HYPERTENSION	Over 140 mm Hg	or	Over 90 mm Hg

FOCUS ON DIETARY CALCIUM AND HYPERTENSION

Low dietary calcium increases BP, and supplemental calcium helps reduce BP. Dietary calcium of 1,200–1,500 mg per day can reduce systolic and diastolic BP.

FOCUS ON TABLE SALT

Table salt is overused by many people globally, and in some countries such as the United States, individuals consume more than twice the recommended amount of salt per day. While most healthy adults should eat less than 2,300 mg of sodium per day, the actual average person eats 2,900–4,300 mg per day. Other products used at the dinner table that contain high levels of sodium include soy, fish, and sweet-and-sour sauces.

FOCUS ON CORONARY ARTERY DISEASE AND STROKE

CAD is the most common cause of death in patients receiving treatment for hypertension. Ischemic or hemorrhagic stroke is a common outcome of insufficiently treated hypertension. Even so, effective control of hypertension is able to prevent most complications and also prolongs the life of the patient.

Test Your Knowledge

1. In which groups of people is hypertension most prevalent?
2. What are the common causes of secondary hypertension?
3. What are the effects of alcohol and smoking upon hypertension?

MYOCARDIAL INFRACTION

Myocardial infarction (MI), or *heart attack*, is the irreversible necrosis of the heart muscle because of prolonged ischemia. According to the Centers for Disease Control and Prevention (CDC), approximately 805,000 cases of MI occur annually in the United States. Heart disease continues to be the leading cause of death in the United States, with approximately 383,000 deaths per year. Gender and racial or ethnic disparities in MI diagnoses are becoming more evident. Although there have been improvements in diagnostic codes, clinically distinguishing the types of MI remains a challenge. A lack of blood flow can damage or destroy part of the heart muscle (see Figure 14.9). This is usually the result of a blockage in one or more of the coronary arteries, caused by a buildup of plaque in the arteries. If the blood and oxygen supply is cut off, muscle cells of the heart begin to be damaged and start to die. Irreversible damage begins within 30 minutes of blockage. The result is that the heart muscle, affected by the lack of oxygen, no longer functions normally.

Inherited or genetic risk factors cannot be changed, but can be improved with medical management and lifestyle changes. Acquired risk factors are caused by activities that we choose, and can be managed through lifestyle changes and clinical care. African-Americans and women have higher rates of mortality from MI. They are more likely to be younger, present with other comorbidities, and often receive fewer novel therapies with respect to type of MI. This is expected to continue into the future. It is estimated that 45.1% of the US population will have some form of heart disease by 2035. Unless the prevalence of heart disease is better controlled and significantly reduced, total direct medical care costs related to heart disease are expected to increase from $318 billion to $749 billion. Today in the United States, someone has an MI every 40 seconds.

The classic symptoms of a heart attack are chest pain and shortness of breath. The most common symptoms include pain in the chest, back, jaw, and the left arm that lasts more than a few minutes, or that goes away and then returns. There is often pressure in the chest, dyspnea, anxiety, nausea, vomiting, fainting, and tachycardia. The most common cause of a heart attack is CAD. Eventually, an area of plaque can rupture. A blood clot can form around the plaque and block the artery. A less common cause of heart attack is a severe spasm of a coronary artery. The spasm cuts off blood flow through the artery. Several health conditions, lifestyle, aging, and family history can increase risks. About 50% **of all Americans** have at least one of the three key risk factors for heart disease: high BP, high blood

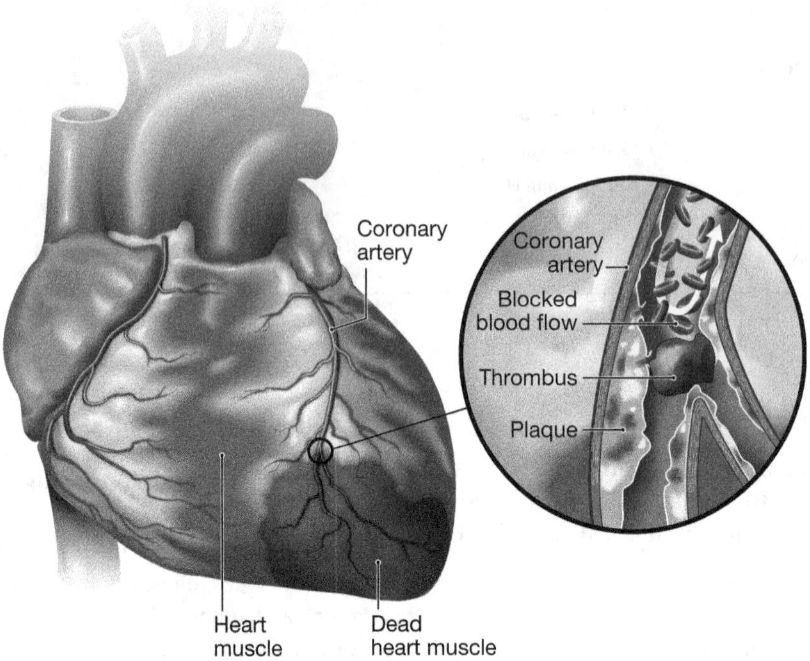

FIGURE 14.9 Illustration showing healthy heart muscle, an area of dead muscle, and a myocardial infarction.

cholesterol, and smoking. Some risk factors cannot be controlled, such as age or family history.

Diagnosis of a heart attack includes checking BP, pulse, and temperature. Tests to diagnose a heart attack include the following:

- *Electrocardiogram (ECG or EKG)* – the first test done to diagnose a heart attack, which records electrical signals as they travel through the heart. Electrodes are attached to the chest and sometimes the arms and legs, using an adhesive backing. Signals are recorded as waves displayed on a monitor or printed on paper. An ECG can show if a heart attack has occurred or is occurring.
- *Blood tests* – certain heart proteins slowly leak into the blood after heart damage from a heart attack. Blood tests can be done to check for these proteins, which are known as cardiac markers.
- *Chest X-ray* – shows the condition and size of the heart and lungs.
- *Echocardiogram* – sound waves (via ultrasound) create images of the moving heart. This test can show how blood moves through the heart and heart valves. An echocardiogram can help identify whether an area of the heart has been damaged.
- *Coronary catheterization (angiogram)* – a long, thin tube called a catheter is inserted into an artery, usually in the leg, and guided to the heart. Dye flows through the catheter to help the arteries show up more clearly on images made during the test.
- *Cardiac CT or MRI* – these tests create images of the heart and chest. Cardiac CT scans use X-rays. Cardiac MRI uses a magnetic field and radio waves to create images of the heart. For both tests, the patient usually lies on a table that slides inside a long tube-like machine. Each test can be used to diagnose heart problems. They can help show the severity of heart damage.

Each minute after a heart attack, more heart tissue is damaged or dies. Urgent treatment is required to restore blood flow and oxygen levels. Oxygen is given immediately. Specific heart attack treatment depends on whether there is a partial or complete blockage of blood flow. Medications to treat a heart attack include the following:

- ***Aspirin*** – reduces blood clotting. It helps keep blood moving through a narrowed artery. If a patient calls 911, chewing aspirin is recommended. Emergency medical providers may give the patient aspirin immediately.
- ***Thrombolytics or fibrinolytics*** – help break up any blood clots that are blocking blood flow to the heart. The earlier a thrombolytic drug is given after a heart attack, the less the heart is damaged, and the greater the chance of survival.
- ***Other blood-thinning medications*** – heparin may be given by IV or injection. It makes the blood less sticky and less likely to form clots.
- ***Nitroglycerin*** – this medication widens the blood vessels. It helps improve blood flow to the heart. Nitroglycerin is used to treat sudden chest pain (angina). It is given as a pill under the tongue, as a pill to swallow, or as an injection.
- ***Morphine*** – given to relieve chest pain that does not resolve with nitroglycerin.

- ***Beta-blockers*** **–** slow the heartbeat and decrease BP. Beta-blockers can limit the amount of heart muscle damage and prevent future heart attacks. They are given to most people who are having a heart attack.
- ***ACE inhibitors*** **–** lower BP and reduce stress on the heart.
- **Statins –** help lower unhealthy cholesterol levels. Too much bad (low-density lipoprotein, or LDL) cholesterol can clog arteries.

When a patient has had a heart attack, a surgery or procedure may be done to open a blocked artery. Surgeries and procedures to treat a heart attack include the following:

- **Coronary angioplasty and stenting –** to open clogged heart arteries. It may also be called PCI. Some stents are coated with a medication that helps keep the arteries open.
- **Coronary artery bypass surgery –** open-heart surgery. A surgeon takes a healthy blood vessel from another part of the body to create a new path for blood in the heart. The blood then goes around the blocked or narrowed coronary artery. CABG may be done as an emergency surgery at the time of a heart attack. Sometimes it is done a few days later, after the heart has recovered somewhat.

Cardiac rehabilitation is a personalized exercise and education program that teaches ways to improve heart health after surgery. It focuses on exercise, a heart-healthy diet, stress management, and a gradual return to usual activities. Most hospitals offer cardiac rehabilitation. The program typically continues for a few weeks or months after the patient returns home. People who attend cardiac rehab after a heart attack generally live longer and are less likely to have another heart attack or related complications. It is important to avoid or limit foods with high levels of saturated fat, trans fats, salt, and sugar. Instead, whole grains, fruits, vegetables, and lean proteins such as fish and beans are recommended.

STROKE

Strokes involve a loss of blood flow to part of the brain, which damages brain tissue. They are caused by blood clots and broken blood vessels in the brain (see Figure 14.10). The brain needs constant glucose and oxygen. Autoregulation of vascular resistance maintains a nearly constant flow of blood, even though there are large ranges of BP and intracranial pressure. When blood flow to the brain is reduced, survival of tissues is based on the length of time of the ischemia, collateral circulation, and blood flow. The brain mostly depends on oxidative metabolism to generate adenosine triphosphate (ATP), which is a compound present in all living tissue. It has a low capacity for *glycolysis*, except for glucose delivered by the blood circulation.

There are three different types of stroke: ischemic stroke, hemorrhagic stroke, and transient ischemic attack (TIA). **An ischemic stroke** is caused by a blockage cutting off the blood supply to the brain, and is the most common type of stroke. **A hemorrhagic stroke** is caused by bleeding in or around the brain. **A transient ischemic attack** is also known as a mini-stroke. It is the same as a stroke, except that the symptoms only last for a short amount of time. This is because the blockage that stops the blood getting to the brain is temporary.

Approximately 15 million people suffer a stroke globally every year. Of these, 5 million die and another 5 million are permanently disabled. The countries with the highest rates of fatal strokes include Kiribati, Mongolia, Lesotho, Solomon Islands, Mozambique, Vanuatu, Myanmar, Montenegro, Central Africa, and Micronesia (see Figure 14.11). Hypertension contributes to over 12.7 million strokes globally. Europe averages

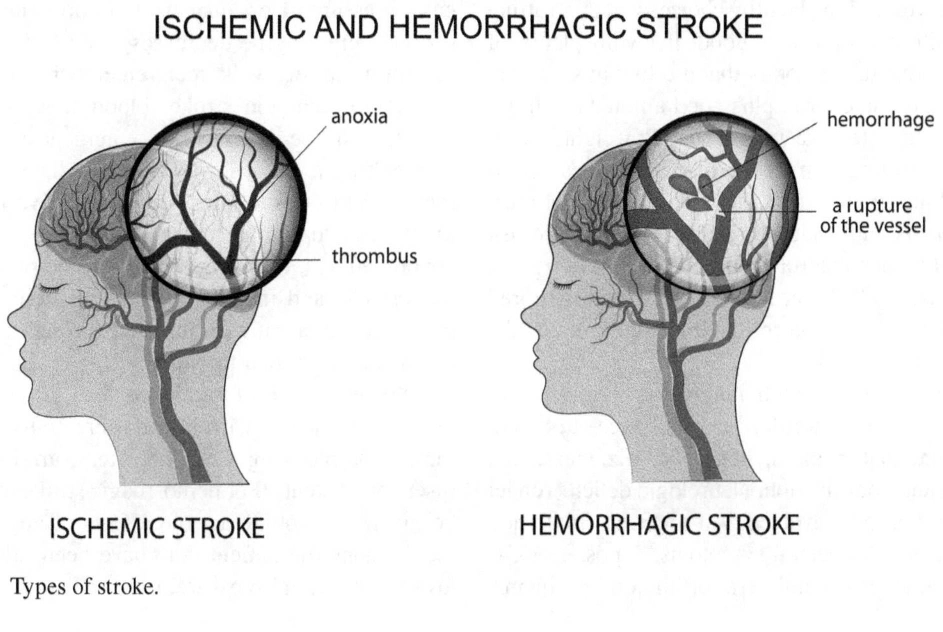

FIGURE 14.10 Types of stroke.

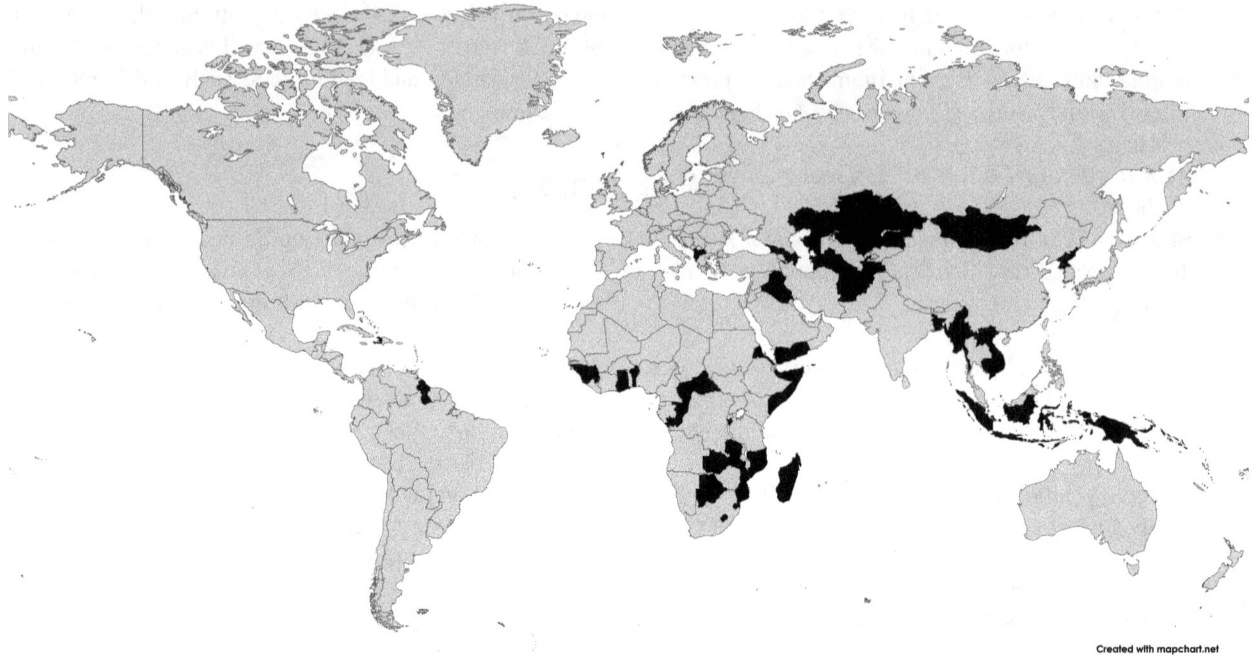

FIGURE 14.11 Countries with the highest rates of fatal strokes.

about 650,000 stroke deaths per year. Stroke is the third leading cause of death in the United States, after heart disease and cancer. It is the most prevalent cause of disability and death due to neurologic disease. Of the forms of stroke, 80% are ischemic and 20% are hemorrhagic. According to the *Internet Stroke Center*, more than 140,000 people die every year in the United States from stroke. About 795,000 strokes occur overall, with 600,000 being first attacks, and 185,000 being recurrent attacks. Nearly 75% of all strokes occur in people over the age of 65. Stroke death rates are higher for African-Americans than for any other group. The cost impacts of stroke in the United States alone are more than $34 billion annually.

The five leading causes of a stroke include hypertension, hypercholesterolemia, smoking, obesity, and diabetes. Prevention involves making healthy choices and controlling underlying health conditions. A good diet with plenty of fresh fruits and vegetables, foods that are low in saturated fats, trans fat, and cholesterol, plus good amounts of high-fiber foods are suggested. Keeping a healthy weight is very important in preventing a stroke, so regular physical activity is needed. Smoking must be avoided, and alcohol must be limited. Patients with underlying conditions that are risk factors for stroke must control their conditions as directed by their physicians. Cholesterol levels must be monitored regularly, and BP must be controlled. It is important to take all medications as directed.

Stroke occurs suddenly with numbness, weakness, or paralysis of the **contralateral** limbs and face, **aphasia**, confusion, visual disturbances, headache, dizziness, and loss of balance and coordination. Neurologic deficits reflect the brain areas that are involved. An anterior circulation stroke usually causes unilateral symptoms. A posterior circulation stroke may cause unilateral or bilateral problems, and is more likely to affect consciousness, usually when the basilar artery is involved. There are sometimes systemic or autonomic disturbances, such as hypertension or fever. A sudden and severe headache suggests a subarachnoid hemorrhage. Impaired conscious or eventual coma, often with chronic headache, nausea, and vomiting suggests increased intracranial pressure. This can occur 48–72 hours after a significant ischemic stroke, but earlier with many hemorrhagic strokes. Fatal brain herniation may develop. Complications of strokes include aphasia, spasticity, confusion, depression, sleep problems, incontinence, pneumonia, and swallowing dysfunction, which can lead to aspiration, dehydration, or undernutrition. Patient immobility can result in deconditioning, sarcopenia, thromboembolic disease, pressure ulcers, urinary tract infections, and contractures. There may be decreases in daily functions, such as the ability to see, walk, feel, remember, speak, and think.

For an ischemic stroke, blood flow must be quickly restored to the brain, with emergency IV medications to break up a clot within 4–5 hours. The gold standard is recombinant **tissue plasminogen activator** (TPA), also known as alteplase or tenecteplase. Emergency endovascular procedures, if needed, must also be performed as soon as possible, and include medications delivered directly to the brain via a catheter inserted through an artery in the groin, which is then threaded to the brain, and removal of the clot with a **stent retriever**, also via a catheter. Other procedures include carotid endarterectomy, which removes the plaque blocking a carotid artery, **angioplasty**, and the insertion of stents. For hemorrhagic stroke, medications can be given that counteract the effects of any blood-thinning medications the patient may have been taking, drugs that lower intracranial pressure, lower BP, prevent blood vessel spasms, and prevent seizures. If the area of the bleeding is large, surgery may be needed to remove the blood, relieve intracranial pressure, and repair blood vessel problems. If there is an aneurysm, surgical clipping is done to clamp the base of it to keep it from bursting. Coiling (endovascular embolization) via catheter is the placement of tiny detachable coils into an aneurysm to fill it, causing blood to clot. Surgery can also be used to remove a small arteriovenous malformation if it is accessible. Finally, stereotactic radiosurgery can be done, using multiple beams of highly focused radiation to repair blood vessel malformations.

FOCUS ON OBESITY AND STROKE

Obesity is one of the most important risk factors for stroke. The relative risk for ischemic stroke is increased by 22% in overweight individuals when the body mass index (BMI) is between 25 and 30. If the BMI is 30 or more, there is an increased risk of 64% for hemorrhagic stroke.

Test Your Knowledge

1. What are the three types of stroke?
2. What are the manifestations of a stroke?
3. What are the complications of strokes?

KEY TERMS

Adipokine

Aneurysms

Angina pectoris

Angioplasty

Aphasia

Arcus senilis

Atheromas

Biliary cirrhosis

Contralateral

Diabetic dyslipidemia

Dyslipidemia

Embolism

Epistaxis

Fatty streak

Foam cells

Glomerulonephritis

Hepatosplenomegaly

Inflammasome

Intermittent claudication

Ischemia

Kawasaki disease

Parenchymal

Paresthesia

Pheochromocytoma

Polycystic renal disease

Pyelonephritis

Renin–angiotensin system

Saphenous veins

Stable angina

Stent retriever

Systemic lupus erythematosus

Tendinous xanthomas

Thrombosis

Tissue plasminogen activator

Unstable angina

Variant angina

Vasoconstriction

Vessel bifurcations

CLINICAL CASE STUDIES

Clinical Case Study 1

A 56-year-old woman was evaluated about her risk factors for cardiovascular disease. Though she was of normal weight, she had hypercholesterolemia and hypertension, and continued to smoke cigarettes whenever she felt stress. Her father had died of an acute myocardial infarction when he was 45 years old. The physician discussed lifestyle changes, which she agreed to, and starting her on statin medications, which she refused. A clinical nutritionist was referred to the patient, and a study was made of her diet, which included too many saturated fatty acids and insufficient fiber. The patient was advised to replace butter with vegetable oil-based margarine and to replace white bread with wholegrain bread. Her LDL cholesterol was reduced but still elevated after only two months. Since the patient did not want to take statins, her diet was changed again, and the vegetable oil-based margarine was replaced with a plant-based margarine. Her LDL reduced even more but not enough, and the patient finally agreed to taking low doses of statins, which lowered her cholesterol.

CRITICAL THINKING QUESTIONS

1. What are the avoidable risk factors related to atherosclerosis and cardiovascular disease?
2. For what conditions or patients are statins used as preventive therapy?
3. What does the treatment of cardiovascular disease involve?

Clinical Case Study 2

A 53-year-old truck driver has been a smoker since college, smoking just less than two packs per day. As he drives across the country, he usually eats potato chips and other snacks, and often drinks soda since the caffeine it contains helps him stay alert. Many of his meals are at fast food restaurants. He gets little exercise due to having to drive for many hours per day. As a child, his parents would be angry with him if he didn't finish everything on his plate, and his eating habits still reflect his upbringing. Over the last several years, his weight continued to increase, reaching 260 pounds. Family history reveals that his father had a mild heart attack that resulted in open-heart surgery on two coronary arteries as part of a coronary arterial bypass graft. One day while driving, he experienced heartburn and chest tightness, so he went for a medical checkup. The physician found that the patient had hypertension, hypercholesterolemia, and hypertriglyceridemia. He was referred to a registered dietitian nutritionist to discuss diet and lifestyle changes initially, prior to being started on medications.

CRITICAL THINKING QUESTIONS

1. What can high triglyceride levels and extremely high LDL cholesterol levels cause?
2. What does hypertension involve and how is obesity implicated?
3. Why would the patient in this scenario be at increased risk for a stroke?

Clinical Case Study 3

A 70-year-old man has had type 2 diabetes mellitus for 11 years, which he manages with dietary restrictions and metformin. A year previously, he had a myocardial infarction and was recently hospitalized for heart failure. He also takes atorvastatin and daily aspirin. The patient is referred to a registered dietitian, who discusses his usual diet habits, and decides to start him on the DASH diet for better heart health. The patient is also instructed to increase his physical exercise to 40 minutes per day for four days out of each week. Resistance training is also started since he has diabetes. After two months, with blood tests revealing that his condition needs better management, another drug, called empagliflozin, is added to the patient's regimen. This, along with his lifestyle changes, results in better management of his health condition.

CRITICAL THINKING QUESTIONS

1. Is diabetes mellitus a significant secondary cause of dyslipidemia?
2. How does increasing exercise and improving overall health result in many positive changes in the body?
3. How do the symptoms of myocardial infarction and other conditions develop?

Clinical Case Study 4

A 42-year-old African-American man has had a long history of poorly controlled hypertension. The patient admits to sometimes ignoring his condition and the recommendations of physicians. He has experienced related nosebleeds, headaches, and palpitations. The patient has not enjoyed the adverse effects of medications such as hydrochlorothiazide and beta-blockers. He has never smoked and seldom drinks alcoholic beverages. Family history reveals that his mother had hypertension. The patient is prescribed lisinopril and nifedipine.

CRITICAL THINKING QUESTIONS

1. How common is hypertension in various racial or ethnic groups?
2. What is the description of primary hypertension?
3. What does the prevention of hypertension require?

Clinical Case Study 5

A 65-year-old woman presented to the emergency department with blurred vision, confusion, loss of balance, and difficulty speaking. She was transferred to the intensive care unit. Laboratory tests revealed a prolonged prothrombin time, and elevated fibrinogen levels. There was central facial palsy on the left side, dysarthria, and facial drop, as well as total paralysis of the ipsilateral upper and lower limbs. A CT scan revealed lesions consistent with those of an ischemic stroke.

CRITICAL THINKING QUESTIONS

1. What causes an ischemic stroke?
2. How does a stroke occur?
3. What are the complications of strokes?

STUDY QUESTIONS

1. All of the following are risk factors for atherosclerosis, EXCEPT:
   A. Obesity
   B. Genetics
   C. Hypoglycemia
   D. Smoking

2. Which of the following races (for males) has the highest total cholesterol?
   A. Hispanics
   B. Non-Hispanic whites
   C. Non-Hispanic Asians
   D. Non-Hispanic blacks

3. Which of the following disorders may cause high triglyceride levels in the blood?
   A. Renal failure
   B. Hypothyroidism
   C. Diabetes mellitus
   D. Acute pancreatitis

4. All of the following may cause coronary artery disease, EXCEPT:
   A. Embolism
   B. Hypoalbuminemia
   C. Aneurysm
   D. Atheroma

5. All of the following are causes of secondary hypertension, EXCEPT:
   A. Addison's disease
   B. Sleep apnea
   C. Polycystic renal disease
   D. Pheochromocytoma

6. Which of the following is NOT recommended as a lifestyle change to prevent hypertension?
   A. Weight loss
   B. Reduced dietary potassium
   C. Smoking cessation
   D. Reduced dietary sodium

7. Which of the following is NOT one of the three types of stroke?
   A. Sclerotic
   B. Transient ischemic attack
   C. Hemorrhagic
   D. Ischemic

8. All of the following are complications of stroke, EXCEPT:
   A. Chronic headache
   B. Depression
   C. Hypercalcemia
   D. Spasticity

9. All of the following are clinical manifestations of hypertension, EXCEPT:
   A. Dizziness
   B. Epistaxis
   C. Malignant fever
   D. Vision changes

10. How many people, globally, are affected by uncontrolled hypertension?
   A. 25 million
   B. 75 million
   C. 500 million
   D. More than 1 billion

11. Which of the following does NOT trigger coronary artery spasms?
   A. Cocaine
   B. Hyponatremia
   C. Nicotine
   D. Stress

12. Dyslipidemia can be prevented by eating a diet of all of the following, EXCEPT:
   A. Whole grains
   B. Nuts
   C. Fish
   D. Foods low in zinc

13. An accumulation of lipid-laden foam cells in the intimal layer of an artery is called which of the following?
   A. Fatty acids
   B. Thrombosis
   C. Fatty streak
   D. Stable plaque

14. Which of the following medical terms means "symptomatic ischemia in the coronary arteries"?
   A. Variant angina
   B. Stable angina
   C. Angina pectoris
   D. Unstable angina

15. Which of the following blood vessels are used for coronary artery bypass grafting?
   A. Internal carotid arteries
   B. Femoral veins
   C. Saphenous veins
   D. Brachial veins

FURTHER READING

1. Ashraf, A., and Sunil, B. (2023). *Pediatric Dyslipidemia – A Practical Guide*. Springer.
2. Bakris, G.L., and Sorrentino, M. (2017). *Hypertension – A Companion to Braunwald's Heart Disease,* 3rd Edition. Elsevier.
3. Campbell-McBride, N. (2016). *Put Your Heart in Your Mouth: Natural Treatment for Atherosclerosis, Angina, Heart Attack, High Blood Pressure, Stroke, Arrhythmia, Peripheral Vascular Disease*. Medinform Publishing.
4. Cicero, A.F.G., and Rizzo, M. (2021). *Nutraceuticals and Cardiovascular Disease – An Evidence-based Approach for Clinical Practice (Contemporary Cardiology)*. Humana Press.

5. Corrigan, M.L., Escuro, A.A., and Kirby, D.F. (2013). *Handbook of Clinical Nutrition and Stroke (Nutrition and Health).* Humana Press.
6. Delemos, J., and Omland, T. (2017). *Chronic Coronary Artery Disease – A Companion to Braunwald's Heart Disease.* Elsevier.
7. El Ghoch, M., and El Shamieh, S. (2020). *Nutrition, Genetics, and Cardiovascular Disease.* Journal of Cardiovascular Development and Disease / MDPI.
8. Etherton, P.K., and Burns, J. (2016). *Cardiovascular Nutrition – Strategies and Tools for Disease Management and Prevention.* The American Dietetic Association.
9. Fogacci, F., Cicero, A., and Borghi, C. (2021). *Diets, Foods and Food Components Effect on Dyslipidemia (Nutrients).* Mdpi AG.
10. Franz, M.J., Boucher, J.L., and Franzini Pereira, R. (2016). *Pocket Guide to Lipid Disorders, Hypertension, Diabetes, and Weight Management*, 2nd Edition. Academy of Nutrition and Dietetics.
11. Garg, A. (2015). *Dyslipidemias – Pathophysiology, Evaluation, and Management (Contemporary Endocrinology).* Humana Press.
12. Grundy, S.M. (2022). *Atlas of Atherosclerosis and Metabolic Syndrome*, 5th Edition. Springer.
13. Houston, M.C. (2022). *The Truth about Heart Disease: How to Prevent Coronary Heart Disease and Personalize Your Treatment with Nutrition, Nutritional Supplements, Exercise and Lifestyle Tailored to Your Genetics.* CRC Press.
14. Houston, M.C., and Bell, L. (2021). *Controlling High Blood Pressure through Nutrition, Nutritional Supplements, Lifestyle, and Drugs.* CRC Press.
15. Houston, M.C. (2022). *Personalized and Precision Integrative Cardiovascular Medicine.* Wolters Kluwer.
16. Kaplan, N.M., and Victor, R.G. (2014). *Kaplan's Clinical Hypertension*, 11th Edition. Wolters Kluwer.
17. Lawhon, D. (2022). *The Complete Stroke Recovery Cookbook Guide for Seniors – Healing Through Food, Delicious and Nutritious Receipes for Older Adults.* Lawhon.
18. Muckley, G. (2022). *Dyslipidemia Disorders – Diagnosis and Management of Dyslipidemia.* Muckley.
19. Oyedola, S. (2023). *Mediterranean Diet for Stroke Patients Under 60 – Delicious Meals for Optimal Health for Men and Women – A Heart-Healthy Eating Plan for Stroke Prevention and Improved Quality of Life.* Oyedola.
20. Qureshi, M. (2020). *Stroke: Prevention and Understanding.* Page Publishing, Inc.
21. Rippe, J.M. (2017). *Nutrition in Lifestyle Medicine (Nutrition and Health).* Humana Press.
22. Schaefer, E.J. (2010). *High Density Lipoproteins, Dyslipidemia, and Coronary Heart Disease.* Springer.
23. Serruys, P.W. (2014). *Coronary Atherosclerosis – Current Management and Treatment.* Informa Healthcare.
24. Sinatra, S.T., and Houston, M.C. (2021). *Nutritional and Integrative Strategies in Cardiovascular Medicine*, 2nd Edition. CRC Press.
25. Stanner, S., Coe, S., British Nutrition Foundation, and Frayn, K.N. (2019). *Cardiovascular Disease: Diet, Nutrition and Emerging Risk Factors – The Report of the British Nutrition Foundation Task Force*, 2nd Edition. Wiley-Blackwell.
26. Tappia, P.S., and Blewett, H. (2020). *Nutrition and Cardiovascular Health.* International Journal of Molecular Sciences / MDPI.
27. Von Eckardstein, A., and Binder, C.J. (2019). *Prevention and Treatment of Atherosclerosis – Improving State-of-the-Art Management and Search for Novel Targets (Handbook of Experimental Pharmacology 270).* Springer.
28. Wilcox, C.S., Choi, M., Segal, M.S., Chen, L., and Williams, W.W. (2017). *Handbook of Nephrology and Hypertension*, 7th Edition. Wolters Kluwer.
29. Wilkinson, M.J., Garshick, M.S., and Taub, P.R. (2021). *Prevention and Treatment of Cardiovascular Disease – Nutritional and Dietary Approaches (Contemporary Cardiology).* Humana Press.
30. Zabetakis, I., Lordan, R., and Tsoupras, A. (2019). *The Impact of Nutrition and Statins on Cardiovascular Diseases.* Academic Press.

15 Nutritional Effects on the Endocrine System

OUTLINE

The Endocrine System
Growth Hormone Deficiency
Iodine Deficiency and Goiter
Hypothyroidism
Hypoparathyroidism
Hyperparathyroidism
Hyperglycemia and Diabetes Mellitus
Hypoglycemia
Nutrition and Reproduction in Females
Nutrition and Reproduction in Males
Key Terms
Clinical Case Studies
Study Questions
References

LEARNING OBJECTIVES

After study of the chapter, readers should be able to:

1. Describe the causes of dwarfism and cretinism.
2. Discuss the signs and symptoms of growth hormone deficiency.
3. Explain the differences between simple nontoxic goiter and endemic goiter.
4. Describe the common causes of myxedema coma and Hashimoto thyroiditis.
5. Explain the role of parathyroid hormone in the body.
6. Identify the complications of hyperparathyroidism.
7. Explain the causes of secondary hypothyroidism.
8. Describe the diagnosis of diabetes mellitus.
9. Explain the effects of calcium in the body.
10. Describe factors that increase the blood glucose during acute hypoglycemia.

OVERVIEW

The endocrine system is responsible for regulating appetite, nutrient absorption, storage, and usage, as well as other functions such as reproduction. The endocrine glands include the pituitary, pineal, thyroid, parathyroid, thymus, adrenals, pancreas, ovaries, and testes. They secrete hormones, which are biological molecules that regulate cellular processes in other target tissues. Therefore, they require transportation by the circulatory system. Adequate nutrition is critical for the functioning of all endocrine glands. A protein deficiency impairs gonadal-hormone release, preventing reproduction. Children who are malnourished usually do not produce enough growth hormone and fail to reach normal height for their age group. Unhealthy dietary patterns are linked to obesity and the development of type 2 diabetes. Some minerals and vitamins may involve various endocrine glands, such as iodine, calcium, vitamin D, phosphorus, and magnesium. Iodine deficiency, while rare in Westernized countries, is still a global problem that is linked to goiter. Hypothyroidism is the most common type of thyroid disorder. Hypoparathyroidism results in calcium and phosphorus imbalances, while hyperparathyroidism can result in serious conditions such as osteoporosis, kidney stones, and cardiovascular disease. Hyperglycemia is related with diabetes mellitus, and hypoglycemia is mostly caused by insulin treatments for diabetes.

THE ENDOCRINE SYSTEM

The functions of the endocrine system are closely connected to nutrition. This organ system is responsible for regulating appetite, nutrient absorption, nutrient storage, and nutrient usage, plus other functions such as reproduction. The glands in the endocrine system are the pituitary, thyroid, parathyroid, adrenals, thymus, pineal, pancreas, ovaries, and testes (see Figure 15.1). The glands secrete hormones, which are biological molecules that regulate cellular processes in target tissues, meaning that they require transportation by the circulatory system. Adequate nutrition is critical for the functioning of all endocrine glands. Protein deficiencies impair gonadal-hormone release, preventing reproduction. Athletic teenage girls with very little body fat often do not menstruate. Children who are malnourished usually do not produce enough growth hormone, and fail to reach normal height for their age group. The most popularized connection between nutrition and the functions of the endocrine system is that unhealthy dietary patterns are linked to obesity and the development of type 2 diabetes.

Overconsumption of high-fat and high-sugar foods causes changes in muscle, fat, and liver cells. This leads to a diminished response from the pancreatic hormone called *insulin*. The cells are then called "insulin-resistant". Insulin is released after a meal and induces the liver and other tissues to take up glucose and fatty acids that are circulating in the blood. When cells are resistant to insulin, they do

DOI: 10.1201/b22969-18

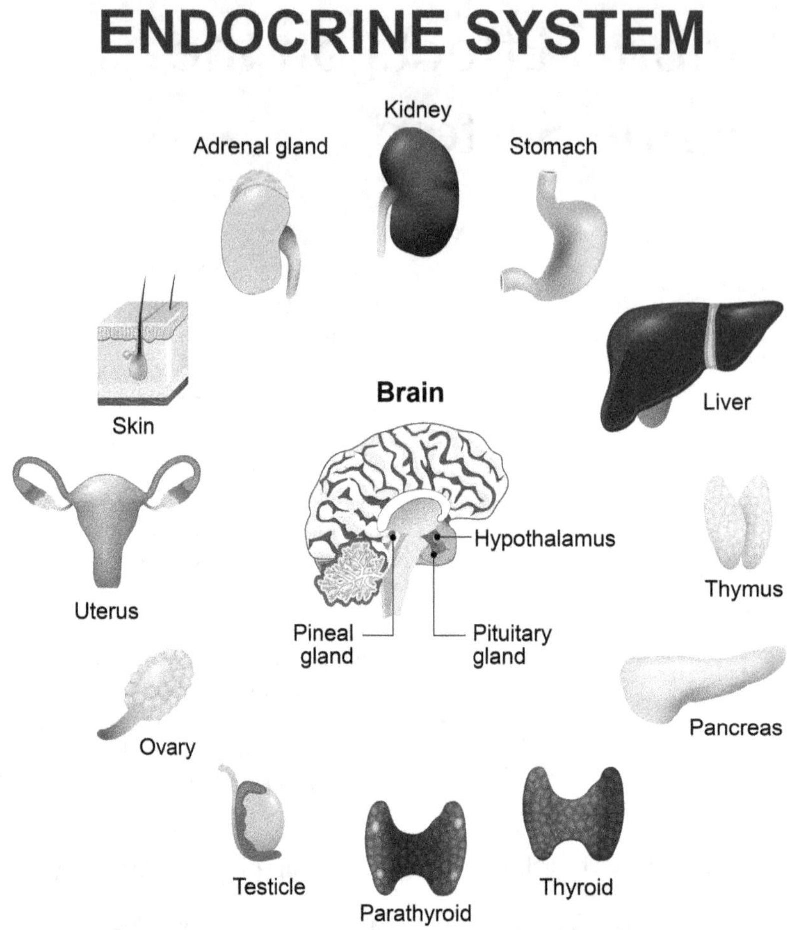

FIGURE 15.1 The endocrine system.

not take up enough glucose and fatty acids. Therefore, glucose and fatty acids remain at high concentrations in the blood. The chronic elevation of glucose and fatty acids in the blood causes damage to other tissues over time. Because of this, people with type 2 diabetes are at an increased risk for cardiovascular disease, kidney disease, nerve damage, and eye disease.

Each gland in the endocrine system releases specific hormones that help control or coordinate many bodily processes. They include the following:

- Pituitary gland – the "master gland"; it influences many other endocrine glands, particularly the thyroid, affecting metabolism, blood pressure, and growth
- Pineal gland – produces melatonin which helps regulate sleep
- Hypothalamus – regulates the pituitary gland in relation to the timing of hormone release
- Thyroid – controls metabolism, heart function, digestive function, mood, plus muscle and bone development
- Adrenal glands – release cortisol (the "stress" hormone)
- Ovaries – produce female sex hormones
- Testes – produce male sex hormones
- Pancreas – controls the release of insulin and glucagon; affects digestion

Because many endocrine glands work together to produce hormones, dysfunction in one gland often causes a cascade of problems throughout the entire endocrine system. Since endocrine hormones affect everything from sleep and metabolism to heart rate and digestion, endocrine disorders can create symptoms throughout the whole body.

Endocrine factors regulate food intake and growth, two related physiological processes critical for proper development of the body. Somatic growth is mainly regulated by growth hormone (GH) and insulin-like growth factors I and II (IGF-I and IGF-II), which act on target tissues such as muscles and bones. Peptidyl hormones produced from the brain and peripheral tissues regulate feeding to meet metabolic demands. The GH-IGF system and hormones regulating appetite are balanced by internal (metabolic) and external (environmental) signals. Among the external signals, the most important are diet availability and composition. Macronutrients and micronutrients act on hormone-producing tissues to regulate the synthesis and secretion of appetite-regulating hormones and hormones of the GH-IGF system. This eventually modulates growth and food intake.

A thorough understanding of how nutrients regulate hormones is essential to design diet formulations that effectively modulate endogenous factors.

GROWTH HORMONE DEFICIENCY

GH is made by the pituitary gland, a small gland at the base of the brain. In children, GH is essential for normal growth, muscle and bone strength, and distribution of body fat. It helps control glucose and lipid levels in the body. Without enough GH, a child is likely to grow slowly and be much shorter than other children of the same age and gender. Growth hormone deficiency (GHD) is also known as **dwarfism** or pituitary dwarfism (see Figure 15.2). Children with GHD have abnormally short stature, but with normal body proportions. GHD can be present at birth or develop later. It can be the result of genetic defects, severe brain injury, or being born without a pituitary gland. Sometimes, GHD can be associated with lower levels of other hormones, such as vasopressin, **gonadotropin hormone, thyrotropin hormone,** or **adrenocorticotrophic hormone**. A lack of GH is often caused by damage to the pituitary gland or the hypothalamus, a part of the brain that controls the pituitary gland. The damage may be due to a tumor, surgery or radiation used to treat the tumor, or to problems with the blood supply to the pituitary gland. A lack of GH can appear either in childhood or in adulthood.

Common symptoms that are present with a diagnosis of GHD include short stature and slowed growth in height in children, as well as low blood glucose levels in infants and toddlers. Children with GHD may have other signs, such as a very small penis in newborn males, or the absence of puberty during teenage years. Babies with severe congenital GHD usually have only a slightly reduced birth length

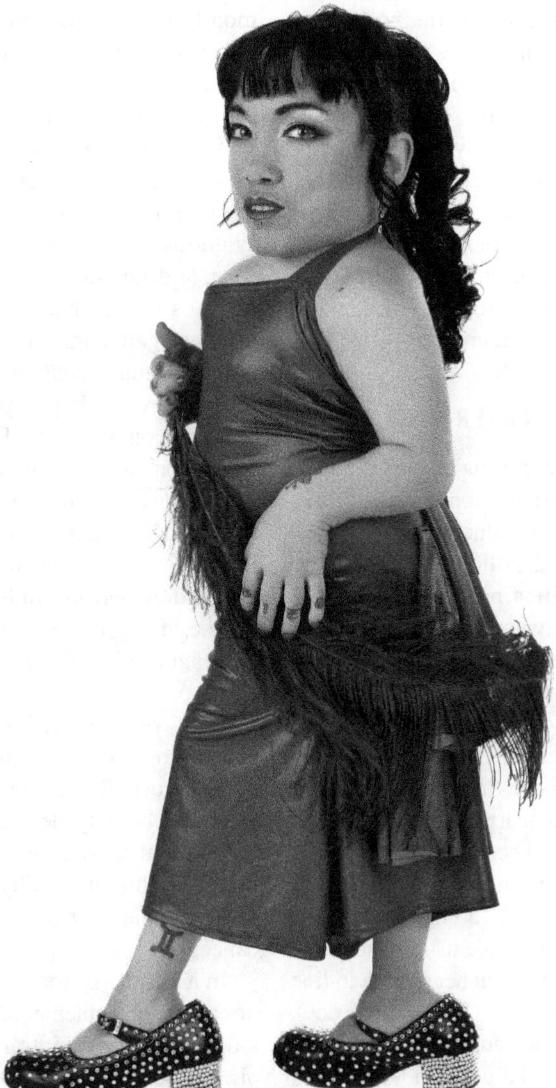

FIGURE 15.2 Pituitary dwarfism.

and may not immediately show signs of slow growth. In these children, low blood glucose can be the primary sign of GHD. Adults with severe GHD may experience an increase in body fat distribution with extra weight around the waist, a decrease in muscle mass and strength, low energy level, abnormalities in cholesterol levels, and increased risk for bone fractures.

Diagnosis depends on the history of patient, with injury that could have harmed the pituitary gland, measurement of GH in the blood, and magnetic resonance imaging (MRI). Once an adult GHD has been confirmed, GHs are injected. Every four to eight weeks and the patient will be monitored. If the patient is receiving too much GH, there will have muscle or joint pain, swelling, pain, or numbness in the hands. Blood cholesterol and bone density will also be monitored. GH therapy should not be given to patients who have active cancer. It also should not be given to patients who are seriously ill as a result of complications from open heart or abdominal surgery, who have multiple injuries from a major accident, or who have breathing problems. Taking GH will not cause an adult to begin growing again. Taking GH can affect the way the body uses insulin, so it is important for anyone who has diabetes to keep their physicians informed, and to be vigilant about monitoring blood sugar levels.

Children who are malnourished usually do not produce enough GH and fail to reach normal height for their age group. The top 20 foods that increase growth hormone are pumpkin seeds, quinoa, black beans, cheese, chicken, broccoli, brown rice, whole milk, mushrooms, beef, oats, cottage cheese, fish oil, kale, spinach, yogurt, lentil beans, cornmeal, wheat germ, and soy (in moderation).

IODINE DEFICIENCY AND GOITER

Iodine deficiency (ID) is considered a major public health problem worldwide affecting all groups of people. Children and lactating women are the most vulnerable categories. At a global scale, approximately 2 billion people are suffering from ID and about 50 million present with clinical manifestations. Iodine is mostly involved in the synthesis of the thyroid hormones known as T4 and T3. It is present in the earth's environment, but in the diet, it is mostly in the form of *iodide*. In an adult, approximately 80% of absorbed iodide is collected by the thyroid gland. In the environment, iodine is present as iodide in seawater. Small amounts enter the atmosphere, then fall back to earth in rain, entering ground water and soil near oceans. Therefore, people living far away from oceans or at higher altitudes have a higher risk for ID. Adequate iodine intake, of 150 mcg per day, is ensured by fortifying table salt with iodide usually about 70 mcg per gram. However, pregnant women need more iodine (220 mcg per day) as do lactating women (290 mcg per day). ID is uncommon in areas where iodized salt is used, yet it is relatively common worldwide. The deficiency develops when intake of iodide is less than 20 mcg per day.

With mild to moderate ID, the thyroid gland is influenced by thyroid-stimulating hormone (TSH). The gland hypertrophies to concentrate iodide inside of itself, causing a colloid goiter. While most patients remain **euthyroid**, a severe ID in an adult can cause **hypothyroidism**, which is also known as *endemic myxedema.* This condition can decrease fertility, or increase risks for stillbirth, spontaneous abortion, as well as prenatal and infant mortality. Severe maternal ID can harm the fetus, causing congenital **cretinism**, low birth weight, impaired mental function, neurological disorders, poor physical development, problems walking, a short stature, and death (see Figure 15.3). Cretinism is a restriction of brain development and growth, characterized by severe mental retardation, hearing problems, loss of speech abilities, muscle spasticity, and short stature.

Simple nontoxic goiter is a benign hypertrophy of the thyroid that may be diffuse or nodular. There is no hyperthyroidism, hypothyroidism, or inflammation. Except in cases of severe ID, thyroid function is normal. The patient is asymptomatic, except for an obvious nontender enlargement of the thyroid. Simple nontoxic goiter is the most common type of thyroid enlargement. It is most often seen at puberty, in pregnancy, or at menopause, but the cause is not usually clear. The understood causes include defects in intrinsic thyroid hormone production, ingestion of foods that inhibit thyroid hormone synthesis (goitrogens such as broccoli, cabbage, cassava, and cauliflower, often in countries with ID), and drugs that decrease thyroid hormone synthesis (compounds that contain iodine such as amiodarone, or drugs such as lithium).

ID is rare in North America, yet is the most common cause of goiter throughout the world (known as **endemic goiter**). Small compensatory elevations in TSH occur, which prevents hypothyroidism, but the TSH stimulation causes a goiter to form. Recurring cycles of stimulation and involution can cause nontoxic nodular goiters. Even so, the actual cause of most nontoxic goiters in locations with sufficient iodine is not understood. Patients may have a history of low iodine intake or overingestion of goitrogens, but this seldom happens in North America. Early in the disease course, the goiter is usually soft, smooth, and symmetric (see Figure 15.4). Over time, multiple nodules and cysts can develop.

Early on, thyroidal radioactive iodine uptake may be normal to high in a normal thyroid scan. Thyroid function tests are usually also normal. With endemic goiter, serum TSH may be only elevated slightly, while serum T4 may be low-normal or slightly low. The serum T3 is usually normal or slightly high. Thyroid ultrasonography is performed to determine if there are any nodules that could suggest cancer.

In areas of ID, the following methods reverse the condition: iodine supplementation of salt, oral administration of iodized oil, annual intramuscular administration of iodized oil, and iodination of water, crops, or **animal fodder**. Any goitrogens that are being eaten should be removed from the diet. Sometimes, suppression of the hypothalamic–pituitary axis with thyroid hormone will block TSH production,

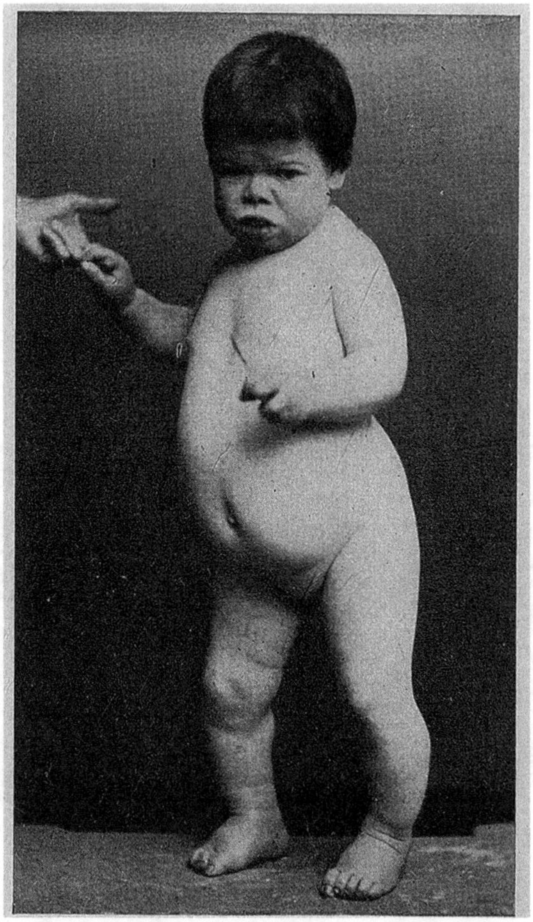

FIGURE 15.3 Cretinism.

stimulating the thyroid. Moderate doses of levothyroxine can be useful in younger patients, to reduce serum TSH to the low-normal range. The moderate doses are 100–150 mcg orally, once per day, based on serum TSH. Levothyroxine should not be used in older patients with nontoxic nodular goiter, since this type of goiter usually does not shrink, and may have autonomic areas that can result in hyperthyroidism. Large goiters sometimes require surgery or iodine-131 in order to shrink the thyroid enough to avoid any problems with respiration, swallowing, or in order to correct cosmetic abnormalities.

Symptoms of ID include enlargement of thyroid glands, a visible goiter, choking, trouble breathing, difficulty swallowing, weight gain, fatigue, thinning hair, dry skin, feeling colder than usual, **bradycardia**, learning problems, and memory difficulties. The diagnosis of ID for people of all ages is usually based on thyroid function tests, plus examination for a goiter, and imaging tests that identify abnormal thyroid function and structure. Every neonate must be screened for hypothyroidism by measuring TSH levels. Infants with ID receive *levothyroxine*, 3 mcg per kg of body weight orally, once per day for one week. They also receive iodide, 50–90 mcg orally, once per day, for several weeks. The euthyroid state is then quickly restored. Children are given iodide, 90–120 mcg once per day, and are also given levothyroxine until they can synthesize T4. Adults receive iodide, 150 mcg once per day, and may also need to receive levothyroxine. Pregnant or breastfeeding women must ingest 250 mcg of iodide once per day. Serum TSH levels are monitored in all patients, until levels normalized to less than 5 milliunits per liter (mU/L).

Iodine is found mainly in animal protein foods and sea vegetables, and to a lesser extent in fortified foods like breads, cereals, seaweed, milk, fish, shellfish, dairy products, eggs, chicken, beef liver, and iodized table salt. A few fruits, like strawberries, cranberries, and pineapple, are an excellent and rich source of iodine.

FOCUS ON IODINE

Iodine is a particularly important microelement, required for normal physical growth during gestation and early life. It is an essential component of the hormones produced by the thyroid gland, of which absence or inadequate levels can cause significant clinical manifestations. ID may increase risk of stillbirths, abortions, perinatal mortality, congenital abnormalities, cretinism, and impaired growth.

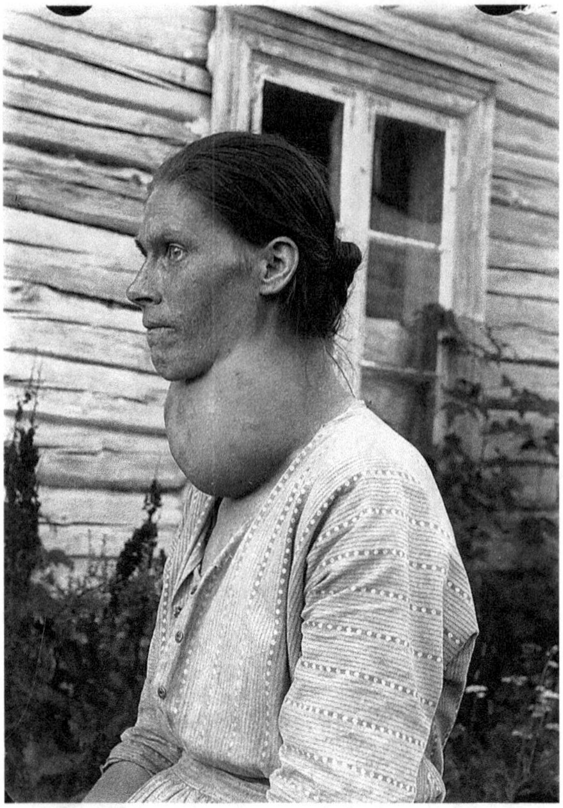

FIGURE 15.4 Goiter.

FOCUS ON IODINE DEFICIENCY IN THE BRAIN

Brain development is a complex process that begins in early pregnancy and goes on for the first years of the newborn's life. This is the reason why the most serious consequences of ID are neurological. Thyroid hormones are essential for a normal neurological development, being involved in myelination, cell differentiation and migration, growth, metabolism, sexual development, and body temperature regulation.

FOCUS ON EXCESSIVE IODINE INTAKE

An iodine excess that develops due to correction of a previous ID, as a higher intake than normal, can also affect the thyroid gland's proper function. This may lead to an autoimmune disease, goiter, hypothyroidism, iodine-induced thyrotoxicosis, or thyroid cancer.

Test Your Knowledge

1. What are the sign and symptoms of cretinism?
2. What are the causes of an endemic myxedema?
3. What are the causes of simple nontoxic goiter?

HYPOTHYROIDISM

Hypothyroidism is a deficiency of thyroid hormone that can occur at any age. However, it may occur more in older adults, because subtle and hard to recognize. Hypothyroidism can be primary or secondary. When thyroid hormone levels become extremely low in adults, it is called **myxedema** (see Figure 15.5). **Primary hypothyroidism** is caused by thyroid disease, while secondary hypothyroidism is caused by disease of the hypothalamus or pituitary gland. Primary hypothyroidism occurs from decreased T4 and T3 secretion from the thyroid gland. The serum T4 and T3 levels are low while TSH is increased. It is usually of autoimmune cause and primarily results from Hashimoto thyroiditis. The condition is often related to a firm goiter, or later on, to a shrunken fibrotic thyroid that has little to no function. The next most common cause is post-therapeutic hypothyroidism – usually after radioactive iodine therapy or surgical removal of the thyroid. Hypothyroidism that occurs due to overtreatment with propylthiouracil, methimazole, and iodide will resolve once therapy is stopped. Other medications, including lithium, beta-blockers, and anesthetic agents, may also cause hypothyroidism.

In patients taking lithium, hypothyroidism can occur, possibly because lithium inhibits hormone release by the thyroid. Hypothyroidism can also occur with use of

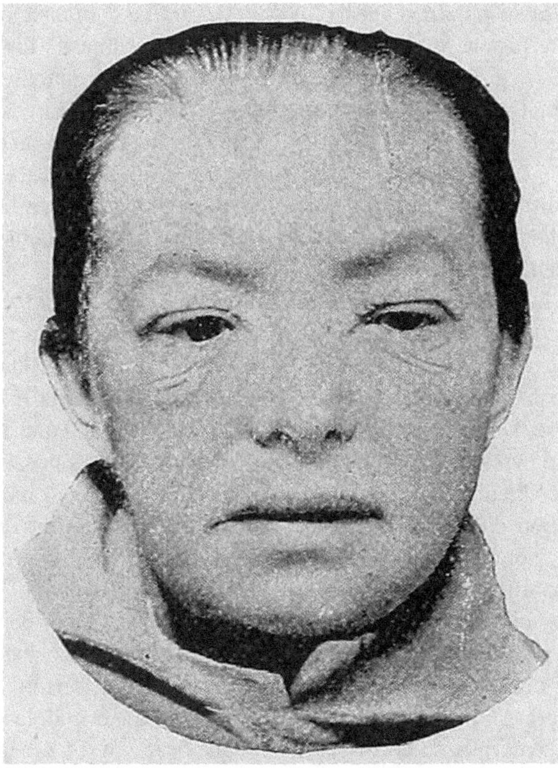

FIGURE 15.5 Myxedema.

amiodarone or other drugs that contain iodine, in people taking interferon-alfa, and those taking checkpoint inhibitors or certain tyrosine kinase inhibitors (for cancer). Hypothyroidism may be due to radiation therapy for cancer of the larynx or **Hodgkin lymphoma**. Incidence of permanent hypothyroidism after radiation therapy is high. Via measurement of serum TSH, thyroid function is evaluated at 6–12 month intervals.

Secondary hypothyroidism develops when the hypothalamus produces too little thyrotropin-releasing hormone (TRH), or the pituitary produces too little TSH. In some cases, deficient secretion of TSH due to deficient secretion of TRH is called *tertiary hypothyroidism*. There is also *subclinical hypothyroidism*, which involves elevated serum TSH even with no or only slight symptoms of hypothyroidism, and normal serum levels of free T4. Subclinical thyroid dysfunction is common, occurring in approximately 15% of older women and 10% of older men, especially when **Hashimoto thyroiditis** is present. If a patient has serum TSH higher than 10 mU/L, there will probably be a progression to overt hypothyroidism with low serum levels of free T4 in the next ten years. Affected patients have a higher risk for hypercholesterolemia and atherosclerosis. Treatment is with levothyroxine, even without symptoms. If a patient has TSH levels between 4.5 and 10 mU/L, levothyroxine is tried if there are symptoms of early hypothyroidism such as depression and fatigue. Levothyroxine is indicated for pregnant women and those who plan to become pregnant, in order to avoid negative effects of hypothyroidism upon the pregnancy and development of the fetus. There should be a yearly measurement of serum TSH and free T4, to assess the condition's progress if it is untreated, or in order to adjust dosages of levothyroxine.

Though signs and symptoms of primary hypothyroidism are often slight, the most common manifestations are fluid retention and puffiness of the eyes, cold intolerance, tiredness, and mental fogginess. There are a variety of organ system manifestations, which include:

- *Metabolic* – slight weight gain due to fluid retention and decreased metabolism, hypothermia
- *Neurologic* – forgetfulness, hand and foot paresthesias. and slowed relaxation phase of the deep tendon reflexes
- *Psychiatric* – depression, personality changes, a dull facial expression, dementia, or frank psychosis known as **myxedema madness**
- *Dermatologic* – hair that is thin, coarse, and dry, skin that is dry, scaly, and thick, **carotenemia** (mostly on the palms and soles due to carotene deposits), and **macroglossia**
- *Ocular* – periorbital swelling from infiltration with hyaluronic acid and chondroitin sulfate, and drooping of the eyelids due to decreased adrenergic drive
- *Gastrointestinal* – constipation
- *Gynecologic* – menorrhagia or secondary amenorrhea

- *Cardiovascular* – bradycardia, enlarged heart mostly due to pericardial effusion, and rarely, hemodynamic distress
- *Other* – pleural or abdominal effusions, hoarse voice, and slow speech

In older patients, symptoms can differ widely. While secondary hypothyroidism is uncommon, it often affects other endocrine organs that are controlled by the hypothalamic–pituitary axis. In females that have hypothyroidism, signs of secondary hypothyroidism include history of **amenorrhea** instead of **menorrhagia**, and some suggestive physical differences. Secondary hypothyroidism involves the skin and hair being dry but not very coarse, skin depigmentation, macroglossia, atrophic breasts, and hypotension. The heart is smaller than normal, and serous pericardial effusions are not seen. Hypoglycemia is common due to concomitant adrenal insufficiency or a deficiency of GH.

Myxedema coma is occasionally called *myxedema crisis.* It is a rare, life-threatening clinical condition that represents severe hypothyroidism with physiologic decompensation. The condition usually occurs in patients with long-standing, undiagnosed hypothyroidism. It is most often precipitated by infection, cerebrovascular disease, heart failure, trauma, or drug therapy. Signs and symptoms of myxedema crisis can include respiratory depression, hyponatremia, hypothermia, confusion, shock, hypoxia, high blood carbon dioxide levels, coma, and seizures. Myxedema crisis can cause death, often due to complications from infection, bleeding, or respiratory failure. It is more common in women and people over the age of 60, and can occur during pregnancy as well.

It is essential to achieve a rapid diagnosis because death is likely without quick treatment. The most sensitive diagnostic test is measurement of serum TSH. With primary hypothyroidism there will be decreased feedback inhibition of the intact pituitary. Serum TSH is always high, while serum free T4 is low. With secondary hypothyroidism, both free T4 and serum TSH are low, though the TSH may be normal but with less-than-normal bioactivity. Many patients with primary hypothyroidism have normal circulating levels of T3, likely due to sustained TSH stimulation of the thyroid as it is failing. This causes preferential synthesis and secretion of biologically active T3. As a result, serum T3 is not sensitive for hypothyroidism. Thyroid antibodies are measured in order to rule out Hashimoto thyroiditis.

Thyroid hormone preparations can be used for replacement therapy. These include synthetic preparations of T4 (levothyroxine), T3 (liothyronine), combinations of these, and desiccated animal thyroid extract. The preferred agent is levothyroxine. Maintenance doses are usually 75–150 mcg, orally, once per day. This is based on patient age, body mass index, and absorption potential. In young or middle-aged patients that are otherwise healthy, the starting dose can be 100 mcg or 1.7 mcg per kg orally, once per day. For patients with heart disease, therapy is started in low doses of usually 25 mcg, once per day. This is adjusted every six weeks until a maintenance dose is achieved. This dose may need to be increased for women that are pregnant. It may also need to be increased if drugs that decrease absorption of T4 or that increase its metabolic clearance are also being given. The chosen dose should be the lowest that will restore serum TSH to the mid-normal range, but this is not for patients with secondary hypothyroidism. Therefore, in secondary hypothyroidism, the levothyroxine dose should achieve a free T4 level that is in the mid-normal range.

Liothyronine is not used alone for long-term replacement because it has a short half-life and it causes large peaks in serum T3 levels. Administration of standard replacement amounts results in quickly increasing serum T3, to between 300 and 1,000 nanograms per deciliter (ng/dL) within 4 hours because of its nearly complete absorption. These levels normalize over 24 hours. Also, patients receiving liothyronine are chemically hyperthyroid for several hours (or more) per day. This can increase cardiac risks. When mixtures of T3 and T4 are taken orally, similar serum T3 changes occur, though peak T3 is lower since less T3 is given. Replacement regimens using synthetic T4 show a different serum T3 response. The increases occur slowly, with normal levels being maintained when sufficient doses of T4 are given. Desiccated animal thyroid preparations have varying amounts of T3 and T4. They are not prescribed unless the patient is already taking them and has normal serum TSH. For secondary hypothyroidism, levothyroxine is not given unless there are signs of sufficient cortisol secretion, or cortisol therapy is given, since levothyroxine could result in an adrenal crisis.

Myxedema coma is treated with IV administration of T4, corticosteroids, supportive care, and conversion to oral T4 once the patient is stable. A large initial dose of T4 or T3 is needed. The IV maintenance dose of T4 is 75–100 mcg once daily and for T3 the dose is 10–20 mcg twice per day until T4 can be accepted orally. Corticosteroids help protect against central hypothyroidism. Patients are not rewarmed quickly since this can cause hypotension or arrhythmias. Hypoxemia is common so the partial pressure of oxygen must be monitored. With compromised ventilation, immediate mechanical ventilatory assistance is needed. The precipitating factors must be quickly, correctly treated. Fluid replacement is given carefully, since hypothyroid patients do not excrete water normally. All drugs are given carefully since they are not metabolized as quickly as in healthy patients.

FOCUS ON MYXEDEMA CRISIS

Myxedema crisis often occurs after a long history of hypothyroidism. It is more common during cold winter months. The condition can be triggered by the stopping of hypothyroidism medications, sudden heart attack or stroke, trauma, stress, exposure to cold, infection, and certain drugs that suppress the central nervous system.

FOCUS ON HASHIMOTO'S THYROIDITIS

Hashimoto's thyroiditis, also known as chronic lymphocytic thyroiditis, is the most common cause of hypothyroidism in the United States. It is an autoimmune disorder involving chronic inflammation of the thyroid, and tends to run in families. Over time, the ability of the thyroid gland to produce thyroid hormones often becomes impaired, leads to a gradual decline in function, and eventually, an underactive thyroid (hypothyroidism). Hashimoto's thyroiditis occurs most commonly in middle-aged women, but can be seen at any age. It can also affect men and children.

Test Your Knowledge

1. What are the causes of primary and secondary hypothyroidism?
2. What are the common manifestations of primary hypothyroidism?
3. What are the risk factors for myxedema coma?

HYPOPARATHYROIDISM

Hypoparathyroidism occurs when the parathyroid glands do not produce enough **parathyroid hormone** (PTH). There are four pea-sized parathyroid glands in the neck, behind the thyroid gland (see Figure 15.6). PTH controls the levels of calcium and phosphorus, so insufficient PTH causes abnormal levels of calcium. The most common cause is injury to or removal of all four parathyroid glands. This can accidentally happen during surgery to remove the thyroid. Some people are born without these glands, or the glands do not function for unknown reasons. Hypoparathyroidism is a rare but treatable condition that causes hypocalcemia. The PTH also helps control the levels of phosphorus and vitamin D in the blood and bones. Hypoparathyroidism affects fewer than 200,000 people in the United States.

Calcium is one of the most important and common minerals in the body. Most calcium is used to build and maintain bone strength. It helps muscles contract, helps nerves and the brain work properly, and helps regulate the heart rhythm and blood pressure. Phosphorus is a mineral found in all cells, but it is stored mostly with calcium in the bones. It helps the body use food for energy and assists the kidneys, muscles, heart, and nerves in their proper function. Vitamin D helps the body to absorb calcium from food and functions to keep blood calcium levels in the normal range. Calcium and phosphorus are both electrolytes. Hypoparathyroidism can lead to electrolyte imbalance since it causes low levels of calcium and high levels of phosphorous in the blood. Low levels of magnesium can also cause hypoparathyroidism because the parathyroid glands need magnesium to function properly.

Both adults and children can get hypoparathyroidism. Though it is a rare condition in children, adults are more likely to get hypoparathyroidism from accidental damage to their parathyroid glands from neck or thyroid surgery. Children are more likely to have hypoparathyroidism due to a genetic condition called **DiGeorge syndrome**. Babies born with DiGeorge syndrome do not have parathyroid glands. Therefore, they are unable to make PTH, and have chronic hypoparathyroidism. Approximately 60% of children with hypoparathyroidism have DiGeorge syndrome. Other genetic syndromes associated with deafness and kidney disease can also cause hypoparathyroidism. Certain autoimmune diseases such as type one **autoimmune polyglandular syndrome** causes the immune system to attack the parathyroid glands, which causes chronic hypoparathyroidism. **Addison's disease** and *pernicious anemia* can also cause hypoparathyroidism. In most cases, hypoparathyroidism progresses very gradually, and symptoms can be mild. Many patients have symptoms for years before they are diagnosed. Signs and symptoms of hypoparathyroidism include tingling of the lips, fingers and toes; muscle cramps, tetany, confusion, dry hair, scaly skin, **cataracts**, brittle nails, and arrhythmias.

To diagnose hypoparathyroidism, a patient must have low levels of blood calcium, a low PTH level, and a high

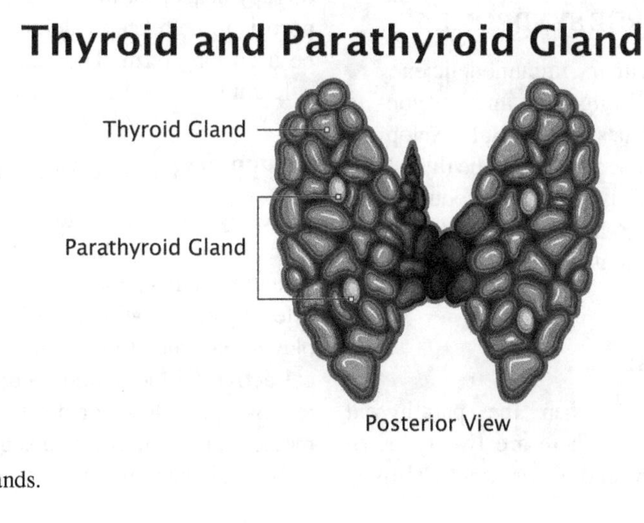

FIGURE 15.6 Parathyroid glands.

blood phosphorus level. A low blood magnesium level may cause a low blood calcium level. Since symptoms are often mild, healthcare providers sometimes "accidentally" find hypoparathyroidism when a routine blood screening shows the patient has low levels of blood calcium. Bone density tests, electrocardiogram, and urinalysis may be done. The goal of treatment is to relieve symptoms and to bring calcium and phosphorus levels in the body back into a standard range. Treatment usually includes:

- **Oral calcium supplements** – as tablets, chews or liquid – can increase calcium levels in the blood.
- **Vitamin D** – high doses, generally in the form of calcitriol, can help the body absorb calcium and eliminate phosphorus. Calcitriol is a prescription form of active vitamin D that is different from the usual supplements you can get without a prescription.
- **Magnesium** – if the level is low and the patient is experiencing symptoms of hypoparathyroidism, supplemental magnesium may be needed.
- **Thiazide diuretics** – if calcium levels remain low even with treatment, or if the amount of calcium in the urine is very high, thiazide diuretics can help decrease the amount of calcium lost through the urine.
- **PTH replacement** – PTH (Natpara) for low blood calcium due to hypoparathyroidism. This is a once-daily injection. Because of the potential risk of bone cancer (osteosarcoma).

The health care provider might recommend that the patient consult a registered dietitian, who is likely to advise a diet that is rich in calcium. This includes dairy products, green leafy vegetables, broccoli, and foods with added calcium, such as some orange juices and breakfast cereals. If there is a need for lower phosphorus, avoid carbonated soft drinks, which contain phosphorus in the form of phosphoric acid, and limit processed foods, meats, hard cheeses, nuts, and whole grains.

FOCUS ON DIGEORGE SYNDROME

DiGeorge syndrome is a primary immunodeficiency disease caused by abnormal migration and development of certain cells and tissues during fetal development. As part of the developmental defect, the thymus gland may be affected and T-lymphocyte production may be impaired, resulting in low T-lymphocyte numbers and frequent infections.

HYPERPARATHYROIDISM

Hyperparathyroidism develops when the parathyroid glands produce too much PTH. There are two types of hyperparathyroidism: *primary* and *secondary*. **Primary hyperparathyroidism** occurs when there is **adenoma**, or in rare cases, a cancerous tumor. An increased risk of developing primary hyperparathyroidism also occurs in patients that have been exposed to radiation from cancer treatment, are taking lithium, or have a long history of calcium and vitamin D deficiencies. **Secondary hyperparathyroidism** occurs in patients with chronic kidney failure, which results in low vitamin D and calcium levels. When calcium levels are too low, the parathyroid glands respond by increasing the production of PTH. This causes the kidneys and intestines to absorb a larger amount of calcium. It also removes more calcium from the bones. PTH production returns to normal when the calcium level goes up again.

Approximately 100,000 people develop hyperparathyroidism in the United States every year. Older women who are post-menopausal are at the highest risk for this condition. In the early stage of hyperparathyroidism, the patient may have no symptoms. However, in mild cases, patients complain about joint pain, muscle weakness, tiredness, loss of appetite, depression, and trouble concentrating. The symptoms of severe hyperparathyroidism include nausea and vomiting, confusion, forgetfulness, polydipsia, polyuria, and constipation. Other problems associated with severe hyperparathyroidism include reduced kidney function, kidney stones, and hypertension. Because the symptoms of hyperparathyroidism can be nonexistent, mild, or common to many other disorders, a diagnosis of hyperparathyroidism can be missed. Often, the condition is discovered through a blood test that is ordered for another condition. Treatments include observation, medications, and surgery, if symptoms are severe or one or more parathyroid glands is enlarged. In mild hyperparathyroidism, when there are no symptoms and blood calcium levels only slightly elevated, observation alone is required. Blood calcium levels and blood pressure must be measured every six months. Kidney function is measured every year, and bone density is measured every one to three years. Surgery is recommended to remove any overactive glands. Medications for hyperparathyroidism include the calcimimetics, hormone replacement therapy, and bisphosphonates. Calcimimetics include cinacalcet and prescription forms of vitamin D. Hormone replacement therapy helps post-menopausal women with signs of osteoporosis to help keep calcium in the bones, but this cannot be used long term. The bisphosphonates prevent a loss of calcium from the bones and can reduce osteoporosis.

HYPERGLYCEMIA AND DIABETES MELLITUS

Hyperglycemia is the technical term for high blood glucose. It happens when the body has too little insulin or when the body cannot use insulin properly. Hyperglycemia affects patients who have diabetes, and several factors can play a role when this occurs. They include food and physical activity, illness, and medications not related to diabetes. Skipping doses or not taking enough insulin or other medication to lower blood sugar also can lead to hyperglycemia. Diabetes mellitus is condition of impaired insulin secretion, with varying degrees of peripheral insulin resistance, which lead to hyperglycemia. Type 1 diabetes was previously called **juvenile diabetes** or *insulin-dependent diabetes*. This chronic condition is signified by the pancreas making little or no insulin, the hormone used to allow glucose to enter cells to produce energy. Type 2 diabetes was previously called *adult-onset diabetes*.

Impaired glucose regulation is an intermediate state between normal glucose metabolism and diabetes mellitus, and becomes more common with aging. It is a serious risk factor for diabetes, and can be present for years before the onset of diabetes. Impaired glucose regulation is associated with a higher risk of cardiovascular disease, though the typical diabetic microvascular complications are not common. For example, albuminuria, retinopathy, or both develop in just 6%–10% of patients (see Chapter 9 for more detailed information).

Diet is a factor in many cases of diabetes. The exposure of infants to dairy products (primarily in cow milk and via the milk protein called **beta-casein**), high nitrates found in drinking water, and low vitamin D consumption increase risks for type 1 diabetes. Exposure to gluten before four months of age, increases islet cell autoantibody production through unknown mechanisms. For type 2 diabetes, plasma glucose levels reach higher levels after eating than in younger adults, primarily after meals that are loaded with carbohydrates. More than 90% of adults with diabetes have the type 2 form. There is impaired first-phase insulin secretion, a loss of pulsatile insulin secretion, increased proinsulin secretion signaling (which indicates impaired insulin processing), and increased islet amyloid polypeptide, which is a protein normally secreted with insulin. Obesity and weight gain are important in determining the insulin resistance of type 2 diabetes. They reflect factors that include diet, exercise, lifestyle, and genetics.

Patients with type 1 diabetes usually have symptomatic hyperglycemia, and sometimes, diabetic ketoacidosis. Patients with type 2 diabetes may present with symptomatic hyperglycemia, but often have no symptoms. The condition is detected as part of routine tests. Sometimes, the initial symptoms are those of diabetic complications, which suggests the presence of the disease for a long time. For some patients, a hyperosmolar hyperglycemic state occurs fist, especially during stress or when glucose metabolism is additionally impaired by corticosteroids or other drugs.

The diagnosis of diabetes is based on fasting plasma glucose levels, **glycosylated hemoglobin A_{1c}** (HbA_{1c}) levels, and sometimes, oral glucose tolerance testing. HbA_{1c} is a type of hemoglobin that is chemically attached to a sugar that increases along with blood glucose. It has a solid relationship with average glucose levels over the preceding three months. Therefore, the diagnostic criteria for diabetes are as follows:

- Diabetes – HbA_{1c} of 6.5% or more
- Prediabetes or risk for diabetes – HbA_{1c} of 5.7%–6.4%

Even so, HbA_{1c} is an indirect measure of blood glucose and values can be false (high or low), and also vary between racial and ethnic groups. Screening for diabetes is done for people that are an increased risk for the disease. People at high risk of type 1 diabetes can be tested for the presence of islet cell or antiglutamic acid decarboxylase antibodies. Risk factors for type 2 diabetes include age of 35 or older, being overweight or obese, a sedentary lifestyle, family history, history of prediabetes, gestational diabetes mellitus or delivery of a high birthweight baby, hypertension, dyslipidemia, history of cardiovascular disease, polycystic ovary syndrome, certain races or ethnicities (African, Hispanic, Asian, or American Indian), fatty liver disease, and human immunodeficiency virus (HIV) infection. Those with risk factors should be screened at least once every three years if plasma glucose levels are normal, and at least every year if results show impaired fasting glucose levels.

Screening for complications of diabetes includes a foot examination, **funduscopic examination**, urine testing for **albuminuria**, and measurement of serum creatinine with a lipid profile. Treatment includes improved diet and regular exercise. For type 1 diabetes, insulin is required. For type 2 diabetes, oral antihyperglycemic, insulin, or a combination of these can be given. For type 1 diabetes, insulin therapy aims at replicating normal patterns of insulin secretion in nondiabetic individuals by using basal-bolus insulin therapy. A longer-acting insulin is used to suppress hepatic glucose production primarily in the fasting state. A shorter-acting insulin is used before meals to control post-prandial glucose levels. Sliding-scale insulin is an option in which varied doses of rapid-acting insulin are given before meals and at bedtime based on plasma glucose levels. For type 2 diabetes, patients that have mildly elevated plasma glucose begin treatment with an improved diet and more regular exercise, followed by metformin.

Patient education is essential, and includes information about the causes of the disease, diet, exercise, medications, self-monitoring methods, how to monitor HbA_{1c}, and information on the signs and symptoms of hypoglycemia, hyperglycemia, and disease complications. Education is reinforced at every physician visit or hospitalization. For type 1 diabetes, carbohydrate counting or the carbohydrate exchange system should be used. Counting involves amounts of carbohydrates in each meal, to calculate the preprandial insulin dose. These ratios are extremely varied between patient and require individualization and regular adjustments. Meals with higher protein or fat content can increase insulin requirements, leading to dose adjustments. A dietitian experienced with diabetes should guide the patient. Nutrition counseling should always complement physician counseling, and include any individuals who prepare meals for the patient. Dietary adjustments are highly individualized and designed to help type 2 diabetes patients to lose weight. Recommendations are based on patient tastes, preferences, culture, goals, and needs that arise from any comorbidities. The diet should be rich in whole foods instead of processed foods. Carbohydrates must be of high quality and contain enough fiber, vitamins, and minerals, while being low in added sugar, fat, or sodium. Low- or very-low-carbohydrate diets can be beneficial, but often not over the long term. For dietary management, it is very important for the patient to be questioned concerning a thorough dietary history that includes timing of meals. This helps identify factors that contribute to poor control. Underlying disorders must be ruled out by physical examination and laboratory testing.

FOCUS ON PRIMARY CAUSES OF DIABETES

Type 1 diabetes is caused by little to no insulin production, due to autoimmune pancreatic beta-cell destruction. This may be triggered by an environmental exposure if the patient is genetically susceptible. Some cases, however, are idiopathic. Type 2 diabetes is caused by insulin resistance, since insulin secretion becomes inadequate. Hepatic glucose production can no longer be suppressed, and peripheral glucose uptake is impaired.

FOCUS ON DIABETES MELLITUS AND DIET

Nutrition is an important component of a healthy lifestyle when patients have diabetes mellitus. It helps keep blood glucose levels in the desired range. Food choices and quantities along with eating times are extremely critical. Most healthy diets include all of the correct food choices for diabetes patients. The foods and drinks that must be limited include anything that is fried, high in saturated or trans fats, high in sodium, or high in sugar. Alcohol intake must be very controlled or cut out completely – no more than one serving per day for women and no more than two servings per day for men.

Test Your Knowledge

1. What are the signs and symptoms of type 1 diabetes?
2. Why is an HbA_{1c} test important to detect type 2 diabetes?
3. Why is patient education essential for controlling type 2 diabetes?

HYPOGLYCEMIA

Hypoglycemia is a condition of low plasma glucose. It can cause sympathetic nervous system stimulation and central nervous system dysfunction. In people taking insulin or antihyperglycemic, hypoglycemia is common. It is defined as a glucose level of 70 mg/dL or lower. Oppositely, hypoglycemia that is not related to exogenous insulin therapy is uncommon, and caused by a variety of disorders or drugs. Most often, symptomatic hypoglycemia is a complication of the use of oral antihyperglycemics and insulin. Normally, the body has many counter-regulatory mechanisms that compensate for low blood glucose. **Glucagon**, epinephrine, cortisol, and GH raise quickly in response to acute hypoglycemia. The threshold for release of these hormones is usually higher than that for hypoglycemic symptoms.

Hypoglycemia can occur in **insulinoma**, fasting, and post-prandial state. Insulinoma is an uncommon neuroendocrine tumor of the insulin-producing beta-cells. Hypoglycemia may also occur along with autoimmune conditions, such as *systemic lupus erythematosus*. As **autoantibodies** bind to insulin or its receptor. The circulating insulin is able to bind to the receptor upon dissociation from the antibodies, and hypoglycemia results. The condition is treated with corticosteroids or immunosuppressants. Non-insulin-mediated causes include adrenal insufficiency and use of drugs such as quinine, gatifloxacin, or pentamidine.

In ill patients, insulin-mediated disorders include exogenous insulin and use of sulfonylureas. Non-insulin-mediated disorders include malnutrition, starvation, cirrhosis, sepsis, end-stage renal disease, advanced heart failure, adrenal insufficiency, and nonislet cell tumor hypoglycemia. For hospitalized patients that are ill, spontaneous hypoglycemia not related to medications has a poor prognosis. **Pseudohypoglycemia** occurs from processing of blood specimens in untreated test tubes that is delayed, since the cells consume glucose over time.

The signs and symptoms of hypoglycemia include sweating, nausea, anxiety, warmth, palpitations, tremulousness, and sometimes, hunger and **paresthesias**. If there is a lack of glucose to the brain, symptoms include headache, blurred or double vision, agitation, confusion, seizures, and coma. For older patients, there may be stroke-like symptoms of aphasia or **hemiparesis**. They are more likely to precipitate an actual stroke, myocardial infarction, or sudden death. Over the long term, diabetic patients may be unaware of hypoglycemic episodes since they no longer experience the autonomic symptoms.

Diagnosis of hypoglycemia is via measurement of blood glucose levels. There are three levels of measurement, as follows:

- *Level 1* – mild – blood glucose is less than 70 mg/dL but at or higher than 54 mg/dL
- *Level 2* – moderate – blood glucose is less than 54 mg/dL
- *Level 3* – severe – assistance from another person is required due to changes in mental or physical status

If the individual is not being treated for diabetes, the diagnosis of hypoglycemia requires confirmation of **Whipple's triad**, or confirmed low blood glucose during a fast. Whipple's triad includes hypoglycemia symptoms, a low plasma glucose level during the time the symptoms occur, and a decrease in symptoms when dextrose or another sugar is administered.

When a healthcare practitioner is present during the symptoms, the patient's blood should be sent for glucose testing in a tube that contains a **glycolytic inhibitor**. When a practitioner is not present, home glucose meters are not reliable to give an accurate diagnosis. Therefore, there is a need for more extensive diagnostic testing. A 48- or 72-hour fast may be required to differentiate the type of hypoglycemia and determine its cause. A 72-hour fast performed in a controlled setting is preferred, though a 48-hour fast is usually adequate. Only noncaloric, noncaffeinated beverages are consumed, with regular plasma glucose measurements.

Treatments include oral sugar or IV dextrose, and sometimes, parenteral glucagon. People at risk for the condition should have glucagon or *dasiglucagon* at home and in places where they regular visit. Trusted family and friends should be able to administer these agents during an emergency. If the patient can eat or drink, fruit juices, sucrose water, glucose solutions, candy or other foods, or glucose tablets can be consumed. Other treatments, for patients not taking antihyperglycemic drugs, include diazoxide, octreotide, and acarbose. Drugs that cause hypoglycemia, including alcohol, must be stopped.

FOCUS ON DIETARY TIPS FOR MANAGING HYPOGLYCEMIA

To manage hypoglycemia, eat small meals every 3–4 hours, avoiding foods high in saturated or trans fats. Choose foods with a low glycemic index score (those that take longer to raise blood glucose levels) such as soybeans, chickpeas, carrots, green peas, or apples. Reduce or eliminate processed sugars, refined sugars, and alcohol. Choose complex carbohydrates over simple carbohydrates, and include lean proteins plus foods high in soluble fibers.

FOCUS ON BRAIN DAMAGE WITH HYPOGLYCEMIA

The human brain is made up of a dense network of neurons, or nerve cells, which are constantly active, even during sleep. To obtain the energy needed to sustain this activity, the brain depends on a continuous supply of glucose from the bloodstream. Therefore, hypoglycemia is very dangerous for the brain and causes neuronal death.

Test Your Knowledge

1. What are the causes of hypoglycemia?
2. What are the signs and symptoms of hypoglycemia?
3. What treatments are available for hypoglycemia?

NUTRITION AND REPRODUCTION IN FEMALES

Anorexia nervosa and bulimia nervosa affect up to 5% of women of reproductive age. These disorders cause amenorrhea, infertility and, in those who do become pregnant, an increased likelihood of miscarriage. Obesity can affect reproduction through fat cell metabolism, steroids, and secretion of proteins (such as leptin and adiponectin). It can also affect reproduction through changes induced at the level of homeostatic factors, such as pancreatic secretion of insulin, androgen synthesis by the ovaries, and sex hormone-binding globulin production by the liver. Obesity-associated anovulation may lead to infertility and a higher risk of miscarriage. Management of anovulation with obesity involves diet and exercise as well as methods to induce ovulation. Many obese women conceive without assistance. However, pregnancies in obese women have increased rates of hypertension, gestational diabetes, large infant size, Cesarean section, plus perinatal mortality and morbidity.

The reproductive system is highly sensitive to influences from the external environment. A common strategy involves timing of conception by *photoperiod* (day length) and/or rainfall, which usually ensures that birth takes place in a season when food and climatic conditions are favorable, such as the spring. Reproduction involves much greater energy expenditure in females than in males. The nourishing of offspring during pregnancy and lactation require the largest expenditure of energy that a female will make in her lifetime. Therefore, the female reproductive system is much more sensitive to disruption than that of the male. Because reproduction involves energy expenditure, it is understood that physiological control mechanisms are linked to those involved with appetite and nutrition. Food is used as a source of energy for various essential and nonessential functions. Very little energy is diverted to the storage of fat. Instead, calories are mobilized from fat stores to maintain energy balance. This means that energy balance regulates reproductive function more than the amount of present fat does.

Undernutrition due to eating disorders may affect ovulation and fertility, alter responses to conventional treatment and assisted reproduction technology. It can also have effects upon pregnancy and the newborn. Relevant eating disorders include bulimia nervosa (excessive eating and compensatory activities such as vomiting or laxative abuse) and anorexia nervosa. Both commonly begin during adolescence, and affect about 3% of young women. Menstrual periods often cease after a 10%–15% decrease in normal body weight. Related mechanisms include altered regulation of gonadotropin-releasing hormone secretion, and changes in the dopaminergic and opioid systems. Amenorrhea is a component of the *female athletic triad*, along with osteoporosis and milder versions of the eating disorders. **Oligomenorrhea** may occur with bulimia nervosa even in women that have a body mass index that is in the normal range. Amenorrhea persists in 30% of patients who regain their normal weight during recovery from anorexia nervosa accompanied by amenorrhea. Women with a history of being anorexic may have more induced abortions. In pregnancy, women with eating disorders have higher rates of **hyperemesis gravidarum**, anemia, impaired weight gain and compromised intrauterine fetal growth. Premature delivery is more likely in underweight women. Rates of Cesarean delivery, post-natal complications, and post-partum depression are higher in mothers with anorexia nervosa. Undernutrition is associated with low birthweight (3,233 g compared to 3,516 g for normal controls).

Although undernutrition is the dominant factor regulating reproductive activity under natural conditions, obesity is an important cause of lower fertility in many modern societies. Adipose tissue is a complex, highly active metabolic and endocrine structure. In addition to adipocytes there are immune cells, connective tissue matrix, nerve tissue, and stromovascular cells. Together, these function as an integrated unit. White and brown fat tissue differ in composition, appearance, and function. White adipose tissue is made up of 60%–85% lipids, and 90%–99% of these lipids are triglycerides. White fat tissue provides heat regulation, body cushioning, and energy storage (via the triglycerides). Brown fatty tissue derives its color from rich vascularization and densely packed mitochondria. The cells are polygonal in shape, have a considerable volume of cytoplasm, and contain many lipid droplets of varying size. The nuclei are round and nearly centrally located. Brown fatty tissue may make up 5% of body weight in neonates, but it disappears by adulthood. It is where nonshivering thermogenesis or metabolic heat production occurs, without rapid contraction of muscles.

FOCUS ON BROWN FAT TISSUE VS WHITE FAT TISSUE

Brown fat breaks down blood glucose and fat molecules to create heat and help maintain body temperature. Cold temperatures activate brown fat, which leads to various metabolic changes. Most fat, however, is white fat, which stores extra energy. Too much white fat builds up when a person is obese. Brown fat foods and compounds that boost activity or induce the browning of white fat include turmeric, green tea, chili peppers, fish oil, resveratrol (a component of red grapes), berberine (a plant chemical), and cinnamon. Other ways to activate brown fat include cold exposure and moderate exercise.

NUTRITION AND REPRODUCTION IN MALES

Nutrition can negatively or positively affect sperm quality. This effect depends on both quantitative and qualitative aspects of a diet. These include the calorie content of each macronutrient (carbohydrates, proteins, and fats), as well as specific fatty acid, carbohydrate, and protein profiles. Unhealthy hypercaloric diets and excessive intake of saturated and trans fatty acids have a negative impact on sperm quality. This means that they also negatively affect the fertilization process. Healthy diets are clearly associated with a better sperm quality. This suggests that nutritional interventions may have a key role in the preservation of male fertility.

Current Western dietary habits generally feature high sugar and fat consumption, with the consequent intake of unbalanced diets containing excessive calories. The Western diet has been a significant contributor to the growing rate of obesity, which has had a large effect upon fertility through changes in hormonal levels, sperm function, and gamete molecular composition. However, the molecular mechanisms responsible for the causal links between obesity and male infertility are not completely clear. Obesity disrupts various components of the hypothalamic–pituitary–gonadal axis, causing hypogonadism. This condition is mainly associated with reduced levels of testosterone and fewer spermatozoa. Increased amounts of adipose tissue cause insulin resistance and have an important role in the development of oxidative stress. Reproductive pathways and sperm function are altered. Hyperinsulinemia and hyperglycemia, the hallmarks of insulin resistance, appear to be responsible for the reduction in sperm glucose uptake and metabolism. Therefore, they have a possible role in the impairment of glycolysis in sperm cells.

KEY TERMS

Addison's disease

Adenoma

Adrenocorticotrophic hormone

Albuminuria

Amenorrhea

Animal fodder

Autoantibodies

Autoimmune polyglandular syndrome

Bradycardia

Carotenemia

Cataracts

Cretinism

DiGeorge syndrome

Dwarfism

Endemic goiter

Euthyroid

Funduscopic examination

Glucagon

Glycolytic inhibitor

Glycosylated hemoglobin A1c

Gonadotropin hormone

Hashimoto thyroiditis

Hemiparesis

Hodgkin lymphoma

Hyperemesis gravidarum

Hypothyroidism

Insulinoma

Juvenile diabetes

Macroglossia

Menorrhagia

Myxedema coma

Myxedema madness

Oligomenorrhea

Parathyroid hormone

Paresthesias

Primary hyperparathyroidism

Primary hypothyroidism

Pseudohypoglycemia

Secondary hyperparathyroidism

Secondary hypothyroidism

Simple nontoxic goiter

Thyrotropin hormone

Whipple's triad

CLINICAL CASE STUDIES

Clinical Case Study 1

A 12-year-old girl was assessed because her growth was slower than that of her peers. She was well below the third percentile for height. Her appetite and weight were normal. Breast development began at eight years of age, but pubic hair development was only slight. The patient had not yet had her first menstrual period. Her birth was full-term. Family history was negative for short stature, endocrine conditions, or autoimmune conditions. Tests revealed low levels of thyroid-stimulating hormone and free thyroxine. She was soon diagnosed with acquired GHD.

CRITICAL THINKING QUESTIONS

1. What is GH essential for?
2. What are the causes of growth hormone deficiency?
3. How does malnourishment in children affect growth hormone production, and what foods can increase this hormone?

Clinical Case Study 2

A 35-year-old African woman complained of cold intolerance, constipation, and tiredness was diagnosed with ID. Because of familial hypertension she always avoided salt in her diet, and also rarely ate fish or consumed dairy products. The patient had no family history of thyroid disease. She was advised to change her diet to include iodized salt and foods that were rich in sodium, but not excessively. Over two months, she improved greatly, with some symptoms lessening.

CRITICAL THINKING QUESTIONS

1. In which global areas do people have a higher risk for iodine deficiency?
2. If a severe iodine deficiency causes hypothyroidism, what are the possible outcomes?
3. What methods reverse iodine deficiency in areas where it is prevalent?

Clinical Case Study 3

A 37-year-old woman with a previous history of fibromyalgia presented to her physician for a regular checkup. She reported that her mother had just been diagnosed with hypothyroidism and asked for thyroid function tests to be included in her blood work. She had experienced some hair loss over the past three months. The test results came back, and her thyroid-stimulating hormone was high, but free T4 was low. A diagnosis of hypothyroidism was confirmed.

CRITICAL THINKING QUESTIONS

1. What are the causes of primary and secondary hypothyroidism?
2. What are the most common signs and symptoms of primary hypothyroidism?
3. What are the signs and symptoms of secondary hypothyroidism in females?

Clinical Case Study 4

A 54-year-old man went to his local emergency department, complaining of fever and cough over more than a week. Examination revealed crackles on auscultation at the bases of both lungs. A chest x-ray revealed patchy, diffuse opacities in both lower lung lobes. Due to the timing of his hospital visit, the patient was tested for SARS-CoV-2 infection, and was positive. He received oxygen therapy and medications to treat the infection. Blood tests revealed hypocalcemia, hyperphosphatemia, and very low serum levels of PTH, confirming a diagnosis of primary hypoparathyroidism. Though the patient had no symptoms of this condition, it was believed to be linked to the infection. The patient received oral calcium supplementation, and his calcium levels improved as symptoms resolved over five days. At one-month follow-up, he had normal levels of serum calcium and serum phosphorus.

CRITICAL THINKING QUESTIONS

1. How does insufficient parathyroid hormone result in altered calcium levels?
2. What are the signs and symptoms of hypoparathyroidism?
3. What are the treatment options for hypoparathyroidism?

STUDY QUESTIONS

1. Which of the following hormone deficiencies may cause dwarfism?
   A. Gonadotropin hormone
   B. Adrenocorticotrophic hormone
   C. Parathyroid hormone
   D. Growth hormone

2. Which of the following is also known as endemic myxedema?
   A. Hypothyroidism
   B. Hypoparathyroidism
   C. Addison's disease
   D. Dwarfism

3. Severe maternal iodine deficiency can cause which of the following conditions?
   A. Dwarfism
   B. Cretinism
   C. Myxedema
   D. Endemic goiter

4. Which of the following is NOT a sign or symptom of myxedema crisis?
   A. Hypothermia
   B. Hypoxia
   C. Renal failure
   D. Seizures

5. Which of the following disorders may cause DiGeorge syndrome?
   A. Hyperparathyroidism
   B. Addison's disease
   C. Hashimoto thyroiditis
   D. Hypoparathyroidism

6. All of the following is part of the treatment for hypoparathyroidism, EXCEPT:
   A. Oral calcium
   B. Vitamin D
   C. Iodized salt
   D. Thiazide diuretics

7. Which of the following foods does NOT contain iodine?
   A. Fish
   B. Orange juice
   C. Dairy products
   D. Strawberries

8. Simple nontoxic goiter is seen in all of the following, EXCEPT:
   A. Pregnant women
   B. Menopausal women
   C. Toddlers
   D. Puberty

9. Which of the following is NOT one of the most common manifestations of primary hypothyroidism?
   A. Weight loss
   B. Puffiness of the eyes
   C. Mental fogginess
   D. Cold intolerance

10. Secondary hypothyroidism can develop when the hypothalamus produces too little of which of the following?
    A. Thyrotropin-stimulating hormone
    B. Thyroxine
    C. Thyrotropin-releasing hormone
    D. Triiodothyronine

11. Which of the following disorders or conditions may cause hyperglycemia?
    A. Insulinoma
    B. Diabetes mellitus
    C. Addison's disease
    D. Systemic lupus erythematosus

12. Glycosylated hemoglobin A_{1C} is elevated in which of the following?
    A. Hemiparesis
    B. Hyperparathyroidism
    C. Diabetes mellitus
    D. Addison's disease

13. Which of the following disorders can lead to an electrolyte imbalance?
    A. Hypoparathyroidism
    B. Primary hypothyroidism
    C. Secondary hypothyroidism
    D. Endemic goiter

14. When calcium levels in the blood are too low, which of the following hormones increases?
    A. T4 and T3
    B. GH
    C. TSH
    D. PTH

15. In which of the following conditions is glucagon administered?
    A. Hypoglycemia
    B. Hypothyroidism
    C. Hyperglycemia
    D. Hypermagnesemia

REFERENCES

1. Agrawal, N.K. (2020). *Goiter: Causes and Treatment.* IntechOpen.
2. Bianco, A.C. (2022). *Rethinking Hypothyroidism: Why Treatment Must Change and What Patients Can Do.* University of Chicago Press.
3. Bonofiglio, D., and Catalano, S. (2020). *Effects of Iodine Intake on Human Health.* Nutrients / MDPI.
4. Brandi, M.L., and Meigs Brown, E. (2015). *Hypoparathyroidism.* Springer.
5. Brito Pateguana, N., and Fung, J. (2020). *The PCOS Plan – Prevent and Reverse Polycystic Ovary Syndrome through Diet and Fasting.* Greystone Books.
6. Burnette, M. (2022). *The Importance of Iodine: Where Iodine Deficiency is Spread and How People Cope with the Issue.* Burnette.
7. Christianson, A. (2021). *The Thyroid Reset Diet – Reverse Hypothyroidism and Hashimoto's Symptoms with a Proven Iodine-Balancing Plan.* Rodale Books.
8. Cicciarello Andrews, L. (2021). *The Complete Thyroid Cookbook – Easy Recipes and Meal Plans for Hypothyroidism and Hashimoto's Relief.* Rockridge Press.
9. Cohen, L.E. (2016). *Growth Hormone Deficiency – Physiology and Clinical Management.* Springer.
10. Cusano, N.E. (2020). *Hypoparathyroidism – A Clinical Casebook.* Springer.
11. Draznin, B. (2016). *Managing Diabetes and Hyperglycemis in the Hospital Setting – A Clinician's Guide.* American Diabetes Association.
12. Falih, S.S., Al-Fartusie, F.S., and Tahir, N.T. (2020). *Growth Hormone Deficiency in Children and Adolescents – A New Clinical Test to Diagnose Growth Hormone Deficiency in Saliva of Patients with Short Stature.* Scholars' Press.
13. Franz, M.J., Evart, A.B., and Franz, M. (2017). *American Diabetes Association Guide to Nutrition Therapy for Diabetes.* American Diabetes Association.
14. Fried, R., and Carlton, R.M. (2018). *Type 2 Diabetes – Cardiovascular and Related Complications and Evidence-Based Complementary Treatments.* CRC Press.
15. Gasparri, G., Camandona, M., and Palestini, N. (2015). *Primary, Secondary, and Tertiary Hyperparathyroidism – Diagnstic and Therapeutic Updates.* Springer.
16. George, F. (2022). *Hypoglycemia Treatment Manual.* George.
17. Kearns, A.E., and Wermers, R.A. (2016). *Hyperparathyroidism – A Clinical Casebook.* Springer.
18. Kellman, R. (2021). *Microbiome Thyroid – Restore Your Gut and Discover the Root Cause of Hidden Thyroid Disease.* Hachette Go.
19. Landry, T. (2018). *The Endocrine Reboot – The 14-day Diet Plan to Reset Your Hormones and Jumpstart Your Journey to Health.* CreateSpace Independent Publishing Platform.
20. Levine, M.A. (2018). *Hypoparathyroidism – An Issue of Endocrinology and Metabolism – Clinics of North America (The Clinics – Internal Medicine Book 47).* Elsevier.
21. Mohamed, A.S. (2015). *Diabetes Mellitus: Types – Mechanisms – Complications.* CreateSpace Independent Publishing Platform.
22. Moini, J., Adams, M., and LoGalbo, A. (2022). *Complications of Diabetes Mellitus: A Global Perspective.* CRC Press.
23. Oguntibeju, O. (2012). *Pathophysiology and Complications of Diabetes Mellitus.* IntechOpen.
24. Opara, E.C., and Dagogo-Jack, S. (2021). *Nutrition and Diabetes*, 2nd Edition. CRC Press.
25. Pappala, A. (2015). *Goiter – Iodine Deficiency Disorder.* Pappala.
26. Pearce, E.N. (2017). *Iodine Deficiency Disorders and Their Elimination.* Springer.
27. Poretsky, L. (2017). *Principles of Diabetes Mellitus*, 3rd Edition. Springer.
28. Robinson, P. (2018). *The Thyroid Patient's Manual: From Hypothyroidism to Good Health (Recovering from Hypothyroidism).* Elephant in the Room Books.
29. Ruggerio, R. (2017). *Do's & Don'ts of Hypoglycemia: An Everyday Guide to Low Blood Sugar Too Often Misunderstood and Misdiagnosed*, 5th Edition. Frederick Fell Publishers, Inc.
30. Stone, M. (2014). *Hypoglycemia – What It Is, What It Isn't, and How to Fix the Root Problem.* CreateSpace Independent Publishing Platform.
31. Sussan, B.E. (2020). *Most Common Iodine Deficiency Symptoms: Goiter, Bradycardia, Fatigue, Cognitive Problems, Weight Gain, Thin Hair, Dry Skin, Infancy Problems, Increased Sensitivity to Cold.* Sussan.
32. Winzant, J. (2021). *Hypoglycemia Diet – A Beginner's Three-Week Step-by-Step Guide to Managing Hypoglycemia Symptoms, with Curated Recipes and a Sample Seven-Day Meal Plan.* Winzant.

16 Nutritional Effects on the Gastrointestinal System

OUTLINE

LEARNING OBJECTIVES

After study of the chapter, readers should be able to:

1. Describe the causes of dysgeusia.
2. Explain the risks for Barrett's esophagus.
3. Describe the signs and symptoms of Plummer–Vinson syndrome.
4. Explain the causes of gastritis.
5. Discuss which populations in the United States are affected by stomach cancer.
6. Describe the causes of Zollinger-Ellison syndrome.
7. Explain the complications of celiac disease.
8. Discuss the causes of Crohn's disease.
9. Explain the characteristics of colorectal, liver, and pancreatic cancers.
10. Describe tropical pancreatitis and its dietary management.

OVERVIEW

The importance of a healthy diet is well understood, and there is a large variety of effects of adequate or poor nutrition upon the gastrointestinal system. All of the structures of this system may be affected by the foods we eat and the lifestyle choices concerning diet that we make. A large number of conditions can result from poor dietary choices, including inflammation, ulcers, diarrhea, malabsorption, and even cancer. The most common gastrointestinal system cancers include those of the esophagus, stomach, colon, rectum, pancreas, and liver. People that consume high amounts of saturated fats, simple refined carbohydrates, and red meat while not eating enough fruits, vegetables, whole grains, and fiber are at a much higher risk for gastrointestinal disorders. Overall, good digestion and the prevention of these disorders require a diet high in whole grains, leafy greens, lean protein, low-fructose fruits, and healthy fats.

DYSGEUSIA

Dysgeusia is a taste disorder in which individuals experience foods as tasting bitter, metallic, sour, or sweet. Some people experience a bad taste in the mouth when not actually eating anything. Others report enjoying foods they previously disliked, or start disliking foods they previously enjoyed. The causes of dysgeusia include zinc deficiency, vitamin B deficiencies, infections, and certain medications. Dysgeusia differs from **ageusia**. As much as 17% of the global population has some type of dysgeusia.

The prognosis of dysgeusia is good since it usually resolves once the underlying cause is treated. However, some conditions such as dementia can only be managed and not actually treated. In those cases, dysgeusia treatment is focused on improving nutrition and appetite. Preventive measures for dysgeusia include avoiding smoking, keeping hydrated, practicing good oral hygiene, and avoiding contact with COVID-19, since this viral infection caused many cases of dysgeusia in people throughout the world.

For dysgeusia, since taste aversions can ruin enjoyment of favorite foods, it is advised that affected individuals should avoid eating favorite foods while the condition is present. When foods seem too bitter, add sweet fruits, honey or sweetener, marinades (pineapple juice, dressings,

DOI: 10.1201/b22969-19

lemon juice, soy sauce, or sweet-and-sour sauces), and if meat tastes too bitter, eat it cold or at room temperature. In place of meat, eat blandly prepared chicken, fish, mild cheeses, eggs, dairy products, or tofu. All of these foods may taste better if prepared in stews or casseroles. When foods taste too sweet, drink the herbal tea called *Gymnema Sylvestra*, which deadens the taste buds to sweet tastes for approximately 20 minutes. It should be held in the mouth for about 5 minutes before eating. Dilute sweet drinks such as fruit juice with water or ice. Avoid sweet fruits. Vegetables may be more appealing. If foods just taste "off" or "bad", drinking water, tea, ginger ale, or fruit juices mixed with club soda may help remove some of these strange tastes. Hard candies, such as sugar-free mints may be helpful, as may sugar-free gum. Starchy foods such as bread, potatoes, rice, and plain pasta may be more acceptable. If added fat is problematic, do not add butter, margarine, or other fatty substances.

ESOPHAGITIS

Esophagitis is characterized by inflammation of the esophagus, which is the structure that connects the pharynx to the stomach. Swallowed food and liquids normally pass through the esophagus. Esophagitis can develop due to many causes. Gastroesophageal reflux disease (GERD) is the most common cause of esophagitis because of the backflow of acid from the stomach, which can irritate the lining of the esophagus. Other causes include chemical injury by alkaline or acid solutions, nonsteroidal anti-inflammatory drugs (NSAIDs), physical injury resulting from nasogastric tubes, alcohol use disorder, stress, allergies, hernia, surgery, chronic vomiting, and infection. Risk factors include pregnancy, smoking, obesity, alcoholism, spinal cord injury, and radiation therapy for chest tumors.

The symptoms of esophagitis include heartburn, nausea, vomiting, abdominal pain, and cough. Esophagitis can have serious consequences that affect the quality of life. If left untreated, esophagitis may develop into a condition called **Barrett's esophagus**. This may increase the risk for esophageal cancer. Esophagitis can be diagnosed by upper endoscopy, biopsy, upper GI series (or barium swallow), and laboratory tests. Treatments for esophagitis are intended to lessen symptoms, manage complications, and treat underlying causes of the disorder. Treatment strategies vary primarily based on the cause of the disorder. For esophagitis, the diet should include soft vegetables and fruits, dairy products, cereals, and crackers. While eating, chew food completely, taking only small bites, and swallowing slowly. This helps avoid excessive pain from the condition. Other acceptable food choices include chutney, rice, chicken, cucumber, oats, yogurt, beans, fish, sprouts, eggs, peas, and tofu. It is important to avoid or limit French fries, onion rings, butter, fatty or fried meats, bacon, ham, ice cream, potato chips, cream sauces, gravies, creamy salad dressings, tomatoes, chocolate, garlic, spicy foods, caffeine, and mint.

ESOPHAGEAL CANCERS

There are several types of esophageal cancers, of which the most common malignant tumor in the proximal two thirds of the esophagus is **squamous cell carcinoma**. In the distal one third of the esophagus, **adenocarcinoma** is the most common. Esophageal cancer makes up nearly 19,000 cases and over 16,000 deaths in the United States every year. Worldwide, squamous cell carcinoma is the most common type of esophageal cancer, but in the United States, adenocarcinoma is approximately twice as common. It is also four to five times more common in African Americans than in Caucasians, and two to three times more common in males than in females.

Primary risk factors for esophageal cancers are excessive alcohol ingestion and use of any type of tobacco products. Additional risk factors include **achalasia**, infection with the human papillomavirus, ingestion of **lye**, esophageal webs caused by **Plummer–Vinson syndrome**, irradiation of the esophagus, and **sclerotherapy**. Though genetic causes are not fully understood, about half of all patients with the autosomal dominant disorder called **tylosis**, also known as *hyperkeratosis palmaris et plantaris*, have esophageal cancer by the age of 45 years.

Adenocarcinoma of the esophagus is more common. Alcohol is not an important risk factor, though smoking definitely contributes to its development. Adenocarcinoma of the distal esophagus is difficult to identify in comparison with adenocarcinoma of the **gastric cardia** that invades the distal esophagus. The majority of adenocarcinomas arise in Barrett's esophagus, which is caused by chronic gastroesophageal reflux disease and reflux esophagitis. With Barrett's esophagus, the mucosa is **metaplastic**, columnar, glandular, and resembles the structure of the intestines. It has a brush border and **goblet cells** that replace the normal stratified squamous epithelium of the distal esophagus as part of the healing phase of acute esophagitis. Obesity is linked to a 16-times higher increased risk of esophageal adenocarcinoma, likely because obesity contributes to reflux.

Metastatic cancer makes up 3% of all esophageal cancers. The cancers most likely to metastasize to the esophagus are melanoma and breast cancer. Others include cancers of the head, neck, lung, stomach, liver, kidney, prostate, testes, and bones. These tumors usually seed the loose connective tissue stroma that surround the esophagus. Primary esophageal cancers, differently, start to develop in the mucosa or submucosa.

In its early stages, esophageal cancer is usually asymptomatic. Dysphagia usually begins as the lumen of the esophagus becomes constricted to less than 14 mm. After first, the patient has problems swallowing solid food, then semisolid food, and finally, liquid food and saliva cannot be swallowed easily. This steady progression indicates a malignant process, and not a spasm, benign ring, or peptic stricture. If chest pain is present, it usually radiates to the back. Nearly all patients lose weight, even though they still have a good appetite. If there is compression of the recurrent laryngeal nerve, vocal cord paralysis and hoarseness may develop.

Nerve compression can lead to hiccups, spinal pain, or **diaphragm paralysis**. Dyspnea may be caused by **malignant pleural effusions** or pulmonary metastasis. If there is intraluminal tumor involvement, it may cause **odynophagia**, vomiting, aspiration, **hematemesis**, iron deficiency anemia, melena, and cough. Fistulas between the esophagus and tracheobronchial tree may lead to lung abscess and pneumonia. Some patients develop **superior vena cava syndrome**, bone pain and **ascites**. Tumors usually metastasize to the lungs and liver, and sometimes to distant areas such as the bones, brain, heart, adrenal glands, kidneys, and peritoneum.

Unfortunately, there are no screening tests for esophageal cancer. If it is suspected, the patient should have endoscopy with biopsy, and cytology (see Figure 16.1). Barium x-rays can show obstructive lesions, but endoscopy is needed to obtain a tissue diagnosis. If esophageal cancer is identified, a computed tomography (CT) scan of the chest and abdomen is needed to determine tumor spread. If there is no metastasis, an endoscopic ultrasonography should be done to determine tumor depth in the esophageal wall as well as regional lymph node involvement. Therapy and prognosis are aided by the findings. Basic blood tests that include complete blood count, electrolytes, and liver function are required.

The prognosis for esophageal cancer is based on staging. Overall, it is poor, with a five-year survival of less than 5%, since many patients are diagnosed once the disease has advanced. If the cancer is restricted to the mucosa, the survival rate is about 80%. This reduces to less than 50% if the submucosa is involved, and 20% if there is extension to the muscularis propria. When the tumor extends to adjacent structures, survival is at 7%, and with distant metastases, less than 3%.

Treatment decisions are based on staging, tumor size and location, and the wishes of the patient. Patients with stage zero, I, or IIa disease respond well to surgical resection, and preoperative chemotherapy and radiation provide more benefits. Those with stages IIb and III have poor survival if they only receive surgery. Response and survival are improved by preoperative radiation and chemotherapy, to reduce tumor volume. If the patient is unable or unwilling to undergo surgery, combined radiation and chemotherapy may still be beneficial, yet either of these treatments on their own is usually not effective. Patients with stage IV cancer need palliative treatments only and should not have surgery. Later, patients are screened via endoscopy and CT (neck, chest, and abdomen) for recurrence, at six-month intervals for three years, and every year thereafter. If Barrett's esophagus is present, the patient must have aggressive long-term treatment for GERD plus endoscopies to assess malignant transformation at 3–12 month intervals, based on the amount of **metaplasia**.

For superficial, early, and noninvasive cancers may be treated with endoscopic mucosal resection or endoscopic submucosal dissection. Surgical widening of the pylorus is also required. Complications may be quite varied, so any

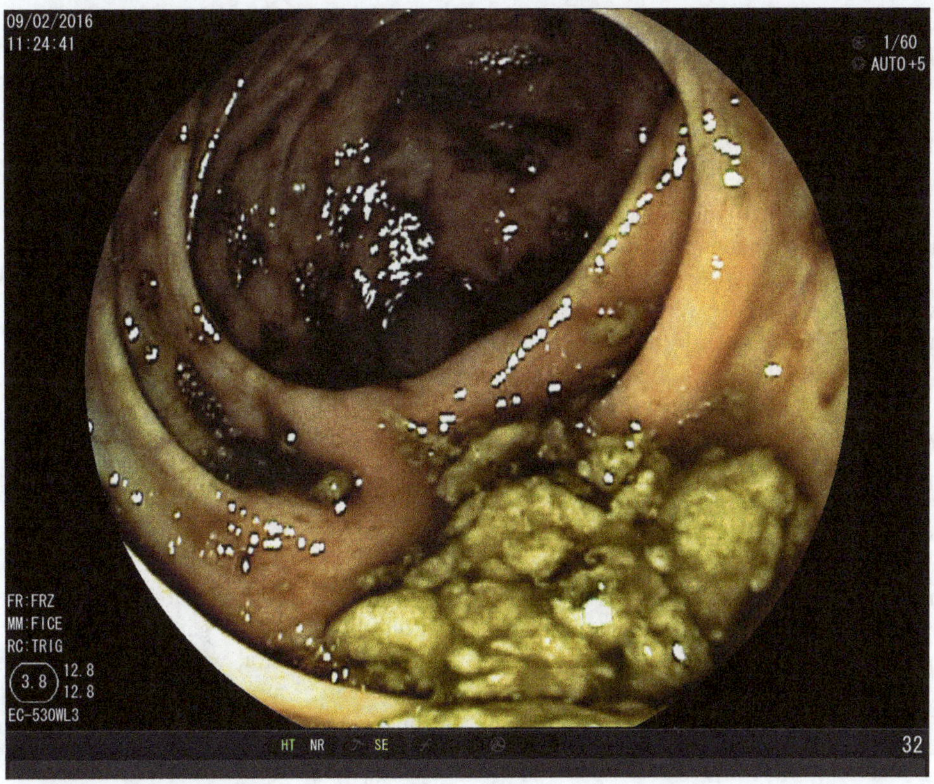

FIGURE 16.1 Endoscopic view of esophageal cancer.

surgical procedure must be determined closely on an individual basis. External beam radiation therapy is usually combined with chemotherapeutic agents such as cisplatin, 5-fluorouracil, mitomycin, doxorubicin, vindesine, bleomycin, and methotrexate. Often, multiple chemotherapeutic agents are combined. Immunotherapy plus chemotherapy is a first-line therapy for advanced esophageal squamous cell cancer. Palliative treatments are directed at reducing esophageal obstructions.

Nutrition for patients with esophageal cancer may be obtained via normal eating or tube feeding, as needed on an individualized basis. A high-calorie, high-protein diet should be followed if the patient is eating less than normal during treatment, to help maintain weight, or if overweight, to lose weight more slowly. The easiest foods that fit these requirement should be chosen. Examples of foods chosen for patients with esophageal cancer, while they are being treated, include beans, chicken salad, eggs, butter, tuna, sunflower seeds, peanut butter, yogurt, ice cream, cottage cheese, shredded cheese, half-and-half, whole milk, cream cheese, sour cream, margarine, oils, mayonnaise, gravy, honey, jam, jelly, chocolate syrup, meal replacement bars, and protein powder. There are also high-calorie, high-protein nutritional supplements in the form of shakes and other types of drinks that may be recommended by nutritionists.

PLUMMER–VINSON SYNDROME

Plummer–Vinson syndrome is a disorder linked to chronic iron deficiency anemia. Small web-like tissue partially blocks the throat and upper esophagus that makes swallowing difficult. Having Plummer–Vinson syndrome may increase the risk of developing esophageal cancer. Also called Paterson-Kelly syndrome and sideropenic dysphagia. The cause of this syndrome is unknown. Genetic factors and nutritional deficiencies may be implicated. The disorder is rare, more common in women than in men, and is linked to esophageal and throat cancers. It is most prevalent between the ages of 19 and 65 years. Signs and symptoms include pallor, glossitis, becoming fatigue easily, tongue atrophy, poor appetite, narrowing of the mouth, increased pigmentation of the mucosa of the mouth, **geophagia**, spoon-shaped nails, **cheilitis**, abdominal pain, **hypochromic microcytic anemia**, and dysphagia. The prognosis of Plummer–Vinson syndrome is excellent since dysphagia and anemia can be effectively treated. However, the prognosis is much worse if there is a related squamous cell carcinoma of the hypopharynx. Prevention involves adequate iron intake, good nutrition, protection against autoimmune processes. If there is a genetic predisposition, the syndrome is not preventable. There is no specific diet that is indicated for Plummer–Vinson syndrome, but foods that are rich in iron are potentially helpful. These include red meats and organ meats, poultry, fish, shellfish, eggs, nuts, dried fruits, whole-meal pasta and bread, iron-fortified bread and breakfast cereals, legumes, dark green leafy vegetables, oats, and tofu.

Test Your Knowledge

1. What is dysgeusia?
2. What are the classifications of esophageal cancers?
3. Which chronic deficiency is linked to Plummer–Vinson syndrome?

GASTRITIS

Gastritis is inflammation of the gastric mucosa. It may be caused by infection with **Helicobacter pylori** (*H. pylori*), NSAIDs, alcohol use, stress, and **atrophic gastritis**. It is classified as either *erosive gastritis* or *nonerosive gastritis*. It is also classified by whether the cardia, body, or antrum of the stomach is involved, and it may be acute or chronic, based on the type of inflammatory cells. Some forms of gastritis involve acid peptic disease and *H. pylori* disease. The term "gastritis" is sometimes applied to nonspecific abdominal discomfort and gastroenteritis. *Acute gastritis* involves polymorphonuclear leukocyte infiltration of the mucosa of the stomach antrum or its body. *Chronic gastritis* involves certain amounts of atrophy or metaplasia. It mostly affects the antrum. If the antrum is mostly affected, there is loss of **G cells** and decreased **gastrin** secretion. If the stomach corpus is involved, there is a loss of the **oxyntic glands**. This leads to reduced acid, pepsin, and *intrinsic factor*.

Proper nutrition for gastritis helps relieve symptoms. Foods to avoid include those that are fried, spicy, or highly acidic. Other troublesome foods include alcohol, carbonated drinks, coffee, fatty foods, pickled foods, and tea. Foods and drinks that may help ease symptoms include whole grains, fruits, vegetables, beans, fish, lean meats, noncarbonated drinks, and caffeine-free drinks. Probiotics may be needed to help with stomach complications caused by *H. pylori*. Probiotic foods include kombucha, yogurt, kimchi, and sauerkraut. Eating smaller, more frequent meals may help ease symptoms. Some types of gastritis make it more difficult to absorb iron or vitamin B12 in small intestine, which can lead to deficiencies. Therefore, mineral or vitamin supplements may be needed.

PEPTIC ULCERS

Peptic ulcer involves erosions or ulcers in the stomach or duodenum (see Figure 16.2). Ulcers can be in various sizes. Erosions are more superficial than ulcers. Most commonly, ulcers develop in middle-aged adults. The majority cases are caused by *H. pylori* infection or by excessive use of NSAIDs. *H. pylori* infection is present in 60% of duodenal ulcers and 40% of gastric ulcers. Cigarette smoking is a proven risk factor, with higher incidence in people that smoke a larger number of cigarettes every day. Moderate alcohol use is not implicated. Signs and symptoms of peptic ulcer are based on patient age and location of the ulcer. Though sometimes asymptomatic, pain is the most common symptom, which is relieved by food or antacids.

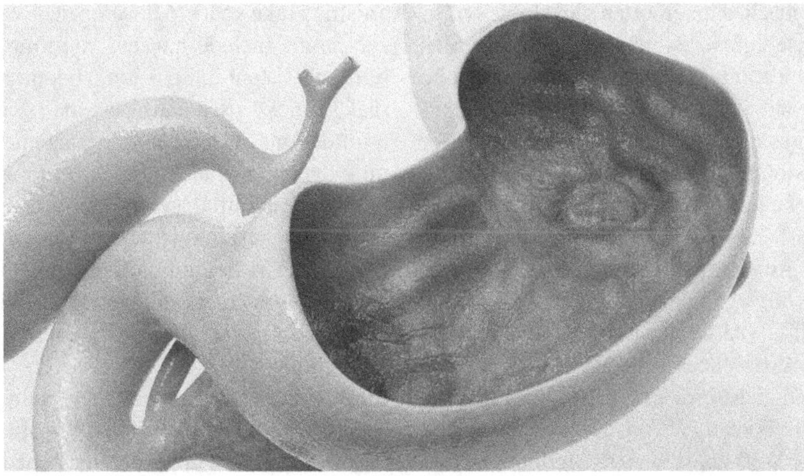

FIGURE 16.2 Peptic ulcer.

It usually recurs chronically. Obstructive symptoms such as bloating, nausea, and vomiting are due to edema and scarring. Duodenal ulcers usually cause pain that is more consistent, usually appearing in the mid-morning hours, relieved by food, but then recurring 2–3 hours after a meal. If a patient is awaked by pain at night, this highly suggests a duodenal ulcer. The diagnosis of peptic ulcer disease is via patient history and endoscopy, and if needed, biopsy, cytologic brushing, CT, or magnetic resonance imaging (MRI). Complications of peptic ulcer include GI hemorrhage and perforation. The prognosis of peptic ulcer is excellent once the underlying cause is successfully treated. Recurrence may be prevented by maintaining adequate hygiene, and by avoiding alcohol, smoking, and NSAIDs. However, recurrence is common, usually occurring in more than 60% of cases.

For peptic ulcers, treatment options include antibiotics, medications that block acid production and promote healing, medications that reduce acid production, antacids that neutralize stomach acid, and medications that protect the linings of the stomach and small intestine. For *H. pylori*, antibiotics may include amoxicillin, clarithromycin, metronidazole, tinidazole, tetracycline, and levofloxacin. They are usually taken for about two weeks along with proton pump inhibitors, and sometimes, bismuth subsalicylate. Proton pump inhibitors (PPIs) block the action of the **parietal cells** that produce stomach acid. They include prescription and over-the-counter options, such as omeprazole, lansoprazole, rabeprazole, esomeprazole, and pantoprazole. However, long-term use of PPIs may increase risks of bone fractures, so calcium supplements may be needed. Histamine (H_2) blockers reduce the amount of stomach acid. They include famotidine, cimetidine, and nizatidine. Antacids neutralize existing stomach acid, to provide rapid pain relief, though side effects can include constipation or diarrhea based on the main ingredients.

The recommended diet for peptic ulcer begins with foods that contain probiotics. These include yogurt, miso soup, kimchi, sauerkraut, kombucha, and tempeh. They help fight *H. pylori* infections and also assist with other treatments. Fiber-rich foods such as apples, pears, and oatmeal help lower the amount of stomach acid, easing bloating and pain. High-fiber diets can even help prevent ulcers from developing. Sweet potatoes are rich in vitamin A, and can help shrink stomach ulcers as well as prevent them. Other foods high in vitamin A include spinach, carrots, cantaloupe, and beef liver. Red bell peppers are rich in vitamin C, which helps heal ulcers. This vitamin is also highly prevalent in citrus fruits, strawberries, kiwis, and broccoli.

The worst food choices for peptic ulcer include milk, because it can prompt the stomach to make more acid, alcohol (ideally, avoiding it completely), fatty or fried foods, spicy foods (for most but not all people), citrus fruits (not for everyone), chocolate (for most but not all people), and too many drinks such as coffee and soda if they contain caffeine.

STOMACH CANCER

Gastric cancer remains one of the most common and deadly cancers worldwide, especially among older males. Stomach cancer mostly affects older people. The average age of diagnosis is 68. About six of every ten people diagnosed with stomach cancer each year are 65 or older. While stomach cancer has become less common in the United States, it is still much more common in some other parts of the world, particularly in East Asia. It remains one of the leading causes of cancer-related deaths in the world. Stomach cancer is the 5th most common neoplasm and the 3rd most deadly cancer, with an estimated 783,000 deaths in 2018. Stomach cancer incidence and mortality are highly variable by region and significantly dependent on diet and *H. pylori* infection. Stomach cancer is caused by a variety of factors, which include *pernicious anemia*, *H. pylori* infection, smoking, being overweight or obese, a diet high in certain foods (pickled, salty, or smoked), chronic alcohol use, surgery for a stomach ulcer, having type-A blood, and family history of gastric cancer.

A person with stomach cancer often develops symptoms late in the disease course, which include early satiety, obstruction, and bleeding. Stomach cancer makes up nearly 28,000 cases and just over 11,000 deaths annually in the United States alone. Cases have declined over recent decades, and stomach cancer is now the seventh most common cause of cancer death. In the United States, the most commonly affected populations include African Americans, Hispanic Americans, and Native Americans. Incidence increases with age, since more than 75% of patients are older than 50 years. However, stomach cancer is common with wide differences between countries. The ten countries with the highest incidence include Mongolia, Japan, South Korea, Tajikistan, China, Kyrgyzstan, Cabo Verde (an island off the West coast of Africa), Bhutan, Iran, and Kazakhstan (see Figure 16.3). Nearly all (95%) malignant tumors of the stomach are *gastric adenocarcinomas*. The World Health Organization has reported a positive link between stomach cancer and the consumption of processed meat. Stomach cancer may be preceded by gastric polyps. Stomach cancer is much more likely if an adenomatous polyp is more than 2 cm in diameter. All polyps discovered during endoscopy should be removed since malignant transformation cannot be detected by inspection.

Affected individuals usually develop gastric cancer at an average age of 38. Women with the stomach cancer also have a high risk for lobular breast cancer. Stomach cancer usually has nonspecific symptoms initially and is often mistaken for a peptic ulcer. Patients are often treated for a stomach acid abnormality, and it is not until later that the symptoms start to change. Early satiety after eating only a small amount of food may indicate that a tumor is obstructing the pyloric region. The cancer is usually slow-growing and may take years to develop. The early warning signs and symptoms include nausea, vomiting, poor appetite, heartburn, persistent indigestion, abdominal pain, upper abdominal fullness after eating a small amount of food, asities, unintentional weight loss, hematemesis, **melena**, and anemia. Secondary anemia may occur after **occult** blood loss. Sometimes, initial symptoms are due to metastasis, and include ascites, and jaundice. Occasionally, the only physical finding is **heme-positive stools**. Later findings include an epigastric mass, enlargement of lymph nodes, hepatomegaly, and a rectal or ovarian mass.

Treatment of stomach cancers is generally **gastrectomy**. After total gastrectomy, vitamin B12 deficiency may develop. The administration of intrinsic factor with vitamin B12 is required. People that have had a partial or total gastrectomy need sublingual, or injections of the vitamin B12. Levels of vitamin B12 that are below 200 picograms per milliliter (pg/mL) may indicate a deficiency.

Overall prognosis for stomach cancer is poor, with five-year survival less than 5%–15% of patients. This is because by the time of presentation, the disease is often very advanced. The five-year survival can be up to 80% if the tumor is only in the mucosa or submucosa. Tumors of the local lymph nodes have a 20%–40% five-year survival. The gastric lymphomas have the best prognosis of the various stomach malignancies.

There is no proven method of preventing stomach cancer, but there are ways to lower the risks for the disease. Keeping at a healthy weight by getting regular physical activity and consuming a good diet is important. Plenty of fresh fruits and vegetables are protective against stomach cancer. Red and processed meats, sugar-sweetened beverages, and highly processed foods should be limited. Avoiding

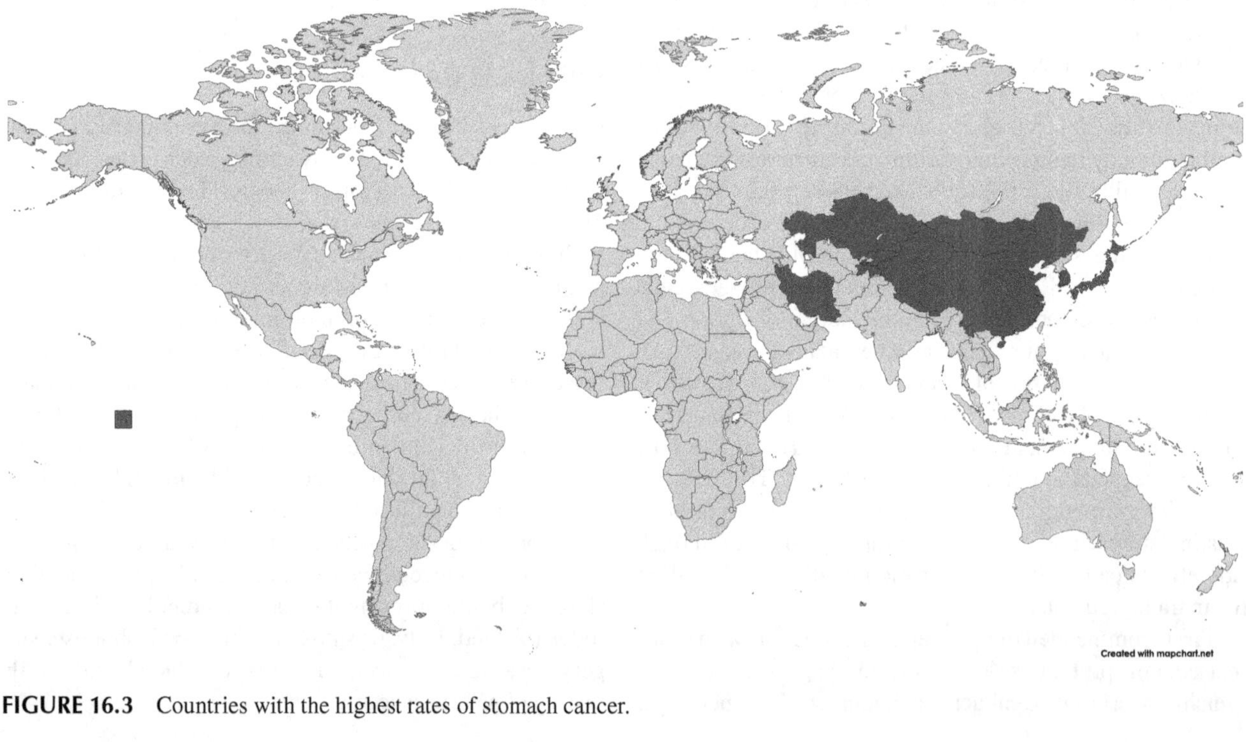

FIGURE 16.3 Countries with the highest rates of stomach cancer.

or limiting alcohol also lowers risks. Dietary supplements and drinking green tea are under study in regards to reducing stomach cancer risks. Smoking increases the risks of stomach cancer. Studies are also ongoing about preventing *Helicobacter pylori* infections. Use of aspirin, ibuprofen or naproxen appears to lower risks for stomach cancer. Dietary modification, smoking cessation, and exercise hold promise in preventing gastric cancer, while genetic testing is helping to achieve earlier diagnoses and greater survival rates.

Test Your Knowledge

1. How common is stomach cancer in the United States compared to worldwide?
2. What is the overall prognosis for stomach cancer?
3. What are the complications of total gastrectomy?

DIARRHEA

Though diarrhea is very common and is caused by many different conditions, it is also linked to deficiencies of protein, niacin, folate, and vitamin B12. The stool is made up of 60%–90% water. In westernized countries, approximately 100–200 grams of stool is excreted per day in healthy adults. In infants, this is 10 g/kg/day, based on how much unabsorbable dietary material is consumed, which is primarily carbohydrates. Diarrhea is defined as a stool weight of more than 200 grams per day, though it is commonly believed that any increased fluidity of the stool signifies diarrhea. Many people that ingest fiber have bulkier, formed stools that are not thought of as diarrhea. If a person frequently passes small volumes of stool, such as accompanying **tenesmus**, this is not diarrhea. Fecal incontinence is also sometimes confused with diarrhea. Also, diarrhea can cause a significant worsening of fecal incontinence. Aside from nutrient deficiencies, other causes of acute diarrhea include the following:

- Viral infections (norovirus, rotavirus)
- Bacterial infections (*Campylobacter, Salmonella, Shigella* species, *Escherichia coli, Clostridioides difficile*)
- Parasitic infections (*Cryptosporidia* species, *Giardia* species, *Entamoeba histolytica*)
- Food poisoning (*Bacillus cereus, Clostridium perfringens, Staphylococci*)
- Drugs (antineoplastic drugs, many antibiotics, caffeine, colchicine, excipients such as lactose as part of elixirs, laxatives, magnesium-containing antacids, prostaglandin analogs, and quinine/quinidine). Some of these drugs also cause chronic diarrhea.

Also, chronic diarrhea can be caused by functional problems such as **irritable bowel syndrome**, dietary factors (fructose, hexitols, sorbitol, mannitol, lactose, magnesium, olestra), **malabsorption syndromes** (carbohydrate intolerance but especially lactose intolerance, *celiac disease*), pancreatic insufficiency, small intestinal bacterial overgrowth, colon adenoma or carcinoma, **carcinoid tumor**, and **mastocytosis**.

The complications of diarrhea include dehydration, electrolyte loss, and sometimes, vascular collapse. This condition can occur quickly when diarrhea is severe, in patients with **cholera**. Severe or chronic diarrhea can cause hypokalemia and hypomagnesemia.

The prognosis for diarrhea is usually good. In most cases, symptoms resolve in a few days. However, prognosis is worsened if diarrhea leads to dehydration, since it can be life-threatening if untreated. Prevention of diarrhea involves adequate consumption of protein, niacin, folate, and vitamin B12. Other measures of preventing diarrhea from different etiologies include safe drinking water, good sanitation, hand washing with soap, exclusive breastfeeding for the first six months of life, good personal and food hygiene, health education about the spread of infection, and the rotavirus vaccination.

For diarrhea, patients should avoid foods that cause the condition to worsen, or that cause cramping or gas. Foods that produce gas include carbonated drinks, beer, beans, cabbage, broccoli, cauliflower, highly spiced foods, and chewing gum. Room temperature foods may be better tolerated than very hot or very cold foods. Fluids and minerals need to be replaced with water, broth, fruit juices, sports beverages, and popsicles. Potassium is needed as part of managing diarrhea, so high-potassium foods include ripe bananas, apricot or peach nectar, potatoes, fish, and meat. It is important to drink fluids between meals in order to avoid dehydration brought on by diarrhea. Small amounts of food should be consumed frequently throughout the day. Fatty foods must be reduced or avoided, such as fried foods, sauces, gravy, salad dressings, and highly spiced foods. All foods with laxative effects must be avoided, including prunes and prune juice. If milk is not a regular part of the patient's diet, it should be avoided while diarrhea is present. It is important to consume well-cooked, tender meats as well as smooth peanut butter.

Test Your Knowledge

1. What are the causes of acute diarrhea?
2. What are the complications of diarrhea?
3. What are the causes of chronic diarrhea?

MALABSORPTION SYNDROMES

Malabsorption is insufficient **assimilation** of foods because of defective digestion, absorption, or transport. It may affect macronutrients, micronutrients, or both. Malabsorption causes excessive excretion of feces, GI symptoms, and nutritional deficiencies. The condition may involve impaired absorption of nearly all nutrients, or be isolated to only certain nutrients. There are three phases of digestion and absorption, though the first one is better explained as *maldigestion* when there is an impairment:

- *Intraluminal hydrolysis via enzymes* – fats, proteins, and carbohydrates are digested, with bile salts enhancing the solubilization of fat
- *Digestion by brush border enzymes* – with uptake of end-products
- *Lymphatic transport of nutrients*

Lipase and colipase, which are pancreatic enzymes, split long-chain triglycerides into monoglycerides and fatty acids. These end-products combine with bile acids and phospholipids, forming **micelles**, which pass through the jejunal enterocytes. The absorbed fatty acids are resynthesized, combining with protein, cholesterol, and phospholipid to form **chylomicrons**. These are carried by the lymphatic system. Medium-chain triglycerides undergo direct absorption. Fats that are not absorbed trap the fat-soluble vitamins and some minerals, resulting in deficiency. Bacterial overgrowth causes **deconjugation** and **dihydroxylation** of bile salts, and fat absorption is limited. When unabsorbed bile salts stimulate water secretion in the large intestine, diarrhea results.

Amylase plus the brush border enzymes on the microvilli, lyse carbohydrates and disaccharides, to form monosaccharides. Unabsorbed carbohydrates are fermented by bacteria in the large intestine, forming carbon dioxide, hydrogen, **methane**, and short-chain fatty acids that include acetate, butyrate, lactate, and propionate. Diarrhea is caused by these fatty acids. The gases that are produced cause bloating and abdominal distention.

Digestion of proteins within the stomach is started by gastric **pepsin**, which also stimulates the release of **cholecystokinin**. The secretion of pancreatic enzymes requires cholecystokinin. The brush border enzyme known as **enterokinase** activates trypsinogen into **trypsin**. This converts many of the pancreatic proteases into their active forms. Proteins are hydrolyzed into oligopeptides by active pancreatic enzymes. The oligopeptides are then directly absorbed, or hydrolyzed into amino acids.

There are many different causes of malabsorption. Celiac disease is an example of a disorder that impairs absorption of most nutrients, vitamins, and trace minerals. Other disorders, such as pernicious anemia, only impairs absorption of certain nutrients. If more than 90% of function is lost, malabsorption is caused by pancreatic insufficiency. Increased luminal acidity, as in **Zollinger-Ellison syndrome**, inhibits digestion of lipase and fat. Cholestasis and cirrhosis reduce bile synthesis in the liver or the delivery of bile salts to the duodenum. Acute infections can cause transient malabsorption. This is probably due to acute superficial damage to the Zollinger-Ellison syndrome and microvilli. Chronic bacterial infections of the small intestine are rare, except for **blind loop syndrome**, systemic sclerosis, and **diverticula**, in which there may be small intestinal bacterial overgrowth. Intestinal bacteria diverticula may consume dietary vitamin B12 and other nutrients, to interfere with enzyme systems and result in mucosal injury.

Unabsorbed substances, especially when there is malabsorption of many nutrients can cause abdominal bloating, diarrhea, gas, and **steatorrhea**. Additional symptoms are due to nutritional deficiencies. The affected individual eats adequate amounts of food yet loses weight. The most common symptom is chronic diarrhea. The hallmark sign of malabsorption is steatorrhea, which occurs when more than seven grams of fat per day are excreted. The stool is bulky, greasy, foul-smelling, and pale in color. In advanced malabsorption, there are severe vitamin and mineral deficiencies. Symptoms are based on the specific nutrient deficiency, as follows:

- *Iron* – hypochromic or microcytic anemia
- *Folate and vitamin B12* – macrocytic anemia
- *Vitamins C and K* – bleeding, bruising, and petechiae
- *Calcium and magnesium* – carpopedal spasm
- *Proteins* – edema
- *Vitamins B1, B2, B3, B6, B12, and folate, iron, niacin* – glossitis
- *Vitamin A* – night blindness
- *Calcium, magnesium, potassium, vitamin D* – pain in the limbs and bones; pathologic fractures
- *Vitamins B1, B2, B12* – peripheral neuropathy

Vitamin B12 deficiency can occur in *blind loop syndrome*, or following an extensive resection of the stomach or distal ileum. With mild malabsorption, iron deficiency may be the only present symptom. Undernutrition may cause amenorrhea. This is an important feature of celiac disease in young women.

For malabsorption syndromes, patients may be put on a special diet of foods that are more easily digested and absorbed, as well as given nutritional supplements. Dietary therapy includes a high-protein, high-calorie, low-fat diet, which will help minimize steatorrhea. Adequate therapy requires monitoring of serum calcium, magnesium, vitamin D, and parathyroid hormone levels, and ideally, 24-hour urinary collections for calcium. Supplementation of these mineral deficiencies requires continual close observation to prevent hypercalcemia. Foods high in calcium include dairy products, soybeans, dark green leafy vegetables, calcium-fortified foods, salmon, figs, flour tortillas, and baked beans. Foods high in magnesium include many of the same choices, as well as nuts, seeds, whole grains, wheat germ, and wheat and oat bran. Foods high in vitamin D include cod liver oil, swordfish, tuna, fortified orange juice, fortified dairy and plant milks, sardines, and beef liver.

FOCUS ON MALABSORPTION SYNDROMES

Malabsorption syndromes are digestive disorders that prevent the body from effectively absorbing nutrients in foods. In most cases, these syndromes result from damage to the mucous lining of the small intestine, which is where most absorption occurs. Malabsorption syndromes can lead to indigestion as well as malnutrition.

FOCUS ON ZOLLINGER-ELLISON SYNDROME

Zollinger-Ellison syndrome is a rare condition in which one or more tumors grow in the pancreas or in the upper part of the small intestine. The tumors are called gastrinomas. These gastrinomas produce large amounts of the hormone gastrin.

Test Your Knowledge

1. What are the three phases of digestion and absorption?
2. Which are the causes of malabsorption?
3. What is the hallmark sign of a malabsorption syndrome?

Celiac Disease

Celiac disease is also known as **gluten enteropathy**. It is an immunologically mediated disease. Celiac disease occurs in people that are genetically susceptible, occurring from an intolerance to gluten. This results in mucosal inflammation and villous atrophy in small intestine, causing malabsorption. The actual sensitivity is to the *gliadin* fraction of gluten (a wheat protein). There are similar proteins in barley and rye. An inflammatory response results in the distinct small-intestine mucosal and villous atrophy.

People of northern European descent are commonly affected. The disorder may affect 1 of every 150 European people (mostly in Ireland and Italy), and as many as 1 of every 250 Americans. However, there are estimated prevalence rates as high as 1 of every 100 people in Northern Africa, Northern India, and Southern Asia. Celiac disease affects 10%–20% of first-degree relatives. Women are affected twice as often as men, with onset usually during childhood, though it can occur later. Risks for celiac disease are higher in people that have **Down syndrome**, lymphocytic colitis, Hashimoto thyroiditis, and type 1 diabetes mellitus.

Signs and symptoms are wide-ranging, with some people being asymptomatic, having signs of a nutritional deficiency, or having extreme GI symptoms. Celiac disease can appear during infancy and childhood, once cereals are introduced into the diet. There will be apathy, failure to thrive, anorexia, generalized **hypotonia**, pallor, abdominal distention, and muscle wasting. The stool is bulky, clay-colored, foul-smelling, and soft. Older children may have anemia or slowed growth. Anorexia, **lassitude**, and weakness are the most common signs in adults. The presenting symptom may be mild, intermittent diarrhea. Steatorrhea can be mild, with 7 grams of fat excreted per day, or severe, up to 50 grams per day. Weight loss may occur, but is usually only slight. The patients often have anemia, angular stomatitis, **aphthous ulcers**, and glossitis (see Figure 16.4). Often, there are signs of calcium and vitamin D deficiencies, including osteomalacia, osteopenia, and osteoporosis. Fertility may be reduced in women and men, and menstrual periods may not occur in affected women. Approximately 10% of patients have dermatitis herpetiformis, an extremely itchy papulovesicular rash. It is distributed symmetrically over the scalp, shoulders, elbows, buttocks, and knees. The rash is often induced by a diet that is high in glutens.

There are complications that can arise from celiac disease. These include **collagenous sprue**, intestinal lymphomas, and **refractory disease**. Between 6% and 8% of patients develop intestinal lymphomas, usually after celiac disease has been present for 20–40 years. There is increased incidence of other GI cancers, such as carcinoma of the esophagus or oropharynx, and small-intestine adenocarcinoma. A gluten-free diet can greatly reduce risks for cancer. This diet consists of whole foods such as fruits, vegetables, meat, and eggs, as well as processed gluten-free foods like gluten-free bread or pasta. If a person has followed this diet for a long time, but then develops symptoms of celiac disease again, an upper endoscopy is usually performed with small-intestine biopsy, with or without capsule endoscopy, to assess the presence of intestinal lymphoma. After adequate treatment and regular medical follow-up, the prognosis for celiac disease is excellent. Those that are not treated or do not respond to treatment may have disease complications or a shortened lifespan. Prevention requires a gluten-free diet to prevent symptoms as well as damage to the small intestine. All foods containing wheat, rye, or barley must be avoided.

Test Your Knowledge

1. Which group of people is mostly affected by Celiac disease?
2. What are the signs and symptoms of Celiac disease?
3. What is the likelihood of cancer in relation to Celiac disease?

Carbohydrate Intolerance

Carbohydrate intolerance involves an inability to digest some carbohydrates because of a lack of one or several intestinal enzymes. This malabsorption syndrome occurs when undigested disaccharides cause an osmotic load to attract water and electrolytes into the intestine. The result is watery diarrhea. As carbohydrates are fermented by bacteria, carbon dioxide, hydrogen, and methane gases are produced. There is excessive flatulence, bloating, distension, and abdominal pain.

Enzyme deficiencies can be congenital, acquired (primary), or secondary. Congenital deficiencies include rare deficiencies of lactase or **sucrase–isomaltase**. *Acquired lactase deficiency*, or *primary adult* **hypolactasia**, is the most common type of carbohydrate intolerance. The lactase levels are high in neonates to allow for digestion of milk. In most ethnic groups, including over 90% of Asians and about 80% of African Americans and Hispanics, levels decrease

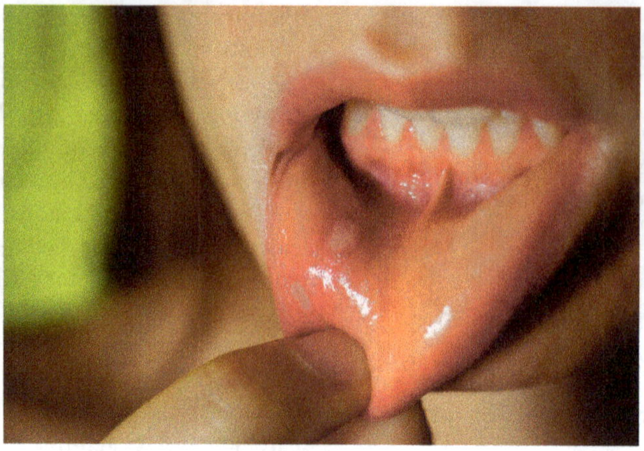

FIGURE 16.4 Aphthous ulcers.

after weaning. This means that older children and adults become unable to digest large amounts of lactose. Between 80% and 85% of Caucasians from Northwest European heritage produce lactase throughout life, and can digest milk or milk products. It has not been determined why the normal state of more than 75% of the global population is labeled as a deficiency. *Secondary lactase deficiency* is caused by damage to the small-intestine mucosa, such as from celiac disease, acute intestinal infections, or **tropical sprue**. In infants, enteric infections or abdominal surgery can be complicated by a temporary, secondary disaccharidase deficiency. When there is recovery from the underlying disease, there will be an increase in the enzyme's activity.

Signs and symptoms of carbohydrate intolerance are nearly the same in all disaccharidase deficiencies. If a child cannot tolerate lactose, diarrhea will occur after ingesting large amounts of milk. The child may not gain weight. Affected adults may have bloating, watery diarrhea, excessive flatus, **borborygmi**, nausea, and abdominal cramps after they ingest lactose. Early in life, children may find that dairy products cause GI problems, so these products are avoided. To cause symptoms, more than 8–12 ounces (250–375 mL) of milk must be ingested. The diarrhea may be so severe that other nutrients are purged before they are able to be absorbed. Symptoms mimic those of irritable bowel syndrome. Prognosis is variable since there is no available cure. Carbohydrate intolerance cannot be prevented since the causes of the enzyme deficiency are unknown.

For carbohydrate intolerance, foods containing high amounts of high-fructose corn syrup, dextrose, and raw sugar should be consumed as sparingly as possible, since they spike insulin levels without providing any solid nutrition. Instead, patients should consume foods that contain more dietary fiber (whole grains, beans, and vegetables). More lean proteins and high-quality fats should be incorporated. Instead of totally restricting carbohydrate intake, it is better to incorporate lean proteins, healthy fats, and fruits and vegetables with high levels of dietary fiber. Healthy fats include olive oil, avocados, nuts, and seeds. These choices slow digestion and absorption, allowing for a more stable rise in blood sugar. Fermented foods such as kefir and sauerkraut, along with probiotic supplementation, are indicated to help the body break down carbohydrates more efficiently. Digestive enzymes are a good option, which assist with carbohydrate metabolism. Bone broth is one of the most healing foods for the gastrointestinal tract.

FOCUS ON CARBOHYDRATE INTOLERANCE

Carbohydrate intolerance is the inability of the small intestine to break down certain carbohydrates efficiently so that they can be used as an energy source. Signs of carbohydrate intolerance include bloating, fatigue, or craving sweet foods after eating a meal. One of the most common forms of carbohydrate intolerance is lactose intolerance.

Test Your Knowledge

1. How does carbohydrate intolerance develop?
2. What is the most common type of carbohydrate intolerance?
3. What is secondary lactase deficiency?

Bacterial Overgrowth Syndrome

Bacterial overgrowth syndrome, also called small intestinal bacterial overgrowth, can be caused by altered intestinal anatomy or GI motility, as well as by a lack of gastric acid secretion. The results of this syndrome can be vitamin deficiencies, malabsorption of fat, and undernutrition. Normally, the proximal small intestine contains mostly gram-positive aerobic bacteria. This low count is regulated by normal **peristalsis** and gastric acid secretion, mucus, an intact **ileocecal valve**, and secretory **immunoglobulin A** (IgA).

Bacterial overgrowth can occur because of anatomic alterations of the stomach, the small intestine, or both

– which promote stasis of the intestinal contents. Conditions causing or requiring anatomic alterations include small-intestine diverticulosis, post-gastrectomy states, **surgical blind loops**, partial obstruction, or strictures. Bacterial clearance can also be impaired by intestinal motility disorders. These may be related to diabetic neuropathy, amyloidosis, systemic sclerosis, hypothyroidism, and idiopathic intestinal pseudo-obstruction. In older people, bacterial overgrowth may be caused by achlorhydria and idiopathic changes in intestinal motility.

The most common bacterial species involved include streptococci, *Bacteroides*, Escherichia, *Lactobacillus*, *Klebsiella*, and *Aeromonas*. Nutrients are consumed by the excessive bacteria, including carbohydrates and vitamin B12. This leads to deprivation of calories and vitamin B12 deficiency. Bile salts are deconjugated by the bacteria. There is failure of micelle formation and a resultant malabsorption of fat. Severe bacterial overgrowth also damages the intestinal mucosa. Diarrhea can be caused by mucosal damage and fat malabsorption. The most common symptom is bloating, but additional symptoms include abdominal discomfort, diarrhea, and excessive flatulence. Diarrhea or steatorrhea may become extreme. Prognosis is variable since the syndrome can recur, and can lead to dehydration and malnutrition without treatment. The syndrome is preventable with accurate diagnosis, treatment, management of underlying conditions that slow gut motility, more exercise, less snacking, avoiding food poisoning, changing the diet to include more plants and nutrients, managing stress, undergoing intestinal massage, and practicing good food safety guidelines.

For bacterial overgrowth syndrome, foods to eliminate include those that fructose, lactose, fructans, galactans, and **polyols**. This means that foods to eliminate include high-fructose corn syrup, agave nectar, honey, soda and other soft drinks, garlic, onions, asparagus, butternut squash, cauliflower, artichokes, beans, apples, dried fruits, sausage, flavored yogurt, ice cream, sweetened cereals, barley, rye, grains, and peas. Foods that are acceptable for bacterial overgrowth syndrome include meat, fish, eggs, gluten-free crackers, oatmeal, unsweetened cereal, spaghetti squash, summer squash, broccoli (in small amounts only), leafy greens, carrots, rice, gluten-free noodles, olives, peanuts, potatoes, pumpkin, quinoa, seeds, blueberries, grapes, oranges, and strawberries.

Crohn's Disease

Crohn's disease is a chronic transmural inflammatory bowel disease. It is also known as *granulomatous ileitis*, *granulomatous ileocolitis*, and *regional enteritis*. In most cases, the distal ileum and colon are affected, though effects can occur anywhere in the GI tract. The disease starts with **crypt** inflammation and abscesses that can progress to tiny focal aphthoid ulcers. These lesions of the mucosa may form deep longitudinal and transverse ulcers along with mucosal edema. As the inflammation undergoes transmural spread, there is lymphedema and thickening of the bowel wall and **mesentery**. The mesenteric fat usually extends onto the serosal surface of the intestine. Significant inflammation may cause hypertrophy of the muscularis mucosae, fibrosis, and the formation of strictures – leading to bowel obstruction. The causes of Crohn's disease are not yet well understood, but recent research suggests that deficiencies of the immune system, as well as hereditary, genetic, and environmental causes must be considered. The disease can occur at any age, it is most prevalent in adolescents and adults between the ages of 15 and 35.

Abscesses commonly occur. Fistulas often extend into nearby structures such as other loops of bowel. The fistulas can extend to the skin of the anterior abdomen or flanks. Aside from intra-abdominal disease, perianal fistulas and abscesses develop in 25%–33% of cases, and are often the most severe aspects of Crohn's disease. There may be non-caseating **granulomas** in the lymph nodes, liver, peritoneum, and all layers of the intestinal wall. Granulomas are not found in about 50% of cases, but they definitely indicate that Crohn's disease is present. Granulomas do not seem to affect the course of the disease. The diseased intestinal segments are sharply demarcated from nearby normal regions, called *skip areas*. This is where the name *regional enteritis* is derived from. Approximately 45% of cases involve the ileum and colon. About 35% of cases involve just the ileum, and about 20% involve only the colon. The rectum is usually unaffected by the disease. If the entire small intestine is affected, the condition is known as **jejunoileitis**. Only rarely are the stomach, duodenum, or esophagus greatly affected.

In affected small-intestine areas, there is an increased risk of cancer. Chronic disease increases long-term risks of colorectal cancer that are equivalent to those of **ulcerative colitis** with the same disease extent and duration. Chronic malabsorption may result in nutritional deficiencies – mostly of vitamins B12 and D. A rare complication is **toxic megacolon syndrome**.

Most commonly, signs and symptoms of Crohn's disease include chronic diarrhea, abdominal pain and tenderness, a sometimes palpable mass or fullness, fever, anorexia, and weight loss. Except for isolated colonic disease that mimics ulcerative colitis, gross rectal bleeding is uncommon. The condition of the abdomen may be similar to acute appendicitis or an intestinal obstruction. About one of every three patients has perianal fissures or fistulas that can be severe. In children, extraintestinal signs and symptoms are often more serious than the GI symptoms. Presenting symptoms include arthritis, anemia, fever of an unknown origin, and growth retardation. Abdominal pain and diarrhea are sometimes not present.

Signs and symptoms are varied when the disease recurs. Pain is the most common symptom with simple recurrence and formation of abscesses. If there is a severe flare-up or abscess, the patient usually has significant tenderness, guarding of the abdomen, rebound, and an overall appearance of toxicity. Stenotic segments may cause bowel obstruction that results in colicky pain, distention, constipation, and vomiting. After any previous surgery, adhesions can also cause bowel obstruction that comes up quickly with no prodrome of fever, malaise, and pain that is usually seen from an obstruction caused by a flare-up. **Pneumaturia** can be caused by an enterovesical fistula. There may be draining of cutaneous fistulas. If the disease is chronic, signs and symptoms may include fever, malnutrition, extraintestinal manifestations of inflammatory bowel disease, and weight loss. There is no single test to diagnose Crohn's disease. However, a combination of tests may help to confirm the diagnosis, including blood tests, stool studies for occult blood, colonoscopy, CT scan, and MRI.

There is currently no cure for Crohn's disease, and there is no single treatment that works for everyone. One goal of medical treatment is to reduce the inflammation that triggers the signs and symptoms. Another goal is to improve long-term prognosis by limiting complications. In the best cases, this may lead not only to symptom relief but also to long-term remission.

The prognosis for Crohn's disease is varied due to intermittent exacerbations and remissions. If the disease is severe, the pain can be frequent and debilitating. Outcomes are improved with careful choices of medications and surgery. Disease-related death is extremely low. The leading cause of excessive disease-related death is GI cancers of the small and large intestines. Often during active Crohn's colitis, thromboembolic complications can lead to death. Approximately 10% of patients are disabled by Crohn's disease and its complications. There is no method of prevention, but symptoms and flare-ups can be minimized by stopping smoking and eating a healthy, low-fat diet.

While there is no special diet proven to help the symptoms of Crohn's disease, some foods cause the condition to worsen, such as foods high in dietary fiber and fat, dairy products, and carbonated beverages. Patient should eat small meals every 3–4 hours, and stay hydrated by drinking small amounts of water throughout the day. When symptoms are not present, they can eat whole grains and a variety of fruits and vegetables. It is important to start new foods one at a time, in small amounts. When symptoms are present, such as diarrhea or abdominal pain, it is important to avoid high-fiber foods, raw and gas-producing vegetables, most raw fruits, and beverages that contain caffeine.

FOCUS ON CROHN'S DISEASE

Crohn's disease can affect any part of the GI tract from the mouth to the anus, but most commonly affects the end of the small intestine and the beginning of the colon. It can also affect the entire thickness of the bowel wall. Crohn's disease often reduces a person's lifespan by at least several years.

Test Your Knowledge

1. How can bacterial overgrowth occur in the GI system?
2. How can Crohn's disease cause bowel obstruction?
3. What are the causes of Crohn's disease?

SHORT BOWEL SYNDROME

Short bowel syndrome is a condition in which the body is unable to absorb enough nutrients from the foods we eat because the patients do not have enough small intestine. Food is pushed through the bowel over an average of 24–72 hours. Muscular peristalsis squeeze food through the different sections, which are separated by sphincters that act as valves. Food stays in one area long enough for a particular type of processing to occur. The small intestine is 6–8 m long and about 2 cm wide. It includes three sections: the duodenum, jejunum, and ileum. Food initially passes from the stomach into the duodenum. As it moves through the other parts of the small intestine, it eventually enters the large intestine. The small intestine absorbs nutrients and much of the liquid from foods. The colon is about 2 m long and 6–7 cm wide. It is made up of the ascending colon, transverse colon, and descending colon, and ends at the rectum and anus. The most important function of the colon is to store, process, and excrete waste. It also absorbs water, vitamins, and minerals.

Short bowel syndrome is malabsorption that is due to extensive resection of the small intestine, usually over 66% of its normal length. Extensive resection may be needed because of Crohn's disease, mesenteric infarction, cancer, congenital anomalies, radiation enteritis, or volvulus. As the jejunum is the main digestive and absorptive area for the majority of nutrients, jejunal resection means that there is a loss of absorptive area. Nutrient absorption is greatly reduced. As a result, the ileum increases the length and absorptive abilities of its villi, slowly improving nutrient absorption.

The ileum is where vitamin B12 and bile acids are absorbed. When more than 100 cm of the ileum is resected, severe diarrhea and bile acid malabsorption occur. There is no way that the remaining jejunum can compensate. As a result, there is malabsorption of vitamin B12, fat, and fat-soluble vitamins. Also, unabsorbed bile acids in the colon cause secretory diarrhea. When the colon is preserved, water and electrolyte losses are greatly reduced. If the terminal ileum and ileocecal valve are resected, this predisposes to small intestinal bacterial overgrowth. Prognosis is variable, but the disorder can usually be treated effectively. When this cannot occur, there may be severe, disabling, and life-threatening complications. In patients with many adhesions, such as from radiation enteritis, the syndrome may be prevented by avoiding extensive **enterolysis** and by careful surgical resection.

For short bowel syndrome, it is important to eat six to eight small meals per day, eating and chewing slowly. Once the bowel has adapted, the patient can return to having three meals per day. Chewing foods well helps break them down for easier absorption, and helps prevent any blockages from occurring. Only four ounces of liquids should be consumed with each meal. Drinking larger amounts pushes food through the bowel more quickly, reducing nutrient digestion and absorption. Most liquids should be consumed between meals, at least 1 hour before or after a meal. The meals should be high in proteins (meats, eggs, tofu, dairy products, and nut butters), high in refined or low-fiber complex carbohydrates (white bread, cereals, skinless potatoes, white rice, white pasta), moderate in fats (oils, butter, margarine, mayonnaise, gravy, cream sauces, salad dressings), and low in sugary foods (cookies, cakes, candies, chocolate, soda, instant teas, fruit drinks, corn syrup, molasses, honey, and pancake syrup). Artificial sweeteners are permitted. Sugar-free candies or cough drops containing sugar alcohols (sorbitol, xylitol, mannitol, isomalt) must be limited, since they can have a laxative effect. As far as liquids, at least eight glasses (8 ounces each) should be consumed per day, but very hot or very cold drinks should be avoided. Drinks that do not contain a lot of sugar are preferred, including water, coffee, tea, milk, or juices diluted with water. However, coffee can cause a laxative effect in some people.

FOCUS ON ANTIBODY PRODUCTION IN THE COLON

The large intestine has many lymphoid tissues, which are vital for immunity. They assist with the creation of antibodies that act against the commensal bacteria but may be useful in acting against harmful bacteria, preventing infections. Commensal bacteria act on the host's immune system to induce protective responses that prevent colonization and invasion by pathogens.

COLORECTAL CANCERS

Colorectal cancers are extremely common, making up nearly 148,000 cases and over 53,000 deaths annually in the United States alone. Incidence rises sharply at ages 40–50. More than 50% of cases occur in rectum and sigmoid, with 95% of cases being adenocarcinomas. Less common types include primary colorectal lymphomas, GI stromal tumors, **leiomyosarcomas**, carcinoid tumors, and melanomas. Colorectal cancer is slightly more common in men than women. Colorectal cancers usually occur as transformations within adenomatous polyps, 80% of cases being sporadic and 20% having an inheritable component. Predisposing factors include chronic ulcerative colitis and Crohn's colitis, and cancer risks increase the longer that these conditions persist. Patients with a high incidence of colorectal cancers eat low-fiber diets that are high in animal protein, fat, and refined carbohydrates. The disease spreads by direct extension through the colon wall, hematogenous metastasis, regional lymph node metastasis, and perineural spread (see Chapter 9).

PANCREATITIS

Pancreatitis is either acute or chronic, with *acute pancreatitis* involving inflammation of the pancreas and nearby tissues that resolves. It is usually triggered by alcohol intake and gallstones, in 70% or more cases. Severity may be mild, moderately severe, or severe – based on local complications and transient or persistent organ failure. Acute pancreatitis is common and an extreme healthcare condition. When gallstones cause acute pancreatitis, there is usually increased pressure in the pancreatic duct from obstruction at the ampulla, resulting from a stone, or edema due to the passage of a stone. Abnormal activation of digestive enzymes from the **acinar cells** is caused by ductal hypertension. Toxic effects of bile acid upon the acinar cells may also be causative.

Excessive, alcohol intake, obesity, diabetes, cigarette smoking, and family history increase risks for pancreatitis. Acute pancreatitis has occurred in susceptible patients after only short periods of high intake of alcohol. Low or moderate levels of consumption are related to progression from acute to chronic pancreatitis. The pancreatic acinar cells metabolize alcohol into toxic metabolites, through oxidative and nonoxidative pathways. The cells are predisposed to autodigestive injury, leading to pancreatic *necrosis*, inflammation, and cell death.

Genetic mutations also predispose to pancreatitis. It occurs in 80% of people that carry an autosomal dominant mutation of the cationic trypsinogen gene. There is a clear familial pattern. The gene causing **cystic fibrosis** increases risks of recurrent acute or chronic pancreatitis.

Systemic complications include acute single or multiple organ failure and shock. The affected organs may be in the cardiovascular, respiratory, or urinary systems. Organ failure is based on laboratory and vital sign indicators of respiratory, renal, and cardiovascular impairment. Mortality within one week of acute pancreatitis is usually due to multiorgan failure. Mortality after one week usually occurs from multiorgan failure combined with an infection of pancreatic necrosis, and complications of surgical or endoscopic interventions.

An attack of acute pancreatitis causes regular, intense upper abdominal pain that is bad enough to require parenteral opioids. It radiates through to the back in about half of patients. In alcoholic pancreatitis, it develops over several days, continuing to persist. The pain may be reduced by sitting up and leaning forward. However, it is worsened by coughing, deep breathing, and vigorous movements. Nausea and vomiting commonly occur. The patient is ill in appearance, sweaty, with tachycardia, and tachypnea. There is extreme **postural hypotension**. The patient may be barely alert or conscious. Scleral icterus may be present, due to a bile duct being obstructed by a gallstone or inflammation, plus swelling of the pancreatic head. Ecchymoses of the flanks and of the umbilical region indicate there is extravasation of hemorrhagic exudate. Infection in the pancreas is suspected if the patient is generally toxic in appearance with fever and a raised white blood cell (WBC) count. Severity of the disease is based on organ failure, and local, systemic, or combined complications. Factors that worsen prognosis include patient age above 60 years, comorbidities, obesity, chronic heavy use of alcohol, elevated blood urea nitrogen, elevated hematocrit, pleural effusions, and altered mental status.

Chronic pancreatitis involves histologic changes that are nonreversible and progressive. The two major causes are alcohol use and cigarette smoking. The abdominal pain can be continual or wax and wane. The inflammation is progressive and long-lasting. There is permanent damage and fibrosis scarring of the pancreas. Less common causes of chronic pancreatitis include cystic fibrosis, hereditary pancreatitis, idiopathic, or autoimmune pancreatitis. For example, in India, Indonesia, and Nigeria, chronic pancreatitis occurs in children in young adults, of unknown causes. This is called **tropical pancreatitis**.

The primary symptom is abdominal pain, varying in intensity, with flare-ups lasting for hours or days. Later in the disease course, the pain usually becomes constant. It is usually worse after meals and may be reduced by sitting upright or leaning forward. With progression, the cells that secrete digestive enzymes are destroyed, and the pain may stop. Another primary symptom is pancreatic insufficiency, a decrease in the amount of pancreatic enzymes in the pancreatic fluid. Food is then broken down inadequately. This means that it is malabsorbed, and steatorrhea often results. Undigested muscle fibers are sometimes found in the feces. Inadequate absorption leads to undernutrition, vitamin deficiencies, and weight loss. Complications include pseudocysts, which can bleed or rupture. Those that expand can cause pain, and can block the duodenum or bile ducts. As the cells that secrete insulin are destroyed, diabetes mellitus slowly develops. Chronic pancreatitis increases risks for developing pancreatic cancer. Prognosis is variable, based on clinical scoring systems and laboratory test results. Prevention of pancreatitis involves limiting alcohol consumption, eating a heart-healthy diet, exercising regularly to lose excess weight, avoiding crash diets, and quitting smoking.

For pancreatitis, it is important to eat high-protein foods that are low in animal fats, and contain **antioxidants**. These include lean meats, beans, lentils, clear soups, flax milk, and almond milk. Spinach, blueberries, cherries, and whole grains help protect digestion and fight damaging free radicals. Fruits should be consumed instead of foods with added sugars because people with pancreatitis are at high risk for diabetes. Snacks should include cherry tomatoes, cucumbers, and hummus. Foods to avoid or limit include red meat and organ meats, fried foods, French fries, potato chips, mayonnaise, margarine, butter, full-fat dairy products, pastries, desserts with added sugars, and beverages with added sugars. For patients recovering from acute or chronic pancreatitis, alcoholic beverages must be avoided. Excellent hydration is also needed, so water or electrolyte beverages must be consumed.

FOCUS ON TROPICAL CHRONIC PANCREATITIS

Tropical chronic pancreatitis (TCP) is a juvenile form of chronic calcific nonalcoholic pancreatitis. It is seen almost exclusively in the developing countries of the tropical world. The classical triad of TCP consists of abdominal pain, steatorrhea, and diabetes. The prevalence of tropical pancreatitis is about 126 per every 100,000 people in southern India. Diets high in cassava (tapioca) predispose individuals to the disease.

Test Your Knowledge

1. What causes short bowel syndrome?
2. How does alcohol intake increase risks for pancreatitis?
3. What are the two major causes of chronic pancreatitis?

PANCREATIC CANCERS

Pancreatic cancer, which is mostly *ductal adenocarcinoma*, makes up about 58,000 cases and over 47,000 deaths in the United States every year. The majority of cases are exocrine tumors developing from the ductal and acinar cells, while the minority are pancreatic endocrine tumors. Adenocarcinomas of the exocrine pancreas arise from duct cells nine times more often than from the acinar cells. About 80% occur in the head of the pancreas. They usually appear around age 55 and are two times more common in men than in women. Risk factors include smoking, a history of chronic pancreatitis, the male gender, obesity, and the African-American race. Heredity is also implicated. Alcohol and caffeine consumption does not seem to be direct risk factors, unless consumption is extremely heavy.

A smoker's chance of developing pancreatic cancer decreases after stopping smoking, and nearly returns to the risk level for the remainder of the population after 20 years of being tobacco-free. Risks increase with age, and obesity increases relative risks by about 50%. Chronic pancreatitis is believed to nearly triple the risks for pancreatic cancer. Diabetes mellitus is another risk factor, since type 2 diabetes present for more than ten years has a nearly 50% increased risk.

The signs and symptoms include abdominal pain and weight loss, but these are nonspecific to the disease, until it is later diagnosed because of metastasis. Upon diagnosis, 90% of patients have locally advanced tumors involving retroperitoneal structures, spread to regional lymph nodes, or metastases to the liver or lungs. Severe upper abdominal pain radiation to the back affects most patients, and weight loss is common. When the cancer is in the head of the pancreas, obstructive jaundice leading to **pruritus** occurs in 80%–90% of patients. If the tumor is in the body or tail of the pancreas, there may be splenic vein obstruction, causing splenomegaly, gastric and esophageal varices, and GI hemorrhage. Between 25% and 50% of patients may develop diabetes, leading to polyuria and polydipsia. The cancers can also lead to pancreatic exocrine insufficiency and malabsorption, resulting in bloating, gas, and diarrhea that is watery, greasy, and/or foul-smelling. This results in more weight loss and vitamin deficiencies.

The diagnosis of pancreatic cancers is via CT or MRI/magnetic resonance cholangiopancreatography (MRI/MRCP), followed by endoscopic ultrasonography. Endoscopic ultrasonography with fine-needle aspiration is done for tissue diagnosis and to assess surgical resectability. Routine laboratory tests are also needed to assess the presence of any other conditions. The prognosis varies with stage but is usually poor, with five-year survival being less than 2% of patients. Treatment is with the **Whipple procedure**, adjuvant chemotherapy and radiation therapy (see Figure 16.5). Medications for pain management include transdermal fentanyl, oxycodone, oxymorphone, and for pruritus, cholestyramine.

For pancreatic cancers, it is important to monitor and maintain a healthy weight. Patients must remain hydrated with at least 64 ounces of fluids per day. Small, frequent meals are indicated. High-protein meals are important, including baked, grilled, or boiled lean meats, eggs, nut butters, low-fat dairy products, beans, soy products such as tofu, and protein bars. Protein drinks, bone broths, shakes made from Greek yogurt or high-protein milk, pureed soups, and smoothies are also suggested. It is important to choose foods that are easy to digest, such as chopped, soft, or boiled foods. Essential whole grains are excellent, and include oatmeal, whole grain bread, brown rice, whole grain pasta, bulgur, corn, farro, and quinoa. Whole fruits and vegetables are high in antioxidants, so at least five servings should be consumed per day. Healthy fats include olive and canola oils, avocados, seeds, nuts, and fatty fish. Sweets and added sugars must be limited. Changes in bowel habits may prompt the addition of dietary alterations or the need for supplemental pancreatic enzymes. Regular exercise helps stimulate appetite.

ALCOHOLIC LIVER DISEASE

Alcoholic liver disease is also referred to as *alcohol-related liver disease.* It is caused by too much alcohol consumption over a long period of time. Approximately 8.5% of adults in the United States alone are estimated to have this disorder. Globally, alcoholic liver disease affects an estimated 5.1%–8.6% of the total population. About two times as many men abuse alcohol compared to women. Alcohol is absorbed in the digestive tract, and most of it is metabolized in the liver. During this process, substances are produced that can damage the liver. With increased alcohol consumption, the liver damage is increased. The organ can continue to function for some time because it is sometimes able to recover from mild damage. It can function normally even if approximately 80% of the liver is damaged. If the patient continues to drink, liver damage progresses, and can be fatal. If an individual quits completely, some of the damage can be reversed, improving outlook. The abuse of alcohol causes three types of liver damage, in this order:

- *Accumulation of fat (known as fatty liver or hepatic steatosis)* – sometimes reversible, it occurs in over 90% of people that drink too much alcohol
- *Inflammation (alcoholic hepatitis)* – about 10%–35% of people experience liver inflammation
- *Cirrhosis* – this develops in about 10%–20% of drinkers; a large amount of normal tissue is permanently replaced with scar tissue. The internal structure is disrupted and the liver cannot function normally; there is usually shrinkage of the organ;

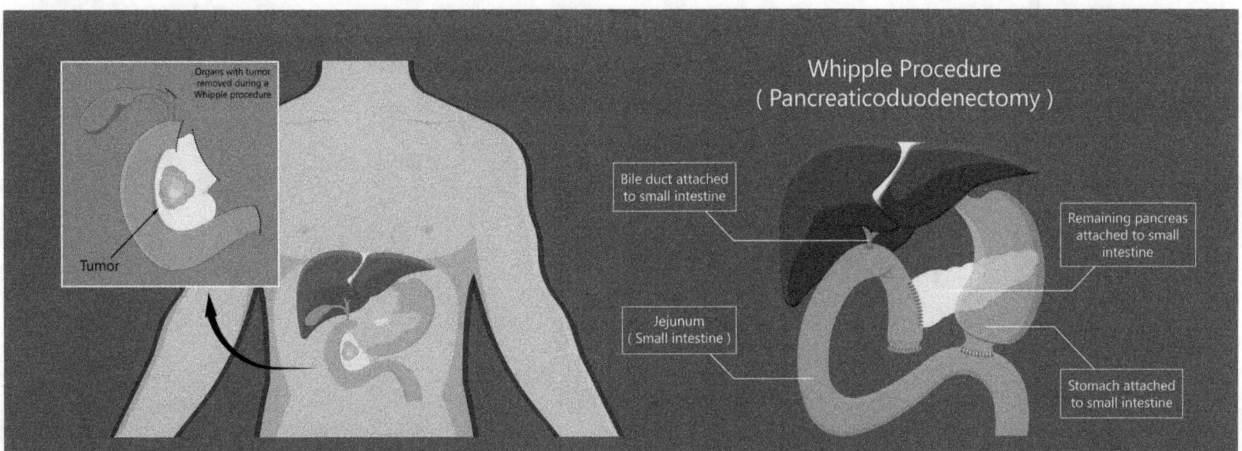

FIGURE 16.5 The Whipple procedure for pancreatic cancer.

symptoms may be limited or identical to those of alcoholic hepatitis; cirrhosis is irreversible (see Figure 16.6).

The complications of cirrhosis include ascites, hepatic portal hypertension, bleeding in the digestive tract, easy bleeding and bruising, and splenomegaly. Alcoholic liver disease is more likely when large amounts of alcohol are consumed for usually more than eight years, in the female gender, with a genetic makeup that increases susceptibility to the disease, and when the individual is obese. One serving of alcohol varies based on the type of drink being consumed.

For men, the daily amount of alcohol should never exceed 1.5 ounces (three cans of beer, three glasses of wine, or three shots of hard liquor). For cirrhosis to develop, men must drink over three ounces of alcohol per day for more than ten years (this would be six cans of beer, six glasses of wine, or six shots of hard liquor). About 50% of men that drink more than eight ounces of alcohol per day for 20 years will develop cirrhosis. Usually, the more alcohol that is consumed over a longer period of time increases risks for alcoholic liver disease. It does not always develop, however, so other factors are believed to be involved. Women are more vulnerable to alcoholic liver disease if they drink about half as much alcohol as men. Their digestive systems may be less able to process alcohol, increasing the amount of alcohol that reaches the liver.

Genetic factors are likely involved because alcoholic liver disease often runs in families. The family members may have the same genes that make alcohol processing less efficient. Obesity also makes liver damage from alcohol more likely. Accumulation of iron in the liver and viral hepatitis C also increase risks. Iron can accumulate because of hemochromatosis (see Chapter 11). Over 25% of heavy drinkers also have viral hepatitis C. Heavy drinking plus viral hepatitis C means risks of cirrhosis are greatly increased. Accumulated iron in the liver or the presence of hepatitis C for over six months increases risks for hepatocellular carcinoma.

Initial symptoms of alcoholic liver disease usually appear when a person is in his or her 30s or 40s, with severe symptoms taking ten years to appear. **Fatty liver disease** is often initially asymptomatic. In 33% of people, it is enlarged and smooth, but not usually tender. As alcoholic hepatitis is developing, symptoms include fever, jaundice, tiredness, and a painful, enlarged liver. Bands of fibrous tissue in the palms can tighten, and the fingers curl (known as *Dupuytren contracture*). The palms may redden, which is known as **palmar erythema**. In the upper body, the skin may develop **spider angiomas**, which are blood vessels that resemble spiders (see Figure 16.7). The salivary glands may enlarge, and there may be muscle wasting. As the peripheral nerves are damaged, there is a loss of sensation and strength. The hands and feet are affected more than the upper arms and legs. Heavy drinkers that are male may develop female body characteristics such as smooth skin, enlarged breasts, and less body hair. Their tests can also shrink.

Pancreatitis may develop, leading to severe abdominal pain and vomiting. Undernourishment can occur because alcohol decreases the appetite without providing any nutrition. Nutrient processing may be abnormal, resulting in deficiencies of folate, thiamin, and other vitamins and minerals. Mineral deficiencies can cause shaking and weakness. Nutritional deficiencies likely cause or worsen peripheral nerve damage. Thiamin deficiency can cause Wernicke encephalopathy and confusion, eye problems, and difficulty walking. Without prompt treatment, Korsakoff syndrome, coma, and death can occur. Korsakoff syndrome involves confusion and memory loss. Anemia may develop since there is bleeding in the digestive tract, or nutrient deficiencies cause poor development of red blood cells. Symptoms may also be due to complications of cirrhosis.

The prognosis for alcoholic liver disease is based on the amount of fibrosis and inflammation. Fatty liver and inflammation can be reversed if the patient stops drinking and there is no fibrosis. Fatty liver is able to be totally resolved within six weeks, but fibrosis and cirrhosis are not reversible.

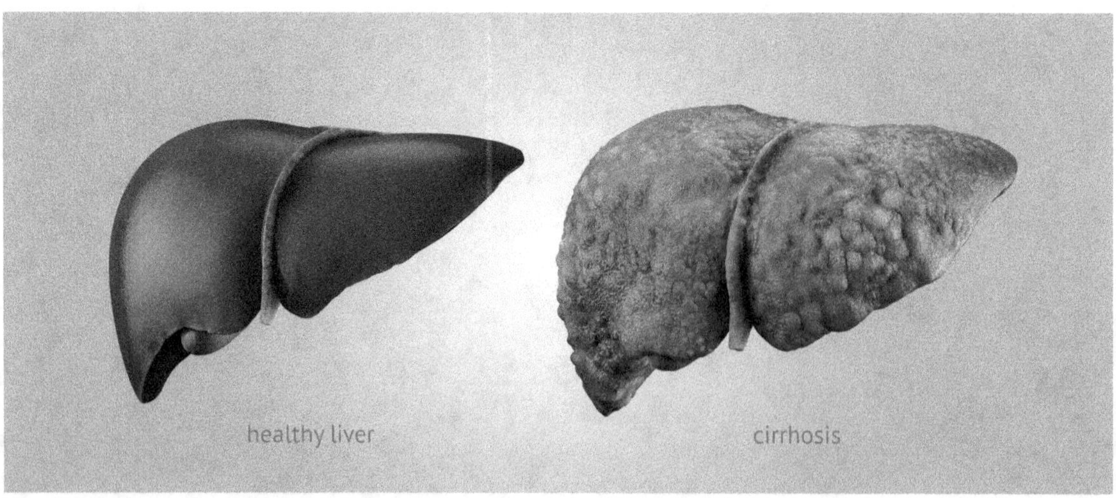

FIGURE 16.6 Cirrhosis of the liver.

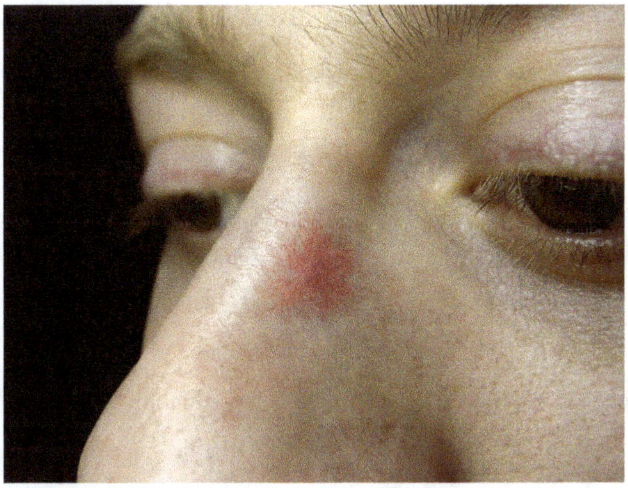

FIGURE 16.7 Spider angiomas.

Biopsies and blood tests can predict the prognosis. Formulas and models that combine various test results are also helpful. The prognosis is worsened once cirrhosis, ascites, and digestive tract bleeding are present. Only 50% of people with these complications survive for five more years. Those that stop drinking alcohol usually live longer than those that continue. The only way to prevent alcoholic liver disease is to avoid all alcohol. The individual should protect against hepatitis C, since it infects the liver and leads to cirrhosis.

For alcoholic liver disease, all alcohol consumption must stop. The diet should consist mostly of nutrient-dense foods, including fruits, vegetables, lean proteins, legumes, nuts, seeds, whole grains, heart-healthy fats, water, coffee, tea, herbs, and spices. Foods to avoid include fast food, convenience meals, canned soups, packaged snacks, margarine, vegetable shortening, fried foods, chips, crackers, pretzels, microwave popcorn, hot dogs, sausage, deli meats, bacon, beef jerky, soy sauce, teriyaki sauce, steak sauce, spaghetti sauce, and raw or undercooked foods (meat, poultry, eggs, fish, oysters, or mussels).

FOCUS ON ALCOHOLIC LIVER DISEASE

Alcoholic liver disease can cause three types of liver damage, which usually occur in the following order: fatty liver, inflammation (alcoholic hepatitis), and scar tissue the replaces normal liver tissue (cirrhosis). Almost everyone who drinks too much alcohol develops a fatty liver. Inflammation usually resolves after stopping drinking, but there can still be permanent damage. Once there is scar tissue, it never resolves, even if all alcohol consumption is stopped.

Test Your Knowledge

1. What is cirrhosis of the liver, and what are its complications?
2. What is fatty liver disease and its signs and symptoms?
3. What are the complications of cirrhosis?

LIVER CANCERS

Liver cancers may be primary or secondary. Primary liver cancer is usually *hepatocellular carcinoma*, with other types being uncommon or rare. They include *fibrolamellar carcinoma*, *cholangiocarcinoma*, *hepatoblastoma*, and *angiosarcoma*. The first signs of the disease are usually nonspecific, which delays the diagnosis, leading to a poor prognosis. For some localized cancers, resection is possible. Resection or liver transplantation may prolong survival.

Hepatocellular carcinoma usually occurs because of cirrhosis, and is common in areas of the world where hepatitis B virus (HBV) and hepatitis C virus (HCV) infections are prevalent. There are more than 42,000 new cases and over 30,000 deaths annually in the United States. Overall, liver cancers are about three times more common in men than in women. Outside of the United States, this cancer is more common in East Asia and sub-Saharan Africa, paralleling the prevalence of chronic HBV infection. Other disorders that cause hepatocellular carcinoma include hemochromatosis and noncirrhotic nonalcoholic steatohepatitis. Environmental carcinogens also play a role. The most common symptoms include abdominal pain, weight loss, right upper quadrant mass, and unexplainable deterioration. Diagnosis is via measurement of **alpha-fetoprotein** (AFP) and imaging via PET-CT, ultrasound, or MRI. Hepatocellular carcinoma is suspected if there is an enlarged liver, unexplained decompensation of chronic liver disease, and imaging tests detecting a mass (especially if the patient has cirrhosis). Treatments are based on staging. Options for treatment include liver transplantation, surgical resection, ablative treatments, radiofrequency ablation, and medications (sorafenib, lenvatinib, regorafenib, and nivolumab). Systemic immunotherapies are quickly evolving, and include medications such as atezolizumab and bevacizumab.

Fibrolamellar carcinoma is a variant of hepatocellular carcinoma, with a morphology of malignant hepatocytes that are enmeshed in lamellar fibrous tissue. It is most common in young adults, with no link to preexisting cirrhosis, HBV, HCV, or other known risk factors. The level of AFP is rarely elevated. It has a better prognosis than hepatocellular carcinoma, with many patients surviving for several years after tumor resection.

Cholangiocarcinoma originates within the biliary epithelium, and is most common in China where infestations with liver flukes may be implicated. It is less common in other regions than hepatocellular carcinoma but may have some histologic similarities. Primary sclerosing cholangitis increases its risks greatly, and the prognosis is usually poor. In the few cases of isolated hilar cholangiocarcinomas that are less than 2 cm in diameter, and treated with adjuvant brachytherapy, liver transplantation has been more and more successful.

Hepatoblastoma is rare, but a highly common primary liver cancer in infants and children especially if they have a history of familial adenomatous polyposis. The cancer is usually found because of overall health deterioration, and a right upper quadrant mass. Diagnosis may be aided by elevated AFP levels and abnormal imaging test results.

Angiosarcoma is rare, and linked to chemical carcinogens such as industrial vinyl chloride.

Liver metastases (secondary liver cancers) are cancerous tumors that have spread to the liver from another part of the body. These tumors can appear shortly after the original tumor develops, or even months or years later. They may spread from the GI tract, breasts, lungs, and pancreas. They are actually more common than primary liver cancers, with similar symptoms. Diagnosis is with ultrasonography, spiral CT with contrast, or MRI with contrast. Treatment is usually palliative chemotherapy and radiation therapy.

Nutrition can be an important part of dealing with liver cancers. Eating a well-balanced diet before, during, and after cancer treatment may help patients feel better, maintain strength, and speed up recovery. Strict dieting is not recommended during cancer treatment. Losing weight can lower the energy level and decrease the ability to fight infection. Frequent small meals will ensure that the patient's body is getting enough calories, protein, and nutrients to tolerate treatment. Smaller meals may also help to reduce treatment-related side effects such as nausea. Protein helps the body to repair cells and tissues. It also helps the immune system to recover from illness. Fruits and vegetables offer the body antioxidants, which can help fight against cancer. It is important that patients choose a variety of colorful fruits and vegetables to get the greatest benefits. They should eat a minimum of five servings of whole fruits and vegetables daily. Fresh fruits and vegetables may need to be cooked for patients with a weakened immune system.

KEY TERMS

Achalasia
Acinar cells
Adenocarcinoma
Ageusia
Antioxidants
Aphthous ulcers
Ascites
Assimilation
Atrophic gastritis
Barrett's esophagus
Blind loop syndrome
Borborygmi
Carcinoid tumor
Cheilitis
Cholecystokinin
Chylomicrons
Collagenous sprue
Crohn's disease
Crypt
Cystic fibrosis
Deconjugation
Diaphragm paralysis
Dihydroxylation
Diverticula
Down syndrome
Dysgeusia
Enterokinase
Esophagitis
Fatty liver disease
G cells
Gastrectomy
Gastric cardia
Gastrin
Geophagia
Gluten enteropathy
Goblet cells
Granulomas

Helicobacter pylori

Hematemesis

Heme-positive stools

Hypochromic microcytic anemia

Hypolactasia

Hypotonia

Ileocecal valve

Immunoglobulin A

Irritable bowel syndrome

Jejunoileitis

Lassitude

Leiomyosarcomas

Malabsorption syndromes

Mastocytosis

Melena

Mesentery

Metaplasia

Metaplastic

Methane

Micelles

Odynophagia

Oxyntic glands

Palmar erythema

Pancreatitis

Parietal cells

Peptic ulcer

Peristalsis

Pleural effusions

Plummer–Vinson syndrome

Pneumaturia

Polyols

Postural hypotension

Refractory disease

Sclerotherapy

Spider angiomas

Squamous cell carcinoma

Steatorrhea

Sucrase–isomaltase

Superior vena cava syndrome

Surgical blind loops

Tenesmus

Toxic megacolon syndrome

Tropical pancreatitis

Tropical sprue

Trypsin

Tylosis

Zollinger-Ellison syndrome

CLINICAL CASE STUDIES

Clinical Case Study 1

A 77-year-old woman was diagnosed with stomach cancer, specifically an adenocarcinoma of the body of the stomach. Her initial complaint had been about one month of intermittent chest pressure that radiated to her back, though a cardiac-related cause was ruled out. An upper endoscopy revealed the stomach tumor, without any evidence of metastatic disease. The patient did not drink alcohol or smoke and had no family history of stomach cancer, though her brother died of colon cancer that metastasized to his liver. Surgery was indicated, and about 80% of the patient's stomach was removed. The gastrointestinal tract was reconstructed via a Roux-en-Y gastrojejunostomy. The patient recovered from surgery. Follow-up treatments included chemotherapy and radiation therapy. The patient was cancer-free over six months of monitoring.

CRITICAL THINKING QUESTIONS

1. How common is stomach cancer in older people?
2. What are the causes of stomach cancer?
3. What types of foods should be limited in order to possibly prevent stomach cancer?

Clinical Case Study 2

A 22-year-old man was taken to the emergency department by his girlfriend, because of nausea, vomiting, and abdominal pain. A CT scan revealed ileal thickening and a small bowel obstruction. The patient was hospitalized, but developed diarrhea and rectal bleeding. A colonoscopy revealed ulcerations of the ileum and colon, and Crohn's disease was diagnosed. A small bowel study with barium contrast revealed that stenoses and ulcerations extended over the distal 30 centimeters of the ileum. Treatment was started with medications, which relieved the abdominal pain and bleeding. The diarrhea took longer to correct, but ultimately was successfully treated.

CRITICAL THINKING QUESTIONS

1. How does Crohn's disease develop?
2. What are the causes of Crohn's disease?
3. What should patients with Crohn's disease eat when symptoms are not present, and when symptoms are present?

Clinical Case Study 3

An 81-year-old man was admitted to the local hospital. His main complain were general malaise, loss of appetite, and weight loss. A full physical examination and an abdominal contrast-enhanced CT scan revealed occlusive cancer of the descending colon with liver metastasis. The exam also revealed swelling of the adjacent lymph nodes and numerous liver masses. Histopathological examination of the biopsy sample revealed the cancer to be adenocarcinoma. The patient was put on a fasting regimen after hospitalization, and parenteral nutrition. Medications were started, which lead to decreased tumor marker levels and allowed the patient to resume oral intake after five cycles were completed. The medications included folinic acid, fluorouracil, oxaliplatin, and panitumumab. A follow-up CT scan performed six months later revealed nearly a complete response to the treatments, and no surgical intervention was needed.

CRITICAL THINKING QUESTIONS

1. How common are colorectal cancers?
2. What is the diagnosis of colorectal cancer based on?
3. What type of diet is required for a colorectal cancer patient?

Clinical Case Study 4

A 59-year-old man complained of generalized weakness, and yellowing of his skin and sclera. Examination revealed mild epigastric tenderness. Tests revealed elevations of tumor markers and bilirubin. A pancreatic head mass was discovered with low level biliary obstruction. There were small visible cysts in the left liver lobe. The pancreatic mass was about 4×3 cm in size. Pancreatic cancer was diagnosed, and there were no distant metastases. The tumor was specifically classified as an adenocarcinoma.

CRITICAL THINKING QUESTIONS

1. What are the risk factors for pancreatic cancer?
2. What are the signs and symptoms of pancreatic cancer?
3. What dietary changes are required to manage pancreatic cancer?

Clinical Case Study 5

A 66-year-old woman with history of cirrhosis due to alcohol abuse was found to have a lesion in the liver that was consistent with hepatocellular carcinoma. A PET-CT scan indicated there was no extrahepatic disease. The diagnosis was confirmed by a biopsy using ultrasound-guided percutaneous needle puncture. Tests revealed elevated alpha-fetoprotein. The liver cancer was in an early stage. Transcatheter arterial chemoembolization was undertaken, but the alpha-fetoprotein levels continued to increase.

CRITICAL THINKING QUESTIONS

1. What is primary liver cancer usually discovered to be?
2. What are the most common symptoms of liver cancer?
3. What are the options for treatment?

STUDY QUESTIONS

1. Which of the following is NOT a cause of dysgeusia?
   A. Vitamin D deficiency
   B. Zinc deficiency
   C. Vitamin B deficiency
   D. Certain medications

2. All of the following are risk factors for esophageal cancer, EXCEPT:
   A. Excessive alcohol ingestion
   B. Smoking tobacco products
   C. Achalasia
   D. Vitamin B12 deficiency

3. In which of the following conditions is there a small web-like tissue partially blocking the throat and upper part of the esophagus, making swallowing difficult?
   A. Short bowel syndrome
   B. Blind loop syndrome
   C. Plummer–Vinson syndrome
   D. Malabsorption syndrome

4. The loss of the oxyntic glands in the stomach corpus may lead to a decrease in which of the following?
   A. Intrinsic factor
   B. Vitamin B12 absorption
   C. Gastrin
   D. Cholecystokinin

5. Which of the following is NOT one of the worst food choices for peptic ulcer?
   A. Milk and fatty foots
   B. Alcohol and soda
   C. Fiber-rich foods
   D. Fried foods

6. All of the following are early warning signs and symptoms of stomach cancer, EXCEPT:
   A. Weight gain
   B. Heartburn
   C. Vomiting
   D. Abdominal pain

7. Which of the following enzymes can split long-chain triglycerides into monoglycerides and fatty acids?
   A. Pepsin
   B. Enterokinase
   C. Amylase
   D. Lipase

8. Chronic bacterial infections of the small intestine are common in all of the following conditions, EXCEPT:
   A. Blind loop syndrome
   B. Systemic sclerosis
   C. Diverticula
   D. Gastritis

9. Which of the following is also known as gluten enteropathy?
   A. Hypolactasia
   B. Celiac disease
   C. Jejunoileitis
   D. Crohn's disease

10. Granulomatous ileitis is also known as:
    A. Crohn's disease
    B. Short bowel syndrome
    C. Tropical pancreatitis
    D. Spider angioma

11. Which of the following is NOT a risk factor for pancreatic cancer?
    A. Obesity
    B. Gender
    C. Alcohol consumption
    D. Smoking

12. Which of the following is NOT a risk factor for pancreatitis?
    A. Diabetes
    B. Down syndrome
    C. Excessive alcohol consumption
    D. Cigarette smoking

13. Risks for celiac disease are high in people that have all of the following conditions, EXCEPT:
    A. Down syndrome
    B. Hashimoto thyroiditis
    C. Hypothyroidism
    D. Lymphocytic colitis

14. Which of the following foods should NOT be eliminated during treatment for bacterial overgrowth syndrome?
    A. Galactans
    B. Fructans
    C. Polyols
    D. Vitamin B12

15. Which of the following viral infections can cause hepatocellular carcinoma?
    A. Hepatitis C
    B. Hepatitis A
    C. Hepatitis E
    D. Hepatitis D

FURTHER READING

1. Adams, D.B., Cotton, P.B., Zyromski, N.J., and Windsor, J.A. (2017). *Pancreatitis: Medical and Surgical Management.* Wiley-Blackwell.
2. Caleb, H. (2022). *The Book on Diarrhea Diet – The Best Meal Plan.* Caleb.
3. Capellan, L.G. (2020). *The Gastritis Healing Book – A Comprehensive Guide to Heal Gastritis and Restore Your Stomach Health.* Capellan.
4. Corrigan, M.L., Roberts, K., and Steiger, E. (2018). *Adult Short Bowel Syndrome – Nutritional, Medical, and Surgical Management.* Academic Press.
5. DiBaise, J.K., Parrish, C.R., and Thompson, J.S. (2021). *Short Bowel Syndrome.* CRC Press.
6. Gasbarrini, G. (2008). *Malabsorption Syndrome (Digestive Diseases).* S. Karger.
7. Golanna, M. (2022). *Fructose Intolerance Diet – A Beginner's Two-Week Step-by-Step Guide to Managing Fructose Intolerance, with Sample Fructose-Free Recipes and a Meal Plan.* Golanna.
8. Gottschall, E. (2020). *Breaking the Vicious Cycle: Intestinal Health Through Diet.* The Kirkton Press.
9. Green, P.H.R., and Jones, R. (2020). *Celiac Disease – A Hidden Epidemic*, 4th Edition. William Morrow Paperbacks.
10. Ishiguro, E., Haskey, N., and Campbell, S. (2018). *Gut Microbiota: Interactive Effects on Nutrition and Health.* Academic Press.
11. Jeffrey, D. (2022). *Stomach Cancer: The Complete Guide on How to Cure Stomach Cancer – Everything from Diagnosis till Recovery.* Jeffrey.
12. Maloney, C. (2016). *The Colon Cancer Diet.* Hygeian Publishing.
13. Manbacci, M. (2019). *The Comprehensive Guide to Crohn's Disease: All You Need to Know About Crohn's Disease from Diagnosis to Management & Treatment (Autoimmune Disease).* Manbacci.

14. Marx, J. (2018). *Victory Over Cancer! Volume 2 – Acid Reflux and Esophageal Cancer.* Marx.
15. Palau, V. (2022). *Gastritis Diet Plan – What to Eat and What to Avoid.* Palau.
16. Purdy, M. (2020). *The Microbiome Diet Reset – A Practical Guide to Restore and Protect a healthy Microbiome.* Rockridge Press.
17. Regan, K., and Siebecker, A. (2018). *The SIBO Diet Plan – Four Weeks to Relieve Symptoms and Manage SIBO.* Rockridge Press.
18. Robillard, N., and Eades, M.R. (2013). *Irritable Bowel Syndrome – Fast Tract Digestion: Diet that Addresses the Root Cause, Small Intestinal Bacterial Overgrowth without Drugs or Antibiotics.* Self-Health Publishing.
19. Scholes, A. (2020). *The Anti-Cancer Diet – All You Need to Know.* Scholes.
20. Siquini, W., Ridolfo, R., Stortoni, P., and Feliciotti, E. (2015). *Total, Subtotal and Proximal Gastrectomy in Cancer: A Color Atlas.* Springer.
21. Strealy, N. (2013). *The Diarrhea Dietitian: Expert Advice, Practical Solutions, and Strategic Nutrition.* Strategic Nutrition Publishing.
22. Sunohara, K. (2020). *The Essential Diet for Diverticulitis – A Three-Stage Nutrition Guide to Manage and Prevent Flare-Ups.* Rockridge Press.
23. Sussman, N.L., and Lucey, M.R. (2019). *Alcoholic Liver Disease, An Issue of Clinics in Liver Disease (Clinics Review Articles).* Elsevier.
24. Tariq, J. (2019). *Stomach Ulcer Diet – Home Remedies for Curing Sour Stomach, Nausea, and Peptic Ulcers.* Tariq.
25. Tepper, B.J., and Tomassini Barbarossa, I. (2020). *Taste, Nutrition and Health.* Mdpi AG.
26. Thompson, E. (2021). *Gastritis Diet and Recipes – The Complete Guide to Curing Gastritis With an Exclusive Seven-Day Anti-Inflammatory Food Plan For Beginners and Workers.* Thompson.
27. Travis, D. (2015). *My Real-World Guide for Eosinophilic Esophagitis – A Guide to Helping Children, Parents, and Anyone Else Navigate Through the Thoughts and Feelings Associated with Eosinophilic Esophagitis.* CreateSpace Independent Publishing Platform.
28. Zibdeh, N. (2018). *The Complete Acid Reflux Diet Plan – Easy Meal Plans and Recipes to Heal GERD and LPR.* Rockridge Press.

17 Nutritional Effects on the Integumentary System

OUTLINE

General Appearance: Skin
- Energy Deficiency
- Pellagra (Niacin Deficiency)
- Skin Abnormalities (Vitamin C and K Deficiency)

Dermatitis (Zinc Deficiency)
Nutrition and Discoloration of the Skin
Skin Abnormalities (Vitamin D Deficiency)
Xerosis (Omega-3 Fatty Acid Deficiency)
Severe Dermatitis (Omega-6 Fatty Acid Deficiency)
Hair and Nail Abnormalities (Protein, Iron, and Selenium Deficiency)
Key Terms
Clinical Case Studies
Study Questions
Further Reading

LEARNING OBJECTIVES

After study of the chapter, readers should be able to:

1. Describe the three layers of the skin.
2. Explain energy deficiency and its related skin symptoms.
3. Describe the signs and symptoms of pellagra that affect the skin.
4. Discuss skin abnormalities in vitamin C deficiency.
5. Explain the signs and symptoms of zinc deficiency.
6. Describe the causes of discoloration of the skin.
7. Identify the skin abnormalities of vitamin D deficiency.
8. Compare the differences between omega-3 fatty acid and omega-6 fatty acid.
9. Describe the effects of omega-3 fatty acid deficiency in the body.
10. Explain iron deficiency and its effect on the nails.

OVERVIEW

Good nutrition has a vast amount of effects upon the integumentary system. For example, diets high in vitamin C and low in fats and carbohydrates are linked with less skin wrinkling, age-related skin dryness, and skin thinning. Essential fatty acids contribute to skin health as well. Omega-6 fatty acids promote healthy skin growth, while omega-3 fatty acids help to prevent dry skin. Poor nutrition increases risks for fatty acid deficiencies that lead to skin and hair abnormalities. Antioxidants such as beta-carotene and vitamins A, C, and E can reduce damage caused by free radicals, which harm skin cells and cause the signs of aging. Minerals such as zinc, copper, and selenium play additional roles in maintaining skin health. Basically, skin, hair, and nail health begin with good nutrition. In order for nails to grow and develop properly, many different nutrients are needed. Good hydration and adequate amounts of protein, as well as zinc, calcium, iron, phosphorus, and the vitamins A, B, C, D, and E are needed.

GENERAL APPEARANCE: SKIN

According to the American Skin Association, the skin (along with the hair and nails) acts as the body's protective covering and prevents pathogens from entering. The skin supports all other body parts and helps maintain our immune systems. The skin also aids in regulating body temperature via the sweat glands. It also interacts with the nervous system to detect pain, pressure, heat, and cold. Exposure to the ultraviolet rays of the sun results in the manufacture of vitamin D by the skin, which is essential for skin health. The general appearance of healthy skin is smooth, with no breaks in the surface, warm (but not hot or reddened), and neither dry, flaky, moist, or wrinkled. Normal skin should also not be excessively oily, and should not have any severe sensitivity. The pores should only be barely visible, and the complexion should not be pale.

The skin is the body's largest organ. Its three layers are the **epidermis**, **dermis**, and subcutaneous layer (see Figure 17.1). The epidermis is paper-thin, and its outermost layer is made up of dead cells that are continually flaking or washing off, to be replaced by new cells manufactured in the lower portion of the epidermis. The cells move upward toward the outside of the skin, and as they do this, they harden and die. The complete cycle takes about 28 days. The epidermis contains **melanocytes**, which are cells that contain melanin – the pigment that provides skin color, which is determined by the amount of melanin. An individual with more melanin has darker skin. The middle layer the dermis contains blood vessels, nerves, **hair follicles**, and sweat and oil glands. About 90% of the thickness of the skin is made up by the dermis, which contains collagen and elastic fibers that provide strength and elasticity. The deep subcutaneous layer is mostly made up of fatty tissue, but additionally contains blood vessels and nerves. The fat provides insulation against extreme heat and cold, while cushioning the

DOI: 10.1201/b22969-20

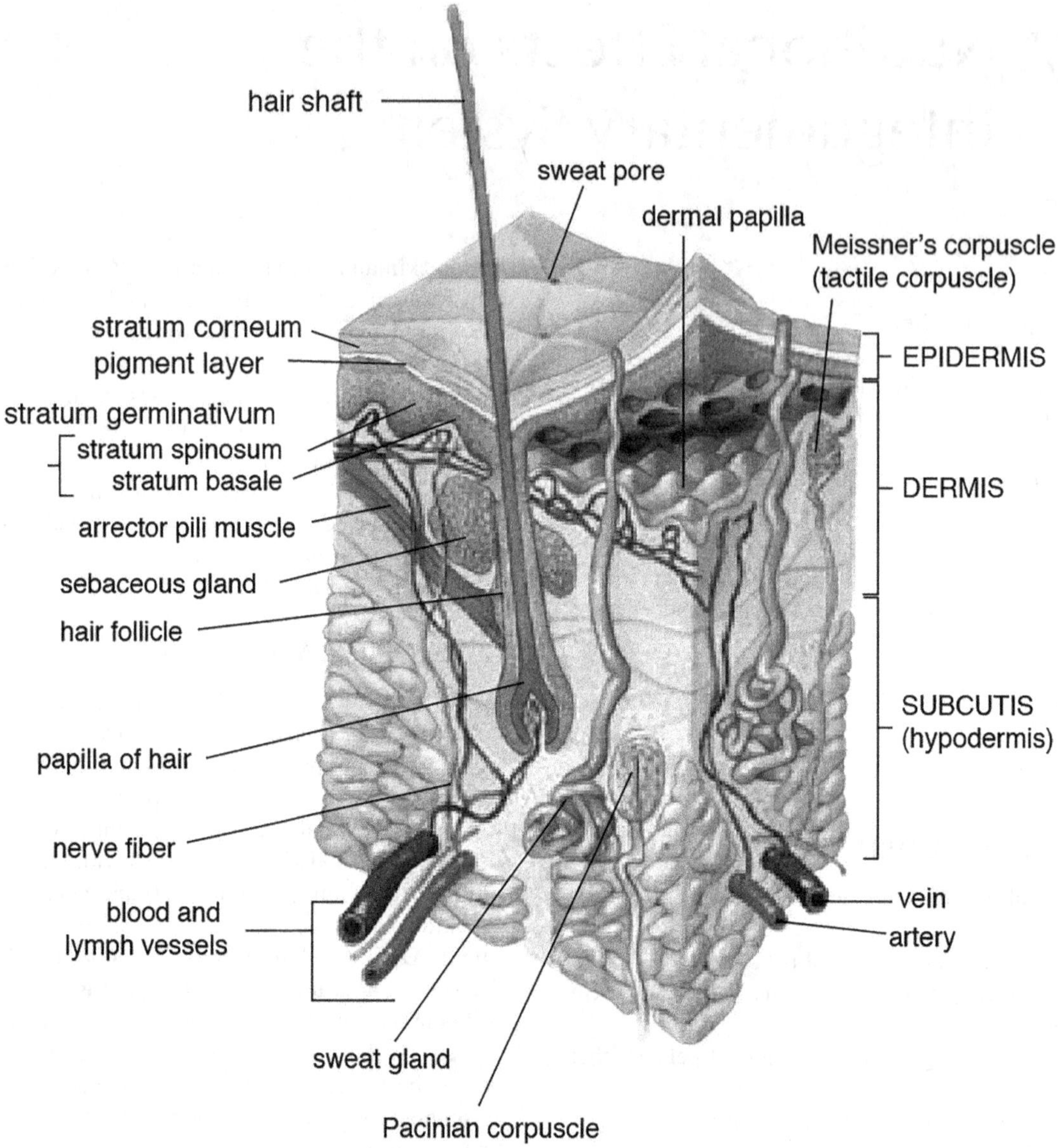

FIGURE 17.1 The layers of the skin.

body against injuries. Factors that can worsen the general appearance of the skin, hair, and nails include excessive consumption of alcohol, smoking, piercings, lack of exercise, excessive use of hair care products, poor hygiene, protection of the **nail cuticles**, excessive use of nail polish or nail glue, excessive use of artificial sculptured nails, poor nutrition, dehydration, stress, excessive exposure to ultraviolet light, and tattoos.

FOCUS ON NUTRITION-RELATED SKIN AGING

Generally, high-fat diets cause more rapid aging of the skin because they result in skin oxidative stress, producing inflammatory damage. There is also a link between sugar and food processing methods such as grilling, and frying. Foods that speed up skin aging include French fries, white bread and sugar, margarine, processed meats, excessive amounts of dairy products, caffeine, alcohol, corn or sunflower oil (used in high-heat cooking), rice cakes, and anything containing high fructose corn syrup.

Energy Deficiency

An individual with any form of energy deficiency, such as *protein-energy undernutrition (PEU)*, often develops signs of obvious wasting, which include edema, hair loss, and skin atrophy. The dry form of PEU is *marasmus*, which causes weight loss and depleted fat and muscle. The wet form of PEU is *kwashiorkor*, which is less common than marasmus. In kwashiorkor, the cell membranes leak, and

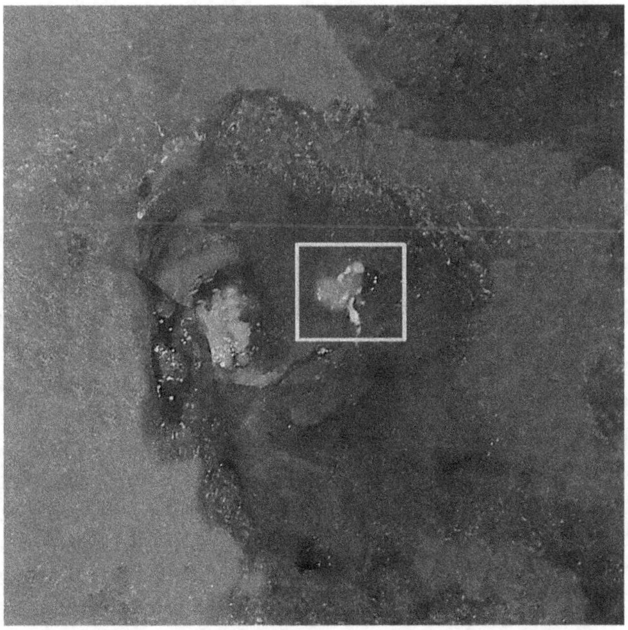

FIGURE 17.2 Decubitus ulcers.

there is extravasation of intravascular fluid and protein, causing peripheral edema. Over time, energy deficiencies cause the skin to become thin, dry, pale, cold, and it also loses elasticity. The hair is dry and falls out more easily than normal. In older patients, the risk for **decubitus ulcers** increases (see Figure 17.2). The skin may become yellowed because of jaundice. In infants, marasmus may cause the skin to become loose and thin, hanging in folds. Kwashiorkor may cause the skin to become dry, thin, and wrinkled. It can also become hyperpigmented and fissured, eventually becoming hypopigmented, friable, and atrophic. Skin in various areas can be affected at different times. The severity of an energy deficiency may be partially assessed by responses to skin antigens. Protein-energy undernutrition, marasmus, and kwashiorkor were discussed in greater detail in Chapter 7.

Test Your Knowledge

1. What are the three layers of the skin?
2. What factors can worsen the general appearance of the skin?
3. How do energy deficiencies affect the skin over time?

Pellagra (Niacin Deficiency)

Pellagra results from a dietary niacin deficiency, and is not common in developed countries. In the early 1900s, it affected over 3 million Americans and killed over 100,000, until scientists discovered that their diets were poor in niacin. Earlier (in the late 1800s) pellagra affected more than 100,000 people in Italy.

There are primary and secondary niacin deficiencies. *Primary niacin deficiency* is caused by very low intake of niacin as well as tryptophan. This is most common in areas where the corn called *maize* makes up a large part of the diet (India and Africa). The bound niacin that is in maize is not taken up by the gastrointestinal (GI) tract unless it has been treated with *alkali*, such as is done in the preparation of tortillas. Corn protein is likewise low in tryptophan. There is a high incidence of pellagra in India, in people that eat **millet** that has a high content of *leucine*. Therefore, it is believed that an amino acid imbalance may actually contribute to the deficiency. Primary niacin deficiency is often accompanied by protein and B vitamin deficiencies as well. *Secondary niacin deficiency* may be caused by cirrhosis, alcoholism, or diarrhea. Pellagra may occur along with carcinoid syndrome and **Hartnup disease**. *Pellagra* is manifested by the *three Ds*: dermatitis, diarrhea, and dementia.

Primary pellagra is caused by insufficient dietary niacin and tryptophan, while *secondary pellagra* is due to an inability to use niacin normally. Pellagra has been prevalent in countries that did not use the lime water-soaking process when preparing corn-based foods, including Europe, sub-Saharan Africa, Indonesia, China, and the United States (primarily, poorer people in Mississippi, Alabama, and South Carolina). Another reason for pellagra developing is that corn-based diets, such as in South America, contain very little tryptophan. During the US epidemic, severe dementia forced many people to be confined to mental institutions. There were outbreaks of pellagra during the 2000s in Angola, Zimbabwe, and Nepal. Isolated cases have occurred in the Netherlands and Denmark. The diagnosis of pellagra is based on symptoms, assisted by urinalysis. There is also pellagrous encephalopathy, which is discussed in greater detail in Chapter 13.

Pellagra involves symptoms that affect the skin, mucous membranes, gastrointestinal tract, and central nervous system. If advanced, there may be a symmetric rash that is photosensitive, glossitis, stomatitis, diarrhea, and mental abnormalities. The symptoms may be individual or occur in various combinations. The skin lesions may be of various types, but are usually bilaterally symmetric (see Figure 17.3). Their distribution, at pressure points or on areas of skin that receive more sun exposure, is more characteristic of the disease than the actual type of lesions. There may be a glove-like distribution on the hands known as **pellagrous glove**, or a boot-shaped distribution on the feet and legs known as **pellagrous boot**. Sun exposure causes facial lesions that have a butterfly shape and a **Casal necklace**. The mucous membranes of the mouth, vagina, and urethra may be affected. Acute deficiency of niacin results in glossitis and stomatitis. With disease progression, tongue and oral mucous membranes may turn red. There is then mouth pain, increased salivation, and tongue edema. Ulcerations often appear under the tongue, on the lower lip mucosa, and opposite the molar teeth.

Pellagra is clinically diagnosed, based on the characteristic symptoms occurring at the same time. A dietary history indicating a lack of niacin and tryptophan aid in the correct diagnosis. Confirmation is from treatment with niacin that improves the symptoms. Laboratory confirmation involves finding a decreased urinary excretion of N1-methylnicotinamide (NMN). Since multiple deficiencies often occur, a balanced diet – especially with riboflavin and pyridoxine – is required. Nicotinamide is usually used for treatment since it does not cause burning, flushing, itching, or tingling the way that nicotinic acid does. Nicotinamide is given in daily oral doses.

FOCUS ON PELLAGRA

The word "pellagra" comes from the Italian words for skin ("pelle") and rough ("agra"). This describes the most obvious feature of the disease – the rough appearance of the skin that resembles severe sunburn in areas exposed to sunlight.

Test Your Knowledge

1. What are the "three Ds" of pellagra?
2. What are the causes of primary and secondary niacin deficiency?
3. Which skin changes are seen with pellagra?

Skin Abnormalities (Vitamin C and K Deficiency)

The antioxidant properties of vitamin C and its role in collagen synthesis make this vitamin a vital molecule for skin health. Dietary and topical ascorbic acid have beneficial effects upon skin cells. However, the effects of vitamin C in the skin are not well understood due to limited research. Cutaneous manifestations of scurvy result from declines in collagen synthesis, leading to disruption of connective tissue and blood vessel fragility. Early symptoms in the skin include a thickening of the **stratum corneum** and spots of small subcutaneous bleeding. As scurvy progresses, wound healing is impaired due to the loss of mature collagen, which allows wounds to remain open. Skin lesions caused by vitamin C deficiency are resolved with adequate intake of vitamin C.

In developed countries, severe vitamin C deficiency that results in scurvy is not common, but the deficiency can be part of general undernutrition. Scurvy involves hemorrhages, and abnormal formation of **osteoid** and **dentin**. The skin symptoms of vitamin C deficiency include **petechiae**, rash, **ecchymoses**, hyperkeratosis, corkscrew hairs, and impaired wound healing. Other symptoms include fatigue, depression, gingivitis, and internal bleeding. In infants and children, there may be impaired bone growth. Dietary sources of vitamin C include citrus fruits, tomatoes, broccoli, potatoes, strawberries, and sweet peppers. Vitamin C is of greater need in people with fever, inflammation, diarrhea, *achlorhydria*, hyperthyroidism, iron deficiency, cold or heat stress, burns, and protein deficiency. People that smoke or have just had surgery also require more vitamin C. Some amount of dietary vitamin C is destroyed by cooking or when infant formulas are sterilized.

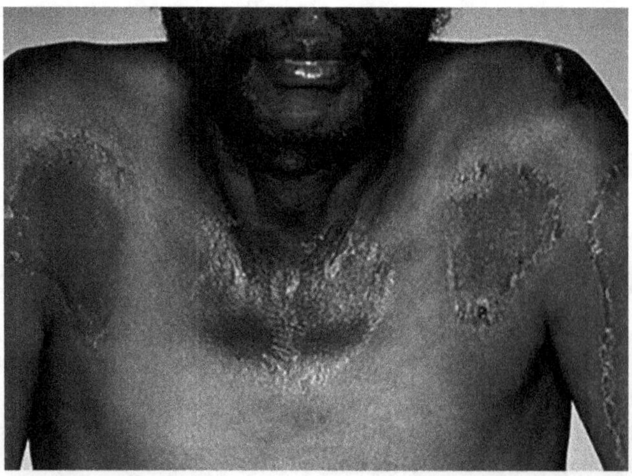

FIGURE 17.3 Pellagra.

After a few months of vitamin C deficiency, there may be scurvy-like symptoms that include **follicular hyperkeratosis**, coiling of the hair, and perifollicular hemorrhages. The gums may be purple, swollen, friable, and spongy, bleeding easily when the deficiency is severe (see Figure 17.4). Wounds heal slowly and can tear back open easily. Spontaneous hemorrhages may occur, often as skin ecchymoses in the lower limbs, or as bulbar conjunctival hemorrhage. Diagnosis is usually clinical, based on the signs and symptoms. Hyperkeratotic hair follicles that have surrounding hyperemia or hemorrhage are characteristic signs. There is usually nonspecific gum bleeding, conjunctival hemorrhage, petechiae, and ecchymoses. Sufficient fruits and vegetables in the diet, as well as vitamin C supplements, prevent deficiency. Once diagnosed with vitamin C deficiency, treatment is with oral ascorbic acid three times per day.

Vitamin K plays an important role in blood clotting. It helps prevent excessive bleeding both inside and outside of the body. Vitamin K deficiency is rare in adults because many of the foods we eat contain adequate amounts of vitamin K1, and because the body manufactures vitamin K2. The human body also adequately recycles its existing supplies of vitamin K. However, certain conditions and some drugs can interfere with vitamin K absorption and creation, making it possible to become deficient. Vitamin K deficiency is caused by very low intake, fat malabsorption, or use of coumarin anticoagulants. This deficiency is most common in breastfed infants, and impairs blood clotting. *Hemorrhagic disease of the newborn* is most common between one and seven days after birth. There is a later form of the disease that occurs in infants between 2 and 12 weeks old – usually those that are breastfed and not given vitamin K supplementation. Dietary vitamin K deficiency is not common in healthy adults since the vitamin is so prevalent in green vegetables and since normal gut bacteria synthesize menaquinones (*vitamin K2).*

Signs and symptoms of vitamin K deficiency include bleeding, easy bruising, and oozing of blood from incisions or puncture wounds. Hemorrhagic disease of the newborn and late hemorrhagic disease in infants can cause cutaneous, GI, intrathoracic, and intracranial bleeding. Blood coagulation studies help to confirm the deficiency, with the prothrombin time is elevated while other clotting features are normal. The deficiency is also prevented by administration of phytonadione. Vitamin K is also discussed in Chapter 10.

Test Your Knowledge

1. What are the skin symptoms of vitamin C deficiency?
2. In which age group is vitamin K deficiency most prevalent?
3. What are the signs and symptoms of vitamin K deficiency?

DERMATITIS (ZINC DEFICIENCY)

Zinc deficiency can result in skin changes that look like eczema at first. There may be cracks and a glazed appearance on the skin, often found around the mouth, groin, and hands. The rash does not get better with moisturizers or steroid creams or lotions.

Zinc is mostly present in the bones, teeth, hair, skin, liver, muscles, leukocytes, and testes. It is a component of hundreds of enzymes in the body. Zinc absorption is reduced by high-fiber diets and when whole-grain bread is consumed in large quantities. However, zinc deficiency is not common in healthy individuals. *Secondary zinc deficiency* can occur in patients with diabetes mellitus, chronic kidney disease, **sickle cell disease**, liver disease, malabsorption, after weight loss, alcohol use disorder, surgery, severe burns, head injury, sepsis, and use of diuretics. A maternal zinc deficiency can cause low birth weight and fetal malformations. In children and adults, dermatitis is a significant outcome of zinc deficiency, followed by impaired wound healing, hair loss, impaired immunity, anorexia, night blindness, anemia, and lethargy.

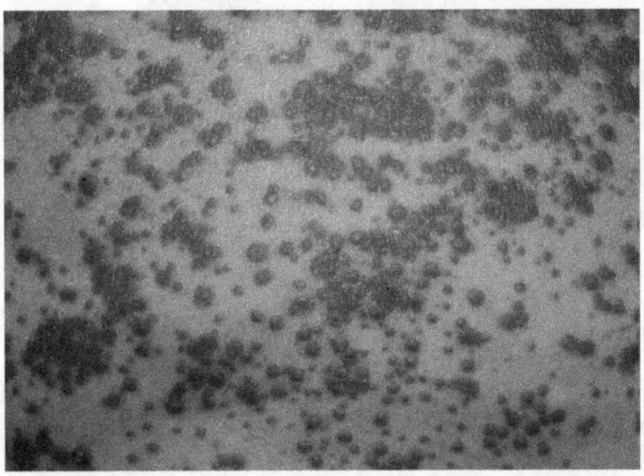

FIGURE 17.4 The effect of vitamin C deficiency on the gums.

Source: Shutterstock

Zinc deficiency is suspected based on the common signs and symptoms, though a clinical diagnosis may be difficult since these are often nonspecific. Zinc deficiency may be mimicked by deficiencies of biotin, riboflavin, or essential fatty acids. Low albumin levels are common with zinc deficiency, but they make serum zinc levels hard to interpret. The deficiency is treated with elemental zinc orally per day. The **autosomal recessive** disorder called **acrodermatitis enteropathica** causes zinc malabsorption, with psoriasiform dermatitis around the eyes, nose, and mouth as well as on the buttocks, perineum, toes, soles, fingers, palms, and nail beds. There may also be hair loss and nail infections. Signs and symptoms often occur after an infant is weaned off of breast milk, but zinc supplementation is usually able to quickly reverse the condition. Zinc deficiency is also discussed in Chapter 11.

NUTRITION AND DISCOLORATION OF THE SKIN

Skin discoloration is defined as any change in the natural color of the skin. It can occur for a variety of reasons. The skin can turn lighter or darker or can gain a tinge of red, orange, yellow, blue, or green. The most common form of skin hyperpigmentation is **melasma**, which involves dark brown or grayish patches on the face, and is due to a deficiency of folic acid (see Figure 17.5). Melasma is most common during pregnancy or when a woman is taking birth control pills. It is usually temporary, and can be reduced by increasing consumption of folic acid. While the problem can be embarrassing, the appearance of dark patches of skin does not usually indicate a serious medical condition.

Some changes in skin color are caused by changes in nutrition. Some can be treated through changes in the diet. While diseases or hormonal imbalances cause some instances of skin discoloration, certain nutrients missing from the diet can be a factor. A temporary change in skin color can be the result of overdosing on beta-carotene, a type of vitamin A. This nutrient can cause the skin to become orange or red when taken in excess. Too much copper in the diet can cause discoloration in skin since it boosts melanin production. The orangish yellow discoloration is a result of excess beta-carotene in the blood from consuming foods like carrots, squash, sweet potatoes, cantaloupe, or dried apricots.

Treating skin discoloration using nutritional supplements and dietary changes is possible in some cases. Adding folic acid to the diet often helps reduce skin discoloration. This nutrient can be found in leafy greens, nuts, liver and whole grains as well as in supplement

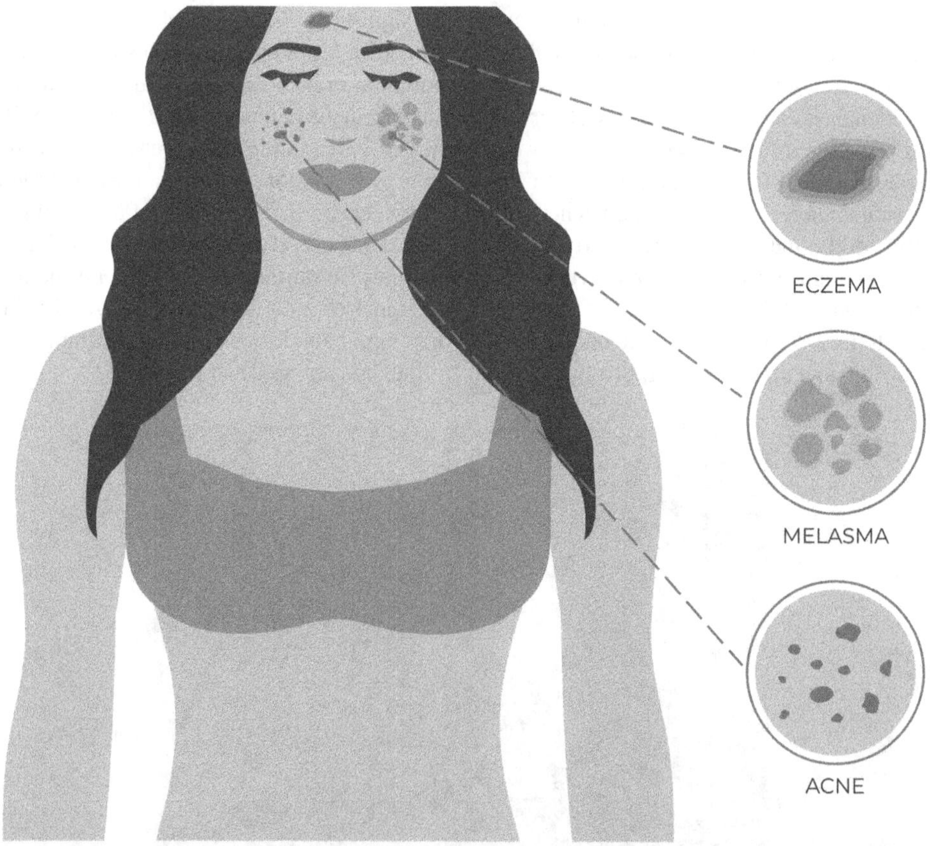

FIGURE 17.5 Melasma on the face.

Source: Shutterstock

form. Fresh fruit, vegetables, mushrooms, yeast, and molasses are good sources of **para-aminobenzoic acid** (PABA). The PABA amino acids are nutritional remedies for skin discoloration. Adding certain herbs and spices to the diet can also be helpful. Dandelion and watercress can be added to salads to provide extra folic acid and to provide protective antioxidant and phytochemical components that fortify and protect skin color.

FOCUS ON HYPERPIGMENTATION

Some factors that may trigger excess melanin production include genetics, age, hormones, sun exposure, inflammation, and skin injuries. Excess melanin production results in hyperpigmentation, which can be managed through diet by consuming foods that promote healing, reduce inflammation, and do not provoke hormonal changes.

FOCUS ON MELASMA IN WOMEN

Many women first see these blotchy patches and freckle-like spots on their face during pregnancy or when they start taking birth control pills. Melasma is so common during pregnancy that it's sometimes called the "mask of pregnancy." Women who have medium to dark skin tones are most likely to develop melasma. When melasma appears, it can cause tan, brown, grayish brown, or bluish gray patches and freckle-like spots. These usually appear on certain areas of face like the cheeks, forehead, chin, and above the upper lip. While less common, melasma can develop on the arms, neck, or elsewhere.

Test Your Knowledge

1. What causes secondary zinc deficiency?
2. What are the most common forms of skin discoloration?
3. How are nutritional supplements and diet used in the treatment of skin discolorations?

SKIN ABNORMALITIES (VITAMIN D DEFICIENCY)

Insufficient exposure to sunlight can lead to a vitamin D deficiency. This impairs bone mineralization and can result in rickets or osteomalacia. Vitamin D deficiency is relatively common worldwide. It is recommended that direct sunlight exposure to the arms, legs, face, arms, and hands occurs for 5–15 minutes for at least three days out of each week. In the diet, the vitamin is mostly found in fish liver oils and salt water fish. In some developed countries, milk and other types of foods are fortified with vitamin D. Human breast milk contains low levels of the vitamin. With age, vitamin D levels can decrease as skin synthesis declines. Use of sunscreen and darker skin pigmentation also reduce skin synthesis of the vitamin.

Vitamin D is metabolized in the liver and converted to the active hormone form, calcitriol, by the kidneys. Vitamin D and its related analogs are used to treat psoriasis, hypoparathyroidism, and renal osteodystrophy. A deficiency of vitamin D may result in the skin becoming red, dry, and itchy. It is also linked to the development of skin rashes. The deficiency may be suspected based on known history of insufficient sunlight exposure or dietary intake, signs and symptoms of bone or muscle conditions, and characteristic bone changes discovered in x-rays, and blood tests for measuring vitamin D. Correction of the deficiency is based on correcting calcium and phosphate deficiencies as well as administration of supplemental oral vitamin D. Vitamin D deficiency is also discussed in Chapter 10.

XEROSIS (OMEGA-3 FATTY ACID DEFICIENCY)

Omega-3 fatty acids are important for every cell in the body. They are an energy source that helps keep the body functioning normally. These fatty acids, which include *linolenic acid*, are found in large quantities in anchovies, bluefish, herring, salmon, sardines, sturgeon, lake trout, and tuna. Another form of the fatty acids is found in walnuts, flaxseed, canola oil, soybean oil, and chia seeds. There are also prescription formulations of omega-3 fatty acids available. **Xerosis**, also known as *xeroderma*, is dry skin related to an omega-3 fatty acid deficiency. There is delayed shedding of the superficial skin cells, leaving behind fine **white scales** (see Figure 17.6). Additionally, there are risk factors for xerosis, which include dry or cold climates, older age, atopic dermatitis, and frequent bathing with harsh soaps. On the hands, severely dry skin can become inflamed, leading to **eczema**. For treatment, the skin must be kept moist, yet bathing frequency should decrease and only warm water should be used. Skin moisturizes are indicated, especially immediately after bathing. They decrease transepidermal water loss. The thicker moisturizers, including those that are petrolatum- or oil-based, are better than those that are water-based. However, water-based lotions are often preferred by patients in warmer climates. Moisturizers often contain alpha-glycolic acids, ceramides, or beta-glycolic acids. Alpha-glycolic acids include glycolic, lactic, and pyruvic acids. Ceramides are composed of **sphingosine** and a fatty acid. An example of a beta-glycolic acid is salicylic acid, which is a keratolytic medication. Patients are advised to increase fluid intake and use room humidifiers. If eczema develops, topical corticosteroids may be needed to decrease inflammation and maintain the skin barrier.

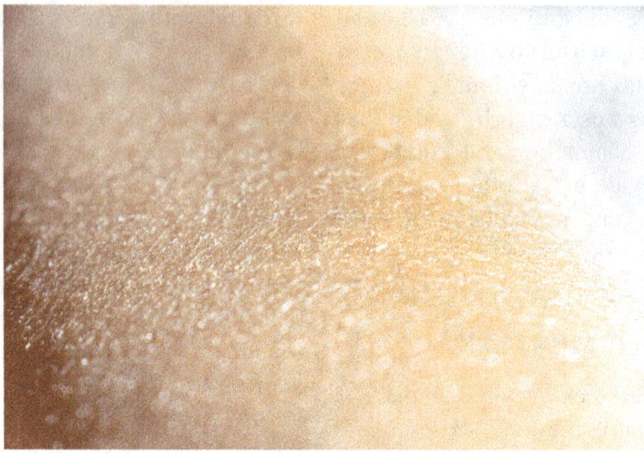

FIGURE 17.6 White scales on the skin signifying xerosis (xeroderma).

SEVERE DERMATITIS (OMEGA-6 FATTY ACID DEFICIENCY)

Omega-6 fatty acids are found in vegetable oils, nuts, and seeds. These fatty acids, which include *linoleic acid*, help protect against a variety of skin symptoms. When they are deficient in the body, the skin may be severely dry, scaly, flaky, cracked, peeling, lacking in a normal healthy appearance, bumpy, dull in certain patches, oily, irregular, thick, or callused. Some individuals develop **cradle cap** or dandruff. The hair may be dry, dull, brittle, or unable to be combed easily. The fingernails may be soft, frayed, split, brittle, dull, or may grow very-slowly. The eyes, mouth, and throat may often be dry. There may be excessive ear wax, excessive thirst, eczema, asthma, hay fever, hives, stiff or painful joints, cravings for fatty foods, and in women, a lack of vaginal lubrication, menstrual-like cramps, and premenstrual breast aches or tenderness.

Good dietary sources of omega-6 fatty acids include flaxseed, hempseed, grapeseed oil, pumpkin seeds, raw sunflower seeds, pine nuts, pistachios, borage oil, evening primrose oil, black currant seed oil, and acai. Omega-6 fatty acids reduce low-density lipoprotein (LDL) (bad) cholesterol and risks for type 2 diabetes mellitus. They help maintain bone health, stimulate hair growth, regulate the reproductive system, reduce nerve pain, reduce mastalgia, relieve premenstrual syndrome symptoms, regulate metabolism, strengthen brain function, and ensure normal growth. However, the omega-6 fatty acids must be taken in the correct quantities because overconsumption can result in increased risks for heart disease, cancer, bronchial asthma, arthritis, and depression.

FOCUS ON OMEGA-6 FATTY ACIDS

Like omega-3 fatty acids, the omega-6 fatty acids are essential fatty acids that are required by the body, but which the body is unable to manufacture. Omega-6 fatty acids are much more prevalent in the average person's diet than omega-3 fatty acids. It is important to understand that foods containing much more omega-6 fatty acids should be consumed in small quantities – such as fried and processed foods containing corn, cottonseed, or soybean oil.

FOCUS ON THE MEDITERRANEAN DIET

The Mediterranean diet has a healthy balance between omega-3 and omega-6 fatty acids. Studies show that people who follow a Mediterranean-style diet are less likely to develop heart disease. The Mediterranean diet does not include much meat, which is high in omega-6 fatty acids, though grass fed beef has a more favorable omega-3 to omega-6 fatty acid ratio. The diet emphasizes foods rich in omega-3 fatty acids, including whole grains, fresh fruits and vegetables, fish, olive oil, garlic, as well as moderate wine consumption.

Test Your Knowledge

1. How can vitamin D deficiency occur?
2. In which foods is linolenic acid found in large quantities?
3. In the proper quantities, what do omega-6 fatty acids help reduce?

HAIR AND NAIL ABNORMALITIES (PROTEIN, IRON, AND SELENIUM DEFICIENCY)

In order for hair and nails to grow and develop properly, many different nutrients are needed. Eating adequate protein is important for hair growth because hair follicles are mostly made of protein. A lack of protein in the diet has been shown to promote hair loss. Biotin is essential for the production of a hair protein called keratin, which is why biotin supplements are often marketed for hair growth. Vitamins and minerals from food play an important role in the hair follicle growth cycle, and in cellular turnover. Good hydration and adequate amounts of vitamins A, B, C, D, E, zinc, calcium, iron, and phosphorus are needed. Some of the best foods for hair growth are foods that have high nutritional value, such as eggs, leafy greens, soybeans, sweet potatoes, avocados, sweet peppers, nuts, beans, oysters, and fatty fish. Deficiencies in nutrients can affect hair health. Consuming a diet lacking the right nutrients can lead to hair loss. The speed of hair growth is based upon genetics, gender, age, and hormones. It may be reduced by nutrient deficiencies due to anorexia or anemia, zinc deficiency, and hormonal fluctuations related to menopause, polycystic ovaries, or thyroid disease. Many of the metabolic requirements of **follicle cells** such as minerals and vitamins must be satisfied for optimal hair growth. Iron deficiency may cause the hair to become dry and dull, and it may even fall out in some cases. Iron plays a key role not only in helping the body perform its appropriate bodily functions, but also aids in hair growth and strengthening. Nutrient deficiencies tend to not lead to permanent hair loss, however. Once the appropriate amount of vitamins is consumed again, hair should begin to regrow. Protein deficiency causes the hair to become thin and the nails to become brittle.

Essential fatty acids, like those found in fish oil or flax seed oil, can also help moisturize and strengthen nails. In addition to diet, there are many other things people can do to keep their nails healthy and strong. Good hygiene is important to keep nails infection-free. Infections can change the shape of the nail bed and cause deformities. Infected nails also break very easily, become discolored, and grow slowly. Overusing nail polish or nail polish remover and other chemicals can also cause damage, as well as dry and weaken the fingernails. Keeping your hands and fingernails well-hydrated with a good moisturizer can also help your nails be strong and appear healthy. In advanced iron deficiency anemia, the nails become brittle and spoon-shaped (see Figure 17.7). Iron assists the body in producing hemoglobin so that the red blood cells can carry enough oxygen to the cells, helping them grow and to be repaired. This also includes the cells that help with hair growth.

Selenium supports various *selenoproteins* that have a known role in maintaining healthy hair and nails. In many cases, common problems such as brittle nails or hair that splits at the ends may be corrected with a selenium supplement. Expensive nail-strengthening formulas and hair cures can be avoided by simply taking extra selenium to see how that affects the condition. Besides contributing to the health of hair and nails, selenium protects against cell damage, infections, and is involved in reproduction as well as the metabolism of thyroid hormones.

FOCUS ON IRON DEFICIENCY AND HAIR LOSS

The rate of hair growth varies between individuals. On average, hair grows around 15 cm (about 6 inches) per year. If hair is not growing sufficiently, there are a number of factors that can cause it, such as an iron deficiency. Therefore, an iron supplement might be able to correct the problem.

FOCUS ON DEFICIENCIES AFFECTING THE HAIR AND NAILS

Poor hair and nail health are usually signs of various nutritional deficiencies. Since the hair and nails are mostly made up of protein, a deficiency affects them in many ways. Iron deficiency has the potential to cause traditional male- and female-pattern hair loss, as well as spooning of the nails. Selenium supports *selenoproteins* that help maintain the hair and nails, so deficiency definitely affects the health of both of these components of the integumentary system.

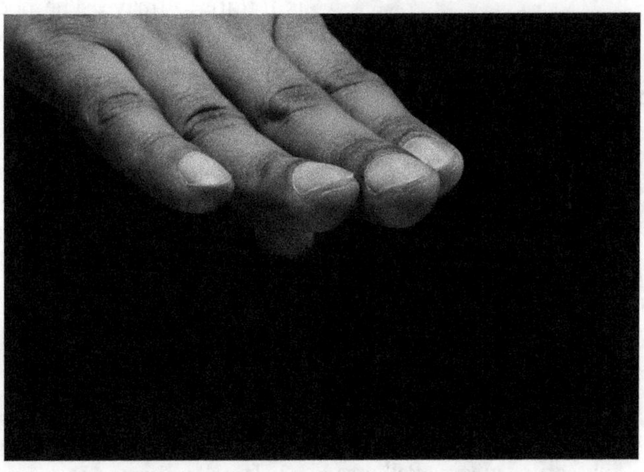

FIGURE 17.7 Brittle spoon-shaped nails due to advanced iron deficiency anemia.

KEY TERMS

Acrodermatitis enteropathica
Autosomal recessive
Casal necklace
Cradle cap
Decubitus ulcers
Dentin
Dermis
Ecchymoses
Eczema
Epidermis
Follicle cells
Follicular hyperkeratosis
Hair follicles
Hartnup disease
Melanocytes
Melasma
Millet
Nail cuticles
Osteoid
Para-aminobenzoic acid (PABA)
Pellagrous boot
Pellagrous glove
Petechiae
Sickle cell disease
Sphingosine
White scales
Xerosis

CLINICAL CASE STUDIES

Clinical Case Study 1

A 29-year-old woman went to her physician because of obvious darkening and thickening of the skin of her neck and upper trunk. She also had symmetrical erythema and scales on the neck and arms, as well as mouth soreness. The lesions got larger after any sun exposure and began to itch and burn. Her dietary history revealed a large consumption of maize, and testing revealed low serum niacin. Pellagra was diagnosed. The patient was started on vitamin B complex supplementation, two times per day. She was educated about changing her diet to consume more fish, vegetables, and nuts. Within one week, her condition started to improve, and by one month, it was completely resolved.

CRITICAL THINKING QUESTIONS

1. What are the descriptions of the dermatitis, diarrhea, and dementia that result from pellagra?
2. How can insufficient dietary niacin be compensated for?
3. What substance is used for the treatment of pellagra?

Clinical Case Study 2

A 22-year-old woman presented with brown lesions on her face, concentrated on her cheeks, forehead, nose, and chin. The lesions had well-defined margins and were worse after any sun exposure. The patient had recently become pregnant with her first child and was excited about being a mother. Examination revealed that the patient did not have a bacterial or fungal infection, so a diagnosis of melasma was given. The patient was told that her condition would probably resolve on its own after she delivered her baby.

CRITICAL THINKING QUESTIONS

1. Which deficiency is linked to melasma?
2. When does melasma most commonly occur?
3. Is melasma permanent or temporary?

Clinical Case Study 3

A ten-month-old infant was brought to his pediatrician by his mother because he has not met normal developmental and growth milestones, though his breastfeeding is normal. No solid foods have yet been introduced. He was in the 50th percentile for height and weight at two months of age, but now is below the 3rd percentile for weight, and is at the 3rd percentile for length. The initial diagnosis is failure to thrive. The pediatrician instructs his mother to start solid foods while breastfeeding continues, plus a formula is added to pumped breast milk to increase the caloric intake. Over several months of monitoring, a diagnosis of rickets is made. The infant is started on vitamin D and calcium carbonate supplementation as well as iron sulfate and zinc. By two years of age, he reaches the 45th percentile for weight and the 30th percentile for height. The supplementation continues as the patient continues to grow and develop.

CRITICAL THINKING QUESTIONS

1. How does rickets result from a vitamin D deficiency?
2. In which dietary sources is vitamin D mostly found?
3. How is vitamin D deficiency suspected in a patient?

Clinical Case Study 4

A 57-year-old man was evaluated because of rough, dry, and scaly skin, dry and dull hair, and nails that were brittle. He also had raised patches on his skin. Tests revealed that he had lower than normal levels of omega-6 fatty acids. When discussing the situation, the physician found that the patient never consumed foods that are high in omega-6 fatty acids because he disliked their taste, such as tofu, walnuts, and peanut butter. Since he was a vegan, he ate no meat of any kind, including chicken or pepperoni (both high in omega-6). A referral to a clinical nutritionist prompted changes in his diet that would naturally normalize his omega-6 fatty acid levels. Foods that were added (that the patient enjoyed) include safflower oil, hempseeds, sunflower seeds, avocado oil, almonds, and cashews.

CRITICAL THINKING QUESTIONS

1. What are the common skin changes caused by omega-6 fatty acid deficiency?
2. Aside from the skin and hair, what other symptoms may develop from omega-6 fatty acid deficiency?
3. Why must omega-6 fatty acids be taken in the correct quantities?

STUDY QUESTIONS

1. All of the following are able to worsen the general appearance of the skin, hair, and nails, EXCEPT:
   A. Smoking
   B. Excessive exercise
   C. Poor nutrition
   D. Stress

2. Which of the following foods do NOT speed up skin aging?
   A. White bread
   B. Caffeine
   C. Dry fruit
   D. Rice cakes

3. Which of the following is a sign or symptom of pellagra?
   A. Diarrhea
   B. Fever
   C. Headache
   D. Vomiting

4. Secondary zinc deficiency may occur in patients with all of the following diseases, EXCEPT:
   A. Sickle cell disease
   B. Liver disease
   C. Stroke
   D. Malabsorption

5. The middle layer the dermis contains all of the following, EXCEPT:
   A. Melatonin
   B. Blood vessels
   C. Nerves
   D. Hair follicles

6. Xeroderma occurs because of which food deficiency?
   A. Vitamin C
   B. Selenium
   C. Niacin
   D. Omega-3 fatty acid

7. Acrodermatitis enteropathica may be caused by malabsorption of which of the following minerals?
   A. Zinc
   B. Iron
   C. Selenium
   D. Calcium

8. All of the following factors may cause discoloration of the skin, EXCEPT:
   A. Folic acid deficiency
   B. Excessive copper in the diet
   C. Niacin deficiency
   D. Excessive beta-carotene

9. An excess of which of the following may trigger hyperpigmentation of the skin?
   A. Melanin
   B. Vitamin C
   C. Vitamin B12
   D. Melatonin

10. Omega-6 fatty acid deficiency may result in all of the following, EXCEPT:
    A. Dry mouth
    B. Hay fever
    C. Fatty liver
    D. Cradle cap

11. All of the following foods contain Omega-3 fatty acids, EXCEPT:
    A. Salmon
    B. Carrots
    C. Tuna
    D. Soybeans

12. Which of the following foods can be reduced by Omega-6 fatty acids?
    A. LDL cholesterol
    B. HDL cholesterol
    C. Estrogen
    D. Insulin

13. Which of the following can help moisturize and strengthen the nails?
    A. Vitamin C
    B. Iron supplements
    C. Fish oil
    D. Bananas

14. Which of the following nutrient deficiencies may cause brittle spoon-shaped nails?
    A. Zinc
    B. Selenium
    C. Iron
    D. Copper

15. All of the following nutritional deficiencies may cause hair loss, EXCEPT:
    A. Protein
    B. Fatty acids
    C. Vitamin E
    D. Zinc

FURTHER READING

1. Bailey, G.H. (2019). *The Etiology and Prevention of Pellagra*. Wentworth Press.
2. Banuelos, G.S., Lin, Z.Q., Ferreira Moraes, M., Guimaraes Guilherme, L.R., and Rodrigues, A. (2015). *Global Advances in Selenium Research from Theory to Application*. CRC Press.
3. Barroa, S. (2013). *Diseases, Diagnosis and Treatment (Volume 9: The Integumentary System – Epidermis, Dermis, Subcutaneous and Appendages)*. Barroa.
4. Burka Wild, D. (2014). *The Skin, Tongue, and Nails Speak – Observational Signs of Nutritional Deficiencies*. Unique Perspective Press.
5. Chive Suzzen, B. (2021). *Zinc Deficiency Symptoms – Acne, Eczema, Xerosis, Alopecia, Oral Ulceration, Stomatitis, Night Blindness, Impaired Immune System, Diarrhea, and Behavioral Abnormalities*. Chive Suzzen.
6. Council M.L., Sheinbein, D., and Cornelius, L.A. (2016). *The Washington Manual of Dermatology Diagnostics*. Lippincott, Williams, and Wilkins.
7. Farrukh, M. (2022). *Vitamin Deficiencies: Food and Health*. Farrukh.
8. Fields, L., and McLaughlin, C. (2022). *Hair Food – Recipes to Promote Positive Hair Health and Hair Loss Restoration*. Well of Wisdom Publishing House.
9. Fischer, K. (2018). *Eczema Detox – The Low-chemical Diet for Eliminating Skin Inflammation*. Exisle Publishing.
10. Forse, R.A. (2018). *Diet, Nutrition, and Immunity (Revivals Series)*. CRC Press.
11. Gay, J. (2018). *On Varicose Disease of the Lower Extremities and Its Allied Disorders, Skin Discoloration, Induration, and Ulcer*. HardPress.
12. Georgeou, G. (2020). *The Healthy Skin Diet – Recipes and Four-Week Eating Plan to Support Skin Health and Healing At Any Age*. Murdoch Books.
13. Hamilton, C. (2020). *Eating Habits for Healthy Skin*. TLC Publications Ltd.
14. Heid, G. (2018). *Iron Deficiency: Detect Iron Deficiency and Treat It Effectively*. Heid.
15. Helsloot, L. (2017). *The Complete Guide to Healthy Hair – A Three-step Program to Heal Your Hair*. Green Fit bvba.
16. Institute of Medicine of the National Archives. (2014). *Dietary Reference Intakes for Energy, Carbohydrate, Fiber, Fat, Fatty Acids, Cholesterol, Protein, and Amino Acids*. National Academies Press.
17. Luyase, N. (2021). *Vitamin C Deficiency Symptoms: Dry Skin, Malaise, Bruising Easily, Bone Pain, Chronic Inflammation, Recurrent Infections, Bleeding Gums, Swollen Joints, Poor Appetite, Poor Weight Gain*. Luyase.
18. Luyase, N. (2021). *Vitamin K Deficiency Symptoms: Nose Bleeding, Dark Stools, Heavy Menses, Blood in Vomit, Easy Bruising, Bleeding Gums, Joint Pain, Hematuria, Paleness or Yellowing of Skin, Blood Clots Under the Nails*. Luyase.
19. Mayor, J. (2022). *Dermatitis Diet – Skin Health Meal Receipes to Reverse Dry Skin, Itchiness, and Bumps*. Mayor.
20. McNamara, R.K. (2013). *The Omega-3 Fatty Acid Deficiency Syndrome: Opportunities for Disease Prevention*. Nova Biomedical.
21. Morton, R. (2016). *Zinc Deficiency: Etiology, Screening Methods and Health Implications (Nutrition and Diet Research Progress)*. Nova Biomedical.
22. Nartey, M. (2016). *The ABCs of Healthy Skin, Hair, and Nails*. CreateSpace Independent Publishing Platform.
23. Patterson, J.W. (2013). *Practical Skin Pathology: A Diagnostic Approach (Pattern Recognition Series)*. Churchill Livingstone.
24. Schoenfeld, P. (2018). *The Collagen Diet – Rejuvenate Skin, Strengthen Joints, and Feel Younger by Boosting Collagen Intake and Production*. Ulysses Press.
25. Seager, R. (2014). *Vitamin D Deficiency and Prevention of Chronic Diseases*. Seager.
26. Sillitoe, H. (2019). *Radiant – Eat Your Way to Healthy Skin*. Kyle Books.
27. Sordillo, L.A., and Sordillo, P.P. (2021). *Biophotonics, Tryptophan and Disease*. Academic Press.
28. Zev, C. (2022). *Dermatitis Treatment Handbook: Everything You Must Know about Dermatitis, Its Treatment, Diagnosis, Causes, Symptoms, Precautions and Prevention*. Zev.

18 Nutritional Effects on the Musculoskeletal System

OUTLINE

LEARNING OBJECTIVES

After study of the chapter, readers should be able to:

1. Explain the signs and symptoms of insufficient dietary protein.
2. Identify risk factors that increase muscle cramps.
3. Discuss the causes of osteoporosis and osteomalacia.
4. Describe the common features of sarcopenia.
5. Identify the causes of rhabdomyolysis.
6. Explain the outcomes of muscle ischemia.
7. Describe the causes of carpopedal spasm.
8. Explain the role of osteoclasts, osteoblasts, and calcitonin in bone mass.
9. Identify the amount of calcium needed per day to help prevent osteoporosis.
10. Discuss the treatment of osteomalacia.

OVERVIEW

Inadequate dietary protein intake may lead to muscle injury. Calcium and vitamin D work together, and are needed for bone health, but also to help muscles work properly. The absence of dietary calcium and vitamin D causes the body to remove these nutrients from the bones and teeth for use. Porous bone tissue results and the bones become brittle and weak. Calcium and phosphate are bound together as a crystal-like mineral, embedded into the collagen protein framework of bones as they grow and develop. The combination of minerals and protein in bones gives them strength and rigidity so that they can protect soft tissues, and provide a rigid framework to support movement. Muscle strength is important for determining risk for falls. Bone loss has long been recognized as a consequence of aging. Sarcopenia is the gradual loss of skeletal muscle mass and strength that occurs with advancing age. Aging is characterized by a progressive decline of muscle mass and function. Bone loss is widespread in older people. Sarcopenia and osteopenia or osteoporosis are associated with adverse outcomes including falls, fractures, functional decline, frailty, and mortality. Nutrition and exercise are important environmental factors that can influence musculoskeletal development, by maintaining peak bone and muscle mass as well as strength.

PROTEIN DEFICIENCY AND MUSCLE INJURY

Protein deficiency refers to low protein levels in the blood. It can occur when there is insufficient dietary protein to meet the body's needs. For example, a diet that severely restricts protein consumption can cause the condition. Deficiency also occurs if the body cannot effectively digest and absorb dietary proteins because of a medical condition. The digestion of proteins breaks them down into amino acids, which aid in function and growth. Therefore, protein is a macronutrient that is important for healthy, strong muscles, bones, hair, and nails. Since there is no mechanism that allows for excess amino acids to be stored in the body, they must be continually supplied in the diet. Insufficient protein can lead to a variety of signs and symptoms, which include:

- Reduced muscle mass
- Reduced immunity and increase infections
- Edema
- Slower wound healing
- Preeclampsia during pregnancy

Protein deficiency in infants and children may have different effects such as lightening of the skin and hair, sometimes in small patches. Preterm infants born with hypoproteinemia have higher risks for severe neurological injury and death.

Current adult guidelines recommend that adults have 10%–35% of their daily calories from protein, but even this amount is considered low by many experts. Though most vegetarian diets supply enough protein since legumes, nuts, and seeds are consumed, protein levels do become too low in some people. Medical conditions that may cause protein

DOI: 10.1201/b22969-21

deficiency include AIDS, anorexia nervosa, cancer, chronic obstructive pulmonary disease (COPD), **amyloidosis** and other gastrointestinal (GI) conditions, and renal failure. About one billion people throughout the world have protein deficiency, often because of limited access to good quality foods. In the United States, even with adequate food supplies, up to 33% of adults over age 50 do not have sufficient daily protein intake. Requirements for protein intake vary, based on age, gender, and physical activity. Most adults should consume 5.5 ounces of protein per day, which is 38.5 ounces per week. About 26 ounces out of this total amounts should come from eggs, meat, and poultry. About eight ounces should come from seafood, and about five ounces from nuts, seeds, and soy products. For vegetarians, there should be 3.5–5.5 ounces or daily protein, based on total caloric intake. This is nearly evenly split between beans, lentils, peas, soy products, nuts, and seeds. There should be about three to four ounces of eggs consumed every week. Three ounces of protein is about as large as the palm of an adult's hand. Ways to increase protein intake include adding foods such as cheese, Greek yogurt, nut butters, oats, and quinoa.

Since the body's muscles are the largest reservoir of protein, insufficient dietary protein causes the body to pull protein from the skeletal muscles in order to preserve more important tissues and functions. Muscle wasting occurs over time. Even moderate protein insufficiency – especially in the elderly – may cause muscle wasting. Increased protein intake may slow natural age-related muscle degeneration. After muscle injury, protein intake that is appropriate for the type and extent of the injury can trigger muscle repair and maintenance. It can also improve insulin sensitivity and speed up wound healing. Muscle injury causes **myoglobin** to be released into the bloodstream and causes kidney damage as well as **myoglobinuria**.

FOCUS ON PROTEIN DEFICIENCY AND EFFECTS UPON MUSCLES

When dietary protein is insufficient, the body takes protein from the skeletal muscles to preserve more important tissues and functions. As a result, a lack of protein leads to muscle wasting over time. Even a moderate protein insufficiency may cause muscle wasting, especially in older adults. The muscles undergo microscopic tears when there is a lack of protein and they are used during exercise or strength training.

Test Your Knowledge

1. What are the signs and symptoms of insufficient dietary protein?
2. What medical conditions may cause a protein deficiency?
3. What is the breakdown of muscle tissue called, and what are its causes?

SARCOPENIA

Sarcopenia is also known as age-related, voluntary muscle wasting. It is a common feature of **frailty**, along with weakness, slowed motor function, exercise intolerance, weight loss, frequent falls, immobility, frequent worsening of chronic diseases, and incontinence. Sarcopenia actually begins when a person is in his or her 30s, as muscle mass starts to decrease, which is a continual process (see Figure 18.1). To reduce or prevent frailty and the likelihood of sarcopenia, exercise and a healthy diet are recommended. Older adults that engage in regular aerobic exercise, via walking, running, or swimming, have increased life expectancy and less functional decline, compared to sedentary adults. Even mood and cognitive function may be improved. Weight training is able to help increase bone mass, and reduce risks for falling and bone fractures. A healthy diet can prevent risks for contributing diseases that make an individual become frail. These include breast and colon cancers, obesity, osteoporosis, and undernutrition. Good diets can also reduce morbidity and mortality.

Symptoms of sarcopenia include weakness and loss of **stamina**. Physical activity declines, which results in further muscle shrinkage. It is believed that with aging, there is a reduction in nerve cells that send signals from the brain to the muscles, initiating movement. There are also lower concentrations of growth hormone, and testosterone. Older people have less ability to convert proteins into energy. Muscle mass is also affected by not getting enough calories or proteins every day.

Various diets are able to prevent frailty and sarcopenia. Low-fat diets and only moderate alcohol intake may decrease risks for cardiovascular disease. A reduced sodium diet can lower blood pressure. High-calcium diets and calcium supplementation help maintain bone density and reduce risks of fractures. High-fiber diets can prevent colon cancer, and have beneficial effects upon serum lipids. Adequate intake of vitamins and minerals can prevent bone loss, falls, fractures, and chronic diseases.

The best treatment for sarcopenia is exercise – primarily, resistance training or strength training, which increase strength and endurance. Resistance training uses *resistance bands*, and can help the neuromuscular system and hormones. It can improve the ability to convert protein to energy in only two weeks. It is important to work with an experienced physical therapist or trainer to develop an exercise plan.

FOCUS ON SARCOPENIA

Physically inactive people can lose 3%–5% of their muscle mass every decade after the age of 30. Even active people lose some muscle loss. Any loss of muscle is important because it reduces strength and mobility. Sarcopenia usually happens more quickly around the age of 75, but it can speed up as early as age 65 or as late as age 80.

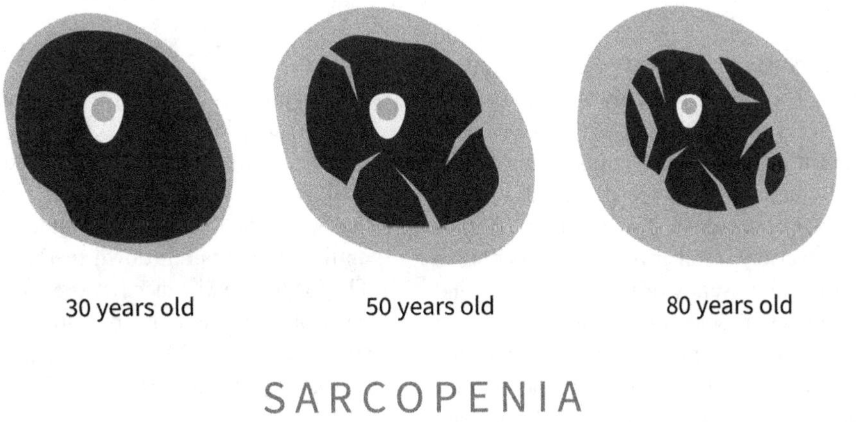

FIGURE 18.1 Sarcopenia over various ages.

MUSCLE INJURY

Injuries to skeletal muscles, the soft tissues that are attached to bones that allow for movement, can be painful and disruptive to everyday life. Thankfully, many muscle injuries are mild and can be addressed at home or at a reputable immediate care center. The four main types of skeletal muscle injuries and the symptoms they may cause are described below.

Muscle Strain

A muscle strain is a microscopic injury to a muscle or tendon. A mild strain usually refers to an overstretching of tissue, while a more severe strain may cause a partial or complete tear that is visible on an imaging test. Most strains are mild and occur in the hands, elbows, legs, and ankles. Common signs and symptoms of a mild muscle strain include tenderness, pain, muscle spasms, bruising, swelling, weakness, and limited range of motion in the affected area. Muscle strains are very common and can affect anyone, although people who frequently exercise or play sports have the highest risk. Fortunately, many mild muscle strains can be addressed at home by resting and icing the affected area.

Muscle Tear

A muscle tear is also referred to as a "pulled muscle," and is a severe strain that causes a muscle or tendon, along with its blood vessels, to tear partially or completely. It is a more extensive injury that requires prompt treatment from a medical professional. It usually takes a significant amount of force to cause a muscle tear, such as during a motor vehicle accident or contact sports injury. Signs and symptoms commonly involve sudden, intense pain along with weakness, swelling, and bruising. Areas of the body that are most susceptible to muscle tears include the neck, shoulders, lower back, and hamstrings.

Rhabdomyolysis

Rhabdomyolysis is the breakdown of skeletal muscle fibers. It is a rare condition that requires emergency medical treatment, and can be fatal, or result in permanent disability. Rhabdomyolysis occurs when muscle fibers die and release of intracellular muscle components, including myoglobin, creatine kinase (CK), aldolase, and lactate dehydrogenase, as well as electrolytes, into the bloodstream and extracellular space. Rhabdomyolysis ranges from an asymptomatic illness with elevation in the CK level to a life-threatening condition associated with extreme elevations in CK, electrolyte imbalances, acute renal failure, and disseminated intravascular coagulation. It largely affects people who routinely perform intense physical activity and work in hot environments. Examples of high-risk individuals include construction workers, firefighters, first responders, professional athletes, and farmers. Common signs and symptoms of this condition include muscle cramps or aches, fatigue, weakness, and dark urine. Factors that can cause rhabdomyolysis include the following:

- Extremes of body temperature
- Ischemia of muscle tissue
- Low phosphate levels
- Long surgical procedures
- Seizures or muscle tremors
- Severe physical exertion
- Severe dehydration
- Trauma or crush injuries
- Use of cocaine, amphetamines, statins, or heroin

Muscle Contusion

A muscle contusion is also known as a muscle bruise or hematoma. It results from a forceful, blunt impact, such as getting hit with a baseball. While this impact does not break the skin, it crushes underlying muscle and can cause significant bruising, swelling, pain, and reduced range of motion. Most muscle contusions can be managed at home with self-care measures like periodic rest and ice therapy. Rarely, surgery may be necessary to relieve pressure that can build from internal bleeding and swelling.

MUSCLE CRAMPS

Muscle cramps are involuntary and painful contractions of one or several muscles. They occur suddenly for brief periods of time. A muscle cramp is commonly referred to as a *charley horse*. It can occur during rest or sleep, but most often during or after exercise. Leg cramps at night usually affect the calf muscle and cause plantar flexion of the foot and toes. Cramps can be mimicked by a variety of other disorders. **Dystonias** cause muscle spasms that are usually of longer duration, and often recur. Spasms affect muscles of the face, neck, and hands. **Tetany** causes muscle spasms that are also more sustained. There may be repetitive, short twitches of the muscles that are usually bilateral and diffuse. *Muscle ischemia* can happen during exertion. In patients with the peripheral arterial disease, **claudication** may occur. This may cause calf pain, but it is due to insufficient blood flow to the muscles. Benign idiopathic leg cramps usually occur at night with unknown cause. Factors that increase risks for muscle cramps and may make them worse include the following:

- Dehydration
- Drugs
- Electrolyte abnormalities, such as low levels of magnesium or potassium
- Metabolic disorders
- Neurologic disorders
- Removal of excessive fluid during dialysis

Patient history must include descriptions of the duration, frequency, location, triggers, and symptoms of the cramps. Symptoms related to neurologic or muscle disorders include stiffness, pain, weakness, and loss of sensation. Any factors that may contribute to dehydration, or to fluid or electrolyte imbalances must be documented. These include diarrhea, vomiting, excessive exercise and sweating, use of diuretics, recent dialysis, and pregnancy. Amenorrhea, menstrual irregularity, and pregnancy can be related. Weakness can be linked to neurologic disorders.

Muscle cramps can be prevented in a variety of ways. These include gently stretching muscles prior to exercising or going to sleep, drinking plenty of fluids after exercise containing potassium, not exercising right after eating, avoiding smoking, and caffeine.

FOCUS ON RHABDOMYOLYSIS

Rhabdomyolysis is a syndrome characterized by muscle necrosis and the release of intracellular muscle constituents into the blood circulation. Muscle pain and myoglobinuria may be present. The severity of illness ranges from asymptomatic elevations in serum muscle enzymes to life-threatening disease associated with extreme enzyme elevations, electrolyte imbalances, and acute kidney injury.

FOCUS ON STRETCHING

The *runner's stretch* involves standing with one leg forward and bent at the knee while the other leg is behind and the knee is straight. Placing the hands on a wall help maintain balance. Both heels remain flat on the floor. The knee of the front leg is bent some more until a stretch is felt down the back of the other leg. The longer the distance between the feet and the more the front knee is bent, the greater the stretch. Each stretch is held for 30 seconds, then repeated five times. Then, the procedure is repeated for the other leg.

Test Your Knowledge

1. When does sarcopenia begin?
2. Which factors increase risks for muscle cramps?
3. How can muscle cramps be prevented?

HEAT CRAMPS

Heat cramps are painful and spasmodic muscle cramps. They are most common after exercising heavily in an environment that is hot and humid. They occur in physically fit individuals that perspire profusely and replace lost water – but not sodium. This causes hyponatremia. Heat cramps are most common in athletes, during training for the military, and in people that work in engine rooms or as miners, roofers, and steel workers. The cramps come on quickly, usually in the arms and legs. Cramps can start during or after exercise. The hands and feet may become incapacitated by **carpopedal spasm** and severe pain. The cramps may last for minutes to hours. Diagnosis is based on patient history and physical evaluation.

Heat cramps can be immediately relieved by firm and passive stretching. Affected people should rest in an environment that is cool. Fluids and electrolytes must be replenished orally, with salted water or commercial sports drinks. If oral repletion is not possible and rapid relief is needed, 0.9% saline solution can be injected IV. Heat cramps can be prevented by sufficient condition, getting adapted to a hot and moist environment before exercising, and managing sodium balance in the body.

NUTRITION FOR HEALTHY BONES

During the adolescent years, bone grows rapidly until peak bone mass is achieved. *Peak bone mass* refers to the greatest mass, strength, and density of bones that can genetically accumulate. Bone building increases steadily during adolescence, reaches its peak in early adulthood, and then starts to decline later in life. By age 18, about 90% of peak bone mass has been achieved. Most young women and men reach their maximum bone density by their late 20s. Although genetics determine 60%–80%

of peak bone mass, lifestyle choices, including diet and physical activity, are also predictors of bone accumulation during growth.

Physical activity and nutrition are essential to achieving peak bone mass. Many studies addressing nutrition and bone health in children have concluded that inadequate nutrition, particularly insufficient intake of calcium and vitamin D during growth periods, may negatively affect peak bone mass. Malnutrition that occurs with eating disorders has also been shown to have a direct effect on bone mass development. In young individuals with anorexia nervosa, bone loss can be detected after only six months of illness. Deficits can remain even after weight gain recovery. The severe deficiency of nutrients that occurs with anorexia results in a reduction of bone formation, as well as increased bone resorption. Even nutrient deficits from short-term fasting, over four days or longer, results in a marked decrease of bone formation markers in normal, healthy young people. Achieving peak bone mass cannot be emphasized enough. It has been shown that achieving peak bone mass during the adolescent years could significantly delay the onset of osteoporosis by 13 years, reducing the risk of osteoporotic fractures later in life.

By the age of 40, we all slowly begin to lose bone mass. However, as with adolescents aiming to achieve peak bone mass, quality nutrition and regular exercise also help adults avoid the severe bone loss that leads to osteoporosis. A recent study examining the effects of diet on bone health found that postmenopausal women who ate a Mediterranean diet were less likely to suffer from hip fractures. The Mediterranean diet is well known for its emphasis on foods that include fish, vegetables, fruits, legumes, whole grains, nuts, seeds, and olive oil. Meat, cheese, and sweets are very limited. This study highlights how an overall healthy diet may be more important in supporting bone health than focusing on the intake of any single nutrient. This is because the matrix of bone is mineralized with calcium and phosphate, which in turn gives strength to its structure. Calcium is also important for muscle contraction, heartbeat regulation, nerve impulse transmission, regulation of blood pressure, and immune system function. 99% of the calcium in the body is stored in the bones. Unfortunately, when there is not enough calcium in the diet, the body pulls calcium from the bones to support these other functions. Without adequate calcium, bones become weak and fragile.

Osteoporosis

Osteoporosis is a major public health problem, affecting millions of individuals. Dietary intake is an important modifiable factor for bone health. Inadequate intake of nutrients important to bone increases the risk for bone loss, and subsequent osteoporosis. The process of bone formation requires an adequate and constant supply of nutrients, such as calcium, protein, magnesium, phosphorus, vitamin D, potassium, and fluoride. However, there are several other vitamins and minerals needed for metabolic processes related to bone, including manganese, copper, boron, iron, zinc, vitamin A, vitamin K, vitamin C, and the B vitamins. Although the recommended levels of nutrients traditionally related to bone were aimed to promote bone mass and strength, the recommended levels of the other nutrients that also influence bone were different parameters. Today we know that they may not be optimal for bone health, because of recent epidemiological studies and clinical trials.

Osteoporosis is a progressive metabolic bone disease. There is decreased bone mineral density, comparing bone mass per unit of volume. The process of osteoporosis is shown in Figure 18.2. The bone structure deteriorates over time. Skeletal weakness results in fractures with only minor or non-apparent trauma. Mostly, the fractures occur in the wrist, hip, thoracic and lumbar spine. In the human body, bone is formed and resorbed continually. These processes are extremely balanced. **Osteoblasts** manufacture the organic matrix of bones and then mineralize them. **Osteoclasts** resorb bone and are regulated by parathyroid hormone, **calcitonin**, estrogen, *cytokines*, vitamin D, and **prostaglandins**.

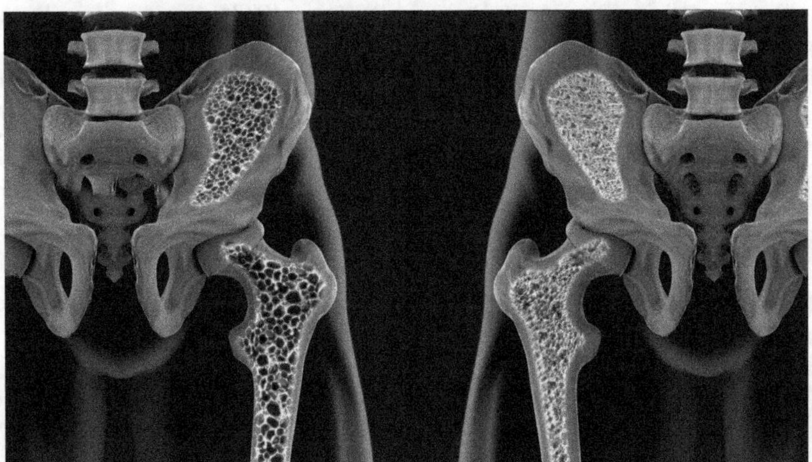

FIGURE 18.2 The process of osteoporosis.

Peak bone mass occurs between the ages of 25 and 30. By age 40 the body begins to lose bone mass. However, to avoid severe bone loss over time, proper nutrition and regular exercise are helpful. Men have higher bone mass than women. The bone mass plateaus for about ten years as bone formation is nearly equal to bone resorption. However, after this, bone loss occurs at about 0.3%–0.5% per year. Starting with *menopause*, bone loss occurs five to seven per years. Then, bone loss slows down again. The majority of cases bone loss occur in postmenopausal women and older men. Conditions that accelerate bone loss may also include gonadal insufficiency, decreased intake of calcium, low vitamin D levels, certain medications, and hyperparathyroidism. Some patients have insufficient intake of calcium during adolescence, and they never achieve their peak bone mass. The primary mechanism of bone loss is increased resorption of bone. This causes decreased bone mass and microarchitectural deterioration.

Fragility fractures are rare in children, adolescents, premenopausal women, or men under age 50 with normal gonadal function and no identified secondary cause. Risk factors for osteoporosis include immobilization, being sedentary on a regular basis, and a low body mass index. Predisposing factors for bone loss include poor dietary intake of calcium, magnesium, phosphorus, and vitamin D. Use of tobacco and alcohol negatively affects bone mass. Family history of osteoporosis – especially a parental history of hip fracture – increases risks.

At least 1,000 mg of elemental calcium should be consumed daily. For postmenopausal women and older men, and during pubertal growth 1,200 mg per day of elemental calcium, including in the diet recommended. For the best results, calcium intake should come from foods. Supplements are to be used if dietary intake is not sufficient. Supplements are usually calcium carbonate or calcium citrate. These are both absorbed well if taken with meals, but calcium citrate is better absorbed if the patient has **achlorhydria**. Calcium is best taken in divided doses, of 500–600 mg, two or three times per day. Vitamin D supplements are recommended to be taken as 600–800 units per day, though those that are deficient in vitamin D may need more. Supplemental vitamin D is usually cholecalciferol (the natural form of the vitamin), though the synthetic form (ergocalciferol) is also acceptable.

FOCUS ON NUTRITIONAL DEFICIENCIES AND OSTEOPOROSIS

Calcium and vitamin D deficiencies can lead to osteoporosis in older adults. In the case of calcium deficiency, a high phosphorus content can damage bone tissue. Also, low serum levels of vitamin D reduce bone density and increase the risk of fracture. Additionally, high protein intake results in calcium excretion and loss of bone mass. A healthy diet contains at least 1,200 mg per day of calcium and 600 International Units of vitamin D.

FOCUS ON IRON DEFICIENCY AND OSTEOPOROSIS

It is important to remember that bone formation is slower than bone resorption. Therefore, a prolonged condition of iron deficiency could result in bone loss, and increase risks for osteoporosis, with significant impacts upon public health.

FOCUS ON DIETARY EFFECTS UPON BONE HEALTH

Diets high in refined sugar have been shown to impair bone growth and mechanical strength. Drinking carbonated soft drinks containing phosphates and coloring has been shown to interfere with calcium metabolism. It is also well known that salt, especially abundant in processed foods, increases the excretion of calcium through the urine. Excessive caffeine, such as four or more cups of coffee a day, can result in loss of calcium and magnesium, predisposing you to higher risk of fractures.

Test Your Knowledge

1. When do heat cramps most commonly occur, and in which individuals are they most common?
2. Where do most osteoporosis-related fractures occur?
3. How much calcium is needed per day to help prevent osteoporosis?

OSTEOMALACIA

Osteomalacia in adults is primarily caused by vitamin D deficiency. Hypocalcemia, caused by vitamin D deficiency, results in increased production of parathyroid hormone (PTH). This causes hyperparathyroidism, followed by increased absorption, bone mobilization, and renal conservation of calcium. Phosphate excretion is increased. Therefore, serum calcium levels may be normal, but due to hypophosphatemia, there is impaired bone mineralization.

People that have chronic kidney disease can develop osteomalacia since renal production of 1,25-dihydroxyvitamin D is decreased and phosphate levels are higher than normal. Hepatic dysfunction may interfere with production of active metabolites of vitamin D. Osteomalacia predisposes all adults to fractures. Elderly people may have hip fractures from only slight trauma. Bone demineralization, mostly of the spine, hip, wrist, and lower extremities appears on x-rays. The fibrous lamellae can be seen. Incomplete areas of demineralization, appearing similar to ribbons, are visualized in the cortex. These areas are classified as **Looser zones**, **Milkman syndrome**, and **pseudofractures**.

The most common symptoms of osteomalacia are pain in the bones and hips, bone fractures, and muscle weakness. Patients can be cured by administration of 1,600 units of vitamin D3 orally once per day. Serum calcium and phosphate increase. Serum **alkaline phosphatase** decreases in about ten days. By the third week of treatment, sufficient calcium and phosphate have been deposited in the bones so that they appear on x-rays. After approximately one month, doses can usually be slowly reduced to the common maintenance levels of 600 units daily. If there is tetany, vitamin D is supplemented with IV calcium salts for as long as one week. Some elderly patients require vitamin D3, 1,000 to more than 2,000 units per day, to maintain sufficient levels. This dose is higher than the recommended daily allowance for older adults, but the current upper limit for vitamin D is 4,000 units per day. Higher doses of vitamin D2 (25,000 to 50,000 unite per week or month) have been prescribed. Vitamin D3 is now preferred over vitamin D2 because it is stronger.

Since osteomalacia related to defective vitamin D metabolite production is resistant to vitamin D, it does not respond well to normally effective doses. Endocrinologic evaluation is needed since treatment is based on the actual defect that is present. When the 25-hydroxy vitamin D production is defective, vitamin D3, 2,000 units, is given per day. If the patient has a kidney disorder, he or she often needs 1,25-dihydroxyvitamin D (calcitriol) supplements. Calcium or phosphate supplements are also needed for treatment, depending on the individual case. Braces can be worn to reduce or prevent bone irregularities. In severe cases, surgery is required to correct bone deformities.

FOCUS ON OSTEOMALACIA

Osteomalacia, the adult form of rickets, refers to significant bone softening, usually due to a severe vitamin D deficiency. In older adults, osteomalacia commonly leads to fractures. Untreated, osteomalacia can also result in severe deformities. With today's treatments, improvements can occur in a few weeks, though complete bone healing takes approximately six months. Osteomalacia affects about one of every 1,000 people worldwide.

Test Your Knowledge

1. How does osteomalacia develop in adults?
2. Where does the bone demineralization of osteomalacia usually occur?
3. How much daily vitamin D3 can be curative for osteomalacia?

BONE FRACTURES

The bones provide the architectural framework for all soft tissues and organs held inside the body. They help us to walk, run, and perform many different motions and activities. The bones are necessary for the production of blood cells. They store many minerals, especially calcium. While strong, bones have a certain amount of flexibility and can bend to some degree when outside force is applied. However, when the force applied is too excessive, the bone will break, which is known as a *bone fracture.*

Bone fractures are a very common injury and can affect anyone, at any age. If you are older than 50 or have a family history of osteoporosis, a bone density screening is required. Fractures are usually caused by traumas like falls, car accidents, or sports injuries. Some medical conditions and repetitive forces such as running can increase the risk for experiencing certain types of fractures. There are many different types of fractures. A specific fracture type depends on the pattern, the cause, and the area of the body.

The classifications of bone fractures include: greenstick, transverse, comminuted, spiral, **pathological**, **longitudinal**, compound, depressed fracture, and **stress fractures** (see Figure 18.3). An **avulsion fracture** occurs when a muscle or ligament pulls on a bone, causing it to fracture. A **greenstick fracture** occurs when a bone bends and cracks, instead of breaking completely into separate pieces. A greenstick fractures occur in children younger than ten years of age. The most common cause of a greenstick fracture is a fall. The majority of greenstick fractures occur in the arms, when children attempt to catch themselves as they fall.

Transverse fractures occur when a bone is broken perpendicular to its length. The fracture pattern is a straight line that runs in the opposite direction of the bone. Transverse

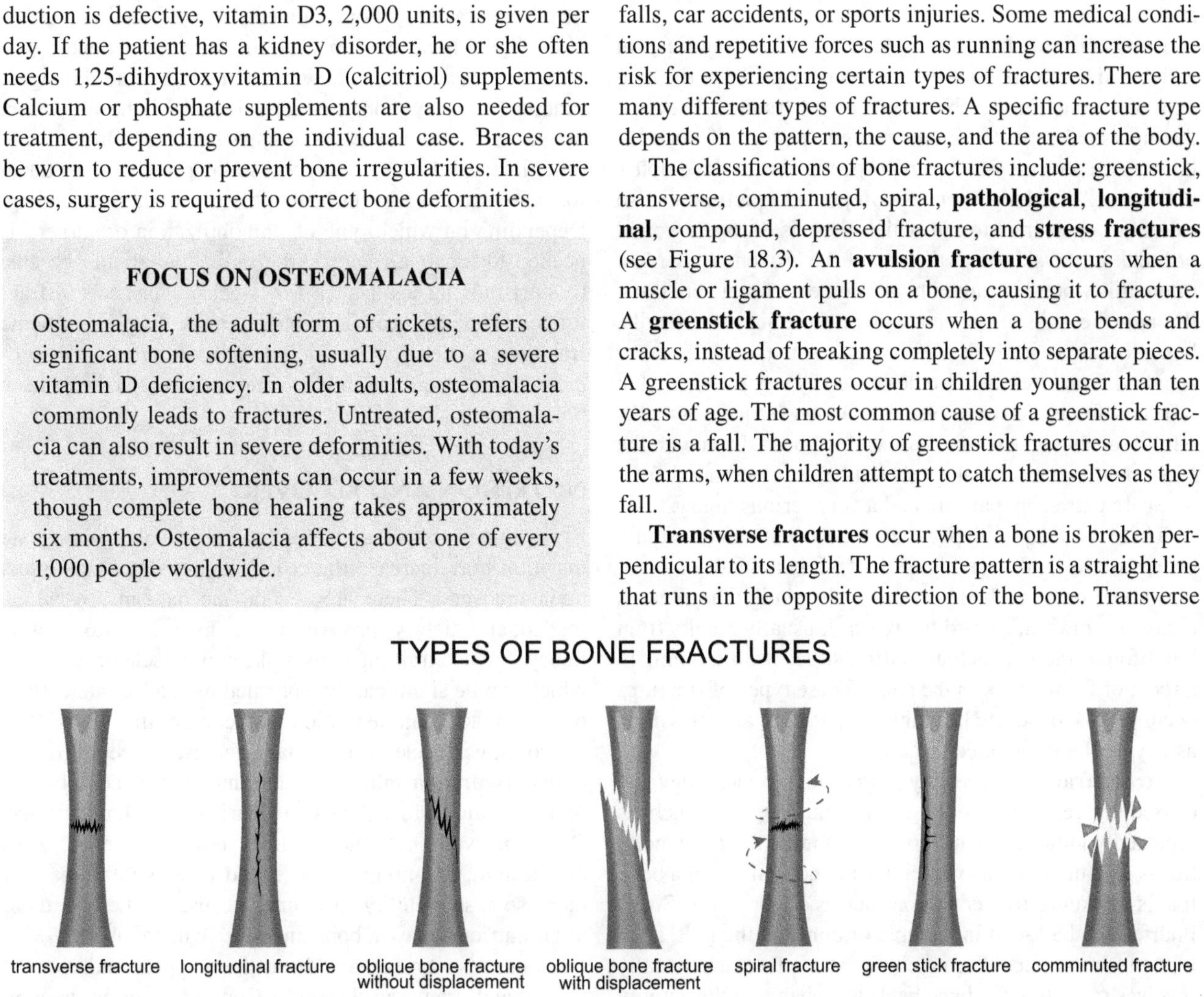

FIGURE 18.3 Types of bone fractures.

fractures can happen to any bone in the body, but usually affect longer bones after a trauma, such as a fall or accident. A **comminuted fracture** is a break of the bone into more than two fragments. Since considerable force and energy is required to fragment a bone, fractures of this degree occur after high-impact trauma, such as in vehicular accidents. Spiral fractures happen when a bone is broken with a twisting motion. They create a fracture line that wraps around the bone and looks like a corkscrew. Spiral fractures are serious bone fractures, because the bone is broken into complicated patterns. They sometimes splinter, making a spiral fracture very difficult to treat.

Pathologic bone fractures occur in patients with chronic disorders, and may have negative effects on the density of bones. With weak bones, there is a higher chance for fractures, even without any direct impact. Pathologic bone fractures are caused by disorders such as bone cancers, osteoporosis, cerebral palsy, muscular dystrophy, spinal muscular atrophy, spina bifida, and renal disease. Factors that increase the risks for pathologic bone fractures include: vitamin D, calcium, and protein deficiency. Lack of physical activity and mobility, sex or growth hormone disruptions, and being underweight or overweight are other factors.

Longitudinal fractures are uncommon injuries, in which a **diaphyseal fracture** line occurs parallel to the long axis of a bone, in the absence of direct trauma. They are distinguished from the more common pattern of horizontal stress fractures, which run perpendicular to the diaphyseal cortex of a long bone. A **compound fracture** is also called an open fracture, in which there is an open wound or break in the skin near the site of the broken bone. Most often, this wound is caused by a fragment of bone breaking through the skin at the moment of the injury. Generally, bones break as a result of force or trauma, such as a car accident. Fractures can also be caused by less traumatic but repeated force. For example, if a person frequently walks while wearing a heavy backpack, the repeated force on the legs could cause a crack in their fibulas. Compound fractures are extremely painful, and a very serious injury.

There is also a **depressed fracture**, which usually occurs in the skull (see Figure 18.4). It is a break in a cranial bone, or a crushed portion of the skull. The bone is depressed inward, toward the brain. It usually results from blunt force trauma, such as getting struck with a hammer, a rock, or from a kick in the head. These types of fractures occur in 11% of severe head injuries, and are also classified as a type of comminuted fracture.

Stress fractures are tiny cracks in a bone. They are caused by repetitive force, often from overuse, such as repeatedly jumping up and down or running long distances. Stress fractures can also develop from normal use of a bone that is weakened by a condition such as osteoporosis. Stress injuries can be found in the tibia or bones of the foot, heel, hip, and lower back. Treatment for stress fractures usually involves rest while the bone heals and changing the activity level to prevent another injury.

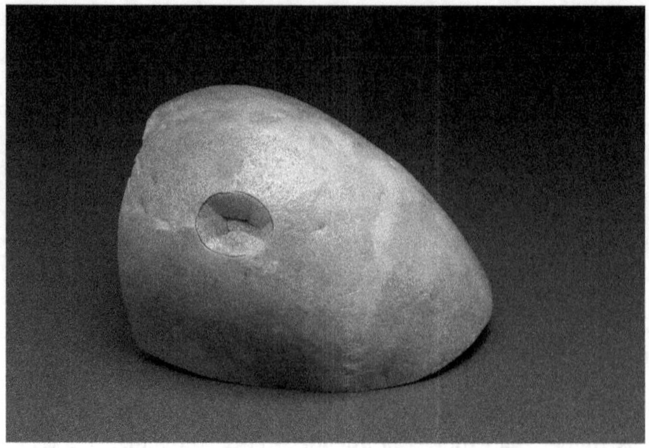

FIGURE 18.4 Depressed fracture of the skull.

Overall, the signs and symptoms of bone fractures include pain, swelling, tenderness, bruising, inability to move, discoloration of the skin, and deformity. The risk of a bone fracture is greatly increased if an individual has osteoporosis. Osteoporosis causes more than one million bone fractures each year in the United States.

X-ray, MRI, CT scans, and bone scans are used to confirm bone fractures. For treatment, immobilization must be done. Some bone fractures require surgery, depending on the type of fracture and how badly the bones are damaged. Fracture surgery complications include bone infection, malunion, nonunion acute compartment syndrome, and other internal damage. Over-the-counter medications taken for pain, such as aspirin or ibuprofen, can cause bleeding. Depending on which type of immobilization or surgery is needed to repair a fracture, the individual should be able to start moving again in a few weeks. More severe fractures can take a year or longer to heal. To prevent some fractures, a diet rich in calcium and vitamin D will promote bone strength. Weightbearing exercise also helps keep bones strong.

NUTRITION AND RECOVERY

Even among active and healthy individuals, inadequate nutrition may increase the risk of injury due to its effect upon recovery. There are several mechanisms by which inadequate dietary protein intake may lead to muscle injury. Intense training causes skeletal muscle breakdown, which can be significantly worsened by inadequate dietary protein. Inadequate hydration may compromise blood flow to working muscle, which may increase susceptibility to injury. Hydration influences the amount and composition of joint fluid, which helps to nourish articular cartilage. Deficiencies in nutrients such as potassium, iron, zinc, magnesium, chromium, copper, and various vitamins may increase susceptibility to injury because of the role these micronutrients play in bone and muscle metabolism.

Connective tissues are those that support and connect tissues and organs in the body. Connective tissue is comprised of two protein compounds: collagen and elastin.

Collagen is the most abundant protein in the human body and is the substance that holds the entire body together. It is found in the bones, muscles, skin, and tendons, where it forms a scaffold to provide strength and structure. Elastin is a highly elastic protein in connective tissue that allows tissues such as the skin and ligaments to resume their shape after stretching or contracting. Both collagen and elastin are easily damaged by inflammation. This can result in a number of different outcomes, ranging from skin wrinkles to auto-immune connective tissue diseases such as rheumatoid arthritis. Because connective tissue is what holds our bones and muscles together, it is essential for joint integrity. As a result, athletes and anyone with a physically demanding lifestyle need to look after their connective tissue to prevent degradation and resultant injuries or joint conditions, such as arthritis and tendon injuries. Overall, eating a diet low in grains and sugar, and high in bone broths, good quality protein from meats and eggs, lots of vegetables, unpasteurized fermented vegetables, kombucha, berries, fruit, and healthy fats keeps the connective tissues healthy. The body relies on nutritional intake to maintain musculoskeletal health. Good nutrition aids in recovery and prevention, as it is required to build and repair healthy connective tissue. In addition to good nutrition, things like stress, lack of sleep and exposure to environmental toxins all affect hormone levels, resulting in increased cortisol, decreased glucose absorption into cells, and therefore, an inability to manufacture glucosamine. Achieving optimal musculoskeletal health requires more than just eating right, it relies on many good lifestyle choices.

Aging is characterized by a progressive decline of muscle mass and function, which is called *sarcopenia.* Also, bone loss is widespread among older people. Sarcopenia and osteopenia or osteoporosis are associated with several adverse outcomes including falls, risk of fractures, functional decline, frailty, and mortality. The life-course approach to prevent or delay functional decline has become very popular in recent years. Regarding musculoskeletal health, there is suggestive evidence that taking appropriate action during critical or sensitive periods of life in which biological reserves are built up may influence the rate of functional decline in the later stages of life. A life-course approach to musculoskeletal health should take place during early life when plasticity allows easier attainment of the peak of the musculoskeletal system in relation to environmental stimuli. The rate of the subsequent decline will depend on the peak previously reached. Nutrition and physical exercise are important environmental factors that can influence musculoskeletal development by favoring and maintaining the highest degree of bone and muscle mass and strength. Body composition changes occurring across the lifespan and strategies based on nutrition and physical exercise to support musculoskeletal health, as well as minimizing losses during older life, are described below.

Most adolescents do not eat enough foods that promote bone and muscle health. To develop and maintain strong bones, their diets should include plenty of calcium-rich foods, such as low-fat dairy foods and green leafy vegetables. Vitamin D, which is made in the skin when it is exposed to mild doses of sunlight, helps the body to absorb calcium. Vitamins A and C also are necessary for proper bone development.

Bone is remodeled throughout life. Old bone is removed and new bone is formed. During childhood and adolescent years, new bone is added faster than old bone is removed. As a result, bones become larger and denser. Bone formation occurs faster than bone removal until about age 30. After this age, breakdown of bone begins to occur at a faster rate than bone formation. Bone loss accelerates with age and can be particularly rapid in women in the years around menopause. This can lead to osteoporosis, in which the bones become porous. This condition, in which bones are not rebuilt as quickly as they are broken down, means that they are more likely to fracture. Adolescents can help prevent osteoporosis later in life by including enough calcium in their diets, and by exercising.

KEY TERMS

Achlorhydria
Alkaline phosphatase
Amyloidosis
Avulsion fracture
Calcitonin
Carpopedal spasm
Claudication
Comminuted fracture
Compound fracture
Depressed fracture
Diaphyseal fracture
Dystonias
Frailty
Greenstick fracture
Longitudinal fractures
Looser zones
Milkman syndrome
Myoglobin
Osteoblasts
Osteoclasts
Osteomalacia
Pathologic bone fractures
Prostaglandins
Pseudofractures
Rhabdomyolysis

Sarcopenia

Stamina

Stress fracture

Tetany

Transverse fractures

CLINICAL CASE STUDIES

Clinical Case Study 1

A 21-year-old man presented to the emergency department with bilateral leg pain and dark discoloration of his urine. He had been engaged in intense aerobic exercises. Blood tests revealed a highly elevated creatine kinase, acute kidney injury, and disseminated intravascular coagulation. A double-incision bilateral fasciotomy with debridement was performed, to relieve the compartment syndrome occurring in both of the patient's legs. Kidney function deteriorated, resulting in several sessions of hemodialysis. After three weeks, the patient was discharged, have had been diagnosed with exercise-induced rhabdomyolysis.

CRITICAL THINKING QUESTIONS

1. What is rhabdomyolysis?
2. When does rhabdomyolysis occur and who does it largely affect?
3. Which factors can cause rhabdomyolysis?

Clinical Case Study 2

A 71-year-old man underwent surgical resection of bile duct tumor that left him bedridden during recovery. He became severely malnourished and very weak. His medical history included cerebral infarction without paralysis, hypertension, and duodenal ulcers. Over about five months, he lost 22 pounds (10 kilograms). Limited strength training for his upper body muscles was started for five days per week, for 20 minutes each time. Lower-limb training was started to prevent loss of skeletal muscle. As the patient's nutrition improved, the strength training regimen was increased. By day 100 of his therapy, he was able to stand without assistance, so walking training was begun. He received daily nutrition, enterally and orally. By day 200, he was nearly as strong as he was prior to his surgery.

CRITICAL THINKING QUESTIONS

1. What options are recommended to reduce or prevent the likelihood of sarcopenia?
2. What is the best treatment for sarcopenia?
3. Which medications are under study for sarcopenia?

Clinical Case Study 3

A 77-year-old woman had surgical reduction and internal fixation of a left displaced femur fracture, after slipping and falling in her bathroom. Her most recent dual x-ray absorptiometry (DXA) was six months previously, which had poor result at the femoral neck and lumbar spine. She was started on calcium twice daily and 1,000 units of cholecalciferol at the time of the DXA. She was also assessed for other drug options that could help increase her bone mineral density and reduced the likelihood of any additional osteoporotic bone fractures.

CRITICAL THINKING QUESTIONS

1. Where do most fractures related to osteoporosis occur in the body?
2. How do fragility fractures often occur?
3. What are the most cases of osteoporosis classified as?

Clinical Case Study 4

A 35-year-old woman presented with a history of general bone pain, muscle weakness, and gait disturbance. Vitamin D-deficient osteomalacia was diagnosed based on laboratory tests, which indicate high serum alkaline phosphatase, high intact PTH, and low 25-hydroxyvitamin D levels. Symptoms improved after oral active vitamin D and calcium were administered. Plain x-rays revealed that the patient had a pseudofracture in the left inferior pubic rami. At 12 months of follow-up, the patient's symptoms had been resolved and her serum levels had been normalized.

CRITICAL THINKING QUESTIONS

1. What are the primary causes of osteomalacia?
2. What does osteomalacia predispose all adults to?
3. How can osteomalacia be cured?

Clinical Case Study 5

An 11-year-old boy went skiing with his family, during which he fell backward, landing mostly on his outstretched right hand. The coccyx region of his back and his right wrist became very sore. He was taken to his pediatrician, who found tenderness over the radial dorsal aspect of the right wrist. An x-ray revealed a slight greenstick fracture. The boy's wrist was immobilized with a cast, and the fracture healed totally within six weeks.

CRITICAL THINKING QUESTIONS

1. When do greenstick fractures occur?

2. What is the most common cause of a greenstick fracture, and in which part of the body do they usually occur?
3. Is a greenstick fracture a type of compound fracture?

STUDY QUESTIONS

1. Which of the following is NOT a sign or symptom of protein deficiency?
   A. Slower wound healing
   B. Preeclampsia
   C. Decreased infection
   D. Muscle atrophy

2. Which of the following body organs contains the largest reservoir or protein?
   A. Bones
   B. Muscles
   C. Liver and heart
   D. Bone marrow

3. Which of the following is a serious medical condition that can be fatal or result in permanent disability?
   A. Sarcopenia
   B. Muscle claudication
   C. Tetany
   D. Rhabdomyolysis

4. Which of the following is the best treatment of sarcopenia?
   A. Stopping smoking
   B. A high-fat diet
   C. Exercise
   D. Administration of growth hormone

5. All of the following may cause muscle spasms, EXCEPT:
   A. Osteoporosis
   B. Tetany
   C. Dystonia
   D. Claudication

6. Which of the following manufacture the organic matrix of bones?
   A. Osteoclasts
   B. Prostaglandins
   C. Osteoblasts
   D. Calcitonin

7. In which of the following age groups is bone mass at its peak?
   A. 15–20
   B. 20–25
   C. 25–30
   D. 40–45

8. All of the following are predisposing factors for bone loss, EXCEPT:
   A. Low calcium intake
   B. Low vitamin B12 intake
   C. Low magnesium intake
   D. Low phosphorus intake

9. All of the following can accelerate bone loss, EXCEPT:
   A. Hypocalcemia
   B. Gonadal insufficiency
   C. Hyperparathyroidism
   D. Low vitamin D levels

10. Which of the following disorder may cause osteomalacia?
    A. Chronic kidney disease
    B. Chronic liver disease
    C. Heart failure
    D. Crohn's disease

11. How many units of vitamin D3 should be given per day to patients with osteomalacia?
    A. 500
    B. 1,000
    C. 2,000
    D. 3,500

12. Which of the following is the most common fracture in children younger than ten years of age?
    A. Transverse
    B. Longitudinal
    C. Open
    D. Greenstick

13. Which of the following describes a tiny crack in a bone?
    A. Greenstick fracture
    B. Stress fracture
    C. Longitudinal fracture
    D. Comminuted fracture

14. Which of the following is NOT a common symptom of osteomalacia?
    A. Fever
    B. Infection
    C. Pain
    D. Vomiting

15. All of the following disorders may cause pathologic fractures, EXCEPT:
    A. Chronic pancreatitis
    B. Cerebral palsy
    C. Bone cancer
    D. Muscular dystrophy

FURTHER READING

1. AAOS, Armstrong, A., and Hubbard, M.C. (2018). *Essentials of Musculoskeletal Care (American Academy of Orthopaedic Surgeons, American Academy of Pediatrics)*, 5th Edition. Jones & Bartlett Learning.
2. Camacho, P.M. (2019). *Metabolic Bone Diseases: A Case-Based Approach.* Springer.
3. Cesari, M., and Marzetti, E. (2020). *Nutrition for Musculoskeletal Health.* Nutrients / MDPI.
4. Clarkson, H.M. (2014). *Musculoskeletal Assessment: Joint Motion and Muscle Testing*, 3rd Edition. Wolters Kluwer / Lippincott, Williams, & Wilkins.
5. Correa, J. (2018). *94 Muscle Cramp Reducing Meal and Juice Recipes – Stop Muscle Cramps Fast by Eating Vitamin Specific Foods.* Correa.
6. Cruz-Jentoft, A.J., and Morley, J.E. (2021). *Sarcopenia*, 2nd Edition. Wiley Blackwell.
7. Denegar, C.R., Saliba, E., and Saliba, S. (2015). *Therapeutic Modalities for Musculoskeletal Injuries*, 4th Edition. Human Kinetics.
8. Dowd, J. (2022). *The Vitamin D3 Cure, Dietary Supplement for Rickets, Osteomalacia, Osteoporosis, Arthritis, Eczema, Kidney Failure, Healthy Muscle Function, and Immune Support.* Lulu.com.
9. Driskell, J.A., and Wolinsky, I. (2014). *Nutritional Assessment of Athletes (nutrition in Exercise and Sport)*, 2nd Edition. CRC Press.
10. Horvai, A., and Link, T. (2014). *Bone and Soft Tissue Pathology: A Volume in the High-Yield Pathology Series.* Saunders/Elsevier.
11. Ives, S. (2022). *Nutrition and Athletic Performance.* Nutrients/MDPI.
12. Kearns, A.E. (2021). *Mayo Clinic on Osteoporosis – Keep Your Bones Strong and Reduce Your Risk of Fractures.* Mayo Clinic Press.
13. Kelly, L., Bryman Kelly, H., and MacDonald Baker, S. (2016). *The Healthy Bones Nutrition Plan and Cookbook – How to Prepare and Combine Whole Foods to Prevent and Treat Osteoporosis Naturally.* Chelsea Green Publishing.
14. Lohman, T., Going, S., Houtkooper, L., Metcalfe, L., Antoniotti-Guide, T., Lisse, J., and Farrell, V. (2017). *The BEST Exercise Program for Osteoporosis Prevention*, 4th Edition. Human Kinetics.
15. Meynial-Denis, D. (2019). *Sarcopenia: Molecular, Cellular, and Nutritional Aspects – Applications to Humans.* CRC Press.
16. Nguyen, V. (2022). *Muscle Food – The Ultimate Muscle Building Nutrition Guide on What to Cook and Eat to Bulk Up (Weight Loss and Muscle Gain Book 4).* Nguyen.
17. Peterson Kendall, F., Kendall McCreary, E., Geise Provance, P., McIntyre Rodgers, M., and Romani, W.A. (2014). *Muscles – Testing and Function with Posture and Pain*, 5th Edition. Lippincott, Williams, & Wilkins.
18. Roberts, K. (2019). *Osteoporosis Diet – Your Complete Guide to Prevent and Reverse Bone Loss Using Natural Remedies, Diet, and Exercise without Medication.* The Fruitful Mind.
19. Travers, J. (2021). *Bone-Strength Plan – How to Increase Bone Health to Live a Long, Active Life.* Orange Hippo!
20. Watkins Bales, C., Locher, J.L., and Saltzman, E. (2014). *Handbook of Clinical Nutrition and Aging, 3rd Edition (Nutrition and Health).* Humana Press.
21. Wold, L.E., Unni, K.K., Sim, F.H., Sundaram, M., and Adler, A. (2014). *Atlas of Orthopedic Pathology, 3rd Edition (Atlas of Surgical Pathology).* Saunders / Elsevier.

19 Nutritional Effects on Cancer

OUTLINE

LEARNING OBJECTIVES

After study of the chapter, readers should be able to:

1. Describe how consuming certain foods may increase risks for cancer.
2. Explain the links between consumption of excessive alcohol and liver diseases.
3. Discuss the signs and symptoms of cirrhosis.
4. Explain the links between red meat and colon cancer.
5. Describe the links between dietary fat and breast cancer.
6. Identify the causes of hepatocellular carcinoma.
7. Explain the risk factors of breast cancer.
8. Describe the links between dietary fat and prostate cancer.
9. Explain cancer cachexia.
10. Discuss the alterations in taste and smell in patients with cancer.

OVERVIEW

The development of cancer leads to organ destruction and impaired function, culminating in cachexia and death. In cachexia, there are many metabolic and physiologic alterations, including weakness, anorexia, weight loss, compromised immune function, and depletion and translocation of normal body components, resulting in a condition that resembles malnutrition. To combat the effects of cancer upon the body, an extremely healthy diet is required. Nutritional interventions must be implemented as soon as cancer is diagnosed and must be individualized to the needs of each patient. The effects of lifestyle choices such as alcohol and dietary components such as red meat, sodium chloride, and fat need to be closely assessed, since they have a clear impact on certain types of cancers. Also, patients should be educated that cancer can result in changes in appetite such as early fullness, as well as alterations of taste and smell which also affect proper nutrition.

DIET AND CANCER

The risk of developing cancer is linked to the consuming of certain food substances. Diets high in fat are linked to an increased risk of breast, colon cancers, and possibly prostate cancer. Alcoholics have a much higher risk of developing cancers of the head, neck, and esophagus. Diets high in smoked or pickled foods, or high in meats cooked at high temperatures increase risks for stomach cancer. Overweight or obese individuals have higher risks for cancers of the breast, colon, endometrium, esophagus, and kidneys. Overall risks for cancer can be reduced by consuming a diet that is high in fruits, vegetables, and whole grains. Sugary drinks should be avoided, and calorie-dense foods should be limited. Another suggested dietary component is a variety of legumes such as beans. Beef, pork, lamb, and processed meats should be limited. Alcoholic beverages should be limited. Salty foods and foods that are processed with table salt must be limited. Supplements should not be used to protect against cancer because proven benefits are extremely limited. New mothers should breastfeed exclusively for up to six months, and then add other foods and liquids. This is the safest way to protect infants from cancer. Cancer survivors must always follow dietary recommendations after they have been treated.

ALCOHOL AND HEPATOCELLULAR CARCINOMA

In the United States and other Westernized countries, alcohol consumption is relatively high. Approximately 8.5% of US adults have an alcohol use disorder over any one-year period. The male-to-female ratio is nearly 2:1. Liver disorders that occur in those with an alcohol use disorder usually occur in the following sequence:

- Fatty liver – more than 90%
- Alcoholic hepatitis – 10%–35%
- Cirrhosis – 10%–20%

Hepatocellular carcinoma may develop in patients with **cirrhosis**, primarily if there is coexisting iron accumulation.

DOI: 10.1201/b22969-22

Primary risk factors for alcohol-related liver disease include the quantity consumed and for how long (eight years or longer), gender, genetic and **metabolic traits**, and obesity. In susceptible individuals, there is usually a linear relationship between the amount and duration of alcohol consumption and the development of liver disease. Alcohol content is calculated as the milliliters (mL) of each beverage, multiple by the contained percentage of alcohol. This is broken down as follows:

- In 45 mL of an 80-proof alcoholic drink, which contains 40% alcohol, the alcohol content is 18 mL, with each mL containing approximately 0.79 g of alcohol
- Values vary, but the percentage of alcohol is 2%–7% for most beers, and 10%–15% for most wines – a 12-ounce glass of beer contains approximately 5–20 g of alcohol; a 5-ounce of wine contains approximately 12–18 g of alcohol; a 1 ½-ounce shot of hard liquor contains about 14 g of alcohol

For men that drink more than 40 g of alcohol per day for ten or more years, the risk of liver disease is greatly increased. This is equivalent to 2–8 cans of beer, 3–6 glasses of wine, or 3-6 shots of hard liquor, per day.

For development of cirrhosis, alcohol consumption must usually be more than 80 g per day for over ten years. Consumption exceeding 230 g per day for 20 years increases the risk for cirrhosis by approximately 50%. Even so, only some chronic abusers of alcohol develop liver disease. Therefore, variations in intake do not completely explain variations in susceptibility, so there must be other factors involved. Women have a higher susceptibility to alcohol-related liver disease, even after figuring in generally smaller body size. Women need just 20–40 g of alcohol per day to be at risk for liver disease, which is half the amount for men. Women have less **alcohol dehydrogenase** in their gastric mucosa, so more intact alcohol reaches their livers, which may increase risks.

Alcohol-related liver disease is often familial. This suggests that genetic factors may be present, such as a deficiency of **cytoplasmic enzymes** that eliminate alcohol. Nutritional status is also important, since diets high in unsaturated fats and the presence of obesity increase susceptibility. Other risk factors for alcoholic liver disease include iron accumulation in the liver, which is not always related to iron intake, and concurrent hepatitis C virus (HCV).

Alcohol, also known as *ethanol*, is easily absorbed from the stomach, yet most is absorbed from the small intestine. Alcohol cannot be stored by the body. Small amounts are degraded as they move through the gastric mucosa, yet most is catabolized within the liver. This occurs primarily by alcohol dehydrogenase (ADH), followed by cytochrome P-450 2E1 (CYP2E1) and the microsomal enzyme oxidation system (MEOS). Via the ADH pathway, metabolism of alcohol involves these components:

- The cytoplasmic enzyme ADH oxidizes alcohol into **acetaldehyde**; genetic **polymorphisms** result in certain individual differences in blood alcohol levels between people, even with the same amount of intake; however, these polymorphisms do not account for the susceptibility to alcohol-related liver disease
- The mitochondrial enzyme *acetaldehyde dehydrogenase* (ALDH) oxidizes acetaldehyde into acetate; if a person consumes alcohol on a chronic level, the formation of acetate is increased; Asian people have lower levels of ALDH, making them more susceptible to the toxic effects of acetaldehyde, such as facial flushing; these effects resemble those of the drug *disulfiram*, which inhibits ALDH
- Hydrogen is generated by these oxidative reactions; it converts nicotinamide-adenine dinucleotide (NAD) to the reduced form known as nicotinamide-adenine dinucleotide hydrogen (NADH); this increases the **redox potential** (NADH/NAD) in the liver
- Fatty acid oxidation and gluconeogenesis are inhibited by the increased redox potential; this promotes fat accumulation within the liver

Triglycerides accumulate in the liver cells due to decreased export of fat from the liver and increased input of fat. Fat accumulation in the liver may predispose the individual to further oxidative damage. Alcohol alters the permeability of the gastrointestinal tract (GIT). This increases absorption of **endotoxins** released by gastrointestinal (GI) bacteria. The liver can then no longer detoxify endotoxins, so liver macrophages called **Kupffer cells** release free radicals, which increase the oxidative damage. Oxidative stress is increased by a variety of factors, which include:

- Alcohol-related hypermetabolism in the liver
- Lipid peroxidative damage from free radicals
- Fewer protective antioxidants such as **glutathione** and vitamins A and E; this is caused by alcohol-related undernutrition
- Acetaldehyde and other alcohol oxidation products binding to liver cell proteins, to form **neoantigens** and cause inflammation
- White blood cell (neutrophil) accumulation, which are attracted by the lipid peroxidative damage and neoantigens

Oxidative damage is aggravated by any hepatic iron that is present. The iron may accumulate in alcohol-related liver disease via ingesting fortified wines that contain iron. Usually, iron accumulation is only slight, but the condition must be differentiated from hereditary *hemochromatosis*.

Cell necrosis and **apoptosis** cause loss of hepatocytes. Further attempts at regeneration cause **fibrosis**. **Stellate cells** line the sinusoids (blood channels) of the liver. They proliferate, transforming into myofibroblasts, to produce excessive collagen and extracellular matrix. Then, the sinusoids narrow to limit blood flow. The terminal hepatic venules are narrowed by fibrosis. This compromises perfusion in the liver, contributing to **portal hypertension**. Significant fibrosis is related to attempted regeneration, causing liver nodules. Eventually, cirrhosis develops.

If cirrhosis is compensated for, there may be no signs or symptoms. In most cases of cirrhosis, the liver is small in size, but if it is enlarged, there must be a consideration of **hepatic steatosis** or **hepatoma**. Signs and symptoms may include an appearance of fatigue, fever, undernourishment, jaundice, right upper quadrant pain, **hepatomegaly** with tenderness, **hepatic bruit**, ascites, portosystemic encephalopathy, variceal bleeding, liver failure with hypoglycemia, **coagulopathy**, portal hypertension, GI bleeding, splenomegaly, intrapulmonary arteriovenous shunting with hypoxemia, cyanosis, **clubbing** of the fingers, acute renal failure due to decreasing renal blood flow, and hepatocellular carcinoma (see Figure 19.1). The carcinoma may develop in 10%–15% of patients that have alcohol-related cirrhosis. For patients with cirrhosis that are stable, it is recommended that liver ultrasonography, with or without measurement of **alpha-fetoprotein** (AFP), be done every six months to screen for hepatocellular carcinoma. Coexisting iron accumulation or chronic hepatitis C increases the risks for hepatocellular carcinoma.

Hepatocellular carcinoma is the most common form of *primary liver cancer*, with more than 42,000 new cases and over 30,000 deaths annually in the United States. These include *intrahepatic bile duct cancers*. Approximately 75% of these liver cancers are hepatocellular carcinoma. Overall, liver cancer is about three times more common in men compared to women. It is more common in countries outside the United States, especially in Eastern Asia and sub-Saharan Africa. The presence of the hepatitis B virus (HBV) increases the risk for hepatocellular carcinoma by more than 100 times in HBV carriers. Other causes of hepatocellular carcinoma include cirrhosis caused by chronic HCV infection and hemochromatosis. The cancer can also develop along with non-cirrhotic non-alcoholic steatohepatitis. Patients that have cirrhosis because of other conditions are also at a higher risk. Environmental carcinogens, such as foods contaminated with fungal aflatoxins, also are causative – mostly in subtropical areas of the world.

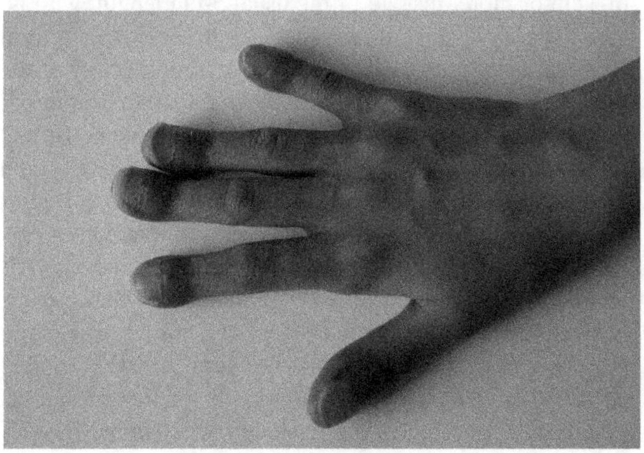

FIGURE 19.1 Clubbing of the fingers.

With cirrhosis, signs of hepatocellular carcinoma include abdominal pain, a right upper quadrant mass, weight loss, and deterioration from no obvious cause. Some patients develop a fever. Sometimes, the first sign is bloody ascites, **peritonitis**, or shock, related to tumor hemorrhage. Some patients have a hepatic **friction rub** or bruit. Systemic metabolic complications may include **erythrocytosis**, hypoglycemia, hypercalcemia, or hyperlipidemia.

Diagnosis is based on AFP measurement and imaging studies. Between 40% and 65% of diagnosed patients have much higher AFP levels. Lower values are not as specific and may occur with hepatocellular regeneration, such as in hepatitis. Initial imaging may be contrast-enhanced computed tomography (CT), magnetic resonance imaging (MRI), or ultrasonography. A definitive diagnosis is done via liver biopsy guided by CT or ultrasonography. After diagnosis, chest CT without contrast, imaging of the portal vein with MRI or contrast-CT (to exclude thrombosis), and bone scans may be performed – mostly if the AFP is highly elevated.

Today, screening programs are identifying more and more hepatocellular carcinomas. Ultrasonography can be done every 6 or 12 months. For obese patients, ultrasonography is alternated with MRI or CT, since obesity reduces ultrasonography sensitivity. Individuals with chronic HBV are often screened even if they do not have cirrhosis. When a patient has one tumor less than 5 cm in size, or three tumors less than 3 cm in size, without vascular invasion, and AFP under 500 mcg/L, transplantation of the liver is indicated and is often curative. For some patients with singular tumors smaller than 5 cm and no portal hypertension, surgical resection may be curative, giving five-year survival rates of 60%–80%. Other options include ablative treatments such as **radiofrequency ablation**. Drugs include sorafenib, regorafenib, and nivolumab. Immunotherapies include atezolizumab, bevacizumab, and combinations of both.

FOCUS ON PREVENTION OF HEPATOCELLULAR CARCINOMA

Aside from avoiding, reducing, or quitting the use of alcohol, incidence of hepatocellular carcinoma may also be reduced by administration of the HBV vaccine, treating chronic HCV, and early detection of hemochromatosis.

Test Your Knowledge

1. How often should screening for hepatocellular carcinoma in patients with alcoholic-related cirrhosis be conducted?
2. With cirrhosis, what are the signs of hepatocellular carcinoma?

RED MEAT AND COLON CANCER

A high consumption of red meat is linked to an increased risk of colon cancer. Individuals that consume at least five ounces of red meat per day are about 33% more likely to develop colon cancer than those who eat less than one ounce per day. Consumption of white meat such as chicken does not affect risks for colon cancer, and a high consumption of fish reduces risks by about 33%. High consumption of red meat as well as processed meats is linked to a substantial increase in risks for cancer of the lower colon and rectum. Long-term consumption of large amounts of fish and poultry appears to be protective.

There are several theories as to why red meat is linked to higher rates of colon cancer. The first states that **heterocyclic amines**, which are produced during high-temperature cooking of red meat, are to blame. Another theory states that preservatives such as *nitrates* are causative because the body converts them to a carcinogenic form known as *nitrosamines*. However, fresh red meat is also linked to colon cancer, so preservatives may not be entirely causative. A third theory states that diets high in red meat result in high levels of *N-nitroso compounds*, which are potentially cancer-causing chemicals. These compounds may induce DNA changes that lead to cancer.

Large amounts of red meat can produce genetic damage to the colon cells over just a few weeks. If the body's mechanisms of DNA repair fail, cells can experience malignant transformation. Prevention of colon cancer is based on reduced caloric intake, regular exercise, avoiding tobacco products, limiting alcohol intake, good amounts of calcium from dairy products, vitamin D, fruits, vegetables, whole grains, fish, low-dose aspirin, and regular colon cancer screening tests based on age, family history, and risk factors. Red meat should always be considered a "side dish" for meals and not the main focus. Just two 4-ounce portions per week are suggested, and the meat should be lean, with excess fat trimmed away, and not charred on a grill. Processed, cured, and salted meats must be limited as much as possible. The main protein sources should be fish, chicken, and turkey (without the skin), accompanied by protein sources such as beans.

There are nearly 148,000 cases of colon cancer in the United States annually, and over 53,000 deaths – mostly in people between 40 and 50 years of age. In elderly people, the incidence of colon cancer is increased. Over 50% of cases occur in the rectum and sigmoid colon, with 95% being **adenocarcinomas**. Colon cancer is slightly more common in men. About 5% of patients have more than one cancer at the same time. Most cases result when adenomatous polyps undergo transformation, with 80% of cases being sporadic and 20% being inherited. Predisposing factors include chronic **ulcerative colitis** and Crohn's disease. Carcinogens are mostly produced by bacterial action upon dietary substances or secretions from the biliary tract or intestines. Colon cancer spreads via direct extension through the colon wall, **hematogenous** metastasis and regional lymph node metastasis.

Colon adenocarcinomas grow slowly, with symptoms occurring much later that are based on tumor location, type, size, and any complications. Obstruction of the right colon occurs later in the disease course, with occult bleeding. Some patients only experience fatigue and weakness from severe anemia. Some tumors can be palpated through the abdominal wall before any other signs and symptoms occur. The left colon is more often obstructed by tumors, resulting in colicky abdominal pain or complete obstruction, streaking or mixing of the stool with blood, focal pain and tenderness, or in rare cases, diffuse peritonitis. If the cancer is only in the rectum, there is usually bleeding with defecation. Obvious hemorrhoids, known diverticular disease, or coexisting cancers must be ruled out. There may be tenesmus or a feeling of incomplete evacuation. If there is perirectal involvement, pain is common. Sometimes, initial signs and symptoms include ascites, hepatomegaly, or supraclavicular lymph node enlargement.

Diagnosis of colon cancer is based on colonoscopy, fecal occult blood testing, and less often, flexible sigmoidoscopy, fecal DNA testing, and CT colonography. Patients with a family history of a first-degree relative with colon cancer before age 60 should have a colonoscopy every five years, starting at age 40, or ten years before the age in which the relative was diagnosed (whichever is first). Diagnostic tests include colonoscopic biopsy, CT scans to evaluate tumor growth and spread, and genetic testing.

The prognosis for colon cancer is based on stage. The five-year survival rates are quite different, as follows:

- Nearly 90% – if limited to the mucosa
- 70%–80% – if there is extension through the colon wall
- 30%–50% – if there are positive lymph nodes
- Less than 20% – if there is metastatic disease

The treatment of colon cancer is surgical resection, sometimes combined with chemotherapy, radiation, or both. A surgical cure is attempted in 70% of patients that present without metastatic disease. For rectal cancer, the sphincter can be saved via surgical resection if there is a distal margin of 1 cm or more, instead of the usual 5-cm length, with no significant risk of local recurrence or decreased long-term survival. If there is liver metastasis, resection of 1–3 of the metastatic lesions is recommended for certain non-debilitated patients as a follow-up procedure. Chemotherapy improves survival by 10%–30% if there are positive lymph nodes. Surveillance colonoscopy is done one year after any surgery or after a clearing preoperative colonoscopy. Another colonoscopy is done three years later if no polyps or tumors have been found. After that, surveillance colonoscopy is done every five years. If curative surgery is not possible or there are dangerous surgical risks, limited palliative surgery may be done, but the median survival is seven months. Medications include capecitabine, irinotecan, oxaliplatin, bevacizumab, cetuximab, panitumumab, or floxuridine, sometimes in combination.

FOCUS ON SCREENING FOR COLON CANCER

For average-risk patients, screening for colon cancer should begin at age 45, continuing until age 75. For those over 75, screening choices are individualized, based on overall health and previous screening history. Screening may involve colonoscopy (every ten years) and annual fecal occult blood testing. Flexible sigmoidoscopy should be done every five years (or every ten years if done with fecal immunochemical tests), CT colonography every five years, or fecal DNA testing with fecal immunochemical tests every three years.

Test Your Knowledge

1. What amount of red meat consumption increases risks for colon cancer?
2. How prevalent is colon cancer?
3. What are the statistics on colon cancer-related death?

SALTY DIET AND STOMACH CANCER

There is a definite link between high-salt foods and stomach cancer, including foods such as meat, fish, and vegetables that are preserved by salting. Many traditional foods in countries such as Japan and Korea are preserved by the use of salting and fermentation, instead of the refrigeration methods preferred by many Westernized countries. Large amounts of salt infuses the foods in the preservation process, resulting in damage to the stomach lining and the development of lesions that may lead to stomach cancer. Infection with the bacteria known as ***Helicobacter pylori*** also damages the stomach lining, which may be worsened by the presence of excessive salt. Much dietary salt is "hidden" in foods, so people may be unaware of just how much they are consuming. With the global population eating outside of the home more often, and cooking less, the proportion of dietary salt is increasing. In the United States, the limit for dietary salt is less than 2.3 g per day. It is important to understand the table salt levels in common everyday foods that are not normally considered to be "salty", such as breads and soups. The top ten foods that contain the highest average amounts of salt are as follows:

- Pizza – 640 mg
- Soups – 600–700 mg
- Sandwiches – 600 mg
- Burritos and tacos – 274–985 mg
- Cold cuts and cured meats – 214–590 mg
- Cheese – 174 mg
- Savory snacks (chips, popcorn, pretzels, snack mixes, crackers) – 120–418 mg
- Breads and rolls – 117 mg
- Fried chicken – 100 mg
- Eggs and omelets (based on how they are prepared) – 62–95 mg

In the United States, there are about 27,000 cases and 11,000 deaths from stomach cancer, making it the seventh most common cause of cancer death. It is most common in African-Americans, Hispanic-Americans, and Native Americans. Incidence increases with age since more than 75% of patients are age 50 or older. Gastric adenocarcinoma makes up 95% of malignant stomach tumors, with less common forms including localized **gastric lymphomas** and **leiomyosarcomas**. Worldwide, stomach cancer is the second most common type of cancer in Japan, China, Chile, and Iceland. Risk factors also include autoimmune atrophic gastritis, smoking, and genetics. Gastric **polyps** can be precursors, with multiple adenomatous polyps being most likely to become cancerous.

Symptoms of stomach cancer include **dyspepsia**, early satiety, **dysphagia**, weight loss, reduced strength, massive **hematemesis**, **melena**, secondary anemia from occult blood loss, jaundice, ascites, heme-positive stools, epigastric masses, lymph node enlargement, and hepatomegaly. There may be pulmonary, central nervous system, or bone metastasis. Diagnosis includes endoscopy with biopsy, followed by CT and endoscopic ultrasonography. Screening with endoscopy is used for Asian populations, but this is not as common in the United States. Prognosis is usually poor, with a five-year survival of only 5%–15%, since most patients present once the disease is already advanced. However, when the stomach cancer is only within the mucosa or submucosa, five-year survival may be up to 80%. If the local lymph nodes are involved, survival is 20%–40%. If more widespread, it is usually fatal within one year.

Treatment is with surgical resection, sometimes accompanied with chemotherapy, radiation, or both. Treatment is heavily based on staging. Most or all of the stomach and adjacent lymph nodes are usually removed. Resection of locally advanced regional disease provides a ten-month median survival compared to only three to four months without resection. For metastasis or extensive nodal involvement, palliative treatments are usually done.

FOCUS ON STOMACH CANCER NUTRITION

The best diet for stomach cancer involves protein-rich foods. These include lean meats (chicken, fish, turkey), eggs, low-fat dairy products (milk, yogurt, and cheese or dairy substitutes), nuts and nut butters, beans, and soy products. Processed foods must be minimized in the cancer patient's diet. These include bacon, sausage, deli meats, candy, packaged snack foods, and sweetened beverages such as soda.

Test Your Knowledge

1. How is dietary table salt linked to stomach cancer?
2. In which countries does stomach cancer occur the most?
3. What are the symptoms of stomach cancer?

DIETARY FAT AND BREAST CANCER

There are known links between dietary fat and certain cancers such as breast cancer. However, for adults, the percentage of calories consumed from total fat does not appear to be significantly linked to higher cancer risks. Animal fat intake is correlated to higher breast cancer risks. Premenopausal women that consume foods high in animal fat have a 40%–50% higher risk of breast cancer compared to women that eat less animal fat. The findings suggest that red meat and high-fat dairy products may contain factors such as hormones, which increase risks for breast cancer. In European studies, lower breast cancer risks are related to high intake of monounsaturated fats (primarily olive oil).

In the United States, breast cancer is the second leading cause of cancer for women in most racial or ethnic groups, except for Hispanic-American women, in which it is the leading cause of cancer death. There are nearly 282,000 new annual cases of invasive breast cancer, nearly 50,000 new cases of in situ breast cancer, and nearly 44,000 deaths from the disease. Male breast cancer only makes up about 1% of all cases of the disease, with over 2,600 new cases and over 500 deaths. While the manifestations, diagnosis, and treatment methods are the same, men usually develop breast cancer at a later stage of life.

For American women, there is an approximate 12% lifetime risk for breast cancer, mostly after age 60, with risk of death being about 10% within five years after diagnosis. Factors that may increase risks include age, family history, gene mutations, personal or gynecologic history, breast changes, lobular carcinoma in situ, use of oral contraceptives, hormone therapy, radiation therapy, smoking, and alcohol use. Most breast cancers are epithelial tumors developing from cells that line the ducts or lobules. **Ductal carcinoma in situ** (DCIS) makes up about 85% of cases. Lobular carcinoma in situ (LCIS) is often multifocal and bilateral, and may be classic or pleomorphic. Invasive carcinoma is usually adenocarcinoma, with 80% being the infiltrating ductal type. *Inflammatory breast cancer* is a form that grows quickly, is highly aggressive, and is often fatal. **Paget disease** is a type of DCIS that extends into the skin over the nipple and **areola**.

Breast cancer invades locally, spreading through regional lymph nodes, the bloodstream, or both. It metastasizes primarily to the lungs, liver, bones, brain, and skin. Some tumors recur earlier, and tumor markers are often able to predict recurrence. Estrogen and progesterone receptors promote DNA replication and cell division when certain hormones bind to them, so they may be useful in treating tumors that have these receptors.

Signs and symptoms of breast cancer include a palpable mass, breast enlargement or thickening, breast pain, skin changes, **erythema**, an "orange peel" appearance of the breast, nipple discharge, abdominal pain, jaundice, dyspnea, breast asymmetry, fixation of a mass to the chest wall or overlying skin, and satellite nodules or ulcers of the skin. Women should begin monthly self-breast examinations at age 20. They should also be screened for breast cancer via three-dimensional mammography, clinical breast examination, and MRI for high-risk patients. Screening mammography usually starts at ages 40–50, repeated every two years until age 75.

Diagnosis of breast cancer involves screening by mammography, ultrasonography, and biopsy that analyzes the presence of estrogen receptors, progesterone receptors. After diagnosis, a multidisciplinary evaluation is usually done to plan treatment. There may be a need for bone scanning, abdominal and chest CT. Grading is based on histologic examination of biopsied tissues. Staging follows the tumor-nearby lymph nodes-metastasis (TNM) classification. Breast cancer patients should avoid becoming pregnant once treatments begin. The long-term prognosis of breast cancer is based on staging. The five-year survival rate is as follows for the various breast cancer stages:

- Localized (primary site only) – 99%
- Regional (in regional lymph nodes only) – 85.8%
- Unknown – 57.8%
- Distant (metastasized) – 29%

A worsened prognosis is based on younger patient age, non-Hispanic African-American racial or ethnic group, larger primary tumors, high-grade tumors, lack of estrogen and progesterone receptors, presence of the HER2 protein, and presence of breast cancer (BRCA) gene mutations.

Treatments for breast cancer include surgery, radiation therapy (in most cases), and systemic therapy with endocrine therapy, chemotherapy, or both. Mastectomy is removal of the entire breast, and may be described as *skin-sparing*, *nipple-sparing*, *simple*, *modified radical*, and *radical*. The radical form is rarely done unless the cancer has invaded the pectoral muscles. Breast-conserving surgery is based on tumor size and the required margins, and may be described as *lumpectomy*, *wide excision*, or *quadrantectomy*. During mastectomy and breast-conserving surgery, the axillary lymph nodes are usually evaluated via *axillary lymph node dissection (ALND)* or *sentinel lymph node biopsy (SLNB)*. The SNLB method is now usually done first. Impaired lymphatic drainage of the ipsilateral arm often happens after ALND or SLNB as well as after radiation therapy. Any lymphedema must be treated by specially trained therapists.

Reconstructive procedures include *prosthetic* and *autologous* reconstruction. In prosthetic reconstruction, a silicone or saline implant is introduced, sometimes after use of a tissue expander. With autologous reconstruction, there is a muscle flap or muscle-free flap transfer. The muscles most often used in muscle flap transfer are the latissimus dorsi, gluteus maximum, or lower rectus abdominis muscles. *Contralateral prophylactic mastectomy* is an option for breast cancer patients if there is a genetic mutation that results in a high risk of the cancer reoccurring in the other breast. After breast-conserving surgery, radiation therapy greatly reduces local recurrences and can improve overall survival for most patients. Chemotherapy or endocrine therapy can delay or prevent recurrence in nearly all patients and can prolong survival for some. Postmenopausal patients with estrogen receptor-negative tumors have the most benefits from adjuvant chemotherapy. For estrogen receptor-positive tumors, predictive genomic tests for primary breast cancer can determine risks and whether combination chemotherapy or endocrine therapy alone will be indicated. The majority of breast cancers in American women are of the estrogen receptor-positive/progesterone receptor-positive/HER-negative form.

Generally, combination chemotherapies are more effective than single drugs. Options include doxorubicin, cyclophosphamide, paclitaxel, filgrastim, pegfilgrastim, trastuzumab, pertuzumab, and endocrine therapies such as tamoxifen or aromatase inhibitors. Metastases require immediate evaluation, with treatments based on the hormone-receptor status of the tumor, length of disease-free interval from remission to manifestations of metastases, the number of metastatic sites and organs affected, and the patient's menopausal status. Endocrine therapies, anti-HER2 drugs, tyrosine kinase inhibitors, radiation therapy, palliative mastectomy, and intravenous bisphosphonates are all options.

FOCUS ON DIETARY FAT AND BREAST CANCER

Increased consumption of total and saturated fats are positively associated with the development of breast cancer. Although some fat is necessary in the diet, too much can lead to cancers, as well as heart disease, obesity, and other health problems. An important consideration is that women with breast cancer that continued to have high *trans-fat* intake have an increased risk of all-cause mortality that is between 45% and 78%.

Test Your Knowledge

1. What is the impact of animal fats in the diet upon premenopausal women in relation to breast cancer?
2. How does breast cancer progress?
3. What are the diagnostic procedures for breast cancer?

DIETARY FAT AND PROSTATE CANCER

Prostate cancer is the second leading cause of cancer death in American men, after lung cancer. Dietary fat may play a significant role in developing the cancer. Diets high in animal fat are linked to prostate cancer, since they may boost testosterone levels. There is also a link between saturated fat and a higher chance of advanced prostate cancer and related death, yet there is no connection to early-stage prostate cancer. In one large study, the primary sources of saturated fat included beef, margarine, and dairy products such as butter and whole milk. Some people may have higher amounts of the hormone known as *insulin-like growth factor 1*, which is implicated in cancer growth. Ongoing studies are focusing on how inflammation, hormone imbalances, and a buildup of lipids from a high-fat diet contribute to prostate cancer.

Adenocarcinoma of the prostate gland is the most common cancer in men age 50 or older. In the United States, there are nearly 249,000 cases and over 34,000 deaths per year. Incidence increases with each decade of age, and autopsies reveal this cancer to be present in 15%–60% of men between 60 and 90 years of age. About one of every six men is diagnosed with prostate cancer. The median age at diagnosis is 72, with more than 75% occurring in men over age 65. There is an African-American predominance. Less common is sarcoma of the prostate, and when it occurs, it is usually seen in children. Other infrequent subtypes include ductal transitional carcinoma, squamous cell carcinoma, and undifferentiated prostate cancer. A possible premalignant histologic change is known as **prostatic intraepithelial neoplasia**. Hormones contribute to the development of adenocarcinoma but not to the other subtypes.

Prostate cancer is usually of slow progression, often without symptoms until it has advanced. At that point, symptoms include **hematuria**, straining, hesitancy, weak or intermittent urine stream, incomplete emptying, terminal dribbling, renal colic, flank pain, renal dysfunction, bone pain, pathologic fractures, or spinal cord compression. Prostate cancer is diagnosed by screening via digital rectal examination and a **prostate-specific antigen** (PSA) test, needle biopsy. Sometimes, a prostate-specific membrane antigen-based positron emission tomography/computed tomography (PET/CT) scan is done. Screening is usually done every year for men age 50 or older, but may be started earlier for those who are at high risk.

Prognosis, especially when localized or regional, is very good. Long-term local control or a cure is often possible. However without early treatment, patients with high-grade, poorly differentiated cancer have a poor prognosis. Metastatic prostate cancer is incurable, carrying a median life expectancy of one to three years in general. For localized cancer, surgery, radiation therapy, or active surveillance is done. For cancer outside of the prostate, treatments include palliation with hormonal therapy, radiation therapy, or chemotherapy. For some men with low-risk cancers, active surveillance without treatment is done. Treatments are guided by PSA levels, grade and stage of the tumor, patient age, any coexisting disorders, life expectancy, and patient preferences. Radical prostatectomy (removal of the prostate with the **seminal vesicles** and regional lymph nodes) is considered best for patients less than 75 years of age with a tumor that is only within the prostate. Other treatments include **cryotherapy**, standard external beam radiation therapy, **hypofractionation**, and **brachytherapy**. For metastatic prostate cancer, hormonal therapy is effective for a limited amount of time. For complications due to bone metastases, denosumab or zoledronic acid can be used.

FOCUS ON "GOOD FATS" TO PREVENT PROSTATE CANCER

Monounsaturated omega-9 fatty acids and polyunsaturated omega-3 fatty acids are the fats recommended to be included in men's diets in order to prevent prostate cancer. The omega-9 fatty acids come from avocados, almonds, hazelnuts, pecans, pistachios, extra-virgin olive oil, almond oil, canola oil, and macadamia nut oil. The omega-3 fatty acids come from cold-water fish (salmon, sardines, black cod, trout, herring) and seeds (flaxseed, chia seeds, hemp seeds, and pumpkin seeds).

Test Your Knowledge

1. What are the links between dietary fat and prostate cancer?
2. What are the "good fats" that may help prevent prostate cancer?
3. How is increased age related to prostate cancer?

INCREASED APPETITE

Cancer patients often worry about weight gain, as a possible side effect of treatment. Weight gain can occur because of eating behaviors that are triggered by chemotherapy-related symptoms, use of corticosteroids, and inactivity. Chemotherapy may cause nausea, but also can cause increased appetite and cravings for sweet foods and carbohydrates. Patients do not have to cut sugar out of the diet completely, and there are healthy alternatives that help curb cravings. Fresh fruit is recommended whenever a craving for sugar develops. For patients experiencing fatigue and an overall lack of physical activity, light walking should be incorporated into the daily routine to combat weight gain from inactivity. Corticosteroids often increase appetite and cause the body to retain extra sodium, which often results in fluid retention. Potassium-rich foods such as bananas, cantaloupe, and kiwi can help retain potassium and less excess fluid. Decreasing dietary sodium also helps. Instead of eating three large meals every day, cancer patients should eat six smaller meals. This allows them to feel fuller over the hours and avoid hunger peaks that lead to cravings and overeating. Refined carbohydrates should be avoided, and whole grains should be consumed instead, including proteins, which extend the feeling of fullness. It is important to remain hydrated as well. Registered dietitians should be consulted to assist in a personalized diet plan, and to establish goals and strategies.

Also, having extra weight when cancer treatments begin can affect prognosis for breast, ovarian, and colon cancers. If weight is gained during treatment, it is important to discuss this with a physician and other healthcare team members. Hormone therapy adds, blocks, or removes hormones to affect cancer cell growth, and low levels of hormones can cause weight gain. Hormone therapy is most commonly used for breast and prostate cancer. Some chemotherapy drugs cause edema, while others temporarily lower metabolism or result in treatment-induced menopause in women, associated with changes in hormones and weight gain. Regarding increased appetite, it is important to be mindful of how you eat, follow prescribed eating plans, eat foods with lower fat and fewer calories, and only eat when you are hungry, avoiding food during activities such as watching television or working on a computer. Regularly scheduled meal times are important.

ALTERATIONS IN TASTE AND SMELL

Before, during, or after cancer treatments, changes to taste and smell regarding food are common. This may affect which foods can be consumed and enjoyed, and may contribute to loss of appetite and weight loss, leading to malnutrition. Taste, smell, and the texture of food help us to enable us to experience flavor. Cancer itself can affect the senses and cause changes prior to treatment beginning. Treatments can affect the senses and damage nerves that connect to the brain. Chemotherapy may damage the **taste buds** and affect nerve endings, causing an individual to not be able to feel hot and cold foods the same as before. Radiation therapy to the head and neck can damage taste buds as well as the salivary glands. Surgery to the mouth or nose can affect the tongue, sinuses, and salivary glands. Sometimes the amount of saliva is reduced, resulting in **xerostomia**. A dry mouth can affect the sense of taste, and if chronic, can cause mouth infections and tooth decay, which further affect sensations. Some cancer treatments cause *mucositis*, damaging the cells lining the mouth and GI tract, which can cause mouth ulcers that increase sensitivity to anything that is hot, cold, salty, spicy, or acidic. Health condition, time of meals, and locations of meals (such as hospitals) also affect feelings about food. Sometimes, a person no longer likes a certain type of food simply due to environmental changes.

Cancer may cause foods to have no flavor, altered flavor, to taste metallic, to seem bitter, or to be too sweet. When the cancer reduces the sense of smell, taste is often also impaired. Some people become overly sensitive to certain odors, or they seem to smell different. Some odors cause nauseousness, and there can also be perceptions of odors that other people do not smell. Foods may seem dry and difficult to chew or swallow. They can start to taste like "cardboard" (extremely bland). Sometimes, individuals become less sensitivity to certain food types, or foods may suddenly taste too spicy, seem to be prickly, or seem to be cold. Some foods become preferred or disliked, regardless of how they were perceived before. There may be less interested in food, and it may be difficult to eat sufficient quantities. There may be cravings for certain types of food. If something negative was experienced while eating a favorite food, in the future that food may be disliked. Most taste and smell changes are temporary, based on treatments. Chemotherapy is able to alter taste and smell immediately in some patients, but this usually resolves over time. Sometimes, it takes several months for taste and smell to return. Radiation therapy may cause longer-term problems with taste and smell, especially when the salivary glands are compromised.

FOCUS ON CANCER AND ITS EFFECTS ON TASTE AND SMELL

Certain types of cancer, and its treatment, definitely alter our senses of taste and smell. Common causes include tumors of the head and neck area, and resultant radiation to that area. Other factors include certain kinds of chemotherapy and targeted therapy. Some treatments cause mouth sores or dryness. Also, some medications used to help reduce side effects and other non-cancer problems can also negatively impact the senses of taste and smell.

Test Your Knowledge

1. What treatments can increase appetite in cancer patients?
2. How can the sense of taste be affected by cancer treatments?
3. What happens to the sense of smell because of therapies to treat cancer?

EARLY SATIETY

Early satiety means a feeling full early or poor appetite, which is often due to cancer treatments such as chemotherapy or the cancer itself. It can lead to drastic weight loss without careful management. Appetite stimulants are often needed. Some cancer patients are able to only eat a few bites of food before feeling full. Early satiety compromises the cancer patient's ability to get enough nutrition. All cancer patients, therefore, should meet with a nutritionist or registered dietician before and throughout their treatments, to help maintain health through appropriate dietary alterations. Protein-rich and other higher calorie foods may be needed, including the following:

- Protein drinks – using powdered protein supplements mixed in fruit, milk, and/or yogurt
- Dairy products
- Eggs
- Meat

Caloric supplementation may also be needed, before and during treatment. Nutritional support may be administered into the patient's veins via *parenteral nutrition*, or directly into the intestines via enteral nutrition. These methods are of most benefit to patients undergoing stem cell transplantation (see Figure 19.2).

Total parenteral nutrition (TPN) delivers nutritionally adequate solutions into the veins. It is used for those who cannot eat, and is often beneficial in perioperative settings when the cancer patient has severe malnutrition. Long-term use of TPN is contraindicated during chemotherapy since it is not as beneficial. Enteral nutrition is done if the patient cannot ingest, chew, or swallow food, but can still digest and absorb nutrients. Appetite stimulants help maintain adequate calorie and nutrient intake, and include dronabinol, megestrol acetate, and dexamethasone. Dronabinol is produced in a laboratory, and is a version of natural marijuana, and not only stimulates appetite but blocks receptors involved in nausea and vomiting caused by chemotherapy. Megestrol acetate is a progesterone that improves appetite in patients with advanced cancer, and is approved for palliative treatment of advanced breast and endometrial cancer. Dexamethasone is a corticosteroid that is only indicated for short-term use due to its ability to cause myopathy (muscle weakness and other changes in muscle tissue).

CANCER CACHEXIA

Cachexia occurs in up to 80% of people with advanced cancer, based on the cancer type and how well the patient responds to treatment. Cachexia is implicated in up to 30% of cancer deaths, often due to muscle loss-related heart or respiratory failure. When severe, the accompanying physical deterioration can result in weakness, fatigue, being unable or unwilling to eat, and very alarming appearance changes. This greatly affects the patient's ability to handle the tasks of everyday life. Mental health issues include worrying, excessive stress, anxiety, and mental anguish. These issues often impact the family and friends of the cancer patient as well.

Though there are no effective treatments for cachexia, there have been studies resulting in a medication that helps patients maintain lean muscle mass, which is crucial for daily living and the ability to tolerate treatments. Other experimental drugs are now being tested in human studies. Cachexia is most common in people with advance lung and pancreatic cancer, but is also commonly occurs along with head, neck, colon, ovarian, and liver cancers. With cachexia, there is a loss of 5% or more of body weight over six months, accompanied by symptoms such as reduced strength and increased fatigue. Patient assessments include analysis of lean muscle mass, body mass index, nutritional status, symptoms, effects upon quality of life, and treadmill tests to assess physical function. Many patients benefit from **gait training** to improve walking and related movements. Another area of improvement is *core strength*.

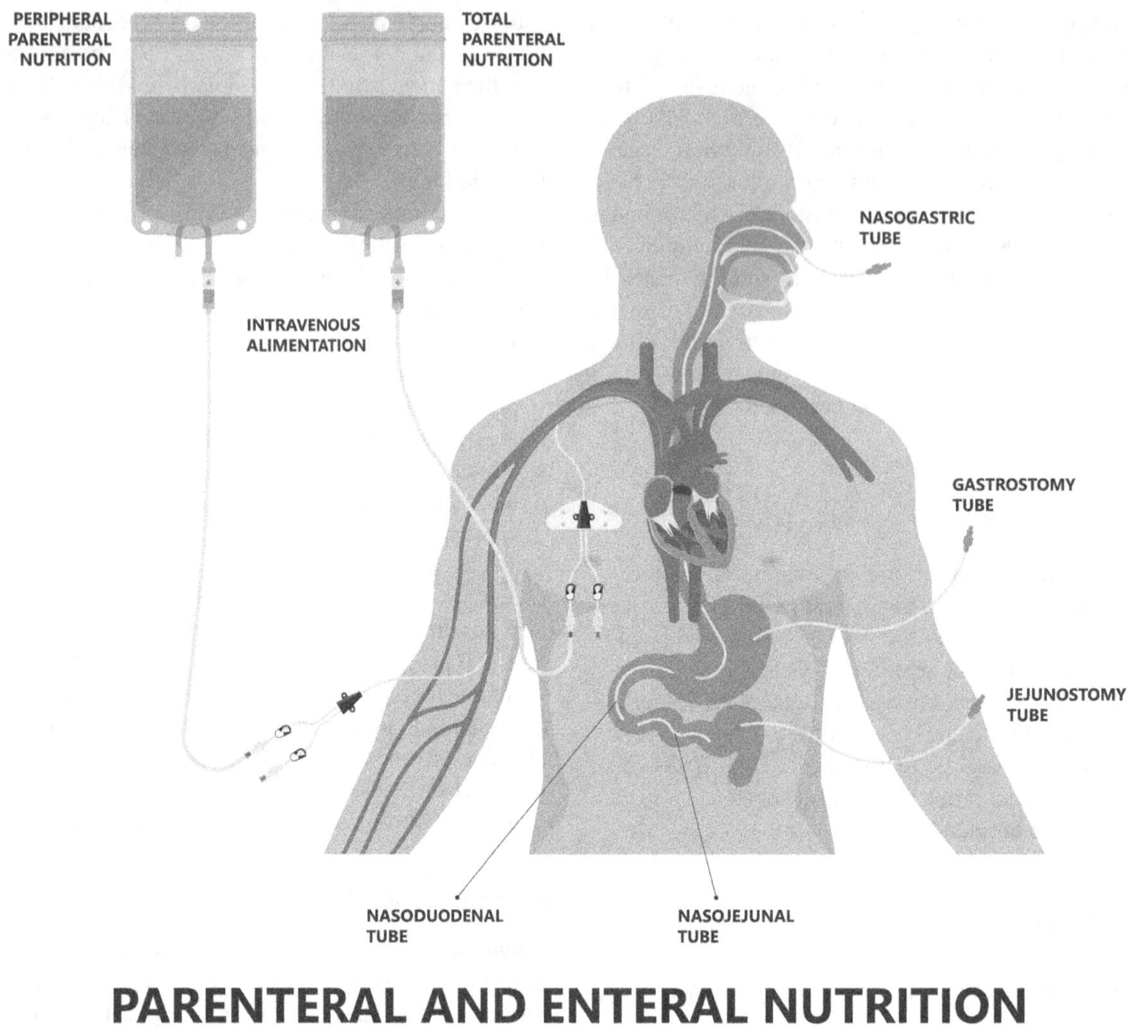

FIGURE 19.2 Parenteral and enteral nutrition.

The widespread inflammation that often accompanies cancer is believed to be the main force that initiates and sustains cachexia. There are disruptions in how the muscle and fat cells make and use energy. The body's metabolic balance becomes disrupted, and the muscle and fat cells break down faster than they can be replenished. Inflammation influences levels of many cytokines, which influence **sarcopenia** and the desire to eat, draining the body of energy. The cytokine called *interleukin-6* is a primary factor in the cycle of tumor growth and cachexia because of "communication" between tumors, fat, and muscle. The bones are repositories of factors that induce inflammation and muscle loss. A bone-produced protein may contribute to muscle loss in patients with ovarian cancer. A protein called **lipocalin 2** may fuel cachexia in those with pancreatic cancer. Malfunctioning mitochondria and deterioration of the nerves supporting skeletal muscle fibers may also play a role in cachexia.

A cytokine called *growth differentiation factor 15* is produced by liver cells, kidneys, and intestines, and directly contributes to appetite. It does this by binding to a protein produced in the area of the brain involved in appetite control. An experimental drug that targets this protein may be able to completely reverse the wasting that occurs with cachexia. This drug is now being tested in human subjects. Though there are no approved drugs for cachexia in the United States yet, Japan approved a drug called *anamorelin* in 2021. It mimics the effects of the hormone called *ghrelin* and stimulates the desire to eat. In people with cachexia, the effects of ghrelin appear to be impaired. Therefore, anamorelin acts in ways similar to ghrelin to increase appetite. Clinical trials of anamorelin proved that in people with advanced lung cancer and cachexia, it helped them to increase lean body mass, appetite, and the ability to eat more food at each meal. However, because the intended goals for the drug were to also increase hand strength in patients, which it failed to do, it was rejected by regulators in the European Union for use in member countries. Further study is ongoing.

FOCUS ON CACHEXIA IN THE CANCER PATIENT

Cachexia is a wasting syndrome in which the body loses fat and muscle, usually because of chronic inflammation caused by cancer. The three stages of cachexia are *precachexia* (loss of less than 5% of body weight), *cachexia* (loss of more than 5% of body weight), and *refractory* (in which treatments are no longer managing the cancer and the prognosis for survival is three months or less).

Test Your Knowledge

1. What is the definition of "early satiety" in relation to cancer or its treatments?
2. What are the forms of feeding that may help provide adequate nutrition to cancer patients?
3. What is believed to be the main force that initiates and sustains cachexia in cancer patients?

KEY TERMS

Acetaldehyde

Adenocarcinomas

Alcohol dehydrogenase

Alpha-fetoprotein

Apoptosis

Areola

Brachytherapy

Cirrhosis

Clubbing

Coagulopathy

Cryotherapy

Cytoplasmic enzymes

Ductal carcinoma in situ

Dyspepsia

Dysphagia

Endotoxins

Erythema

Erythrocytosis

Fibrosis

Friction rub

Gait training

Glutathione

Helicobacter pylori

Hematemesis

Hematogenous

Hematuria

Hepatic bruit

Hepatic steatosis

Hepatocellular carcinoma

Hepatoma

Hepatomegaly

Heterocyclic amines

Hypofractionation

Kupffer cells

Lipocalin 2

Melena

Metabolic traits

Neoantigens

Paget disease

Peritonitis

Polymorphisms

Polyps

Portal hypertension

Prostatic intraepithelial neoplasia

Prostate-specific antigen

Redox potential

Sarcopenia

Seminal vesicles

Stellate cells

Taste buds

Ulcerative colitis

Xerostomia

CLINICAL CASE STUDIES

Clinical Case Study 1

A 58-year-old woman had been diagnosed with colon cancer that had metastasized to her liver. She presented for management of weight loss, since she had lost 22% of her body weight over the past six months. Her most significant symptoms were loss of appetite, drowsiness, and shortness of breath. The patient was treated for a vitamin D deficiency, started on a home exercise program to improve her overall strength, and received nutritional counseling. Radiation therapy was given for her abdominal metastases. Slowly, her weight began to increase, and there was improvement of all other symptoms.

CRITICAL THINKING QUESTIONS

1. What is the prevention of colon cancer based on?
2. Which age groups are mostly affected by colon cancer?
3. What are the five-year survival rates for colon cancer?

Clinical Case Study 2

A 62-year-old man had experienced sharp stomach pains and feelings of fullness over about six months. He believed it to be from a stomach ulcer and tried his best to self-medicate to reduce the symptoms. However, the pain eventually became severe enough that it affected his ability to work. His appetite diminished and he began losing weight, prompting his to finally see his physician. He had lost 16 pounds very quickly. Blood tests and an endoscopy with biopsy were done, revealing stomach cancer. A surgical procedure to remove the tumor was scheduled. After surgery, the patient received chemotherapy and radiation therapy. He could not tolerate enteral feeding, so his physician ordered total parenteral nutrition to be administered.

CRITICAL THINKING QUESTIONS

1. How does large amounts of dietary salt lead to stomach cancer?
2. What is the most common type of malignant stomach tumor?
3. What are the symptoms of stomach cancer?

Clinical Case Study 3

An obese 69-year-old man had developed all of the symptoms of an aging prostate gland. His diet mostly consisted of fatty foods, which he thoroughly enjoyed, with very little fruits, vegetables, or whole grains. He was an African-American man whose father had developed prostate cancer but survived, later dying of a pulmonary condition. His mother had died of breast cancer. A thorough review of the patient's diet showed that he always used whole milk and regular dairy products. Testing revealed that his PSA was highly elevated. An ultrasound revealed enlargement of the prostate gland, and a biopsy was ordered, which confirmed that prostate cancer had developed. Fortunately, the cancer had not spread, so the patient was scheduled for surgical resection.

CRITICAL THINKING QUESTIONS

1. How common is adenocarcinoma of the prostate gland?
2. When symptoms of prostate cancer appear, what do they include?
3. What are the treatment options for prostate cancer?

STUDY QUESTIONS

1. Which of the following liver disorders is NOT related to alcoholism?
   A. Cirrhosis
   B. Alcoholic hepatitis
   C. Hemochromatosis
   D. Fatty liver

2. Which of the following types of viral hepatitis may cause hepatocellular carcinoma?
   A. Hepatitis D virus
   B. Hepatitis A virus
   C. Hepatitis E virus
   D. Hepatitis B virus

3. All of the following are signs and symptoms of cirrhosis, EXCEPT:
   A. Fever
   B. Cardiomegaly
   C. Hepatomegaly
   D. Clubbing of the fingers

4. Which of the following disorders may be caused by foods that are contaminated with fungal aflatoxins?
   A. Hepatocellular carcinoma
   B. Peritonitis
   C. Erythrocytosis
   D. Hypercalcemia

5. Which of the following colon cancers is the most common?
   A. Sarcoma
   B. Ductal carcinoma
   C. Adenocarcinoma
   D. Lobular carcinoma

6. Which of the following infections may cause stomach cancer?
   A. Hepatitis C virus
   B. *Helicobacter pylori*
   C. *Salmonella typhi*
   D. *Haemophilus ducreyi*

7. Which of the following may be affected by Paget disease?
   A. Breast
   B. Colon
   C. Prostate
   D. Stomach

8. Which of the following is the second leading cause of cancer death in American men?
   A. Stomach
   B. Lung
   C. Prostate
   D. Liver

9. Which of the following sites of cancer may affect taste and smell?
   A. Liver
   B. Head
   C. Prostate
   D. Lung

10. Which is the most effective treatment for cachexia?
   A. High carbohydrate diet
   B. Antibiotics
   C. High consumption of fat-soluble vitamins
   D. There is no treatment that is most effective

11. All of the following foods contain high protein, EXCEPT:
   A. Eggs
   B. Meat
   C. Avocado
   D. Yogurt

12. Prostate cancer is more common in which of the following ethnic groups?
   A. African-Americans
   B. Native Americans
   C. Italian-Americans
   D. Hispanic-Americans

13. Which of the following diets may lead to stomach cancer?
   A. A diet high in spicy foods
   B. A diet high in fatty foods
   C. A diet high in salty foods
   D. A diet high in bitter foods

14. All of the following are signs and symptoms of colon cancer, EXCEPT:
   A. Colicky abdominal pain
   B. Ataxia
   C. Severe anemia
   D. Occult bleeding

15. A high consumption of red meat is linked to an increased risk of which of the following cancers?
   A. Colon
   B. Prostate
   C. Breast
   D. Liver

FURTHER READING

1. American Cancer Society, Besser, J., and Grant, B. (2018). *What To Eat During Cancer Treatment*, 2nd Edition. American Cancer Society.
2. Andrews, N. (2022). *Sugar Does Not Feed Cancer – The Complete Guide to Cancer Prevention Nutrition and Lifestyle*. The Oncology Dietitian.
3. Bauman, E., Waldman, H., and Abrams, D.I. (2012). *The Whole-Food Guide for Breast Cancer Survivors – A Nutritional Approach to Preventing Recurrence*. New Harbinger Publications.
4. Bishoy, S. (2022). *Red Meat Increases the Risk of Colon Cancer*. Bishoy.
5. Del Fabbro, E., Inui, A., and Strasser, F. (2012). *Cancer Cachexia (Pocket Books for Cancer Supportive Care)*. Springer Healthcare.
6. Dodson, S., Baracos, V.E., Jatoi, A., Evans, W.J., Cella, D., Dalton, J.T., and Stiner, M.S. (2012). *Muscle Wasting in Cancer Cachexia: Clinical Implications, Diagnosis, and Emerging Treatment Strategies*. Annual Reviews of Medicine.
7. Doris, M. (2020). *Managing Cancer with Alkaline Diet – Scientifically Proven Ways to Prevent and Reverse Cancer*. Doris.
8. Gabbert, H., Beach, K., and Lee, C.M. (2014). *Battling Breast Cancer with Nutrition*. Provenir Publishing.
9. Heber, D., Li, Z., and Liang, V. (2021). *Nutritional Oncology*. CRC Press.
10. Hofbauer, K.G., Anker, S.D., Inui, A., and Nicholson, J.R. (2005). *Pharmacotherapy of Cachexia*. CRC / Taylor & Francis.
11. Jeffrey, D. (2022). *Stomach Cancer – The Complete Guide on How to Cure Stomach Cancer – Everything from Diagnosis to Recovery*. Jeffrey.
12. Kafta, S. (2022). *The Complete Cancer Diet and Nutrition Therapy – Nutritious Anti-cancer Diet Recipes Cookbook for the Newly Diagnosed*. Kafta.
13. Kalamian, M., and Seyfried, T.N. (2017). *Keto for Cancer – Ketogenic Metabolic Therapy as a Targeted Nutritional Strategy*. Chelsea Green Publishing.
14. Karon, Y. (2021). *Signs of Stomach Cancer – Appetite Loss, Weight Loss, Heartburn, Abdominal Pain, Feeling Full Easily, Anemia, Fatigue, Abdomen Swelling, Regular Vomiting, Blood in Stools*. Karon.
15. Katz, R., and Edelson, M. (2017). *The Cancer-Fighting Kitchen – Nourishing Big-Flavor Recipes for Cancer Treatment and Recovery*, 2nd Edition. Ten Speed Press.
16. Katzin, C. (2021). *The Cancer Nutrition Handbook*, 7th Edition. Foundation Resources, Inc.
17. Kushi, M., and Jack, A. (2009). *The Cancer Prevention Diet – The Macrobiotic Approach to Preventing and Relieving Cancer, Revised and Updated 25th Anniversary Edition*. St. Martin's Griffin.

18. Lipsky, S.A. (2017). *Beyond Cancer – The Powerful Effect of Plant-based Eating – How to Adopt a Plant-based Diet to Optimize Cancer Survival and Long-term Health.* Wellness Ink Publishing.
19. Marc, M. (2022). *Alcohol-Related Liver Disease Recovery Manual – Understand to Survive, Manage, Treat, Prevent, Strive and Reverse Symptoms Completely.* Marc.
20. MB Foundation. (2019). *Outsmart Cancer – Defeat Cancer with Vitamin B17, Healthy Nutrition, and Alternative Medicine.* MB Foundation.
21. McLelland, J. (2018). *How to Starve Cancer: Without Starving Yourself.* Agenor Publishing.
22. Nedrow, B. (2022). *Metabolic Flexibility – How to Heal Your Metabolism with a Ketogenic Diet.* Bonnie Nedrow.
23. Noyes, V.O. (2022). *The Truth About Cancer – What You Should Know About Cancer History, Prevention, Treatment, and What to Eat.* Noyes.
24. Oncology Nutrition Dietetic Practice Group. (2019). *Oncology Nutrition for Clinical Practice.* ONDPG.
25. Padilla, L. (2015). *Anti-Cancer Habits & Anti-Inflammatory Nutrition.* Padilla.
26. Quillin, P. (2021). *Beating Cancer with Nutrition: Using Nutrition and Other Modalities to Improve Quality and Quantity of Life for Medically Treated Cancer Patients*, 5th Edition. Nutrition Times Press Inc.
27. Rayman, M., Dilley, K., and Gibbons, K. (2020). *Healthy Eating for Prostate Care.* Kyle Books.
28. Rothenberg, T. (2022). *Cancer Diet for the Newly Diagnosed – An Integrative Guide and Cookbook for Treatment and Recovery.* Rockridge Press.
29. Sammut, J. (2015). *Eat Your Way Out of Cancer – The Alternative Way to Healing the Human Body Using Anti-cancerous Plant Foods.* Blurb.
30. Sears, W., Sears, M., and Van Etten, R. (2022). *Help Heal Yourself from Cancer – Partner Smarter with Your Doctor, Personalize Your Treatment Plan, and Take Charge of Your Recovery.* BenBella Books.
31. Stone, T. (2022). *Starving Breast Cancer with Nutrition – Easy, Latest, Research-based Recipes for Breast Cancer Treatment and Recovery.* Stone.
32. Tedric, J. (2022). *Breast Cancer Patients and Full-Fat Dairy Products.* Tedric.
33. Werner Gray, L., and Hyman, M. (2019). *Cancer-Free with Food – A Step-by-Step Plan with 100+ Recipes to Fight Disease, Nourish Your Body and Restore Your Health.* Hay House Inc.
34. Winters, N., Higgins Kelly, J., and Turner, K. (2017). *The Metabolic Approach to Cancer – Integrating Deep Nutrition, the Ketogenic Diet, and Nontoxic Bio-Individualized Therapies.* Chelsea Green Publishing.

20 Nutritional Effects on Hereditary Metabolic Disorders

OUTLINE

Hereditary Metabolic Disorders
- Amino Acid Metabolism Disorders
- Carbohydrate Metabolism Disorders
- Fatty Acid Metabolism Disorders
- Purine and Pyrimidine Metabolism Disorders
- Lysosomal Storage Disorders

Nutritional Changes to Correct Metabolic Disorders
Enzyme Replacement
Special Diets
Key Terms
Clinical Case Studies
Study Questions
Further Reading

LEARNING OBJECTIVES

After study of the chapter, readers should be able to:

1. List three examples of amino acid metabolism disorders.
2. Describe maple syrup urine disease.
3. Explain the signs and symptoms of phenylketonuria.
4. Describe two examples of urea cycle disorders.
5. Explain the initial signs and symptoms of galactosemia.
6. Discuss the signs and symptoms of glycerol kinase deficiency.
7. Explain purine metabolism disorders and their causes.
8. Describe lysosomal storage disorders.
9. Explain various types of Niemann-Pick disease.
10. Describe the causes of Tay-Sachs disease, Gaucher disease, and Fabry disease.

OVERVIEW

Because of the advent of newborn screening and development of newer and better therapies, more people with inherited metabolic disorders have been identified early than ever before in history. Dietary therapy is the primary treatment for many of these disorders. The goals of dietary therapy are maintenance of normal growth and development, plus the limiting of harmful metabolites. Usually, the problematic metabolite is greatly reduced or totally removed from the diet, then reintroduced in small quantities until blood levels are within normal ranges. These treatments may occur throughout life, and require close monitoring of micronutrient and macronutrient intake. The most serious hereditary metabolic disorders generally include phenylketonuria, Gaucher disease, Krabbe disease, maple syrup urine disease, and Niemann-Pick disease.

HEREDITARY METABOLIC DISORDERS

Hereditary metabolic disorders are also known as *inherited disorders of metabolism* and *inborn errors of metabolism.* The majority of them are caused by mutations in genes that code for enzymes. Any deficiency or inactivity of enzymes results in accumulation of **metabolites**, or enzyme products. There are hundreds of hereditary metabolic disorders. However, most are extremely rare on an individual basis, while collectively they are not rare. Inherited metabolic disorders are usually classified by the **substrate** that is affected. These include the following:

- *Amino acid metabolism disorders* – branched-chain amino acid disorders, methionine metabolism disorders, phenylketonuria, tyrosine metabolism disorders, and urea cycle disorders
- *Carbohydrate metabolism disorders* – fructose metabolism disorders, galactosemia, glycogen storage diseases, pyruvate metabolism disorders, and other carbohydrate metabolism disorders
- *Fatty acid metabolism disorders* – these may involve fatty acid transport and mitochondrial oxidation, glycerol, ketones, peroxisome biogenesis and very long-chain fatty acids, and other disorders of fat metabolism
- *Purine and pyrimidine metabolism disorders* – purine catabolism disorders, purine nucleotide synthesis disorders, purine salvage disorders, hereditary orotic aciduria, dihydropyrimidine dehydrogenase deficiency (inborn error form and pharmacogenetic form), dihydropyrimidinuria, beta-ureidopropionase deficiency, pyrimidine 5' nucleotidase deficiency, and activation-induced cytidine deaminase deficiency (hyper IgM syndrome type II)
- *Lysosomal storage disorders* – inherited metabolic diseases that are mostly caused by genes encoding a lysosomal enzyme; these monogenic disorders involve 40 different acid hydrolases within the lysosomes

DOI: 10.1201/b22969-23

Neonatal screening is regularly done in most Westernized countries such as the United States, to assess the presence of certain inherited disorders of metabolism and other conditions. These include phenylketonuria, tyrosinemia, biotinidase deficiency, homocystinuria, maple syrup urine disease, and galactosemia. Many locations have an expanded screening program covering other inherited disorders of metabolism, including fatty acid oxidation disorders and other organic acidemias. Metabolic defects that mostly cause disease in adults, such as gout or **porphyria**, are specific to certain organs. Examples include congenital adrenal hyperplasia and Wilson disease. Some of the more common diseases include cystic fibrosis and hemochromatosis.

FOCUS ON HEREDITARY METABOLIC DISORDERS

Inherited metabolic disorders are present at birth, and some are detected by routine screening. All 50 states screen newborns for phenylketonuria. Most states also test newborns for galactosemia. However, no state tests babies for all known inherited metabolic disorders.

Amino Acid Metabolism Disorders

Disorders that affect the metabolism of amino acids include maple syrup urine disease, hypermethioninemia, phenylketonuria, tyrosinemia, homocystinuria, argininemia, ornithinemia, and hyperinsulinism-hyperammonemia syndrome. These disorders are autosomal recessive, and all may be diagnosed by analyzing amino acid concentrations in body fluids. The causes of amino acid metabolism disorders include incomplete breakdown of proteins in the digestive system, inherited abnormalities in the biochemical mechanisms of the body, a poor diet, and stress.

Maple Syrup Urine Disease

Maple syrup urine disease (MSUD) is a rare but a life-threatening metabolic disorder, resulting in neurologic and developmental delays. The disease affects an estimated one of every 185,000 infants worldwide. The mortality rates, based on location, range between 21% and 27%. The body becomes unable to process certain amino acids. This causes a harmful buildup of substances in the blood and urine. Normally, the body breaks down protein foods such as meat and fish into amino acids. MSUD is characterized by deficiency of an enzyme complex (branched-chain alpha-keto acid dehydrogenase) that is required to metabolize the three branched-chain amino acids leucine, isoleucine and valine. Symptoms of classic MSUD appear in newborns within 48 hours of birth. In older children, signs of intermediate, **intermittent**, and thiamine-responsive MSUD usually develop before age seven. Signs and symptoms include:

- Urine, sweat, or earwax that smells like maple syrup or burned sugar
- Poor feeding, vomiting, loss of appetite, irritability
- Tiredness and weakness
- Changes in muscle tone – poor muscle tone, muscle tightness/tension
- Abnormal muscle movements, and spasms that cause a backward arching of the head, neck and spine
- Developmental delays
- Eventual seizures, convulsions, respiratory failure, and coma

There must be aggressive management of nutrition that includes protein restriction of leucine, isoleucine, and valine. There is a need to closely monitor **cerebral edema** and acute pancreatitis. Treatment of MSUD also requires dietary thiamin supplementation. There should be an emergency plan for acute illness since it can provoke a metabolic crisis. Finally, liver transplantation may be required. Complications of MSUD include brain damage, neurological problems, and developmental delays. There is an increased risk of attention deficit/hyperactivity disorder (ADHD), anxiety, and depression. Loss of bone mass causes the bones to fracture easily. Pancreatitis develops, especially during crisis states. Chronic headaches occur, caused by an increase in blood pressure in the brain. There may be movement disorders, such as tremors and uncontrolled muscle contractions. Coma and death may be caused by crisis states such as infection, stress, or poor dietary control.

Test Your Knowledge

1. What are the five basic types of hereditary metabolic disorders?
2. What are the causes of amino acid metabolism disorders?
3. What are the complications of maple syrup urine disease?

Methionine Metabolism Disorders

Hypermethioninemia occurs when methionine is not metabolized properly. Individuals with this condition often do not show any signs and symptoms. **Homocysteine** acts as an intermediate in the metabolism of methionine. Defects in the **remethylation** or **transsulfuration** processes can cause homocysteine to accumulate, causing hypermethioninemia. The initial step in methionine metabolism is the conversion of it to **adenosylmethionine**. This requires the enzyme called methionine adenosyltransferase. Classic homocystinuria is an autosomal recessive condition. Since remethylation is intact, some additional homocysteine is converted to methionine, which accumulates in the blood. The disorder affects the muscles, liver, and brain. It is characterized by **psychomotor** development delays, low intelligence quotient (IQ), unusual facial features, neurological problems, and hypotonia, as well as chronic inflammation and fibrosis of the liver. Cases may be asymptomatic until early adulthood, depending on the severity of the mutation. Usually, the eyes and skeleton are affected. Serious neurologic effects may be from thrombosis or a direct effect. Arterial or venous thromboembolic features can occur at any time. Many patients develop lens **subluxation**, intellectual disability, and osteoporosis. Patients are usually of short stature, but can have a **marfanoid habitus**. Classic homocystinuria is diagnosed by neonatal screening for elevated serum methionine. Confirmation is by elevated total plasma homocysteine levels, DNA testing, or both. Treatment is with a low-methionine diet and L-cysteine supplementation, along with high-dose pyridoxine, which is a **cystathionine** synthetase cofactor, of 100–500mg orally per day. When early treatment occurs, intellectual outcome is normal to near-normal. Thromboembolism can be prevented by10mg of oral vitamin C is given per day.

FOCUS ON HYPERMETHIONINEMIA

Hypermethioninemia can occur when methionine is not metabolized normally in the body. It can occur along with other metabolic disorders such as homocystinuria, tyrosinemia, and galactosemia. The disorder can also result from liver disease or excessive dietary intake of methionine (from consuming large amounts of protein or a methionine-enriched infant formula). For most individuals, eating a plant-based diet is usually sufficient to reduce methionine intake.

Phenylketonuria

Phenylketonuria (PKU) is a rare inherited disorder that causes an amino acid called phenylalanine to build up in the body. It may occur in any ethnic group, but is relatively less common in Ashkenazi Jews and African-American people. PKU frequency varies by population. The prevalence in the general U.S. population is approximately 4 cases per 100,000 individuals, and the incidence is 350 cases per every million live births. Approximately 0.04%–1% of the residents in intellectual disability clinics are affected by PKU. The inheritance is autosomal recessive, and in Caucasians, it only occurs in about 1 of every 10,000 births. Excessive dietary phenylalanine is usually converted to tyrosine by phenylalanine hydroxylase. When a gene mutation causes deficiency or absence of phenylalanine hydroxylase, there is an accumulation of dietary phenylalanine, with the brain mostly affected, possibly because of disturbed myelination. Some excess phenylalanine is metabolized to **phenylketones**, excreted in the urine. The amount of enzyme deficiency and severity of hyperphenylalaninemia is varied in patients based on the actual gene mutation.

The majority of children with PKU are normal at birth, developing signs and symptoms slowly over months as phenylalanine accumulates. Since diagnosis and treatment of PKU most often occur shortly after birth due to an abnormal screening test, noticeable signs and symptoms are very rare. The main signs of untreated PKU are severe intellectual disability and behavioral problems. There are also psychoses, an unpleasant "mousy" body odor, eczema, microcephaly, and light skin, hair, and eyes. In most developed countries, neonates are screened for PKU within 24–48 hours after birth via blood tests (see Figure 20.1). Genetic testing is also helpful. Children of families with positive history can be diagnosed prenatally.

Good treatment within the first days of life prevents severe manifestations, but mild cognitive deficits and mental health issues can still occur even when the diet is well-controlled. Treatment started after two to three years may only help to control the extreme hyperactivity and seizures. If a child is born to a mother with poorly controlled PKU during pregnancy, the infant is at a high risk for microcephaly and developmental deficits. Treatment of PKU is with lifelong dietary phenylalanine restriction. Since all natural protein contains about 4% phenylalanine, dietary components must include low-proteins, natural fruits, vegetables,

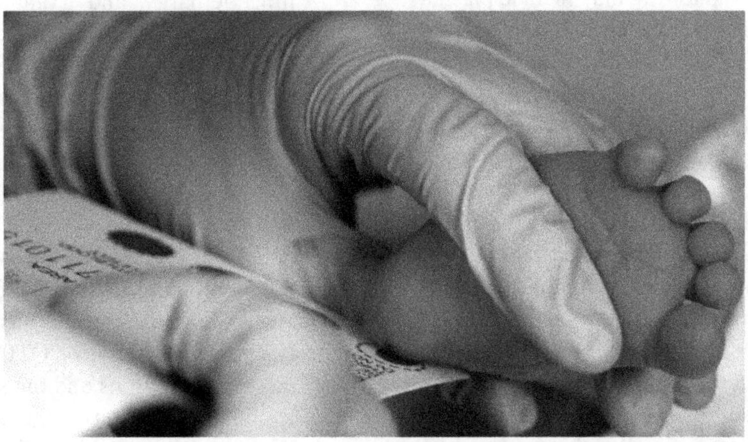

FIGURE 20.1 Blood testing for phenylketonuria.

and certain cereals. There are a variety of commercially-available products designed specifically for infants, children one to eight years of age, and children older than eight years of age. Some amount of phenylalanine is needed for growth and metabolism, but this requirement is met by measured amounts of natural protein from milk or low-protein foods. Frequent monitoring of plasma phenylalanine is required. Dietary planning and management is required for women of childbearing age that have PKU before pregnancy. Tyrosine supplementation is used more often today, since it is an essential amino acid in patients with PKU.

Test Your Knowledge

1. What are the characterizations of classic homo cystinuria?
2. What are the main signs and symptoms of untreated phenylketonuria?
3. What is the required treatment for phenylketonuria?

Urea Cycle Disorders

The **urea cycle disorders** are genetic conditions, which cause ammonia to build up in the blood, creating a toxic and life-threatening situation. The primary forms of these disorders include *argininosuccinic aciduria*, *argininemia*, *Lysinuric protein intolerance*, *ornithinemia*, and *hyperinsulinism-hyperammonemia syndrome.* Inheritance of all these subtypes is autosomal recessive. Argininemia, ornithinemia, and hyperinsulinism-hyperammonemia syndrome are further explained as follows:

- ***Argininemia*** – a urea cycle disorder caused by harmful genetic changes. This is a defective arginase I, resulting in elevated plasma arginine, **diaminoaciduria** (argininuria, cystinuria, lysinuria, and ornithinuria), **orotic aciduria**, and **pyrimidinuria**. Symptoms include anorexia, growth and developmental delay, hyperactivity, irritability, protein intolerance, seizures, spasticity, vomiting, and hyperammonemia. To confirm the diagnosis of argininemia, newborn screening is essential. Follow-up testing may include plasma amino acid analysis, urine orotic acid, and enzyme assay on red blood cells. DNA testing is used for final diagnostic confirmation. Treatment is with a low-protein diet, benzoate, phenylacetate, and liver transplantation. Without treatment, individuals will experience poor growth, stiff muscles, developmental delays, and intellectual disability. Lifespan is normal in most affected individuals, but some may die early from complications of extremely high ammonia.
- ***Ornithinemia*** – a toxic condition occasionally producing localized cerebral swelling, caused by abnormal amounts of **ornithine** in the blood. It is a rare X-linked genetic disorder characterized by complete or partial lack of the enzyme ornithine transcarbamylase (OTC), resulting in elevated plasma ornithine. This is most common type of urea cycle disorder. A severe form of the disorder affects some infants, typically males, shortly after birth. A milder form of the disorder affects some children later in infancy. Both males and females may develop signs and symptoms of OTC deficiency during childhood. Most carrier females are healthy, but may be prone to severe headaches following protein intake. Children and adults with mild forms of the disorder may only have a partial OTC enzyme deficiency. Therefore, a greater tolerance to protein in the diet. Male infants with the severe form of the disorder often have a complete lack of the OTC enzyme. The severe form of OTC deficiency occurs in some affected males anywhere between 24 hours to a few days after birth, usually following a protein feeding. Initial signs and symptoms may include refusal to eat, poor suckling, vomiting, progressive lethargy, and irritability. The disorder may rapidly progress to include seizures, hypotonia, hepatomegaly, and respiratory abnormalities. Affected infants and children may also exhibit edema within the brain. If untreated, infants with the severe form may fall into coma and potentially develop neurological abnormalities. These include intellectual disability, developmental delays, and cerebral palsy. The longer an infant remains in a hyperammonemic coma, the greater the chance neurological abnormalities may develop and become severe. If untreated, hyperammonemic coma may result in life-threatening complications. Some infants and children may have a milder form of OTC deficiency. These infants and children may not exhibit symptoms of OTC deficiency until later during life. If this occurs, it often happens during an episode of illness, and is concurrent with hyperammonemia. Episodes can recur, alternating between periods of wellness. During a hyperammonemic episode, affected children may experience vomiting, lethargy, and irritability. Additional signs and symptoms may include confusion or delirium, hyperactivity, self-mutilation behaviors (such as biting), and ataxia. In some cases the deficiency may not become apparent until adulthood. Adults who have OTC deficiency may exhibit migraines, nausea, **dysarthria**, ataxia, confusion, hallucinations, and blurred vision. The treatment of OTC deficiency is aimed at preventing excessive ammonia from being formed, or from removing excessive ammonia during a hyperammonemic episode. Long-term therapy for OTC deficiency combines dietary restrictions and the stimulation of alternative methods of converting and excreting nitrogen. Dietary restrictions in individuals with OTC deficiency are aimed at limiting the amount of protein

intake to avoid the development of excess ammonia. However, enough protein must be taken in by infants to ensure proper growth. Infants with OTC deficiency are placed on a low-protein, high-calorie diet supplemented by essential amino acids. A high biological value natural protein such as breast milk or cow's milk formulate is combined with an essential amino acid formula.

- **Hyperinsulinism-hyperammonemia syndrome** – the second most common form of congenital hyperinsulinism. Children affected by this syndrome have both fasting and protein sensitive hypoglycemia combined with persistently elevated ammonia levels. Gain of function mutations in the mitochondrial enzyme glutamate dehydrogenase are responsible for this syndrome. Glutamate dehydrogenase is effected in liver, kidney, brain, and pancreatic beta-cells. Patients with this syndrome have an increased frequency of **generalized seizures**, or **absence seizures**, in the absence of hypoglycemia. Symptoms include recurrent hypoglycemia, seizures, asymptomatic hyperammonemia, and hyperinsulinism. Treatment involves prevention of hypoglycemia.

FOCUS ON ORNITHINEMIA AND BUILDUP OF AMMONIA

Ornithinemia is an inherited disorder that causes the buildup of ammonia in the blood. Ammonia is formed when proteins are broken down in the body, and is toxic when its levels become too high. The nervous system is extremely sensitive to the effects of excess ammonia. If untreated, a hyperammonemia coma may result in death. Eating a plant-based diet helps to reduce any dietary-related increases of the condition.

Test Your Knowledge

1. What causes urea cycle disorders to be potentially life-threatening?
2. What are the symptoms of argininemia?
3. What is the description of the most common type of urea cycle disorder?

Carbohydrate Metabolism Disorders

Carbohydrate metabolism disorders are errors of metabolism affecting catabolism and anabolism of carbohydrates. Most of these disorders involve an inability to effectively use metabolites of carbohydrates.

Fructose Metabolism Disorders

Fructose is a monosaccharide present in high concentrations in fruit and honey. It is a constituent of sucrose and sorbitol. Fructose metabolism disorders include galactosemia and glycogen storage diseases, which are further described as follows:

- **Galactosemia** – one of the metabolic diseases that can be identified through newborn screening evaluation. Every state in the United States has or has access to a newborn screening program and is mandated by law to screen for galactosemia. It affects 1 in every 40,000–60,000 newborns around the world. Classic galactosemia occurs in approximately 1 of every 60,000 live births. However, the reported incidence of galactosemia varies geographically from 1 in 30,000 to 40,000 in Europe, to one per million in Japan. The estimated incidence in the United States is 1 in 53,000. Initial signs and symptoms usually present in the first few weeks of life include refusal to feed, vomiting, lethargy, jaundice, **cataracts**, and infection. Infants born with galactosemia need to be put on a special lactose-free diet shortly after birth in order to prevent serious multiorgan involvement and death. If treatment is started after the first ten days of life, the majority of infants with severe or classic galactosemia will die because of a systemic infection. If they do survive the first month of life untreated, they are likely to develop cirrhosis. Even if children receive treatment at an early age, delays in learning and development, as well as speech defects, are common. The specific issues and level of delay varies from child to child, but may include learning disabilities, neurological impairments, and ovarian failure in females. Classic galactosemia occurs when an enzyme called galactose-1-phosphate uridyl transferase is missing or not functional. This liver enzyme is responsible for breaking down galactose into glucose. Galactose is found in breast milk, cow's milk, and other dairy foods. When galactose cannot be changed to glucose, the byproducts such as galactose-1-phosphate, build up in tissues and blood, affecting many parts of the body. Diagnosis is based on a comprehensive review of medical and family history, physical evaluation, and specific biochemical testing. All infants born must be tested on day the second day of life. The only treatment for galactosemia is avoiding foods that contain lactose and galactose.
- **Glycogen storage diseases** – glucose is the main energy fuel for the brain. Maintenance of glucose homeostasis is crucial to meet cellular energy demands in both normal physiological states, and during stress or increased demands. Glucose is stored as glycogen primarily in the liver and skeletal muscle, with a small amount stored in the brain. Liver glycogen primarily maintains blood glucose levels,

while skeletal muscle glycogen is utilized during high-intensity exertion. Brain glycogen is an emergency cerebral energy source. Glycogen storage diseases are rare metabolic disorders involving the inability to properly store or break down glycogen. There are many subtypes, all caused by deficiencies of enzymes involved in glycogen synthesis or breakdown. Type I (**Von Gierke disease**) is the most common type of glycogen storage disease, and accounts for 90% of all glycogen storage disease cases. Type II (**Pompe's disease**) is defined as acid maltase deficiency). Glycogen storage diseases are caused by a genetic enzyme defect that is inherited from both parents. Normally, enzymes help convert glucose into glycogen for storage. Enzymes **phosphorylase kinase** and **glycogen phosphorylase** convert the glycogen back to glucose when quick energy is needed, as in exercise. In a person with a glycogen storage disease, the enzymes are defective, deficient, or absent. Signs and symptoms include hypoglycemia during periods of fasting, poor growth, hepatomegaly, abnormal blood tests, low muscle tone, muscle pain and cramping during exercise, acidosis, and fatigue. Treatment focuses on maintaining adequate levels of blood glucose, ingestion of uncooked cornstarch, frequent meals that are restricted (low sucrose, fructose, and lactose). Infants need to be fed every two hours. Sometimes a high-protein diet is helpful. Calcium, vitamin D, and iron supplements may be needed. Medications include allopurinol to lower lipid levels and prevent kidney disease. Human granulocyte colony stimulating factor can be given for recurrent infections.

Test Your Knowledge

1. What are the initial signs and symptoms of galactosemia?
2. What is the only treatment for galactosemia?
3. What is the most common type of glycogen storage disease?

Fatty Acid Metabolism Disorders

Fatty acid metabolism disorders actually involve a broad classification for genetic disorders that result from an inability of the body to produce or utilize one enzyme that is required to oxidize fatty acids. Fatty acids are the preferred source of energy for the heart. They are an essential energy source for skeletal muscle during extensive exercise. While fasting, most of the body's energy needs must be supplied by fat metabolism. Free fatty acids are metabolized in the liver and peripheral tissue. Glycerol is used by the liver for triglyceride synthesis, or for gluconeogenesis.

Fatty Acid Transport and Mitochondrial Oxidation Disorders

Fatty acid oxidation disorders are a group of inherited metabolic conditions that lead to an accumulation of fatty acids, and a decrease in cell energy metabolism. These disorders result from an inability of the body to produce or utilize an enzyme required to oxidize fatty acids. The enzyme can be missing or incorrectly structured. Therefore, the body is unable to produce energy in the liver and muscles from fatty acid sources. These conditions include **beta-oxidation cycle** disorders and metabolic acidosis, with some causing cardiomyopathy and muscle weakness. Signs and symptoms include extreme sleepiness, behavior changes, irritability, poor appetite, fever, nausea, vomiting, diarrhea, hypoglycemia, **cardiomegaly**, and muscle weakness. Most affected individuals with a fatty acid metabolism disorder can live a normal active life with only simple adjustments to diet and medications. The primary treatment method for fatty acid metabolism disorders is dietary modification, so that blood glucose levels remain regulated. Patients should snack on low-fat, high-carbohydrate nutrients every 2–6 hours. Some affected children and adults can sleep for 8–10 hours through the night without snacking.

Mitochondrial oxidation disorders are a group of clinically **heterogeneous diseases**, commonly defined by lack of cellular energy due to defects of oxidative phosphorylation. They result from pathogenic mutations in nuclear DNA. Mitochondrial oxidation disorders result in a failure of mitochondrial beta-oxidation or the carnitine-based transport of fatty acids into the **mitochondria**. They lead to deficient energy production and hypotonia, and have caused sudden death in infants. There is a decrease in reducing of equivalents for oxidative phosphorylation due to enzymatic reaction of fatty acid oxidation, reduced production of the tricarboxylic acid cycle substrate acetyl-coenzyme A, and reduced production of ketone bodies. These disorders are generally signified by recurrent hypoglycemia, exercise intolerance, and chronic fatigue. Treatment is based on prevention of hypoglycemia, by avoiding fasting.

FOCUS ON THE MOST COMMON FATTY ACID OXIDATION DISORDER

The most common fatty acid oxidation disorder is called medium-chain acyl-CoA dehydrogenase deficiency. An affected individual will become extremely ill if energy demands exceed energy intake, such as during infections or repeated vomiting. Affected children are unable to fast for very long without developing hypoglycemia.

Glycerol Metabolism Disorders

Isolated glycerol kinase deficiency (GKD) is a very rare X-linked disorder of glycerol metabolism characterized biochemically by elevated plasma and urine glycerol levels. Clinically, it is characterized by neurometabolic manifestations, depending on the age of onset, and can be a life-threatening childhood metabolic disorder. GKD has the features of hyperglycerolemia and glyceroluria. Common symptoms include vomiting, lethargy, and hypotonia, which are usually the only symptoms. When GKD is accompanied by Duchenne muscular dystrophy and adrenal hypoplasia congenita, the symptoms can become much more severe. Signs and symptoms visible shortly after birth include **cryptorchidism**, seizures, **strabismus**, metabolic acidosis, hypoglycemia, learning disabilities, **myopathy**, and adrenal cortex insufficiency. GKD can be divided into three distinct forms: infantile, juvenile, and adult. Out of all of these, the infantile form is the most clinically relevant because it leads to developmental delays and adrenal insufficiency. Treatment is most critical if there is adrenal hypoplasia and insufficiency since all deaths from these disorders appear to have been caused by an Addisonian crisis. Glucocorticoids and mineralocorticoids are required. Patients with vomiting, acidemia, and stupor linked to the deficiency or glycerol intolerance syndrome may be placed on a glycerol-restricted low-fat diet, but it is very important to avoid prolonged fasting. Complications vary depending on the type of glycogen storage disease. They can include liver problems, hypoglycemia, growth and developmental delays, as well as lung and heart problems.

Test Your Knowledge

1. What are the signs and symptoms of fatty acid transport disorders?
2. What do mitochondrial oxidation disorders lead to?
3. What are the three distinct forms of glycerine kinase deficiency, and which is most clinically significant?

Ketone Metabolism Disorders

Ketone bodies are circulating metabolites that are primarily formed in the liver. They play a key role in the glucose-sparing energy supply. Ketone bodies are especially important for the brain, which is unable to take up and use fatty acids for energy. These bodies originate from fatty acids and, to a lesser extent, from ketogenic amino acids such as leucine. Disorders of ketone body metabolism present either in the first few days of life or later in childhood, during an infection or some other metabolic stress. With defects of ketogenesis, decompensation leads to encephalopathy, vomiting, and hepatomegaly. Poorly controlled or decompensated diabetes mellitus is the most common pathologic condition causing ketonuria. Ketone metabolism disorders also include metabolic acidosis without ketonuria. Defective enzymes or proteins may cause hypoglycemia, encephalopathy, hepatomegaly, irritability, lethargy, vomiting, ketoacidosis, hyperventilation, intellectual disability, or hypotonia. Treatments include avoidance of fasting, leucine restriction, glucose during acute episodes with careful use of bicarbonate, and a high-carbohydrate diet with some restriction of protein and fat.

Purine and Pyrimidine Metabolism Disorders

The **purines** are a group of molecules used by all cells of the body for many essential biochemical processes. They are important components of cellular energy systems, signaling, and along with the pyrimidines, production of RNA and DNA. The end product of the complete catabolism of purines is uric acid. Inborn errors of purine and pyrimidine metabolism have been documented in 14 different disorders, representing a broad spectrum of clinical manifestations. The following sections explain these disorders.

Purine Metabolism Disorders

Inborn errors of purine metabolism exhibit broad neurological, immunological, hematological and renal manifestations. Purine metabolism disorders are caused by deficiencies of myoadenylate deaminase, adenosine deaminase, purine nucleoside phosphorylase, or xanthine oxidase. Signs and symptoms include exercise-induced myalgias or cramping, severe combined immunodeficiency, lymphopenia, **thymic deficiency**, recurrent infections, **hypouricemia**, developmental delays, ataxia, spasticity, symptomatic stones with hematuria, urinary colic, and urinary tract infections. Treatment options include exercise modulation, bone marrow or stem cell transplantation, enzyme replacement therapy, high fluid intake to reduce likelihood of stone formation, and allopurinol. Affected patients have an enormous overproduction of purines, hyperuricemia, **uricosuria** and all of the complications of gout, including arthritis, **tophi**, renal calculi, and renal failure, which results from the deposition of urate in the renal parenchyma (see Figure 20.2).

FOCUS ON PURINE METABOLISM DISORDERS

Disorders of purine metabolism include hyperuricemia, gout, nephrolithiasis, immunodeficiency, anemia, diseases of the nervous system, and myopathies. Overproduction of uric acid can be severe enough to lead to death.

Purine Salvage Disorders

Purine salvage is a biochemical pathway that recycles partially degraded purine bases to reform purine nucleotides. Purine salvage disorders include Lesch-Nyhan syndrome and adenine phosphoribosyltransferase deficiency. **Lesch-Nyhan syndrome** is a rare, X-linked recessive disorder caused by deficiency of hypoxanthine-guanine phosphoribosyl transferase (HPRT). The degree of deficiency and

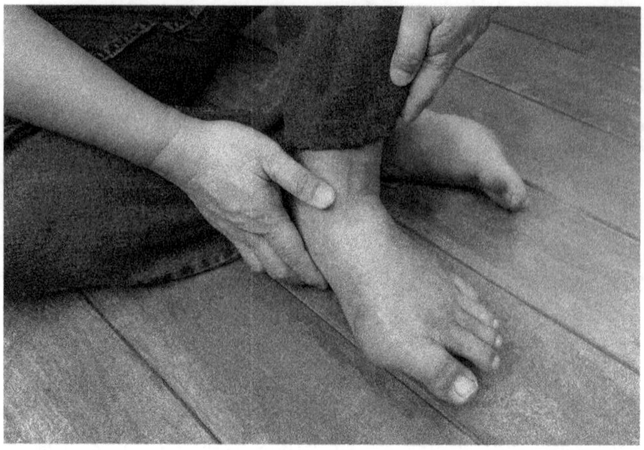

FIGURE 20.2 Tophi related to overproduction of purines.

manifestations vary with the specific mutation. HPRT deficiency results in failure of the salvage pathway for hypoxanthine and guanine. These purines are instead degraded to uric acid. The disease usually manifests between 3 and 12 months of age with the appearance of orange sandy precipitate (xanthine) in the urine. However, it can also occur rarely in adults. The syndrome progresses to central nervous system involvement with intellectual disability, spastic cerebral palsy, involuntary movements, and self-mutilating behavior (particularly biting). Later, chronic hyperuricemia causes symptoms of gout. Diagnosis of Lesch-Nyhan syndrome is suggested by the combination of dystonia, intellectual disability, and self-mutilation. Serum uric acid levels are usually elevated, and confirmation by DNA analysis is done.

Adenine phosphoribosyltransferase deficiency is a rare autosomal recessive disorder that results in the inability to salvage adenine for purine synthesis. Accumulated adenine is oxidized to 2,8-dihyroxyadenine, which precipitates in the urinary tract, causing problems similar to those of uric acid nephropathy such as renal colic, frequent infections, and, if diagnosed late, renal failure. Onset can occur at any age. Treatment options include a low-purine diet, allopurinol, high fluid intake, avoidance of urine alkalinization, and renal transplantation.

Test Your Knowledge

1. What are ketone bodies?
2. What are purine metabolism disorders caused by?
3. What is the meaning of purine salvage?

Lysosomal Storage Disorders

Lysosomal storage disorders are inherited metabolic diseases characterized by an abnormal buildup of various toxic materials in the cells, as a result of the absence or deficiencies of an enzyme, leading to the inappropriate storage of material in various cells of the body. There are nearly 50 of these disorders, and they may affect different parts of the body, including the skeletal muscles, brain, skin, heart, and central nervous system. New lysosomal storage disorders continue to be identified. Most lysosomal storage disorders are inherited in an autosomal recessive manner. Signs and symptoms include pain, numbness, tingling, or burning in the hands and feet, fever, red or purple skin sores, edema in the legs, dyspnea, hearing loss, dizziness, arrhythmia, heart attack, and stroke. While clinical trials are in progress on possible treatments for some of these diseases, there is currently no approved treatment for many lysosomal storage diseases. Lysosomes are spaces inside cells that break down waste products of metabolism. Various enzyme deficiencies inside lysosomes can result in buildup of toxic substances. The following sections explain some lysosomal storage disorders.

Hurler Syndrome

Hurler syndrome is caused by a deficiency of the lysosomal enzyme known as alpha-L-iduronidase, which aids in the breakdown of dermatan sulfate and heparin sulfate. This results in large amounts of **glycosaminoglycans** in the body, which eventually cause the cells to become extremely dysfunctional and then die. Hurler syndrome is signified by abnormal bones in the spine, cloudy corneas, deafness, **claw hand**, stiffness of joints, and developmental delays. While there is no cure for Hurler syndrome, treatment options include enzyme replacement therapy, hematopoietic stem cell transplant, surgical interventions as needed, physical therapy, occupational therapy, speech therapy, respiratory support, hearing aids, medications for pain and gastrointestinal (GI) disturbances, and corneal transplants.

Niemann-Pick Disease

Niemann-Pick is a rare, inherited disease that affects the body's ability to metabolize lipids within cells. These cells malfunction and die. Patients with Niemann-Pick disease have abnormal lipid metabolism that causes a buildup of harmful amounts of lipids in various organs. The disease primarily affects the brain, nerves, liver, spleen, bone marrow, and in severe cases, the lungs. The disease is broken down into types A, B, C, and E. Originally there was a type

D, but research has found that it is a variant of type C. Types A and B are referred to as type 1. Type C is referred to as type 2. Type E is a less common version of Niemann-Pick that develops in adulthood. The risk factors include having other family members with the disease. People of Ashkenazi Jewish heritage develop types A and B. People of Nova Scotia or French-Canadian descent, or Spanish-American descent develop type C. Affected organs, symptoms, and treatments vary based on the particular type of Niemann-Pick disease. However, every type is severe and can shorten a person's life expectancy. The signs and symptoms of the type A form of Niemann-Pick disease are present within the first few months of life and include:

- Swelling of the abdomen from enlargement of the liver and spleen, which usually occurs around three to six months of age
- Swollen lymph nodes
- A cherry-red spot inside the eye
- Difficulty feeding
- Difficulty performing basic motor skills
- Poor muscle tone
- Brain damage along with other neurological problems, such as a loss of reflexes
- Lung disease
- Frequent respiratory infections

The symptoms of the type B form of Niemann-Pick disease usually begin to appear in late childhood or adolescence. Type B does not include the motor difficulty commonly found in type A. The signs and symptoms of type B may include:

- Swelling of the abdomen from enlargement of the liver and spleen, which often begins in early childhood
- Respiratory infections
- Low blood platelets
- Poor coordination
- Mental retardation
- Psychiatric disorders
- Peripheral nerve problems
- Lung problems
- High lipids in the blood
- Delayed growth, or failure to develop at a normal rate, which causes short stature and eye abnormalities

Symptoms of the type C form of Niemann-Pick disease usually begin to appear in children around five years of age. However, type C can appear anytime in a person's life, from birth to adulthood. The signs and symptoms of type C include:

- Difficulty moving limbs
- An enlarged spleen or liver
- Jaundice, or yellowing of the skin after birth
- Difficulty learning
- A decline in intellect
- Dementia
- Seizures
- Difficulty speaking and swallowing
- A loss of muscular functioning
- Tremors
- Difficulty moving the eyes, especially in an up-and-down direction
- Unsteadiness
- Difficulty walking
- Clumsiness
- A loss of vision or hearing
- Brain damage

The symptoms of the type E form of Niemann-Pick disease are present in adults. This type is quite rare and research on the condition is limited, but the signs and symptoms include swelling of the spleen or brain and neurological problems, including swelling within the nervous system.

FOCUS ON NIEMANN-PICK DISEASE

Niemann-Pick disease affects the body's ability to metabolize cholesterol and lipids within the cells. It can affect the brain, liver, spleen, bone marrow, and lungs. Type A occurs mostly in infants and usually causes death within a few years. Type B occurs later in childhood, and many people survive into adulthood. Type C is not as common, but eventually also affects the brain.

Test Your Knowledge

1. What organs of the body can lysosomal storage disorders affect?
2. What are the signs and symptoms of the type A form of Niemann-Pick disease?
3. For all types of Niemann-Pick disease, what cannot be metabolized, and what results from this?

Tay-Sachs Disease

Tay-Sachs disease is a rare genetic disorder that is passed down from parents to their children. It is caused by the lack of an enzyme needed to help break down **gangliosides**, which build up to toxic levels in the brain and spinal cord, affecting nerve cell function. Approximately 1 in every 27 Jews in the United States is a carrier of the gene for Tay-Sachs disease. Non-Jewish French Canadians living near the St. Lawrence River and in the Cajun community of Louisiana also have a higher incidence of Tay-Sachs. For the general population, about 1 in 250 people are carriers. The carrier rate for Tay-Sachs disease is approximately 1 in every 250–300 people. Tay-Sachs disease causes progressive weakness in infants that are only a few months old, and progresses to severe nerve damage. An affected child usually lives only until age four or five.

In the most common and severe form of Tay-Sachs disease, signs and symptoms start to show up at about three to six months of age. As the disease progresses, development slows and the muscles begin to weaken. Over time, this leads to seizures, vision and hearing loss, paralysis, and other major issues. Children with this form of Tay-Sachs disease typically live only a few years. Less commonly, some children have the juvenile form of Tay-Sachs disease and may live into their teen years. Rarely, some adults have a late-onset form of Tay-Sachs disease which is often less severe than forms that begin in childhood.

Tay-Sachs disease is incurable and no treatments slow the disease's progression. Treatment goals are focused on support and comfort. They include medications, respiratory care, nutrition, hydration, physical therapy, occupational therapy, and speech/language therapy. Anti-seizure medications or antibiotics may be required. Chest physiotherapy, exercise, and other techniques may help remove mucus from the lungs. Medications can be used that reduce saliva production. Positioning techniques help reduce risks of mucus accumulation and prevent aspiration pneumonia. Some patients require a feeding tube, either nasogastric or gastrostomy. Physical therapy can delay joint stiffness, and reduce or delay loss of function and pain resulting from affected muscles. Occupational therapists can recommend activities and supportive devices that help with daily functioning. Speech and language therapists can assist with swallowing problems.

Gaucher Disease

Gaucher disease is a rare, inherited metabolic disorder that is classified as a type of lysosomal storage disease known as **sphingolipidosis**. The prevalence of Gaucher disease ranges from 0.70 to 1.75 per 100,000 individuals. However, the prevalence of the disease is higher in individuals with Ashkenazi Jewish ethnicity, with a birth incidence of approximately one in 850. Gaucher disease occurs in 1 of every 50,000–100,000 people in the general population. Type 1 is the most common form of the disorder in Europe, Israel, Canada, and the United States. Splenomegaly and hepatomegaly are observed in about 90% of patients with Gaucher disease Type 1. The fatty substances of the disease can also build up in bone tissue. This weakens bones and increases risks for fractures. It is often mild, and affects children as well as adults. The signs and symptoms include fatigue, anemia, abnormal reduction in the number of platelets, epistaxis, and easy bruising. Treatments for Gaucher disease include medications and surgeries. Enzyme replacement therapy is given on an outpatient basis, intravenously. Medications include miglustat, eliglustat, and osteoporosis drugs. If symptoms are severe and the patient is not a candidate for less-invasive treatments, bone marrow transplant or splenectomy may be required.

Fabry Disease

Fabry disease is an inherited disorder that results from the buildup of the fat known as **globotriaosylceramide** in the cells. The disease is seen in all ethnic, racial, and demographic groups. It is estimated to affect approximately 1 of every 1,500–4,000 males, and approximately 1 of every 20,000 females. The data from newborn screening programs suggests that the incidence of Fabry disease is generally underestimated and may be higher than previously approximated.

Fabry disease starts in childhood, and causes wide-ranging signs and symptoms. Characteristic features include episodes of numbness, tingling, burning or pain in the hands or feet, **angiokeratomas** (usually around the buttocks, groin, umbilicus, or upper thighs), a decreased ability to sweat, heat or cold intolerance, corneal opacity or **corneal verticillata**, GI problems, tinnitus, and hearing loss (see Figure 20.3). Kidney and heart disease as well as strokes may be observed in adulthood. Comprehensive treatment includes IV enzyme replacement therapy or oral **chaperone therapy**, and lifestyle modifications. Enzyme replacement therapies include agalsidase alfa and beta. Antihistamines are often given before these IV infusions to reduce the chance of infusion-related reactions. They are also sometimes given after the infusions. The most popular oral chaperone therapy is migalastat. It

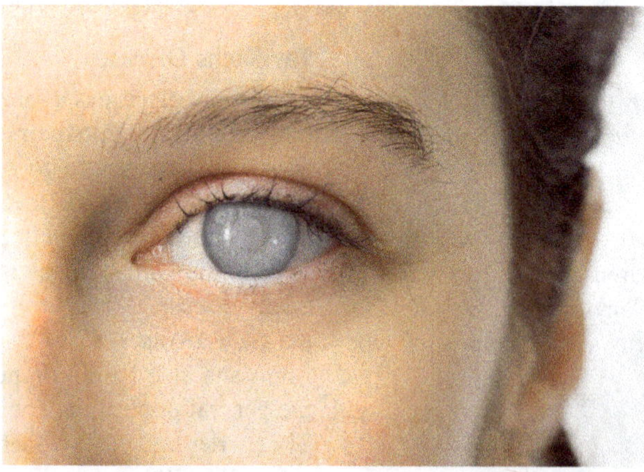

FIGURE 20.3 Corneal opacity in a young girl.

is suitable for patients that have been tested and have gene mutations that will respond. If present, proteinuria is treated along with other therapies, to prolong kidney health.

Krabbe Disease

Krabbe disease is a rare inherited metabolic disorder, in which harmful amounts of lipids buildup in in various cells and tissues, and destroy brain cells. It is also known as *globoid cell leukodystrophy.* Globoid cells break down the protective myelin coating of nerves. It is caused by a deficiency of **galactocerebrosidase**, an essential enzyme for myelin metabolism. The disease usually affects infants (before six months), but can occur in adolescence or adulthood. Krabbe disease causes progressive nerve damage and developmental delays in young children. Occasionally, adults are affected. Additional symptoms include severe deterioration of mental and motor skills, muscle weakness, hypertonia, myoclonic seizures, spasticity, unexplained fever, blindness, difficulty swallowing, and deafness. Medications may be prescribed to help treat pain. Physical therapy may help maintain or increase muscle tone and circulation. In a clinical trial, children that received umbilical cord blood stem cells from unrelated donors, prior to symptom onset, developed little neurological impairment. Bone marrow transplantation may also be helpful.

The outlook for Krabbe disease is poor. It usually results in death, but life expectancy varies based on the age of onset. The average lifespan for children with infantile Krabbe disease is 13 months. Most children with late infantile disease die within two years of the start of symptoms.

FOCUS ON KRABBE DISEASE

Krabbe disease is characterized by globoid cells (which have more than one nucleus), breakdown of myelin coatings, and destruction of brain cells. It is classified as a leukodystrophy, causing severe deterioration of mental and motor skills. The disease is generally fatal, in its infantile form, within a few years. Those with juvenile- or adult-onset Krabbe disease usually have a less severe disease course and live much longer.

Test Your Knowledge

1. How early in life can Tay-Sachs disease be fatal?
2. What age group is primarily affected by Krabbe disease?
3. What are the characteristic features of Fabry disease?

NUTRITIONAL CHANGES TO CORRECT METABOLIC DISORDERS

Metabolic disorders may be caused by a missing enzyme or vitamin that is required for important chemical reactions. There may be abnormal chemical reactions that harm normal metabolic processes. A disease in the liver, pancreas, endocrine glands, or other organs may have a large impact upon metabolism. The final cause of metabolic disorders is a nutritional deficiency. Nutritional changes are based on the causes and are able to correct the metabolic disorders. These changes include the following:

- Enzyme replacement therapy
- Removing lactose, sucrose, and/or glucose from the diet
- Limiting dietary intake of branched-chain amino acids
- Limiting dietary intake of certain forms of protein

For metabolic syndrome, nutritional changes include avoiding white flour, sugary snacks, sugar-sweetened beverages, saturated fats, whole-milk dairy products, many types of baked foods, cured meats, and processed foods (including packaged items and fast food). The diet should be changed to include more vegetables (salad greens, broccoli, peppers, beans, lentils, chickpeas), fruits (raspberries, blackberries, pears), whole grains (whole-wheat breads, barley, oats), and omega-3 fatty acids (nuts, seeds, and fatty fish like salmon and mackerel). Also, drinking plenty of water is essential.

ENZYME REPLACEMENT

Enzyme replacement therapy (ERT) is a medical treatment in which replacement enzymes are given to patient suffering from chronic conditions, due to enzyme deficiencies or malfunctions. Usually, this therapy is done intravenously. The replacement enzyme is administered directly into the bloodstream through a controlled drip of fluids. Replacement enzymes are derived from human, animal, and plant cells. They are genetically modified and processed before being administered. By receiving these enzyme replacements, the body can then perform functions that were previously inhibited. Effectiveness of ERT is varied between patients and conditions, but sometimes it is the only option for treatment. The most common conditions treated by ERT are lysosomal storage diseases. Normally, lysosomes break down proteins and other macromolecules.

SPECIAL DIETS

Maple syrup urine disease requires a protein-restricted diet that limits the amount of branched-chain amino acids. Protein restriction must start as soon as possible after birth in order to promote proper growth and development. *Hypermethioninemia* may require a low-methionine diet. This means avoiding high-methionine food such as turkey, beef, fish, pork, tofu, milk, cheese, nuts, beans, and whole grains such as quinoa. Other foods that should be avoided include crab, shrimp, clams, eggs, green peas, sweet potatoes, lima beans, spinach, sweet corn, avocados, and kiwi. *Phenylketonuria* requires a low-protein diet that completely avoids high-protein foods such as meat, eggs, and dairy products, and controls the intake of many other foods such as potatoes and cereals.

Argininemia and *ornithinemia* require a protein-restricted diet. Foods that are high in protein that need to be avoided or limited include milk, cheese, and other dairy products, meat, poultry, fish, eggs, dried beans and legumes, nuts, and peanut butter. *Galactosemia* is treated with a low-galactose diet, avoiding milk, butter, cheese, ice cream, and other dairy products. For infants with the condition, human breast milk should be replaced with formula that does not contain galactose. *Glycogen storage diseases* are treated with cornstarch at every meal along with complex carbohydrates (as long as they do not contain added sugar, dried fruits, or honey). Low-sugar cereals include puffed rice, Cheerios, Corn Chex, and Rice Krispies. Sugars that are prohibited include agave syrup, fructose, galactose, lactose, high fructose corn syrup, brown sugar, invert sugar, powdered (confectioners') sugar, maple syrup, molasses, raw sugar, sorghum, sorbitol, sugar beets, and sucrose.

Fatty acid transport and mitochondrial oxidation disorders require a fat-restricted diet and supplementation of medium-chain triglyceride oil, and often, docosahexaenoic acid (DHA), which is an essential fatty acid that is crucial for brain, visual, and immune function as well as preventing fat soluble vitamin deficiencies. *Glycerol metabolism disorders* are treated with a low-fat diet, with glucocorticoid replacement when adrenal hypoplasia is present. *Sjögren-Larsson syndrome* requires a diet supplemented with omega-3 and omega-6 fatty acids.

For *Hurler syndrome,* changes to the diet will not prevent the progression of the disease. However, limiting milk, sugar, and dairy products can help with excessive mucus. Overall, a well-balanced diet is important. *Niemann-Pick disease* may benefit from a high-calorie, high-protein, lactose-free, and sucrose-free diet, plus supplementation of L-glutamine, probiotics, omega-3, and coenzymes Q10. *Tay-Sachs disease* may benefit from a ketogenic diet. *Gaucher disease* benefits from an overall healthy diet, with foods rich in vitamin D and calcium. Supplements of these may also be helpful. *Fabry disease* treatment is improved when dietary sodium is limited, dietary protein is adequate, plant protein is increased, and lean meats are adequately consumed. *Krabbe disease* does not appear to benefit from any dietary modifications.

Test Your Knowledge

1. What special diet is used to treat maple syrup urine disease?
2. What foods must be completely avoided with phenylketonuria?
3. What dietary components may be beneficial for Niemann-Pick disease?

KEY TERMS

Absence seizures

Adenosylmethionine

Angiokeratomas

Beta-oxidation cycle

Cardiomegaly

Cataracts

Cerebral edema

Chaperone therapy

Claw hand

Corneal verticillata

Cryptorchidism

Cystathionine

Diaminoaciduria

Dysarthria

Fabry disease

Galactocerebrosidase

Galactosemia

Gangliosides

Gaucher disease

Generalized seizures

Globotriaosylceramide

Glycogen phosphorylase

Glycosaminoglycans

Glycogen storage diseases

Heterogeneous diseases

Homocysteine

Hurler syndrome

Hypouricemia

Intermittent

Krabbe disease

Lesch-Nyhan syndrome

Lysosomal storage disorders

Maple syrup urine disease

Marfanoid habitus

Metabolites

Mitochondria

Myopathy

Ornithine

Orotic aciduria

Phenylketones

Phenylketonuria

Phosphorylase kinase

Pompe's disease

Porphyria

Purine salvage

Purines

Pyrimidinuria

Remethylation

Sphingolipidosis

Strabismus

Subluxation

Substrate

Tay-Sachs disease

Thymic deficiency

Tophi

Transsulfuration

Uricosuria

Von Gierke disease

CLINICAL CASE STUDIES

Clinical Case Study 1

A two-year-old child was evaluated for a significant delay in achievement of milestones, pale skin, very light colored hair, and behavioral problems. Tests revealed a large amount of phenylketones in his urine, and elevated plasma phenylalanine. The boy was diagnosed with phenylketonuria. He was placed on a low phenylalanine diet. His clinical and biochemical responses were monitored with urinary ferric chloride tests. Over time, his condition began to improve significantly.

CRITICAL THINKING QUESTIONS

1. What are the main signs and symptoms of phenylketonuria when it has not been treated?
2. If treatment of phenylketonuria is started after two to three years, what may occur?
3. What will this child's diet need to be throughout the rest of his life?

Clinical Case Study 2

A newborn, after being breastfed, started to develop jaundice, lethargy, bilirubin and conjugated bilirubin. The jaundice continued to worsen. By one week, the newborn had hepatomegaly and acute liver failure, plus compromised blood clotting. She started to lose weight quickly. A metabolic disease was suspected. The feeding of breast milk was stopped and parenteral nutrition was initiated. Slowly, her condition began to stabilize. In two days, results of a newborn screening program indicated that galactosemia was the probable diagnosis. She was started on an amino acid-based formula without lactose or galactose, and she quickly began to improve.

CRITICAL THINKING QUESTIONS

1. Why is it essential to start treatment for galactosemia as quickly as possible?
2. What complications commonly develop from galacto semia?
3. What is galactose found in?

Clinical Case Study 3

A seven-year-old child was brought to the local hospital with abdominal distension, history of intermittent fever, difficulty walking, and respiratory infections. The child had normal development until the age of three years, after which she started falling behind in all developmental aspects. Examination revealed global developmental delays with mild mental retardation. She also had moderate hepatosplenomegaly. Bone marrow examination was done, revealing the presence of Niemann-Pick cells. Lysosomal enzyme studies confirmed a diagnosis of type B Niemann-Pick disease.

CRITICAL THINKING QUESTIONS

1. What is the main difference between type A and type B Niemann-Pick disease?
2. What other signs and symptoms appear in type B Niemann-Pick disease?
3. What does any form of Niemann-Pick disease affect in regard to metabolism?

Clinical Case Study 4

A two-year-old girl was brought by ambulance to the local hospital because of 18 hours of vomiting and worsening lethargy. On examination, her arms and legs were very cold. Her blood glucose was 18.02 mg/dL. She was actively resuscitated, and her blood glucose level only slightly increased to 23.42 mg/dL. When a urine dipstick test was performed, there were ketones and traces of protein present. The patient received two boluses of 2 mL/kg of 10% dextrose solution and was maintained on dextrose saline solution. Though hypoglycemia persisted, the patient stabilized over several days. Her blood glucose attained a range of 68.47 mg/dL to 86.49 mg/dL. Tests result in a diagnosis of medium-chain acyl-CoA dehydrogenase deficiency.

CRITICAL THINKING QUESTIONS

1. What is medium-chain acyl-CoA dehydrogenase deficiency?
2. What happens to an individual with medium-chain acyl-CoA dehydrogenase deficiency?
3. What are fatty acid oxidation disorders?

Clinical Case Study 5

A 45-year-old man was assessed because of hyperuricemia. He previously had recurring nephrolithiasis and chronic gout that did not respond well to treatment. The patient's enzymes were assessed, and it was found that he was deficient in hypoxanthine-guanine phosphoribosyltransferase. Therefore, Lesch-Nyhan disease was diagnosed. Treatment of the hyperuricemia was with allopurinol. To prevent nephrolithiasis, the patient was educated about avoiding dehydration, and to aim on achieving a minimum urine output of 2 liters per day. Urinary alkalinization with potassium citrate was begun. The patient was also referred for genetic counseling.

CRITICAL THINKING QUESTIONS

1. What is Lesch-Nyhan syndrome classified as?
2. What does Lesch-Nyhan syndrome progress to cause?
3. What do the enzyme deficiencies of Lesch-Nyhan syndrome result in?

STUDY QUESTIONS

1. All of the following are examples of amino acid metabolism disorders, EXCEPT:
   A. Phenylketonuria
   B. Pompe's disease
   C. Argininemia
   D. Ornithinemia

2. Von Gierke disease is classified as which of the following?
   A. Glycerol metabolism disorder
   B. Purine metabolism disorder
   C. Lysosomal storage disorder
   D. Glycogen storage disease

3. Which of the following is an example of a purine salvage disorder?
   A. Lesch-Nyhan syndrome
   B. Hurler syndrome
   C. Glycerol intolerance syndrome
   D. Hyperammonemia syndrome

4. Homocysteine acts as an intermediate in the metabolism of which of the following?
   A. Phenylalanine
   B. Ornithine
   C. Methionine
   D. Arginine

5. In which of the following amino acid metabolic disorders may microcephaly plus light skin, hair, and eyes be present?
   A. Hypermethioninemia
   B. Phenylketonuria
   C. Argininemia
   D. Ornithinemia

6. The majority of infants with severe galactosemia will die, if not treated within ten days, because of which of the following?
   A. Systemic infection
   B. Jaundice
   C. Liver failure
   D. Heart failure

7. Which of the following is the most common type of glycogen storage disease?
   A. Pompe's disease
   B. Niemann-Pick disease
   C. Von Gierke disease
   D. Tay-Sachs disease

8. Sphingolipidosis is a classification of which of the following?
   A. Fabry disease
   B. Gaucher disease
   C. Tay-Sachs disease
   D. Krabbe disease

9. Which of the following involves abnormal lipid metabolism?
   A. Pompe's disease
   B. Tay-Sachs disease
   C. Von Gierke disease
   D. Niemann-Pick disease

10. Which of the following is caused by the lack of an enzyme needed to break down gangliosides?
    A. Tay-Sachs disease
    B. Niemann-Pick disease
    C. Gaucher disease
    D. Fabry disease

11. Accumulation of glycosaminoglycans in the blood is caused by which of the following?
   A. Lesch-Nyhan syndrome
   B. Glycerol intolerance syndrome
   C. Hyperammonemia syndrome
   D. Hurler syndrome

12. Which of the following is an X-linked disorder?
   A. Glycerol kinase deficiency
   B. Phenylketonuria
   C. Hypermethioninemia
   D. Maple syrup urine disease

13. Orotic aciduria and diaminoaciduria are caused by which of the following?
   A. Ornithinemia
   B. Galactosemia
   C. Hypouricemia
   D. Argininemia

14. All of the following are signs and symptoms of purine metabolism disorders, EXCEPT:
   A. Thymic deficiency
   B. Myalgia
   C. Lymphopenia
   D. Microcephaly

15. All of the following are lysosomal storage disorders, EXCEPT:
   A. Hurler syndrome
   B. Pompe's disease
   C. Tay-Sachs disease
   D. Niemann-Pick disease

FURTHER READING

1. Amato, A., and Russell, J. (2015). *Neuromuscular Disorders*, 2nd Edition. McGraw-Hill/Medical.
2. Barton, J.C., Edwards, C.O., Phatak, P.D., Britton, R.S., and Bacon, B.R. (2014). *Handbook of Iron Overload Disorders.* Cambridge University Press.
3. Bernstein, L.E., Rohr, F., and Helm, J.R. (2015). *Nutrition Management of Inherited Metabolic Diseases – Lessons from Metabolic University.* Springer.
4. Blau, N., Dionisi Vici, C., Ferreira, C.R., Vianey-Saban, C., and van Karnebeek, C.D.M. (2022). *Physician's Guide to the Diagnosis, Treatment, and Follow-up of Inherited Metabolic Diseases*, 2nd Edition. Springer.
5. Burdge, G.C. (2018). *Polyunsaturated Fatty Acid Metabolism.* Academic Press.
6. Burlina, A.P. (2018). *Neurometabolic Hereditary Diseases of Adults.* Springer.
7. Chiva-Blanch, G., and Cofan, M. (2022). *Dietary Intakes and Metabolic Disorders.* Mdpi AG.
8. Cohen, R. (2023). *Keto Diet for Metabolic Disorders.* Cohen.
9. Dichi, I., and Name Colado Simao, A. (2021). *Nutritional Intervention in Metabolic Syndrome.* CRC Press.
10. Dickens, F., Randle, P.J., and Whelan, W.J. (2014). *Carbohydrate Metabolism and Its Disorders.* Academic Press.
11. Dureja, H., Murthy, S.N., Wich, P.R., and Dua, K. (2022). *Drug Delivery Systems for Metabolic Disorders.* Academic Press.
12. Ebrahimi-Fakhari, D., and Pearl, P.L. (2020). *Movement Disorders and Inherited Metabolic Disorders – Recognition, Understanding, Improving Outcomes.* Cambridge University Press/Medicine.
13. Ekvall, S.W., and Ekvall, V.K. (2017). *Pediatric and Adult Nutrition in Chronic Diseases, Developmental Disabilities, and Hereditary Metabolic Disorders: Prevention, Assessment, and Treatment*, 3rd Edition. Oxford University Press.
14. El-Khoury, A.E. (2017). *Methods for Investigation of Amino Acid and Protein Metabolism.* CRC Press.
15. Ichai, C., Quintard, H., and Orban, J.C. (2018). *Metabolic Disorders and Critically Ill Patients – From Pathophysiology to Treatment.* Springer.
16. Jockers, D. (2020). *Keto Metabolic Breakthrough – A Radical Approach to Reversing Metabolic Dysfunction, Optimizing Nutrient Timing, and Balancing Hormones for Success on a Low-Carb Diet.* Victory Belt Publishing.
17. Kellum, J.A., and Cerda, J. (2012). *Renal and Metabolic Disorders (Pittsburgh Critical Care Medicine).* Oxford University Press.
18. Khan, H., Akkol, E., and Daglia, M. (2022). *The Role of Phytonutrients in Metabolic Disorders.* Academic Press.
19. LaLane, E. (2021). *Easy Ingredients Metabolic Syndrome Diet – Essential Cookbook of Meals You Can Eat to Reverse Inflammation Naturally.* LaLane.
20. Lyon, G., Kolodny, E.H., and Pastores, G.M. (2010). *Neurology of Hereditary Metabolic Diseases of Children*, 3rd Edition. McGraw-Hill/Medical.
21. McGrath, B.M., and Walsh, G. (2005). *Directly of Therapeutic Enzymes.* CRC/Taylor & Francis.
22. Mehta, A.B., and Winchester, B. (2022). *Lysosomal Storage Disorders: A Practical Guide*, 2nd Edition. Wiley Blackwell.
23. Putnam, A.R., and Thompson, K.S. (2022). *Diagnostic Pathology: Nonneoplastic Pediatrics*, 2nd Edition. Elsevier.
24. Pyeritz, R.E., Korf, B.R., and Grody, W.W. (2020). *Emery and Rimoin's Principles and Practice of Medical Genetics and Genomics: Metabolic Disorders*, 7th Edition. Academic Press.
25. Rodriguez, T. (2022). *The Keto Solution for Kidney Disease – Reversing Metabolic Disorders with a Ketogenic Diet.* JumpStart Creative Solutions.
26. Sahota, A., and Taylor, M.W. (2013). *Purine and Pyrimidine Metabolism in Man VIII (Advances in Experimental Medicine and Biology, 370).* Springer.
27. Takahashi, M.P., and Matsumura, T. (2018). *Myotonic Dystrophy: Disease Mechanism, Current Management, and Therapeutic Development.* Springer.
28. Wells, J.C.K. (2016). *The Metabolic Ghetto – An Evolutionary Perspective on Nutrition, Power Relations, and Chronic Disease.* Cambridge University Press.
29. Wesson, D.E. (2016). *Metabolic Acidosis – A Guide to Clinical Assessment and Management.* Springer.

21 Environmental Effects on Nutrition

OUTLINE

LEARNING OBJECTIVES

After study of this chapter, readers should be able to:

1. Describe the effects of environmental change that may reduce the quality and quantity of crops.
2. Discuss how human health and disease can be influenced by the effects of climate.
3. Explain the ways that humans can contact hazardous agents.
4. Identify the most common microorganisms that cause food poisoning.
5. Describe the effects of food pollution in humans.
6. Explain how environmental pollution affects human nutritional status and health.
7. Describe the signs and symptoms of exposure to high levels of lead.
8. Discuss the effects of chronic mercury poisoning in humans.
9. Explain the signs and symptoms of arsenic poisoning.
10. Describe the effects of chronic cadmium exposure in humans.

OVERVIEW

Environmental contamination from a variety of industrial and agricultural chemicals can compromise our nutritional status and health. This may occur directly, or through changes in the diet. Examples of contaminants include heavy metals, organochlorines, and radionucleotides. Environmental factors such as weather, time of day, locations, and advertisements also influence food choices. Soil and water quality and temperature significantly influence food systems via their impact on the production, storage, and transportation of food. Unfortunately, exposure to environmental chemicals is increasing on a global scale, and nutritional status may modify human susceptibility to chemical exposures. There are many different toxicants, and malnutrition can take many forms. Other environmental impacts upon food production include use of resources, production methods required to process foods, and food wastes.

ENVIRONMENTAL EFFECTS ON GLOBAL NUTRITION

The effects of the environment upon global disease are significant, since over 12 million people die every year, in multiple countries, due to living or working in unhealthy environments. In the United States, the Healthy People 2030 initiative focuses on reducing exposures to harmful agents in the air, water, soil, food, and materials – in homes and in workplaces. Environmental agents can cause many different health problems, including respiratory and heart diseases, plus some types of cancer. Lower-income individuals are more likely to live in polluted areas, and to have unsafe drinking water. Children and pregnant women are at increased risk of health problems related to environmental agents. Tracking these agents is important in finding out how and where people are exposed. There is a need for better policies and laws to reduce harmful environmental agents with the goal of preventing serious health problems and deaths.

The effects of environmental change has reduced the quality and quantity of crops, resulting in more food and financial insecurities that lead to malnutrition as well as diet-related non-communicable diseases. These include diabetes mellitus and cardiovascular diseases. The ability to grow enough nutritional foods for the global population may be impaired. Food systems make up approximately 30% of global greenhouse gas emissions, contributing to environmental and biodiversity degradation and deforestation. Unsustainable food systems reduce access to diets that are healthy and affordable. This increases risks for poor health and diseases that are related to diet. Low- and middle-income countries in Africa and Southeast Asia will experience the greatest reductions in food availability, leading to increased deaths attributed to being underweight. Certain grains and legumes will experience a decline in nutritional quality, related to the higher atmospheric carbon dioxide concentrations. This may lead to an increased risk of zinc and iron deficiency. In high-income countries, environmental-related reductions in fruit and vegetable consumption

DOI: 10.1201/b22969-24

are primary risk factors for increases non-communicable diseases and deaths. As of 2020, about three billion people throughout the world could not afford a healthy diet.

HEALTH EFFECTS OF CLIMATE

Human health and disease is influenced by the effects of climate as well as other natural and man-made health stressors. Some of today's existing health threats will worsen as other threats begin to emerge, and not everyone throughout the world is at equal risk. Individual ages, locations, and economic resources must be considered. In the United States, public health is affected by disruptions of ecological, biological, and physical health systems that may originate in this country or outside of it. These disruptions may cause health effects such as cardiovascular and respiratory disease, extreme weather-related injuries and premature deaths, threats to mental health, and changes in the prevalence and distribution of food- and waterborne illnesses, as well as other infectious diseases.

Extreme heat has resulted in large increases in death rates in areas that experience heat waves. Death can occur from heat stroke, related conditions, and diseases of the cardiovascular, respiratory, and cerebrovascular systems. Heat waves are also linked to increased hospital admissions for cardiovascular, kidney, and respiratory disorders. In the United States, summer heat appears to be increasing as climate projections indicate the likelihood of more frequent and intense extreme heat events to come. Even with better forecasting, early warning systems for extreme heat events, and better access to air conditioning, these events still remain a cause of preventable death. Urban populations are projected to have increased vulnerability to heat-related health problems in the future because of **urban heat islands**, the aging population, and increased urbanization. In some areas, milder winters due to an overall warmer climate may reduce health problems and deaths related to cold and snow. The vulnerability to cold weather is based on non-climate factors such as overall health status, housing, and age. Deaths and injuries related to extreme cold events are projected to decline due to climate change, but they are not expected to be of greater significance than the increased heat-related health problems and deaths.

Many forests are now more vulnerable to wildfires since long periods of record high temperatures are related to droughts that contribute to dry conditions. Drought is also linked to dust storms that carry fungal pathogens that cause **coccidioidomycosis** (*valley fever*). A drought also affects agriculture, resulting in food shortages. The smoke from a wildfire contains particulates, carbon monoxide, nitrogen oxides, and volatile organic compounds that have **ozone precursor** effects. These components can greatly reduce the quality of the air, locally and in all areas that are downwind of a wildfire. Smoke exposure increases hospitalizations for respiratory and cardiovascular conditions, as well as visits to emergency departments, medications, and medical visits for lung illnesses. There is an increased need for medications to treat asthma, bronchitis, chest pain, chronic obstructive pulmonary disease (COPD), and respiratory infections. Smoke exposure is associated with hundreds of thousands of annual deaths. Increased heat is projected to increase risks for wildfires and the associated emissions, potentially harming the health of millions of people.

On the other side of the coin, increased events of extreme rain are projected to occur. Increased extreme precipitation and total precipitation have caused severe flooding in various regions. Floods are the second deadliest of all the weather hazards in the United States, killing about 98 people every year, mostly due to drowning. Flash floods and flooding related to tropical storms claim the most lives. Waterborne disease outbreaks also occur over the weeks after heavy rainfall. Water that enters buildings can cause mold contamination with later serious effects that include reduced indoor air quality. Buildings damaged by hurricanes are highly susceptible to water **intrusion**. People living in damp indoor environments have more cases of asthma and other upper respiratory tract symptoms, plus lower respiratory tract infections.

Another consideration is the effect of war upon nutrition. Many wars today are accompanied by mass starvation, and sometimes, starvation is actually used as a weapon. Though this action has been condemned by the United Nations Security Council, it still occurs. The UN demands that countries in conflict allow humanitarian aid workers full access to populations in extreme need, and states that using starvation of civilians as a method of warfare constitutes a war crime. Among the hundreds of millions of people suffering from chronic malnutrition, about 60% live in areas affected by wars and other armed conflicts. When armies deliberately destroy farms, livestock, and other types of civilian infrastructure, entire populations may be threatened. Refugees from war-torn countries are often vulnerable to disease and acute food insecurity. Some armies have trapped people in their homes, depriving them of food and other vital resources until they surrender. In recent years, countries that have experienced war-related food deprivation have included South Sudan, Syria, and Yemen. The best example is the attack by Russia upon Ukraine, which prevented grain from being able to leave the region. Ukraine produces about 50% of the wheat needed by the whole world. The war therefore made food more expensive across the globe, worsening shortages, hunger, and political instability in developing countries such as those in Africa. When Russia relented somewhat and allowed grain shipments out of the region, some of the problem was reduced, and needy countries were able to receive at least some of the food supplies they required.

Test Your Knowledge

1. Because of environmental change, which countries will experience the greatest reductions in food availability?
2. How common is malnutrition in relation to areas involved in wars?

3. How did Russia's attack upon Ukraine affect food availability on a global scale?

TOXICITY OF CHEMICAL AND PHYSICAL AGENTS

Chemical and physical agents can be highly toxic to humans, causing a variety of health and physical hazards. Health hazards include carcinogenicity, irritation, and sensitization, while physical hazards include corrosion, explosibility, and flammability. Understanding chemical toxicity requires a knowledge of chemicals that may be present, either as part of manufacturing processes, or as related impurities and environmental effects. The outcomes of the metabolism of drugs and chemicals after ingestion are highly important. Regarding the skin, percutaneous absorption can be defined as the translocation of surface-applied agents, through the various skin layers, to a location where they can enter the systemic circulation through the dermal microvasculature and lymphatics, or remain in the deeper layers. The rate-limiting barrier to skin absorption is generally believed to be the outermost, nonviable **stratum corneum**.

Exposure to potentially toxic agents occurs when humans have contact with a chemical or physical agent, either directly or via another substance that has become contaminated or has contacted the toxic agent. The place where an agent originates is called the *source*. Chemicals can move through air, soil, and water, can be present on plants or animals, and can find their way into our food sources. The ways that humans can contact hazardous agents are called *exposure pathways*. These include inhalation, ingestion, and skin contact. Factors that play roles in the outcomes of a toxic exposure include the type of chemical or agent, the amount or level an individual was exposed to, the length of the exposure, and how many times the exposure occurred. Young and middle-aged adults generally have fewer adverse health effects after an exposure than fetuses, children, adolescents, and the elderly. Should a toxic agent enter the body and reach the liver and kidneys, any compromise of the functions of these organs could mean that adverse health effects will occur because of an inability to eliminate the toxic agent from the body.

The **potency** and toxicity of a chemical can be affected by its breakdown within the body. Its chemical structure may be changed or metabolized to a substance that is more or less toxic. The amount of a chemical in its **exposure medium** is its concentration, usually reported in parts per million, milligrams per liter, or milligrams per cubic meter. Acute exposure is short-term exposure to a toxic agent, over seconds to a few hours. Chronic exposure is continuous or repeated contact over months to years. Chemicals that leak from landfills can enter our groundwater and contaminate wells or find their way into basements. This can result in chronic exposure. Toxic agents have the ability to affect each and every body system. Delayed health effects can be reversible or permanent, and include examples such as lung disease and cancer.

Food poisoning occurs when people eat contaminated food. Some microorganisms release a toxin, such as bacteria, or fungus. Sometimes the toxic byproducts of these organisms cause food poisoning. Therefore, the body reacts to purge the toxins. Most people recover on their own, but some can become gravely ill. Pregnant women, young children and elderly are more at risk. Food can become contaminated at any stage of production, from harvesting to storage to cooking or preparation. Contamination occurs when food is not:

- Fresh
- Washed well
- Handled in a sanitary way
- Cooked to a safe internal temperature
- Held at proper temperatures
- Refrigerated or frozen promptly

Food and water may be contaminated by bacteria, viruses, parasites, fungi, toxins, and some chemicals. There are more than 250 specific types of food poisoning. Some of the most common microbial causes include:

- ***Salmonella:*** Raw eggs and undercooked poultry are common sources of salmonella poisoning. It can also occur from beef, pork, vegetables and processed foods containing these items. *Salmonella* is the most common bacterial cause of food poisoning in the United States and is responsible for the highest number of hospitalizations and deaths from food poisoning.
- ***E. coli (Escherichia coli):*** Normally live in the intestines of healthy people and most types of *E. coli* are harmless. However, a few strains can cause severe abdominal cramps, bloody diarrhea and vomiting. Usually found in undercooked meat and raw vegetables, *E. coli* bacteria produces a toxin that irritates the small intestine. The **Shiga toxin** is what causes foodborne illness. Most healthy adults recover from *E. coli* illness within a week. Some people, particularly young children and older adults, may develop a life-threatening form of kidney failure called hemolytic uremic syndrome (HUS), which causes destruction of red blood cells, leading to kidney failure. HUS occurs as a complication of a diarrheal infection (usually *E. coli* O157:H7 infection).
- ***Listeria:*** Bacteria in soft cheeses, deli meats, hot dogs and raw sprouts can cause an infection called listeriosis, which is especially dangerous for pregnant women.
- ***Norovirus:*** You can get norovirus by eating undercooked shellfish, leafy greens, and fresh fruits or by consuming food that a sick person prepared. This is the virus most commonly associated with stomach flu.

- ***Hepatitis A:*** Viral hepatitis A can be spread through shellfish, fresh produce or water and ice contaminated by stool. It's not a chronic infection like other hepatitis viruses, but it can affect your liver.
- ***Staphylococcus aureus (staph):*** A staph infection occurs when people transfer the staph bacteria from their hands to food. Foods that are often implicated are meats, poultry, milk and dairy products, salads, cream-filled baked goods, and sandwich fillings. The bacteria can affect many parts of your body.
- ***Campylobacter:*** This common bacterial infection producing severe gastrointestinal (GI) upset can linger for weeks. Usually, culprits are undercooked poultry, meat or eggs, poorly processed meats, contaminated vegetables and raw (unprocessed) milk or water sources. It's also spread by cross-contamination. The condition is generally self-limited, causes bloody diarrhea and is rarely fatal.
- ***Shigella (shigellosis):*** *Shigella* bacteria is most typically found in uncooked vegetables, shellfish and cream or mayonnaise-based salads (tuna, potato, macaroni, chicken). It can cause blood or mucus in your diarrhea, which is why the infection is sometimes called bacillary dysentery.

Cyanogenic glycosides are phytotoxins (toxic chemicals produced by plants) which occur in at least 2,000 plant species, of which a number of species are used as food in some areas of the world. Cassava, sorghum, stone fruits, bamboo roots and almonds are especially important foods containing cyanogenic glycosides. The potential toxicity of a cyanogenic plant depends primarily on the potential that its consumption will produce a concentration of cyanide that is toxic to exposed humans. In humans, the clinical signs and symptoms of acute cyanide intoxication can include: **tachypnea**, hypotension, dizziness, headache, stomach pains, vomiting, diarrhea, mental confusion, cyanosis with twitching and convulsions, followed by a terminal coma. Death due to cyanide poisoning can occur when the cyanide level exceeds the limit an individual is able to detoxify.

FOCUS ON CYANIDE POISONING

Cyanide is a fast-acting poison and lethal. It prevents the cells of the body from using oxygen, and the cells die. Cyanide is more harmful to the heart and brain because these organs require more oxygen. The poison may be a colorless gas or as a crystal form. Cyanide is released from natural substances in some foods. Signs and symptoms occur within minutes and resulting in respiratory failure.

Test Your Knowledge

1. How can potentially harmful chemicals reach the food supply?
2. How does food contamination occur?
3. What are the most common microbial causes of food poisoning?

FOOD POLLUTION

Food pollution is the presence of toxic chemicals and biological contaminants in food that are not naturally present. Though low "background" levels of these agents may be present, food pollution occurs when the levels are highly increased. Outcomes of food pollution include mild to severe illnesses, or serious hormonal or metabolic problems, as well as cancer. Sometimes, serious food poisoning and death occurs. There are over 70 million cases of foodborne illnesses in just the United States every year, resulting in about 5,000 deaths. Any pollutant that comes into contact with food has the potential to pollute it. Vegetables can be contaminated with toxic bacteria from irrigation water, groundwater, or soil. These bacteria may only be destroyed by processed polluted food at very high temperatures. Toxic chemicals can also get into food sources via the following:

- Growing crops in polluted soils, by using solid wastes as fertilizer, or in areas that have polluted groundwater
- Irrigation of crops with polluted water
- Growing crops in areas with polluted air
- Agricultural treatments such as pesticides, insecticides, or **herbicides**
- Agricultural application of sewage sludge or polluted fertilizers that contain ash from power plants
- Consumption of polluted water or food by fish or other creatures
- Poor food processing, packaging, and handling procedures
- Propagation and concentration of pollutants throughout the food chain

Plants can become contaminated with pollutants when they extract them through their roots, along with water and nutrients. Air pollutants may first become deposited on the ground with rainwater, entering plants through their roots. Sources of food pollution are many, including chemicals and microorganisms that contact food while it is grown, processed, or packaged. Risks for food pollution are based on many different factors, which include:

- The type of pollutant – those that are persistent and **bioaccumulative** have higher risks for food pollution since they can accumulate in food over time, resulting in very high concentrations; hormones in foods can also pose serious risks that are not fully understood; it is wise to avoid any food source that contains hormones

- The type of food – fish are more exposed to a wider variety of contaminants; also, certain compounds can accumulate and become concentrated in fish; birds or other animals that eat polluted fish can then become contaminated and transmit the pollution further, throughout the food chain
- The health of individuals – people that are most affected by food pollution include children, the elderly, pregnant women, and people with chronic food diseases or illnesses

Water pollution usually first affects fish, which are then eaten by other animals, which later may be consumed by humans. By the time this pollution reaches humans, it may be greatly increased compared to its original concentrations. Therefore, human intoxication cases may be very serious.

For example, certain species of fish are more often contaminated by mercury, which has three forms (organic, inorganic, and metallic), of which the organic form – especially *methylmercury* – is the most dangerous. Contamination mostly comes from mercury in organic sediment that is transformed into methylmercury by microorganisms. This form is absorbed by the tissues of **fish gills** as they swim, and through their digestive tracts as they feed. Fish that contain higher levels of mercury include shark, ray, swordfish, barramundi, gemfish, orange roughy, ling, king mackerel, tilefish, and Southern bluefin tuna. Areas of the world in which the waters contain the highest levels of mercury include those near eastern Asia (especially around India and China), Europe, the Mediterranean Sea, and around South America.

Another potentially serious problem exists when oil spills into shallow or confined waters. Many species of shellfish are relatively immobile, and because they are filter-feeders, they may not be able to avoid exposures to oil. They also do not have the same enzymes needed to break down contaminants as fish with fins have, which detoxify many oil compounds. Fish eggs in shallow water can be destroyed by oil spills. Other areas of concern are lakes, lagoons, and some shallow-water nearshore areas, where spilled oil naturally concentrates. The type of oil and the timing of its release influence the severity of effects upon fish. Light oils and petroleum products may cause acute toxicity, but this usually is resolved fairly quickly. Heavier oils either do not affect fish significantly, but can kill those of them in larval or spawning stages. Only when testing shows that fish are no longer contaminated should they be sold for human consumption.

For example, in 1989, an oil tanker called the *Exxon Valdez* ran aground in Prince William Sound, Alaska (see Figure 21.1). It spilled 11 million gallons of oil into an ecologically sensitive location. The spill affected over 1,300 miles of coastline, killing seabirds, otters, seals, eagles, whales, and billions of salmon and herring eggs. Even today, species that have not been proven to have recovered from the spill include Killer whales, and birds known as murrelets and pigeon guillemots. Massive protection projects have been created since the spill to help restore the region's species. In 2004, the bulk cargo ship called the *Selendang Ayu* ran aground off of Unalaska Island in western Alaska's Aleutian Islands. The ship broke into two pieces, resulting in a large oil spill. Though not as large as the Exxon Valdez spill, thousands of birds were killed along with a smaller amount of otters.

Microplastics can move through wastewater into the oceans, where they may be consumed by fish and other creatures (see Figure 21.2). This can cause them to accumulate in their bodies, leading to harm to humans if they consume the contaminated creatures. Microplastics are less than 5 mm in length. Larger pieces of plastic can become microplastics as they break down and move through the oceans. Some manufacturers use microplastics in their products, such as in exfoliating products and toothpastes. Any product that lists the word **microbeads** on the label contains microplastics. The closer to the top of the food chain a creature is, the more likely it is to consume significant amounts of microplastics. Smaller creatures eat the microplastics, are consumed by larger creatures, which are consumed by still larger creatures. This allows for microplastic levels to accumulate, finally reaching humans. There is no way to eliminate microplastics from a creature once they are present. There is also no source of wild seafood that is guaranteed to be completely free of microplastics. Potential but not fully proven effects of eating microplastic-contaminated seafood include oxidative stress, neurotoxic effects, endocrine disruption, thyroid damage, and cancer. Additional pollutants that can contaminate the food supply include fertilizer (from water runoff) and other toxic chemicals that are dumped into waters that reach the oceans.

Microplastics have been detected in drinking water – both bottled water and tap water. Hazards include physical particles, chemicals, and microbial pathogens as part of **biofilms**. In drinking water, fragments and fibers are the main particle shapes, and polyethylene terephthalate and polypropylene are the most-detected polymers. Plastics and microplastics can contain unbound **monomers** and additives. Biofilms can include pathogens such as *Pseudomonas aeruginosa, Legionella* species, non-tuberculosis *Mycobacterium* species, and *Naegleria fowleri*. Wastewater and drinking-water treatment systems are effective, however, in removing particles of similar sizes and characteristics as microplastics. Water suppliers and regulators must continue to **prioritize** the removal of microorganisms and chemicals in drinking water.

Since, on average, less than 10% of plastics are recycled annually, the problem of plastic contamination of the food supply is ongoing. About 93% of all bottled water contains traces of microplastics. The most commonly used plastic is *polyethylene terephthalate (PET)*, which may disrupt the

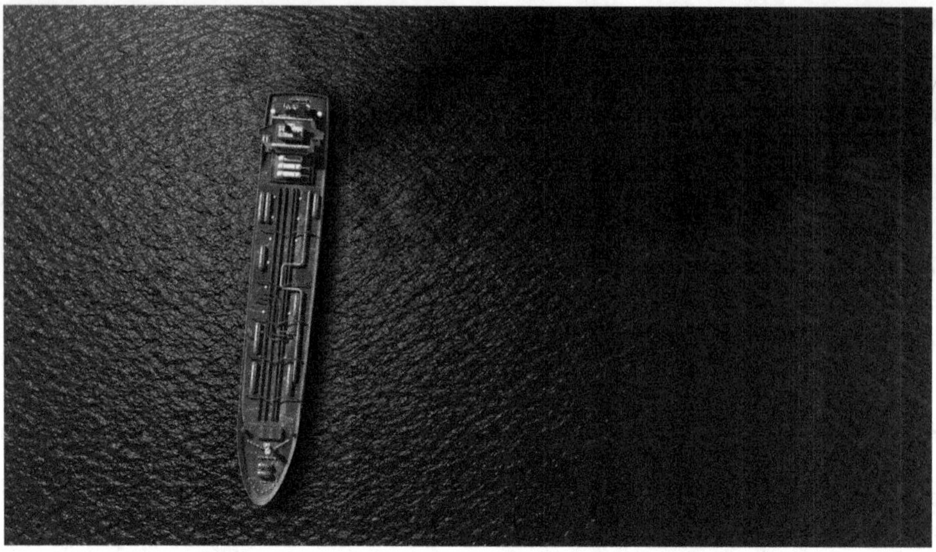

FIGURE 21.1 The Exxon Valdez oil spill.

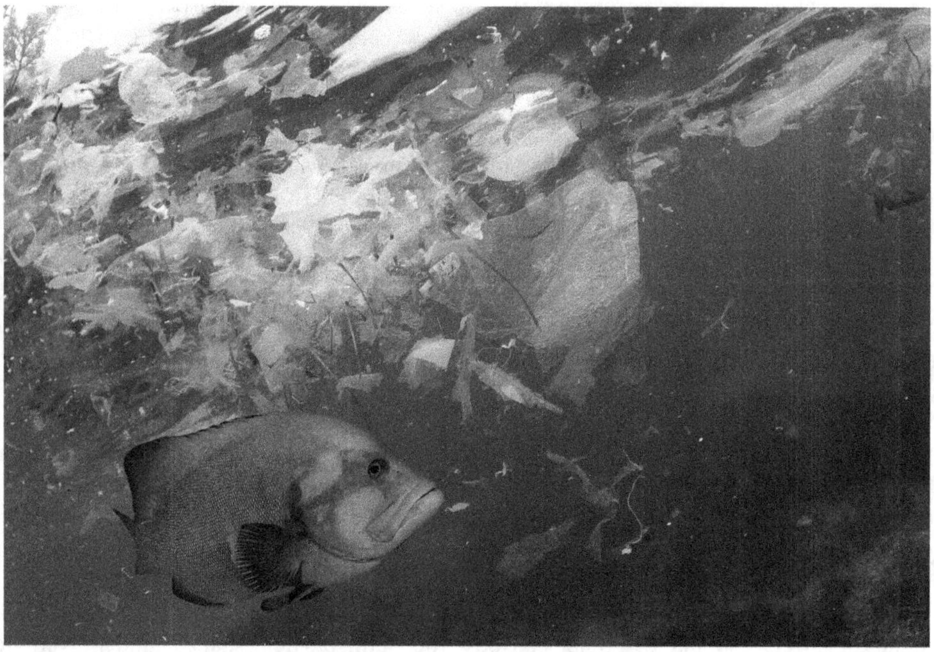

FIGURE 21.2 A fish swimming underneath many microplastics in the ocean.

human endocrine system and its hormones. Another type called *plastic number 7* contains **bisphenol A**, which is linked to fertility issues, altered brain development, cancer, and heart complications. While tap water must be tested to show contaminant levels, it is not mandatory for bottled water to receive the same testing. Therefore, while bottled water costs much more than tap water, it may also be significantly more dangerous to consume. Initiatives are being debated to develop more clean water bills and legislation to better regulate the quality of bottled water on a global scale.

FOCUS ON FUTURE PREVENTION OF FOOD POLLUTION

It has been proposed by experts that growing vegetables in factories, in the future, may be able to eliminate effects of environmental pollution. The process could be computerized to control various factors that affect growth. It is estimated that planting crops and growing them in factories could reduce food pollution by more than 33%.

Test Your Knowledge

1. How can toxic chemicals get into food sources?
2. What factors are the risks for food pollution based on?
3. How can mercury, oil, and plastic harm fish, and eventually, humans?

IMPACT OF NUTRITION ON POLLUTANT TOXICITY

Nutrition can positive and negatively modulate toxicity from exposure to pollution. A diet that is high in pro-inflammatory fats, such as linoleic acid, can increase pollutant toxicity. Diets rich in anti-inflammatory and bioactive components, such as omega-3 fatty acids and **polyphenols**, can reduce toxicant-related inflammation. Nutrition is able to modulate *epigenetic markers* linked to increased disease risks, or to protection against diseases. Overnutrition and undernutrition affect prenatal **epigenetic tags**, which may increase risks of developing disease later in life. Exposure to pollutants alters epigenetic markers, possibly contributing to inflammation and disease. Through epigenetic modulations, pollutants can increase factors in the body that are related to inflammation, cardiac injury, and oxidative damage. Some nutritional components can protect against pollutant-induced inflammation through various types of epigenetic regulation. Overall, exposure to environmental pollutants may increase risks for developing chronic inflammatory diseases, including cardiovascular disease, diabetes mellitus, and metabolic syndrome. Pollutant exposure inhibits negative combined effects with less-than-optimal nutrition, since pollutants and nutritional components can target identical molecular pathways.

The impact of environmental pollution, primarily chronic low exposures of heavy metals, affects the nutritional status and health of livestock as well as humans. Malnutrition inhibits the enzyme system, changes **neurotransmitter** levels, degenerates **myelin** as well as glial and neural elements, lowers intelligence quotient (IQ) scores, and impairs fine and gross motor coordination. The additive impact of undernutrition and adverse effects of heavy metal exposure is becoming a serious threat to health in developing countries. Effects are seen in the **hemopoietic**, renal, and nervous systems of neonates, children, post-partum women, and in those experiencing occupational exposures to pollution. There three main ways in which pollutants and nutrition are interconnected. They include the following:

- Food sources may be the vehicles for delivering toxicants, and can increase exposure and the burden of the toxicants upon the body
- An absorbed toxicant may interact with the nutritional status, to determine the amount of the toxicant that is retained and bioavailable so that it can be harmful
- Once absorbed, nutrients and their metabolism may also interact with the toxicant to determine a specific health outcome – gender and age need to be considered, since that affect nutritional status and toxicant exposure

FOCUS ON MALNOURISHMENT AND POLLUTANTS

Malnourished people, especially women of reproductive age and young children, may be more vulnerable to the negative health effects of food pollutants. It has been established that malnutrition harms so many body systems that any person that encounters environmental pollutants is much more significantly impacted by them. Also, defects in innate and adaptive immune function can contribute to interrelationships between pollution, infection, and undernutrition, resulting in a cycle of recurrent illness.

METALS AND ENVIRONMENTAL POLLUTANTS

Heavy metals such as lead, cadmium, and copper, plus other toxins, can cause a type of chronic **interstitial nephritis**. Some of these metals are well-known pollutants because of their toxicity, high levels in the environment, and their **bioaccumulative** nature. Natural sources include weather effects upon rocks that contain metals, and volcanic eruptions. Anthropogenic sources include mining, plus industrial and agricultural processes. Contamination of water and ecosystems with toxic heavy metals is a significant environmental problem. Heavy metals accumulate in the environment to eventually contaminate food chains. Their bioaccumulation and effects on human health involve fish, rice, and tobacco products. This chapter focuses on the effects of lead, mercury, arsenic, and cadmium.

LEAD

Lead is a metal often used in residential installations, and in metal alloys or chemicals. It is present in pipes, paints, putties, and pesticides. It is one of the heavy metals that can most easily contaminate humans and is extremely harmful to health. Lead is one of the heavy metals that has caused the most harm to the population. Tobacco smoke is another pollutant with a high concentration of this metal. Lead poisoning is known as **plumbism**. It often causes slight symptoms initially, but can later cause acute encephalopathy or irreversible organ damage, usually resulting in cognitive deficits in children. As lead accumulates in the proximal tubular cells, chronic tubulointerstitial nephritis results. Short-term lead exposure causes proximal tubular dysfunction (see Figure 21.3). This includes decreased urate secretion and hyperuricemia, since urate is the substrate for saturnine gout, as well as aminoaciduria and renal glucosuria. People that are at the highest risk include children

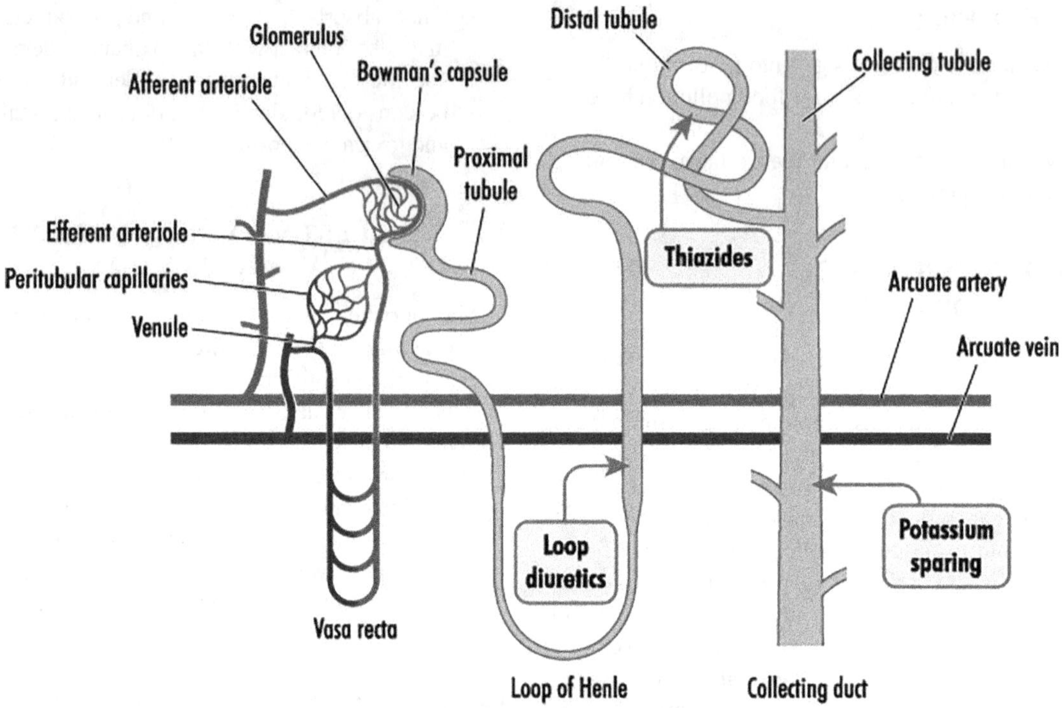

FIGURE 21.3 The structure of a nephron, including the proximal tubule.

exposed to lead paint chips or dust, battery workers, drinkers of high-proof distilled alcohol (moonshine), and welder.

Any child with blood lead levels of more than 5 mcg/dL (0.24 micromole/L) must receive treatment, follow-up testing, serial monitoring, and assessment for vitamin deficiency and overall nutritional status. Symptoms of lead poisoning may include abdominal cramping, constipation, mood changes, and tremors. Exposure to high levels of lead may cause anemia, weakness, plus kidney and brain damage. Very high lead exposure can cause death. Lead can cross the placental barrier, which means pregnant women who are exposed to lead also expose their unborn child. In children, acute lead poisoning may cause decreased attentiveness and irritability, with cerebral edema developing over one to five days. The cerebral edema may cause an ataxic gait, forceful and persistent vomiting, hair loss, altered consciousness, seizures, and finally coma. The encephalopathy may follow several weeks of decreased play activity. Chronic lead poisoning may cause intellectual disability, aggressive behavior disorders, seizure disorders, chronic abdominal pain, anemia, and developmental regression. Adults exposed to lead at their jobs may develop headache, personality changes, abdominal pain, and neuropathy over several weeks or more. There may also be impaired libido, infertility, and in males, erectile dysfunction.

Diagnosis is based on lead levels in blood, abdominal x-rays, and sometimes, x-rays of the long bones of children with suspected chronic exposure. **Burton's line** is a blue-purplish line on the gums that is caused by lead poisoning. It is due to a reaction between circulating lead with sulfur ions released by oral bacterial activity, which deposits lead sulfite at the junction of the teeth and gums. Treatment is based on eliminating the source of lead, such as with whole-bowel irrigation, and chelation (for adults with symptoms plus a high whole blood lead level; and for children with encephalopathy or a high whole blood level). Chelating agents include **succimer**, calcium disodium ethylenediaminetetraacetic acid, and dimercaprol. Measures that reduce risks of household lead poisoning include regular hand washing, regular washing of pacifiers and toys, and regular cleaning of household surfaces.

Children with empty stomachs absorb more lead than children with full stomachs. Foods rich in iron, calcium, and vitamin C help protect children from lead poisoning. This means they should consume meat and seafood, beans, vegetables, eggs, molasses, peanut butter, nuts, whole grains, iron-fortified cereals, fruits, milk and milk substitutes, and calcium-fortified orange juice. Fatty foods must be limited since these can make a child's body absorb lead faster. Eating at fast food limits must be extremely limited. Foods should never be cooked, stored, or served in traditional pottery because it may contain lead. Imported foods stored in leaded cans must be avoided. Mexican candies containing chili powder or tamarind must be avoided because they can contain lead. The effects of plumbism can be worsened as well by diets low in calcium, phosphorus, iron, zinc, and sometimes, copper. Lead appears to have a pro-oxidant stressor effect on red blood cells, causing their accelerated destruction.

FOCUS ON THE FLINT, MICHIGAN WATER CRISIS

A human-made public health crisis (from April 2014 to June 2016) involved the municipal water supply system of Flint, Michigan. Tens of thousands of Flint residents were exposed to dangerous levels of lead. Outbreaks of Legionnaire disease killed at least 12 people and sickened dozens more.

FOCUS ON IRON DEFICIENCY AND LEAD ABSORPTION

Iron deficiency increases the absorption of lead from the stomach and intestines. Prevent iron deficiency by consuming iron-fortified cereals, green leafy vegetables, pureed meats or lean red meats, fish, raisins, dates, prunes, dried beans and peas, skinless poultry, and nuts or sunflower seeds.

Test Your Knowledge

1. What are the three main ways in which pollutants and nutrition are interconnected?
2. Which individuals are at highest risk for lead poisoning?
3. Which foods help protect children from lead poisoning?

Mercury

Mercury is considered to be a highly toxic heavy metal. It can be present naturally in a metallic form (as mercury), or in the form of mercury salts. Mercury is highly volatile. When it is present in the air, we can breathe it in through our lungs or absorb it through our skin. The most dangerous form of exposure is inhaled mercury, since it enters our body, accumulates, and remains for a long time. The effects of mercury compounds upon the body are often extreme. These compounds include ammoniated mercury, bichloride of mercury, calomel, corrosive sublimate, mercurial diuretics, mercuric chloride, and merthiolate. Acute mercury compound poisoning causes burning mouth, salivation, severe gastroenteritis, abdominal pain, colitis, vomiting, anuria, **nephrosis**, and **uremia**. With the alkyl and phenyl mercurials, there are skin burns. Chronic mercury compound poisoning causes **gingivitis**, mental disturbances, and neurologic deficits. For skin contact, soap and water are used during scrubbing. For ingestion, there must be consideration of **gastric lavage**, activated charcoal, and penicillamine or succimer. There must be maintenance of fluid and electrolyte balance, **hemodialysis** for renal failure, and observation for GI perforation.

Elemental mercury poisoning may occur via a liquid form (ingestion or skin contact) and through mercury vapors. For ingestion of the liquid form, there may be no symptoms. If it is injected intravenously, **pulmonary emboli** may develop. Severe **pneumonitis** occurs because of mercury vapor inhalation. There is no treatment needed if the liquid form is ingested. For the IV or vapor forms, only supportive care is needed.

Mercury may contribute to chronic neurological disorders, cardiovascular disease, metabolic syndrome, chronic fatigue, **fibromyalgia**, autoimmune thyroiditis, hypothyroidism, thyroid cancer, **adrenal fatigue syndrome**, digestive disorders, allergies, sleep disorders, and chronic infections. The two minerals most commonly depleted by mercury are magnesium and zinc. Organ meats are nutrient-dense, helping to supply these depleted minerals and vitamins. For example, liver is high in vitamins A and B12, as well as zinc, magnesium, and selenium. Mercuric ions are almost always toxic, which is associated with a high affinity for protein thiol groups. Mercury poisoning is signified by tremors, insomnia, memory loss, neuromuscular effects, headaches, and both cognitive and motor dysfunction. Mercury-related nutritional deficiencies, including those of the long chain polyunsaturated fatty acids, **eicosapentaenoic acid** and **docosahexaenoic acid**, the amino acid methionine, and the trace minerals zinc and selenium influence neuronal function, producing defects in neuronal plasticity.

Arsenic

Arsenic is the most common cause of acute heavy metal poisoning in adults. It is not a metal, but a metalloid (which basically means that it has both metallic and nonmetallic properties). It is released into the environment by industrial processing of chemicals and glasses, and reaches water supplies throughout the world, resulting in marine life being exposed. Arsenic poisoning, or **arsenicosis**, occurs after the ingestion or inhalation of high levels of arsenic, which is carcinogen that is gray, silver, or white in color. Arsenic is extremely poisonous to humans. What makes arsenic especially dangerous is that it has no taste or odor, so exposure can occur without any knowledge by the affected person. Arsenic is a naturally occurring element, found in combination with inorganic or organic substances, to form a variety of different compounds. Inorganic arsenic compounds are present in soil, sediment, and groundwater. These compounds occur naturally, or may be a result of mining, the **smelting** of various ores, and because of industrial use of arsenic. Organic arsenic compounds are mostly found in fish and shellfish. People are usually exposed to inorganic arsenic through drinking water. Water sources in some locations have higher natural levels of inorganic than other areas. Other sources of inorganic arsenic include contaminated soil or wood that was previously preserved with arsenic.

Exposure to arsenic through drinking water is a major public health problem affecting many countries, but it is most severe in low-income countries. There is a wide variation in susceptibility to arsenic toxicity, which is likely related to variations in arsenic metabolism, nutrition status, the body's defense mechanisms, and genetic predisposition. Arsenic induces oxidative stress, which is compounded by arsenic-induced inhibition of several antioxidant systems. There is a link between a low degree of arsenic metabolism and risks of various toxic effects. Arsenic is metabolized in the liver. Administration of ascorbic acid, alpha-tocopherol, plant extracts, flavonoids, polyphenols, and selenium all help to decrease this toxicity. Signs and symptoms of arsenic poisoning include dysphagia, throat constriction, burning GI pain, diarrhea, vomiting, dehydration, GI hemorrhage, pulmonary edema, renal failure, liver failure, and shock. Long-term exposure to arsenic from drinking water and foot can cause cancer, skin lesions, muscle cramps, and tingling of fingers and toes. Arsenic is also associated with cardiovascular disease and diabetes mellitus. In utero and early childhood exposure is linked to poor cognitive development and increased deaths in young adults. Long-term exposure to arsenic can cause more severe symptoms such as darkened skin, constant sore throat, and persistent digestive issues.

Various tests are available to diagnose poisoning by measuring arsenic in the blood, urine, hair, and fingernails. A urine test is the most reliable test for arsenic exposure over the previous few days. Urine testing needs to be done within 24–48 hours for an accurate analysis of an acute exposure. The initial management of acute arsenic intoxication includes gut decontamination and hemodynamic stabilization are. Patients with suspected acute arsenic poisoning generally require rapid stabilization with fluid and electrolyte replacement in an intensive care setting, and the following may be required:

- Aggressive intravenous fluid replacement therapy – this may be life-saving in severe cases
- Gastric lavage – may be useful soon after an acute ingestion to prevent further absorption
- Activated charcoal – though its efficacy is controversial, administration along with a cathartic (such as sorbitol) is frequently recommended
- If profuse diarrhea is present, cathartics should be withheld
- Hemodialysis may be beneficial if there is concomitant renal failure

Chelating agents administered within hours of arsenic absorption may successfully prevent the full effects of toxicity. The patient's nutritional status may play a role in preventing severe health effects. For example, arsenic and selenium may be mutually antagonistic. There have been recent reports that a diet rich in selenium and other antioxidants such as vitamin E helps promote methylation of arsenic, which leads to increased excretion. Methyl donors such as folate may also be of help in arsenic metabolism and excretion. Arsenic-related disease has been shown to increase in individuals who are malnourished or undernourished, possibly due to the decrease in arsenic methylation.

Test Your Knowledge

1. Which foods help to combat mercury poisoning?
2. How can inorganic arsenic affect humans?
3. After a patient with a suspected acute arsenic poisoning is stabilized, what else can be done in regard to treatment?

Cadmium

Cadmium is a metal that is soft, malleable, and bluish-white in its elemental form. While it is a relatively widespread element, it is rarely found on its own as a pure metal. More often, it forms complex compounds in zinc ores. Cadmium is mainly produced through the process of smelting, mining, and refining zinc, lead, and copper. While initially used as a dye for producing shades of yellow, orange, and red, it is most widely used today in nickel-cadmium rechargeable batteries. Cadmium is also found in the following:

- Plating on iron and steel products
- Plastic stabilizers
- Alloy elements for lead, copper, and tin
- Cigarette smoke
- Silver jewelry

Along with being an industrial byproduct, cadmium is a natural component of the earth's crust, and can easily enter the atmosphere, water, and soil. This may happen through volcanic activity, weathering of sediment, or the burning of fossil fuels. It can lead to cadmium being present in sources of drinking water and food, including vegetables, fish, and animals. The foods that are potentially most susceptible to cadmium contamination are mushrooms, shellfish, freshwater fish, dried algae, and potable water.

Cadmium toxicity occurs when high levels of cadmium are inhaled from the air, or contaminated food or water is consumed. In the general population, exposure to cadmium occurs primarily by eating foods grown in contaminated soil. Cigarette smoke is one of the highest sources of cadmium exposure. High levels of cadmium in soil can cause some crops to uptake the heavy metal. The rate of cadmium absorption depends on a whole host of factors, like the crop species, the quality of the soil (pH and salinity), and the presence of other elements. Proximity to certain industrial plants, particularly those involving construction and manufacturing, can also affect soil and sources of water for crops. Smokers may ingest twice the daily amount of cadmium as non-smokers. People breathing in secondhand smoke also take in a higher amount of cadmium, as this is a form of environmental exposure. Ingested cadmium is usually stored in the liver, kidneys, and bones. Eliminating cadmium is a naturally slow process, and it can remain in the human body for decades.

Exposure to cadmium through contaminated workplaces, food, water, or tobacco products cause respiratory diseases, kidney damage, and bone diseases. Cadmium toxicity can affect major aspects of health, though more studies are necessary to fully assess the potential risk to humans and the environment. The general symptoms for acute cadmium poisoning include nausea and vomiting, diarrhea, abdominal pain, and flu-like symptoms. When inhaled consistently over time, cadmium may affect the lungs and breathing. Many studies associate chronic occupational inhalation of cadmium dust and cadmium fumes with an increased risk of respiratory problems, such as **emphysema**, bronchitis, chronic rhinitis, damage to the olfactory epithelium, and COPD (see Figure 21.4).

Cadmium is also classified as a probable carcinogenic agent when inhaled. This suggests that chronic cadmium exposure through inhalation may contribute to lung cancer. The kidneys receive the most damage from chronic cadmium exposure, both via ingestion and inhalation. This is because the kidneys act as a filtration system, removing waste and excess fluid from the body. It can take up to ten years of regular and consistent exposure for cadmium levels to build up enough to cause kidney damage, though animal studies have suggested some subtle changes to renal function even after acute exposure to cadmium. Most commonly, regular cadmium exposure has been linked to progressive renal tubular dysfunction. Some studies suggest that even at lower concentrations, cadmium intake can have severe effects on the kidneys and general renal function. At high concentrations, chronic cadmium poisoning may even cause renal failure, with high serum creatinine and urea. There is also fractional excretion of uric acid and elevated phosphate, as a urine protein-to-creatinine ratio and a urine albumin-to-creatinine ratio. Kidney stones are also more common in populations experiencing excessive cadmium exposure. Cadmium-related bone diseases and skeletal health issues are more often side effects of renal issues, since any damage to the kidneys may cause changes in how calcium and vitamin D are metabolized and absorbed. Severe chronic cadmium poisoning can contribute to bone lesions, including decreased bone density, in later stages. This can eventually lead to **osteoporosis** and **osteomalacia**, which can contribute to certain types of fractures and other effects (see Figure 21.5).

Diagnosis is based on history of occupational exposure to cadmium. Cadmium levels can be measured in blood, urine, hair, nail and saliva samples. Patients with cadmium toxicity require GI irrigation, supportive care, and chemical decontamination, via traditional chelation therapy, using appropriate newer chelating agents and nanoparticle-based antidotes. It has also been recommended to determine the level of food contamination and suspicious areas of exposure. Public education and awareness programs should be considered for exposed individuals, in order to prevent additional cadmium poisoning. Increased levels of urinary beta2-microglobulin may be found during a **radioimmunoassay**, plus increased urinary cadmium levels of 7 mcg/g creatinine or higher.

Treatment focuses on eliminating further exposure. Immediate considerations include evaluation of the airways, breathing, and circulation. The gastrointestinal tract should be irrigated to remove cadmium-containing solutions. Acute or chronic ingestion of cadmium salts is rare, but may lead to death. The lowest lethal dose of cadmium is 5 gr in a person that weighs 154 pounds (70 kg). If emesis has not occurred, gastric lavage is performed soon. A small nasogastric tube must be used. Activated charcoal cannot effectively absorb the cadmium. Hospitalization may help patients exposed to cadmium for evaluating the extent of damage to the liver, as well as the gastrointestinal, urinary, and respiratory tracts. Therefore, supportive therapy is the best choice.

Test Your Knowledge

1. How does cadmium toxicity occur?
2. What are the general signs and symptoms of acute cadmium poisoning?
3. What treatment options exist for cadmium poisoning?

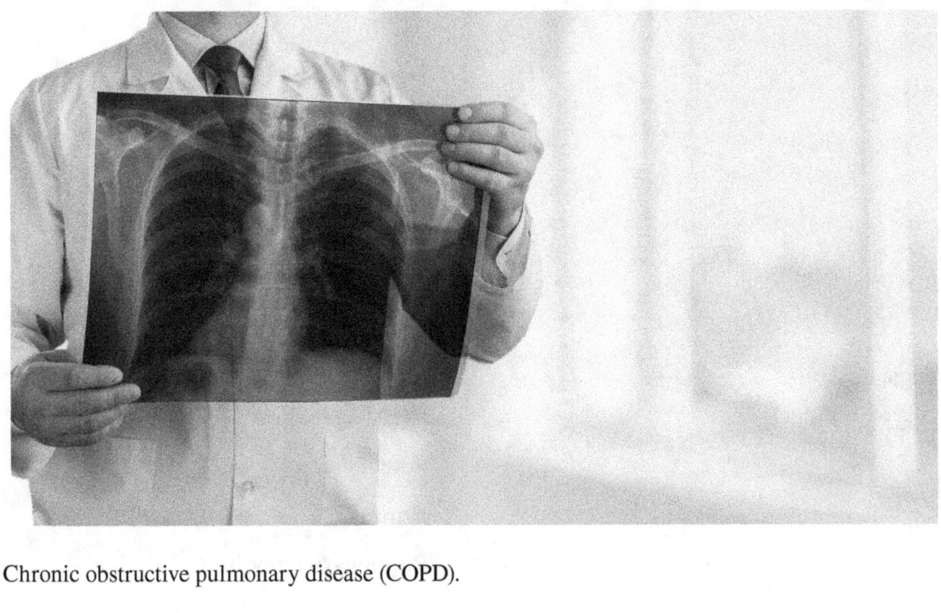

FIGURE 21.4 Chronic obstructive pulmonary disease (COPD).

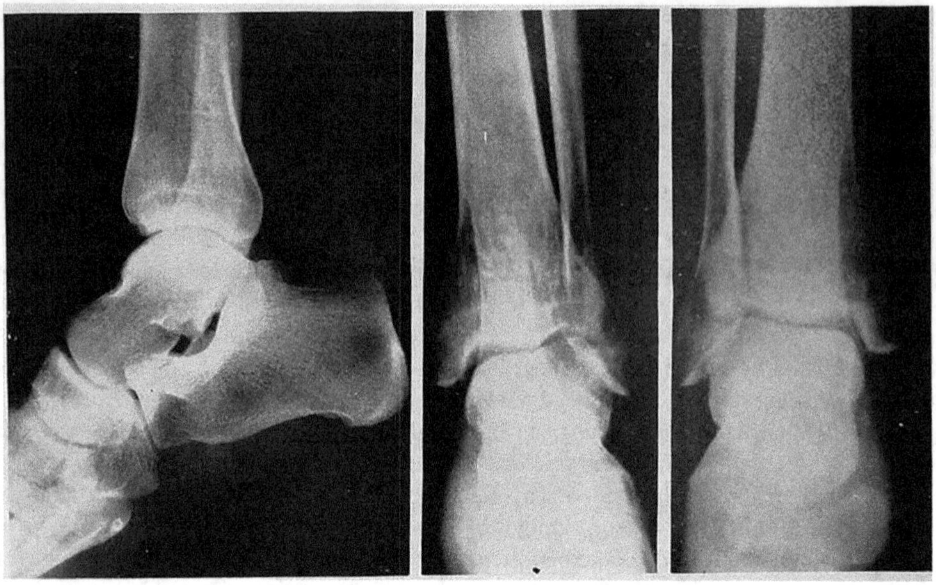

FIGURE 21.5 Decreased bone density, which leads to osteoporosis and osteomalacia, from cadmium poisoning.

FOCUS ON DEFICIENCIES IN RELATION TO CADMIUM TOXICITY

Vitamin C, B1, and B6 deficiencies enhance sensitivity to cadmium toxicity. Vitamin C attenuates oxidative damage and histopathological changes in the lungs and brain, and can also protect the kidneys and testes. Vitamin E also shows protective effects against cadmium in the blood, liver, and brain. Vegetables, fruits, and other edible plants are important dietary sources of these vitamins. Plants that may also be protective include soybeans, garlic, ginger, and onion.

KEY TERMS

Adrenal fatigue syndrome
Arsenicosis
Bioaccumulative
Biofilms
Bisphenol A
Burton's line
Coccidioidomycosis
Creatures
Docosahexaenoic acid
Eicosapentaenoic acid
Epigenetic tags
Exposure medium
Fibromyalgia
Fish gills
Gastric lavage
Gingivitis
Hemodialysis
Hemopoietic
Herbicides
Interstitial nephritis
Intrusion
Microbeads
Microplastics
Monomers
Myelin
Nephrosis
Neurotransmitter
Osteomalacia
Osteoporosis
Ozone precursor
Plumbism
Pneumonitis
Polyphenols
Potency
Prioritize
Pulmonary emboli

Radioimmunoassay

Shiga toxin

Smelting

Stratum corneum

Tachypnea

Urban heat islands

Uremia

CLINICAL CASE STUDIES

Clinical Case Study 1

A 73-year-old grandmother took her grandchildren to a local taco restaurant. The next day, they awoke with abdominal cramping, which led to the development of diarrhea. The grandmother was the worst affected. Her symptoms also included a fever, fatigue, bruising, and decreased urine output. While the grandchildren recovered, she had to be taken to the local emergency department due to the symptoms. Tests revealed her serum creatinine concentration was high and her platelet count was low. A blood smear revealed many red blood cell fragments, with no platelet clumping. The patient was hospitalized and started on hemodialysis. A stool culture was positive for *E. coli*. She was treated but remained hospitalized for two weeks. After discussing the location of the restaurant with authorities, it was soon discovered that the beef they used in their tacos was indeed contaminated with *E. coli*.

CRITICAL THINKING QUESTIONS

1. Where is *E. coli* bacteria usually found?
2. What toxin is produced by *E. coli* bacteria?
3. What is the life-threatening disease that may be caused by *E. coli*, particularly in young children and older adults?

Clinical Case Study 2

A seven-year-old boy was assessed by his pediatrician because of pain in his legs, neck, and abdomen. His appetite had been poor for the last two months, and he had lost about eight pounds. The boy was also very fatigued. When his arms, hands, legs, and feet were palpated, he described sensations of painfulness. Blood tests revealed a high level of mercury. He was given D-penicillamine. Over two months, his abdominal pain was reduced, and the pain in his extremities was also lessened. At this time, his mercury levels were assessed again, and they had nearly returned to normal. Over eight months of follow-up and continued administrations of D-penicillamine, no other symptoms were present.

CRITICAL THINKING QUESTIONS

1. What does acute mercury compound poisoning cause?
2. How can elemental mercury poisoning occur?
3. What symptoms signify mercury poisoning?

Clinical Case Study 3

A 49-year-old man presented with increasing skeletal pain. X-rays of his lumbosacral spine and hip revealed reduced bone density and prominent trabecular markings. He also had impaired renal function with high serum creatinine and urea. The patient's fractional excretion of uric acid and phosphate were elevated, as were his urine protein-to-creatinine ratio and urine albumin-to-creatinine ratio. When questioned about his work history, the patient described having in the silver jewelry industry for several decades. Tests confirmed that he had tubular proteinuria, indicating the likelihood of heavy metal toxicity. Since cadmium is a significant component of working with silver, his blood levels were assessed, and found to be extremely high. The diagnosis was severe cadmium toxicity. This was believed to be due to the cadmium fumes that are released as silver is mixed with cadmium in the process of making silver jewelry.

CRITICAL THINKING QUESTIONS

1. What is cadmium?
2. Where is cadmium most widely used and where is it also found?
3. When does cadmium toxicity occur?

STUDY QUESTIONS

1. Valley fever is caused by which of the following types of pathogens?
   A. Bacterial
   B. Fungal
   C. Viral
   D. Rickettsial

2. Which of the following countries produces about 50% of the wheat consumed throughout the world?
   A. China
   B. Russia
   C. Australia
   D. Ukraine

3. Which of the following individual age groups have fewer adverse health effects after a toxic exposure?
   A. Fetuses
   B. Children
   C. Middle age adults
   D. The elderly

4. Which of the following agents causes the most food poisonings in the United States?
   A. Salmonella
   B. Listeria
   C. Norovirus
   D. Shigella

5. Cyanide poisoning may result in which of the following?
   A. Hepatic failure
   B. Respiratory failure
   C. Renal failure
   D. Stomach perforation

6. Plastics that contain bisphenol A are linked to all of the following, EXCEPT:
   A. Fertility issues
   B. Cancer
   C. Kidney failure
   D. Heart complications

7. Which of the following heavy metal poisonings is also called "plumbism"?
   A. Mercury
   B. Cadmium
   C. Arsenic
   D. Lead

8. Which of the following is NOT a sign or symptom of arsenic poisoning?
   A. Dysphagia
   B. Coma
   C. GI hemorrhage
   D. Pulmonary edema

9. Which of the following minerals are most commonly depleted by mercury?
   A. Magnesium and zinc
   B. Copper and chromium
   C. Manganese and selenium
   D. Iron and iodine

10. Which of the following heavy metals may cause a Burton's line on the gums?
    A. Cadmium
    B. Copper
    C. Lead
    D. Arsenic

11. Severe chronic cadmium poisoning can contribute to which of the following?
    A. Osteoporosis
    B. Liver failure
    C. Heart failure
    D. Encephalitis

12. Which of the following foods is NOT potentially the most susceptible to cadmium contamination?
    A. Freshwater fish
    B. Sweet potatoes
    C. Mushrooms
    D. Shellfish

13. Which of the following is the most common type of acute heavy metal poisoning?
    A. Mercury
    B. Copper
    C. Lead
    D. Arsenic

14. Which of the following is NOT caused by chronic mercury compound poisoning?
    A. Gingivitis
    B. Neurologic deficits
    C. Liver failure
    D. Mental disturbances

15. Which of the following types of mercury contamination is more common?
    A. Organic
    B. Inorganic
    C. Metallic
    D. Nonmetallic

FURTHER READING

1. Bala Dhull, S., Singh, A., and Kumar, P. (2022). *Food Processing Waste and Utilization – Tackling Pollution and Enhancing Product Recovery.* CRC Press.
2. Baudo, R., Glesy, J., and Muntau, H. (2020). *Sediments – Chemistry and Toxicity of In-Place Pollutants.* CRC Press.
3. Birch, C.S., and Bonwick, G.A. (2019). *Mitigating Contamination from Food Processing (Food Chemistry, Function, and Analysis).* Royal Society of Chemistry.
4. Chatoui, H., Merzouki, M., Moummou, H., Tilaoui, M., Saadaoui, N., and Brhich, A. (2022). *Nutrition and Human Health – Effects and Environmental Impacts.* Springer.
5. Cole, J. (2019). *Planetary Health – Human Health in an Era of Global Environmental Change.* CABI.
6. Davis, W.T., Fu, J.S., and Godish, T. (2021). *Air Quality*, 6th Edition. CRC Press.
7. Featherstone, C. (2019). *Food Contamination: Qualitative and Quantitative Analysis.* Syrawood Publishing House.
8. Food and Agriculture Organization. (2021). *Global Assessment of Soil Pollution – Summary for Policymakers.* Food and Agriculture Organization.
9. Galal, T., Hassan, L., and Elawa, O. (2019). *Impact Assessment of Environment Pollution on Economic Food Crops.* Lap Lambert Academic Publishing.
10. Gothandam, K.M., Srinivasan, R., Ranjan, S., and Dasgupta, N. (2023). *Biotechnology for Toxicity Remediation and Environmental Sustainability.* CRC Press.
11. Gubbels, J.S. (2020). *Environmental Influences on Dietary Intake of Children and Adolescents.* Mdpi AG.

12. Hassan Sabry, A.K. (2019). *Pesticides and Food Contamination*. Lap Lambert Academic Publishing.
13. Inamori, Y. (2019). *Microcosm Manual for Environmental Impact Risk Assessment – From Chemicals to Whole Effluent Toxicity (WET)*. Springer.
14. Institut National de Recherche Chimique Applique. (2014). *Pollution by the Food Processing Industries in the EEC*. Springer.
15. Jones, M.D. (2021). *Toxin Nation: The Poisoning of Our Air, Water, Food, and Bodies*. Visible Ink Press.
16. Jungueria Dorta, D., and Palma de Oliveira, D. (2022). *The Toxicity of Environmental Pollutants*. InTechOpen.
17. Kumar Kesari, K., and Kumar Jha, N. (2022). *Free Radical Biology and Environmental Toxicity (Molecular and Integrative Technology)*. Springer.
18. Kumar, V., Dasgupta, N., and Ranjan, S. (2018). *Environmental Toxicity of Nanomaterials*. CRC Press.
19. Li, X., and Liu, P. (2020). *Gut Remediation of Environmental Pollutants – Potential Roles of Probiotics and Gut Microbiota*. Springer.
20. Lichtfouse, E., Schwarzbauer, J., and Robert, Didier. (2014). *Pollutant Diseases, Remediation and Recycling – Environmental Chemistry for a Sustainable World*. Springer.
21. Liu, W. (2022). *Environmental Analysis of Organic Pollutants*. Mdpi AG.
22. Marolla, C. (2017). *Climate Health Risks in Megacities – Sustainable Management and Strategic Planning*. CRC Press.
23. Mihai Grumezescu, A., and Holban, A.M. (2017). *Microbial Contamination and Food Degradation (Handbook of Food Bioengineering 10)*. Academic Press.
24. Nesheim, M.C., Orio, M., Tsai Yih, P., *Food and Nutrition Board, Board on Agriculture and Natural Medicine, and National Research Council. (2015). A Framework for Assessing Effects of the Food System*. National Academies Press.
25. Otuu, C.F., Aloh, O., Shu, E. (2018). *Environmental Pollution and Food Quality – Impact of lead-zinc mining on the quality of four dominant staple foods*. Lap Lambert Academic Publishing.
26. Pan, X., and Zhang, B. (2021). *Environmental Toxicology and Toxicogenomics – Principles, Methods, and Applications (Methods in Molecular Biology, 2326)*. Humana Press.
27. Papadopoulou, P., Marouli, C., and Misseyanni, A. (2019). *Environmental Exposures and Human Health Challenges*. IGI Global.
28. Pizzorno, J. (2018). *The Toxin Solution: How Hidden Poisons in the Air, Water, Food, and Products We Use Are Destroying Our Health – and What We Can Do to Fix It*. HarperOne.
29. Rakesh, S.S., Ramasamy, M., and Veerasawmy, D. (2021). *Microplastics and Food Contamination: Microplastics on Environment*. Lap Lambert Academic Publishing.
30. Rodriguez Bernalde de Quiros, A., Lestido Cardama, A., Sendon, R., and Garcia Ibarra, V. (2019). *Food Contamination by Packaging: Migration of Chemicals from Food Contact Materials*. De Gruyter.
31. Romero-Gonzalez, R. (2022). *Detection of Residual Pesticides in Foods*. Mdpi AG.
32. Sabate, J. (2019). *Environmental Nutrition – Connecting Health and Nutrition with Environmentally Sustainable Diets*. Academic Press.
33. Saxena, G., Kumar, V., and Shah, M.P. (2020). *Bioremediation for Environmental Sustainability – Toxicity, Mechanisms of Contaminants Degradation, Detoxification, and Challenges*. Elsevier.
34. Selendy, J.M.H. (2019). *Water and Sanitation-Related Diseases and the Changing Environment – Challenges, Interventions, and Preventive Measures*, 2nd Edition. Horizon International/Wiley Blackwell.
35. Vandegrift, G.F., Tasker, I.R., and Reed, D.T. (2021). *Environmental Remediation – Removing Organic and Metal Ion Pollutants*. American Chemical Society.
36. Vasanthy, M., Sivasankar, V., and Sunitha, T.G. (2021). *Organic Pollutants – Toxicity and Solutions (Emerging Contaminants and Associated Treatment Technologies)*. Springer.

Part IV

Clinical Treatments and Costs

22 Nutritional Clinical Medicine

OUTLINE

LEARNING OBJECTIVES

After study of this chapter, readers should be able to:

1. Describe the principles of nutritional medicine.
2. Explain the benefits of dietary counseling for patients.
3. Discuss energy balance in obese people.
4. Describe direct and indirect calorimetry.
5. Identify the three main ways to change energy balance.
6. Discuss multidisciplinary nutrition support teams in nutritional medicine.
7. Explain which people have the highest risk for undernutrition.
8. Identify the easiest way to estimate the BMR for men and women.
9. Describe the role of dietitians in hospitals and home care.
10. Discuss the complications in patients receiving long-term home tube feedings.

OVERVIEW

Nutritional clinical medicine has become much more popular in recent decades. It is defined as the science or practice of diagnosis, treatment, and prevention of disease, using food, food supplements, and other nutritional substances. Dietary counseling is a type of assessment that evaluates patients' health needs and determines which diets and lifestyle changes will help them achieve their health goals. Since there is no such thing as a one-size-fits-all diet, individualized diet plans designed by dietitians consider each patient's genes, health status, health priorities, motivations, and lifestyle to personalize a food regimen. Energy balance is the balance of calories consumed through foods and beverages, compared to calories burned though physical activity. Undernutrition is a type of malnutrition that is treated with food being given in slowly increasing amounts, either orally, via tube feeding, or intravenously. In various settings, dietitians provide medical nutrition therapy, educate patients, consult during medical appointments, and interact with caregivers concerning the provision of nutrition to patients.

NUTRITIONAL MEDICINE

Nutritional deficiencies often make health status worse, with or without any present underlying condition. For example, malabsorption that occurs because of celiac disease, **Crohn's disease**, **tropical sprue**, and damage from radiation treatments regularly causes nutritional deficiencies. Many patients, especially those that are older and in acute hospitalization situations, have unsuspected nutritional deficiencies. These conditions often require treatment. Multidisciplinary nutrition support teams may be required, including the combined services of dietitians, physicians, pharmacists, and nurses. Together, these individuals may be able to help clinicians prevent, diagnose, and treat nutritional deficiencies. Also, overnutrition can contribute to a variety of chronic conditions, including hypertension, coronary artery disease, diabetes mellitus, obesity, and cancer. For many hereditary metabolic disorders such as **galactosemia** and phenylketonuria, dietary restrictions are required.

Nutritional evaluation is indicated for patients who are a suspicion of certain deficiencies or toxicities involving essential nutrients, especially for infants and children, or there is insufficient growth and development. Nutritional status should be regularly evaluated as part of clinical examinations for the following:

- Infants
- Children
- Older adults
- Patients taking multiple medications
- Patients with psychiatric disorders
- Patients with systemic disorders lasting more than a few days

General nutritional status is evaluated via patient history, physical examination, and blood testing. If undernutrition is suspected, there may be testing of albumin levels in blood and urine. A body composition analysis is done to estimate the percentage of body fat in the evaluation of obesity, including bioelectrical impedance analysis and

DOI: 10.1201/b22969-26

skinfold measurements. Patient history assesses dietary intake, weight changes, a focused review of body systems, and risk factors for nutritional deficiencies. Dietitians are able to obtain more detailed histories, including lists of foods eaten in the previous 24 hours, and food questionnaires. Food diaries are helpful to record all foods that are eaten. The most accurate record is the *weighed ad libitum diet*. The patient weighs himself or herself and writes down all foods that were consumed.

A complete physical examination includes measurements of height, weight, and distribution of body fat. The body mass index (BMI) adjusts weight for height, and is more accurate than traditional height and weight tables. It includes standards for growth and weight gain, for infants, children, and adolescents. Distribution of body fat is important, since disproportionate abdominal obesity (a waist to hip ratio greater than 0.8) is linked to cardiovascular disorders, cerebrovascular disorders, diabetes mellitus, and hypertension. Measurement of the waist circumference, when the patient has a BMI of less than 35, helps assess if abdominal obesity is present. Risks are higher if the waist circumference is more than 40 inches for a man or more than 35 inches for a woman. Obesity and its complications were discussed in detail in Chapters 8 and 9.

FOCUS ON NUTRITIONAL MEDICINE

Nutritional medicine is based on the principle that nutrients, including the essential micronutrients, are needed for proper functioning of all biochemical processes on which the body depends. During the treatment of symptoms or diseases, dietitians look for underlying causes that are often interrelated with nutritional and environmental factors.

Test Your Knowledge

1. For which patients should nutritional status be regularly evaluated as part of clinical examinations?
2. What is the most accurate type of food diary that a patient can use to record weight changes and food consumption?
3. What type of body fat distribution increases risks for cardiovascular and other health conditions?

DIETARY COUNSELING

Dietary counseling is a process in which specially-trained health professionals help patients make healthy food choices, and form healthy eating habits. It is a therapeutic approach to help patients live healthier, and benefits people of all ages. Dietary counseling can benefit patients in the following ways:

- Management of chronic conditions – including type 2 diabetes mellitus, insulin resistance and hypercholesterolemia. Learning how to choose nourishing foods helps patients have better control of their conditions, and sometimes, can totally reverse them.
- Weight loss – counselors can teach patients how their bodies respond to food choices. Meal plans are created that promote weight loss and wellness. Eating habits are carefully evaluated so that the plan that is created results in positive and lasting changes, and continued weight loss. Dietary counseling succeeds in greater weight loss and long-term results than is seen when patients try to accomplish this on their own.
- Long-lasting healthy habits – learned methods and habits simply last longer with dietary counseling. Better dietary choices are then made. This avoids drastic dietary changes that do not lead to long-lasting changes.
- Improved wellness – counselors focus on all of the patient's needs, and not just the weight loss. Good nutrition improves overall health and wellness. It increases energy, improves sleep, strengthens the immune system, boosts mood, increases concentration, and reduces disease symptoms.
- Better fitness – nutritious meal plans increase muscle mass, build stamina, improve strength, and provide better fitness. Patients learn to avoid trying different diet components and supplements, and are instead guided to the right choices. Specific fitness programs are also recommended to meet the patient's goals.

Many patients see a dietary counselor several sessions, but monthly or yearly follow-ups are also available. Counseling begins with changes that will make the biggest impact, but it is flexible so that it will fit into the patient's lifestyle, with smaller changes continuing to be made.

FOCUS ON DIETARY COUNSELING

Some of the health conditions that benefit from the changes made through dietary counseling include allergies, hypertension, nausea, high cholesterol, obesity, celiac disease, heart disease, diabetes mellitus, hypoglycemia, and irritable bowel syndrome.

INDIVIDUALIZED DIET PLANS

Individualized diet plans are the key to helping people meet health and performance goals. Improved diet results in better health, body fluid composition, and overall living. Diet plans are about weight management as well as creating eating patterns that can be enjoyed and maintained. They reduce stress, save money, and give us more time to enjoy life. Individualization of diet plans is important to increase strength, maintain energy levels, minimize cravings, take into account dietary restrictions, improve food choices, keep people accountable for their dietary choices, and instill confidence.

Individualized diet plans work because they take into account that no two people respond exactly the same the identical food choices. Even between twins, one of them may have a blood glucose spike after eating a specific food, while his or her twin does not have the same spike with the same food. Like glucose, fat levels may not be elevated in the same way after an identical meal between individuals. Diets are never "one size fits all". People that follow diet plans with specific, individualized goals eat healthier than those that do not. The one overall true fact about diet plans is that once they are established, they must be followed. Dieters relapse badly once they stop following a diet that is not individualized for them. Individualized diet plans should not include "forbidden" foods that must be avoided at all costs, because people simply do not adhere to them over the long term.

FOCUS ON PRECISION NUTRITION

Precision nutrition seeks to improve the personalized treatment of diseases and is specific to dietary intake. Individualized diets are based on a patient's DNA, race, gender, health history, and lifestyle habits. These diets assume that each individual may have a different response to specific foods and nutrients. Precision nutrition considers the microbiome, which is also unique to each individual.

Test Your Knowledge

1. In what ways can dietary counseling benefit patients?
2. Why do individualized diet plans work?

ENERGY BALANCE

The concept of energy balance is based on the fundamental thermodynamic principle that energy cannot be destroyed, and can only be gained, lost, or stored. To maintain a stable body weight, energy intake must, over time, equal energy expenditure. An understanding of the physiologic control of energy balance may be useful for designing interventions to tackle the global obesity epidemic. Obesity occurs when the body's energy balance is positive. Human physiology maintains energy balance at high levels of energy intake and expenditure. Strategies to combat obesity should focus on increasing physical activity as food intake is reduced in relation to calories. Prevention of weight gain should be easier than the treatment of obesity. Components of energy balance are interdependent, and weight loss requires major behavior changes.

A calorie is a unit of energy needed to raise one kg of water one Celsius degree. When the same amount of calories are taken in as are burned, the *energy equation* is balanced, and weight is neither gain nor lost. **Positive energy balance** is when energy going into the body is more than energy leaving the body. Obviously, when more calories are taken in than are burned, we gain weight, and the reverse is also true. Regulating the energy equation is difficult, which explains the high rates of obesity in adults and children throughout the world. The basal metabolic rate (BMR) makes up most of our energy needs, which is about 60%–75% of total energy expenditure. Since different body tissues use different mounts of energy, the BMR is influenced by how much muscle body mass is present. Higher BMR levels occur from greater levels of lean body mass. Men generally have more lean body mass than women, so their BMR is usually higher. The BMR also decreases with age, and as lean body mass decreases.

The BMR is influenced by physical activity levels. Those that exercise regularly can increase it by 5%–14%, based on the intensity of the activity. Strength training increases BMR by 5%. The BMR is also increased in growing children, and during pregnancy. However, it decreases in the first trimester, then increases in the last half of the pregnancy. Hormones related to the menstrual cycle cause variations in BMR of about 359 calories, with requirements being highest just before menstruation. Additional factors that cause increased BMR include hyperthyroidism, epinephrine, leptin, fever, climate, illness, and tissue damage. Exercising in temperatures over 86°F increases BMR by approximately 5%. Damage to tissues, such as those caused by burns, increases BMR while the body is repairing itself. The easiest way to estimate BMR is as follows:

- For men – multiply the ideal body weight for height by 11
- For women – multiply the ideal body weight for height by 10

Energy balance is affected by physical activity, body size, amount of body fat and muscle, and genetics. Energy expended by physical activity is the most variable part of our energy needs, varying between individuals, and even between different days. Based on activity, energy needs may be increased by 20%–50% of BMR. The **thermic effect** of food is about 10% of the amount of energy expenditure, and varies by the size of meals and the types of macronutrients that are included. Less energy is needed to metabolize fat than is needed for proteins and carbohydrates. Fat has about 4% thermic effect, so 100 calories of fat would require four calories to utilize the meal. Protein has 15%–20% thermic effect, while carbohydrates have about 25%. Overall thermic effect of a meal varies since most meals do not consist of just one of these macronutrients. Additional factors increase the effect of meals upon metabolism, including caffeine and spicy foods.

Direct **calorimetry** measures heat released from the body, while indirect calorimetry measures the amount of oxygen that is used, since there is a direct relationship between the use of energy and oxygen. Estimated Energy Requirements are used to estimate energy needs of adults. They are within plus or minus 200 calories for men, and plus or minus 160 calories for women. The equations take into account gender, age, physical activity level, body composition, and body size. Pregnant women and children have different sets of energy equations.

FOCUS ON ENERGY NEEDS AND PHYSIOLOGICAL STATES

Energy needs are affected by various physiological states. Anorexia, obesity, pregnancy, and lactation increase energy needs, while people with spinal cord injuries need less energy because they have less physical activity.

The hypothalamus is responsible for hunger regulation and satiety. When energy is needed, the feeding centers of the hypothalamus are stimulated to send the signal of hunger. As people eat, the satiety centers are stimulated, and then signaled to stop eating. Sometimes, certain medications, surgery, and cancers affect satiety centers in the brain, and people either overeat or undereat. Satiety is also affected by stimulation of smell and taste, water content, and fiber content. When we become used to larger food portions, we may perceive that a small portion would not be enough to make us feel full.

A severe **negative energy balance** can be reduced metabolism by bone mass, thyroid hormones, and testosterone level concentration. It leads to weight loss as the body detects an energy deficit and fat reserves are used to make up the difference. When the body determines it is not getting enough energy, it slows down or stops all "non-survival" functions. Excessive fasting greatly reduces the metabolism, and non-survival functions such as the sex drive drop to almost nothing. Oppositely, overeating and lack of exercise may cause hypertension and hypercholesterolemia, insulin resistance, diabetes mellitus, and cancer.

For long-term success, there must be a consistently healthy diet and regular physical activity. Exercise should include strength training to help build and maintain muscle, especially with aging. Muscle mass natural decreases over time, so the number of calories burned while resting also declines. Our energy needs slowly decrease due to loss of muscle mass, so the amount of food needed without gaining weight is less.

Activity **thermogenesis** is the energy expended while moving, which includes structured exercise and non-structured movements such as walking between different locations or doing housework. The most effective way to assess energy balance is to track body weight over extended periods of time such as weeks or months. Body weight can fluctuate widely during one day or week, based on hydration status, glycogen status, and other variables. The average weight over several weeks or months is a good indicator the state of energy balance.

The three main ways to change energy balance are: (1) change food intake, (2) change the amount of structured exercise, and (3) change non-exercise activities (sitting for shorter periods of time, doing more things around the house, and taking stairs instead of elevators or escalators).

FOCUS ON THE REALITIES OF ENERGY BALANCE

It is quite common to overestimate just how many calories are burned from exercise. For example, a person that weighs 150 pounds is able to burn about 190 calories while jogging for 20 minutes. However, if they eat a piece of chocolate cake after dinner (about 300 calories), their jog did not even come close to balancing their energy intake and out take. The key word is "balance".

THE BASICS OF ENERGY BALANCE

When we are in a state of positive energy balance for extended periods of time, the extra energy is stored mostly as fat, increasing adiposity and health risks. When people are in a state of negative energy balance for extended periods of time, the energy debt harms body tissues, often causing impaired performance and increase risks for stress fractures, tendon and ligament damage, and other injuries.

Test Your Knowledge

1. What is the basal metabolic rate?
2. What are the percentages of thermic effect of fats, proteins, and carbohydrates?
3. What happens in the body when there is a severe negative energy balance?

UNDERNUTRITION THERAPY

Dietitians oversee undernutrition therapy, using individualized diet plans, plus the inclusion of fortified foods with extra nutrients, approved snacks between meals, consuming high-calorie drinks, and having food delivered to the home instead of expending energy going shopping. Some patients require supplements to supply extra nutrients, as guided by a healthcare professional. Regular medical appointments are required to assess any changes in diet so that it can be carefully adjusted. For some individuals, if there are problems swallowing, options include nasogastric tubes, percutaneous endoscopic **gastrostomy** tubes, and parenteral nutrition, which will be discussed in detail in Chapter 23. These treatments usually begin in a hospital, but can be continued in the patient's home if the individual is healthy enough. Also, some undernourished people may need help from home care visitors, occupational therapists, meals-at-home services, and speech or language therapists. For severely malnourished children, there may be a need for extremely careful feeding and rehydration, and a normal diet may not be able to be consumed immediately. Hospitalization is often required. Once a certain level of wellness is achieved, the patient can gradually being eating a normal diet, and then can continue to do this after returning home. Treatment is monitored regular to ensure that it is effective. Weight and height measurements are taken, and if improvement is not good, the patient is referred to a specialist.

Treatment of undernutrition at home involves discussions with diet planners and advisers, gradual increase of nutrients, dietary supplements, use of protein bars, regular monitoring of BMI, occupational therapists, various medical specialists, and sometimes, soft or pureed foods. In the hospital, treatment of undernutrition combines the expertise of gastroenterologists, dietitians, nutrition nurses, psychologists, and social workers. Nasogastric tubes, percutaneous endoscopic gastrostomy (PEG), intravenous infusion, or parenteral nutrition may be done if the patient cannot take food via the mouth. Nasogastric tubes are designed for short-term use, for up to six weeks. For undernourished pregnant women, vitamins and minerals may need to be supplemented, such as iron and folic acid.

Undernutrition is what most people think of when the term *malnutrition* is used. It is a deficiency of nutrients due to an inadequate diet or problems absorbing nutrients from foods. Undernutrition may cause visible wasting of muscle and fat, but it also can be unseen. It is possible for an overweight person to be undernourished. Macronutrient undernutrition is a deficiency of proteins, fats and carbohydrates. Without them, or even just one of them, the body begins to break down tissues and shut down nonessential functions in order to conserve energy. The micronutrients (vitamins and minerals), though required in smaller amounts, are still essential.

It is important that therapy for undernutrition begins as soon as possible in order to avoid the immune system shutting down, which increases chances for illness, infection, and reduced healing. Therapy can also prevent cardiovascular conditions, emotional and mental problems, and atrophy of certain areas of the digestive system. Undernutrition therapy must also take into account abnormalities caused by vitamin deficiencies.

FOCUS ON ELDERLY RISKS FOR UNDERNUTRITION

The elderly are at risk for undernutrition because of reduced mobility, institutionalization, reduced appetite, and reduced absorption of nutrients.

Test Your Knowledge

1. For a patient who is able to eat, what does undernutrition therapy involve?
2. If swallowing is difficult, what forms of undernutrition therapy are available?
3. What is protein-energy undernutrition?

THE ROLE OF DIETITIANS IN HOSPITALS AND HOME CARE

The hospital dietitian directs the operation of all kitchens and dining rooms to provide nutritious and well-prepared food for patients. Hospital dietitians also develop diets that are appropriate for patients based on their medical needs. Ideally, the dietitian should be involved within 24 hours of a patient's admission. The patient is evaluated so that a nutrition care plan can be created. The hospital dietitian meets with physicians and other health care professionals to coordinate each patient's medical and dietary needs. Some of them specialize in management of overweight and critically ill patients, including those with cardiovascular disorders, renal disease and diabetes mellitus. Clinical dietitians in nursing care facilities, smaller hospitals, and correctional facilities may manage food service departments. There are some subtypes of dietitians as well. *Corporate dietitians* work in food manufacturing, advertising, and marketing. *Management dietitians* oversee large-scale meal planning and preparation in health care facilities, company cafeterias, prisons, and schools. *Consultant dietitians* work under contract with health care facilities, or in their own private practices.

Without sufficient support at home after being discharged from a hospital, outcomes can worsen, especially for older adults, who have a higher risk of death compared to those that are well-nourished. Home health care is usually less expensive, just as effective, and more convenient as care given in hospitals or nursing homes. Home dietary care also allows for reductions in acute care needs and costs associated with preventable hospital visits. Dietitians help ensure that home care is comprehensive, coordinated, and of high quality. They determine nutritional risks for home care clients and develop individualized care plans. Interventions include nutrition support, medical nutrition therapy, and therapeutic diets.

Nutrition support may include enteral or parenteral nutrition. Dietitians also provide nutrition-related training and education to caregivers so that they can help manage nutrition support. Complications in those receiving long-term home tube feedings include discharge from the tube site, irritated and reddened **stoma**, and granulation tissue. There are common mechanical or technical issues with tubes because of breaking, falling, or plugging. Medical nutrition therapy (MNT) helps treat and manage conditions though individualized nutrition care, and is provided by registered dietitians when referred by a physician. The MNT procedures can reduce complications, and reduce medical costs – especially those associated with type 2 diabetes and chronic kidney disease. The MNT services are partially covered by Medicare Part B, and some related services for diabetes or kidney disease are also covered. Services include initial nutrition and lifestyle assessments, individual or group nutritional therapy services, assistance with managing diabetes-related lifestyle factors, and follow-up visits to assess progress.

Therapeutic diets control intake of foods or nutrients, and are modifications of regular diets to adjust nutrients, texture, food allergies, and food intolerance. Dietitians help monitor the effectiveness of therapeutic diets and also educate patients and caregivers about dietary adherence. This is very important, since diet instructions are more effective when given at home than in a hospital. Home-visit nutrition education by dietitians improves nutritional status and health outcomes for older adults. Dietitians are trained to identify nutrition risk factors in older adults so that quicker, more effective interventions can occur.

FOCUS ON THE ROLES OF DIETITIANS

Dietitians counsel patients on nutrition issues and healthy eating habits, assessing patients' needs, developing and implementing nutrition programs, and evaluating and reporting results. In hospitals, they work with patients and family members to make sure that diets meet individual needs. Their expertise extends to the provision of home care, which often focuses on the needs of elderly patients.

Test Your Knowledge

1. What does the hospital dietitian direct?
2. Which dietary interventions are offered as part of home health care?
3. What are the complications of long-term home tube feedings?

KEY TERMS

Calorimetry

Crohn's disease

Galactosemia

Negative energy balance

Night blindness

Positive energy balance

Stoma

Thermic effect

Thermogenesis

Tropical sprue

CLINICAL CASE STUDIES

Clinical Case Study 1

A 66-year-old man with Crohn's disease, weight loss, and diarrhea visits his gastroenterologist because of feeling weak and being unable to enjoy social activities. He must stay close to a bathroom most of the time, so going outside of his home for any length of time is difficult. The patient wants to make the diarrhea manageable and gain back his weight and strength. The diagnosis is exacerbation of Crohn's disease, with possible malabsorption due to bacterial overgrowth. Antibiotics and pancreatic enzymes are prescribed. The patient is referred to a dietitian, who comes up with a treatment plan of an energy- and protein-enriched diet that is lower in fat, supplementation with vitamin A and vitamin D3, plus antidiarrheal medications with maximal doses of a bile salt binder. Over time, the combined treatments begin to work as the patient gains weight and the diarrhea and undernutrition resolve.

CRITICAL THINKING QUESTIONS

1. Are nutritional deficiencies linked to malabsorption conditions such as Crohn's disease?
2. For which patients should nutritional status be regularly evaluated as part of clinical examinations?
3. What does treatment of undernutrition at home involve?

Clinical Case Study 2

A 71-year-old woman is hospitalized because of a stroke, which had affected her ability to swallow normally. She had recently experienced weight loss because of her condition. Therefore, her health care team puts a percutaneous endoscopic gastrostomy tube in place. A dietitian is consulted so that the patient's nutritional status can be improved, and so that enteral nutrition can be started. The plan is for some oral intake to be offered at the point the patient will be able to handle it. Several months later, she becomes able to eat normally again, and energy and protein needs are being met. She starts physical therapy once per week in order to help regain her strength.

CRITICAL THINKING QUESTIONS

1. What are the available options for individuals that have problems swallowing?
2. How can dietary counseling benefit patients in regard to weight loss?
3. How can a severe negative energy balance lead to weight loss?

Clinical Case Study 3

A 35-year-old man who had moved to the United States from Brazil had been diagnosed with tropical sprue. He was very thin and complained of chronic diarrhea, tongue soreness, **night blindness**, and a feeling of weakness. A few days before, he also had a high fever, which subsided on its own. Blood tests revealed that the patient also had anemia. A dietitian was called in, the patient was immediately started on folic acid, vitamin A, and cobalamin supplements. He was also given tetracycline. Very rapidly, the patient's symptoms were reduced in their severity. Antidiarrheal agents were able to correct the condition. The dietitian also started the patient on iron supplements.

CRITICAL THINKING QUESTIONS

1. What factors influence the body metabolic rate?
2. Why is it important that therapy for undernutrition begins as soon as possible?
3. Is undernutrition directly related to the term "malnutrition"?

STUDY QUESTIONS

1. Which of the following may NOT cause malabsorption?
   A. Crohn's disease
   B. Chronic esophagitis
   C. Tropical sprue
   D. Celiac disease

2. Which of the following is the most accurate method of recording for all foods that are eaten?
   A. Mediterranean diet
   B. Weighed ad libitum diet
   C. Asian diet
   D. Apple watch

3. Which of the following areas of body fat distribution may increase risks for cardiovascular disorders?
   A. Chest
   B. Neck
   C. Buttocks
   D. Abdomen

4. All of the following may benefit patients as part of dietary counseling, EXCEPT:
   A. Long-lasting healthy habits
   B. Improved wellness
   C. Weight gain
   D. Better fitness

5. Individualized diets are based on all of the following patient factors, EXCEPT:
   A. Sexual activity
   B. Lifestyle habits
   C. Gender
   D. Race

6. A calorie is a unit of energy needed to raise:
   A. One pound of water one Fahrenheit degree
   B. One pound of water one Celsius degree
   C. One kilogram of water one Fahrenheit degree
   D. One kilogram of water one Celsius degree

7. Which percentage range of total energy is made up by the basal metabolic rate?
   A. 20%–35%
   B. 40%–50%
   C. 50%–55%
   D. 60%–75%

8. Which of the following is the easiest way to estimate the basal metabolic rate for men?
   A. Multiply body weight for height by 22
   B. Multiply body weight for height by 18
   C. Multiply body weight for height by 11
   D. Multiply body weight for height by 10

9. Indirect calorimetry measures the amount used of which of the following?
   A. Oxygen
   B. Heat
   C. Water
   D. Carbon dioxide

10. A severe negative energy balance can reduce metabolism by all of the following, EXCEPT:
    A. Thyroid hormone
    B. Parathyroid hormone
    C. Testosterone
    D. Bone mass

11. Which of the following is NOT one of the three main ways to change energy balance?
    A. Change food intake
    B. Change the amount of structured exercise
    C. Change medication intake
    D. Change non-exercise activities

12. Undernutrition may cause visible wasting of which of the following?
    A. Muscle and fat
    B. Muscle and bone
    C. Muscle and skin
    D. Muscle and liver tissue

13. Medical nutrition therapy is partially covered by which of the following types of Medicare?
    A. Type D
    B. Type A
    C. Type B
    D. Type C

14. The concept of energy balance is based on which principle
    A. Physiologic
    B. Thermodynamic
    C. Metabolic
    D. Homeostasis

15. Which of the following means positive energy balance?
    A. When energy going into the body is less than energy leaving the body
    B. When energy going into the body is equal to energy leaving the body
    C. When energy going into the body is more than energy leaving the body
    D. When energy leaving the body is more than energy going into the body

FURTHER READING

1. Bansal, M., and Narang, M. (2021). *Pinnacle View of Hospitality in Hospitals.* Bansal Narang.
2. Bauer, K.D., and Liou, D. (2020). *Nutrition Counseling and Education Skill Development*, 4th Edition. Cengage.
3. Bozzetti, F., Staun, M., and Van Gossum, A. (2014). *Home Parenteral Nutrition*, 2nd Edition. CABI.
4. Canter, D.D., and DeYoung-Daniels, R. (2021). *The Profession of Dietetics*, 7th Edition. Jones & Bartlett Learning.
5. D'Adamo, P.J., and Whitney, C. (2016). *Eat Right 4 Your Type – The Individualized Blood Type Diet Solution.* Berkeley.
6. Diamond, E.A. (2014). *Nutritional Medicine: A – Z of Disease & Illness.* Diamond.
7. Feather, A., Randall, D., and Waterhouse, M. (2020). *Kumar and Clark's Clinical Medicine*, 10th Edition. Elsevier.
8. Gaby, A.R. (2016). *Nutritional Medicine*, 2nd Edition. Gaby.
9. Gandy, J. (2014). *Manual of Dietetic Practice*, 5th Edition. Wiley Blackwell.
10. Goday, P.S., and Walia, C.L.S. (2022). *Pediatric Nutrition for Dietitians.* CRC Press.
11. Grodner, M., Escott-Stump, S., and Dorner, S. (2022). *Nutritional Foundations and Clinical Applications – A Nursing Approach*, 8th Edition. Elsevier.
12. Heber, D., Li, Z., and Go, V.L.W. (2021). *Nutritional Oncology.* CRC Press.
13. Herbold, N., and Edelstein, S. (2009). *Dietitian's Pocket Guide to Nutrition.* Jones & Bartlett Learning.
14. Hoffer, A., and Prousky, J. (2011). *Healing with Clinical Nutrition: Nutrient-Rich Food & Nutritional Supplements for Optimum Health, Professional Edition.* CCNM Press.
15. Holli, B.B., and Beto, J.A. (2017). *Nutrition Counseling and Education Skills – A Guide for Professionals*, 7th Edition. Wolters Kluwer.
16. Kaloni Ilunga, I. (2022). *Undernutrition and Nutritional Care in Hospitalized Adults – the Need for the Creation of Food and Clinical Nutrition Services in Hospitals.* Our Knowledge Publishing.
17. Katz, D.L., Essel, K.D., Friedman, R.S.C., Joshi, S., Levitt, J., and Yeh, M.C. (2022). *Nutrition in Clinical Practice*, 4th Edition. Wolters Kluwer.
18. Kim, M., Roth, J., and Bashrat, A. (2019). *Reuniting Over- and Undernutrition, Macronutrients and Micronutrients.* Lap Lambert Academic Publishing.
19. Kubota, T., and Fukuoka, H. (2018). *Developmental Origins of Health and Disease (DOHaD) – From Biological Basis to Clinical Significance (Advances in Experimental Medicine and Biology, 1012).* Springer.
20. Lonsdale, D. (2014). *A Nutritional Approach to a Revised Model for Medicine – Is Modern Medicine Helping You?* Strategic Book Publishing & Rights Agency, LLC.
21. Morton, J.M., Brethauer, S.A., DeMaria, E.J., Kahan, S., and Hutter, M.M. (2019). *Quality in Obesity Treatment.* Springer.
22. Mukherjee, M. (2018). *Under-Nutrition and Vulnerability.* Studium Press.
23. Rippe, J.M. (2019). *Lifestyle Medicine*, 3rd Edition. CRC Press.
24. Seccafien, G. (2019). *The Role of the Dietitian and Nutritionist in the Nursing Home.* Seccafien.
25. Sinatra, S.T., and Houston, M.C. (2022). *Nutritional and Integrative Strategies in Cardiovascular Medicine*, 2nd Edition. CRC Press.
26. Skipper, A. (2014). *Dietitian's Handbook of Enteral and Parenteral Nutrition*, 3rd Edition. Jones & Bartlett Learning.
27. Smith, I.K. (2021). *Fast Burn! – The Power of Negative Energy Balance.* St. Martin's Press.
28. Snetselaar, L. (2006). *Nutritional Counseling for Lifestyle Change.* CRC Press/Taylor & Francis.
29. Sutherland, M. (2023). *The Science of Nutrition and Health.* Sutherland.
30. Vasquez, A. (2016). *Textbook of Clinical Nutrition and Functional Medicine, Volume 1 – Essential Knowledge for Safe Action and Effective Treatment (Inflammation Mastery and Functional Inflammology)*, 4th Edition. International College of Human Nutrition and Function.
31. Winters, N., Higgins Kelley, J., and Turner, K. (2017). *The Metabolic Approach to Cancer – Integrating Deep Nutrition, the Ketogenic Diet, and Nontoxic Bio-individualized Therapies.* Chelsea Green Publishing.

23 Nutritional Therapy

OUTLINE

LEARNING OBJECTIVES

After study of this chapter, readers should be able to:

1. Compare enteral tube nutrition with parenteral nutrition.
2. Explain the polymeric formulas used for enteral tube feeding.
3. Describe the serious complications of enteral tube feeding.
4. Explain nutritional therapy for anorexia nervosa.
5. Identify the most common head and neck cancers.
6. Describe refeeding syndrome and dumping syndrome.
7. Explain nutritional therapy for chronic pancreatitis.
8. Describe types of bone marrow transplantation.
9. Discuss nutritional therapy for acute pancreatitis.
10. Explain nutritional therapy for chemotherapy and radiotherapy.

OVERVIEW

Nutritional therapy is an evidence-based and individualized nutrition process designed to help treat various medical conditions. It can be performed for inpatients and outpatients. Treatment methods can be in the form of IV therapy (total parenteral nutrition), medical foods, tube feeding (enteral nutrition), and oral supplements. Nutritional therapists assist patients with specific health problems through assessment and counseling about their diets. Nutritional therapy is commonly used for dying patients, those with anorexia nervosa, dementia, head and neck cancer, esophageal cancer, pancreatitis, bone marrow transplantation, and for patients receiving chemotherapy or radiotherapy.

ORAL NUTRITIONAL SUPPLEMENTS

Oral nutritional supplements are powerful tools against malnutrition. They provide a concentrated energy source and high levels of nutrition. Though whole foods are usually preferred as much as possible, when eating enough foods are not realistic or possible, oral nutritional supplements are an excellent choice to bring in needed calories. Diseases and conditions that compromise adequate consumption of whole foods include inflammatory bowel disease, severe malabsorption, oral cancer, **short bowel syndrome**, anorexia, dementia, and severe and unintentional weight loss. Even a 10% decrease in caloric intake can weaken the immune system. Almost 50% of all hospitalized people have some amount of malnourishment, so using oral nutrition supplements can be very helpful.

Oral nutritional supplements provide calories, protein, vitamins, and minerals, and can be used as meal replacements. Some of them contain additional fiber, omega-3 fatty acids, prebiotics, and *probiotics*. These supplements are widely available at grocery stores, drug stores, and online. Many oral nutritional supplements provide 100% of the daily recommended intakes (DRIs) for vitamins and minerals within a volume of 1–1.5 liters per day. It is important to remember that DRIs are meant for healthy people, so for specific health conditions, more vitamins and minerals may be required than these supplements provide.

Generally, calories range from one to two calories per mL, with most coming from carbohydrates. These carbohydrates often come from corn syrup solids, and are very sweet – sometimes too sweet. Many of these supplements can be warmed up before drinking but they should never be boiled because it will reduce their nutritious capacities. The protein sources in oral nutritional supplements come from **daisy**, soybean, or pea protein (see Figure 23.1). Nearly all supplements are lactose-free, gluten-free, or both, and may or may not be plant-based. Fat sources may come from corn, sunflower, soy oil, safflower, coconut, palm oil, fish oil, or **medium-chain triglyceride** (MCT) oil. For people that have problems digesting fat, MCT oil-containing supplements may be preferred, to enhance absorption and optimize tolerance.

Fiber and probiotics are important for gut health and a healthy microbiome, yet not all oral nutritional supplements contain them. Most oral nutritional supplements, including those with added fiber, are still considered "low fiber", and below the recommended amount of 25–38 g of fiber per day. While taking oral nutritional supplements, it is still important to get additional fiber from vegetables, fruits, legumes, nuts, seeds, whole grains, 100% ground **psyllium husk**, flaxseeds, or **chia seeds** (see Figure 23.2). The fiber sources in oral nutritional supplements may come from soy fiber, **guar gum**, or **inulin**. It is important to discuss oral

DOI: 12432545124234-27

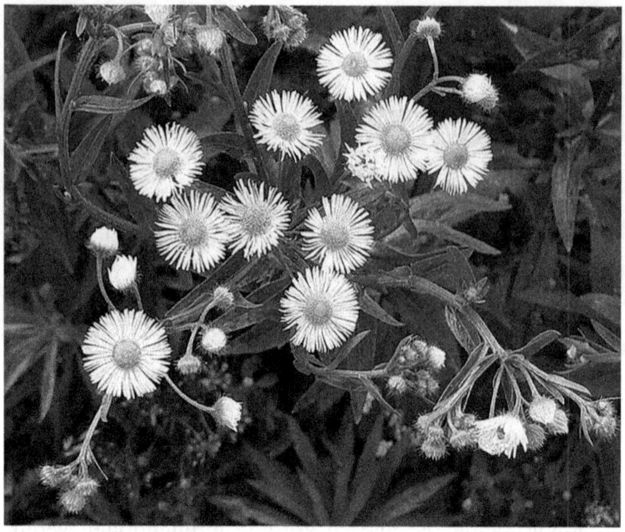

FIGURE 23.1 Daisy flowers.

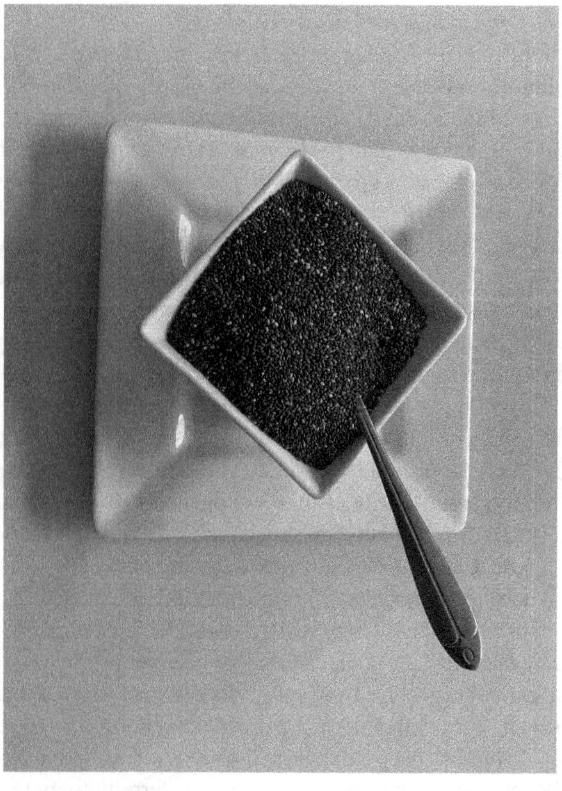

FIGURE 23.2 Chia seeds.

nutritional supplements with or without fiber, with a physician or dietitian. Sweeteners used in oral nutritional supplements include maple syrup, brown rice syrup, corn syrup, corn maltodextrin, glucose syrup, natural sugar, stevia leaf extract, cane sugar, tapioca dextrin, sucralose, fructose, **acesulfame K**, and rice starch. Therefore, it is important to check which sweeteners are present, just like all ingredients, in case of allergies to any of them.

Oral nutritional supplements are generally sterile liquids, but may also be semi-solids or powders. Some of them are specifically indicated for certain conditions, including dysphagia, short bowel syndrome, intractable malabsorption, inflammatory bowel disease, pre-operative preparation of undernourished patients, bowel fistulae, total gastrectomy, and disease-related malnutrition. These supplements may be prescribed for acute illnesses or for long-term chronic conditions. There are also prescription oral nutritional supplements, and individual dietetic assessments take into account nutritional needs, plus taste and texture preferences, so that the prescribed product will be the best that can be tolerated or enjoyed by the patient. The most common types of oral nutritional supplements available include the following:

- Milkshake type – volume 125–200 mL, energy density 1–2.4 kcal/mL, also available with added fiber
- Juice type – volume 200–220 mL, energy density 1.25–1.5 kcal/mL; these products are fat free
- High-energy powders – volume from approximately 125–350 mL, ideally made up with whole milk to provide an energy density of 1.5–2.5 kcal/mL
- Soup type – volume 200–300 mL; some are ready-mixed, while others are powdered that are made up with water or milk to provide an energy density of 1–1.5 kcal/mL
- Semi-solid/dysphagia types – may be thickened liquids (for stage 1 and 2 **dysphagia**) to smooth pudding styles (for stage 3 dysphagia), with an energy density of approximately 1.4–2.5 kcal/mL
- High protein – may be jellies, shots, or milkshake types with 11–20 g of protein, in volumes of 30–200 mL
- Low volume high concentration shots – fat and protein based products, takin in small quantities as "shots", usually 30–40 mL, taken three to four times daily

It is important to mix up the various available flavors in order to avoid taste fatigue. There is an emerging group or oral nutritional supplements designed for people over age 65 who may be at risk of vitamin D deficiency. Others may be good for patients with medical conditions in which fluid and electrolyte balance is important. Patients with short bowel syndrome may not be able to tolerate **hyperosmolar** oral nutritional supplements, since they can cause the patency of a stoma to be reduced.

Oral nutritional supplements should never be prescribed without being monitored, to ensure that they remain appropriate and are being used as prescribed. They may be stopped when dietary intake is sufficient to meet nutritional requirements, the target weight has been reached, the body mass index is within a healthy range, an underlying medical condition has improved sufficiently, or the patient can no longer tolerate them due to taste fatigue.

Test Your Knowledge

1. How can oral nutritional supplements be used to supplement the diet?
2. When taking oral nutritional supplements, how can additional fiber be supplemented?
3. Why do oral nutritional supplements require regular monitoring?

FOCUS ON SOYBEANS

Soybeans are one of the few vegetarian sources of total protein that contain all of the essential amino acids required in the human diet. Soy protein is the primary protein found in soy products, including tofu, tempeh, soy milk, and other soy-based dairy and meat alternatives. It is also found in the form of soy protein powder, which can be used to supplement a workout routine or add more protein to the diet.

ENTERAL TUBE NUTRITION

Enteral tube nutrition is a way of delivering nutrition directly to the stomach or small intestine. Enteral tube nutrition (ETN) is also known as tube feeding or *enteral nutrition*. It is used for patients who cannot ingest enough nutrients by mouth due to being unable or unwilling. Enteral nutrition is better than parenteral nutrition because it offers better preservation of gastrointestinal (GI) structure and function, it is less expensive, and in most cases, it involves less complications such as infections. ETN is specifically indicated for the following conditions:

- Critical illnesses such as burns, which cause metabolic stress
- Inability to take oral feedings because of head or neck trauma
- Liver failure
- Prolonged anorexia
- Severe protein-energy undernutrition
- Coma or **depressed sensorium**

Additional indications include bowel preparation for surgery in a patient that is seriously ill or undernourished, enterocutaneous fistula closure, and small-intestine adaptation after a large intestinal resection, or in disorders causing malabsorption, such as Crohn's disease.

If tube feeding is required for up to four to six weeks, the selected tube is usually of a small internal diameter (caliber) and soft, made of silicone or polyurethane. The tube can be a nasogastric or nasoenteric tube. When the patient has a nasal deformity or injury, and nasal placement would be difficult, an **orogastric** or other oroenteric tube can be put into place. Tube feeding that is needed for more than four to six weeks usually utilizes a gastrostomy or jejunostomy tube (see Figure 23.3). This is put into place endoscopically, radiologically, or surgically. It is chosen based on the capabilities of the physician and the preference of the patient.

Jejunostomy tubes are used if the patient has contraindications to gastrostomy, which include bowel obstruction that is proximal to the jejunum, or gastrectomy. These tubes do not offer any lower risk of tracheobronchial aspiration than gastrostomy tubes, however, even though this is not widely believed by many practitioners. Jejunostomy tubes can be easily dislodged, and are mostly used for inpatients. Feeding tubes are placed via surgery if endoscopic or radiologic placement is unavailable, impossible, or unsafe. For placement, open or **laparoscopic techniques** can be used (see Figure 23.4).

Liquid formulas used for enteral tube feeding commonly include feeding modules and **polymeric formulas**. A feeding formula is a commercially available product. It contains just one nutrient, such as a protein, fat, or carbohydrate. Feeding modules can be used on an individual basis to treat a deficiency, or can be combined with other formulas to totally satisfy nutritional requirements. Polymeric formulas include blenderized food, and commercially available formulas that are milk-based or lactose-free. These formulas usually provide a complete and balanced diet, and for tube or oral feedings, are usually preferred over feeding modules. In hospitalized patients, lactose-free formulas are the

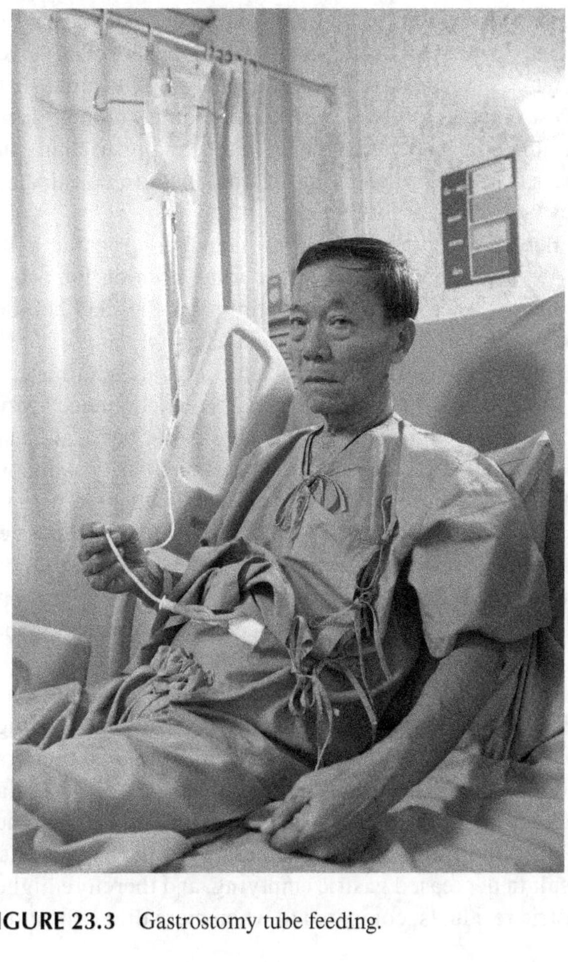

FIGURE 23.3 Gastrostomy tube feeding.

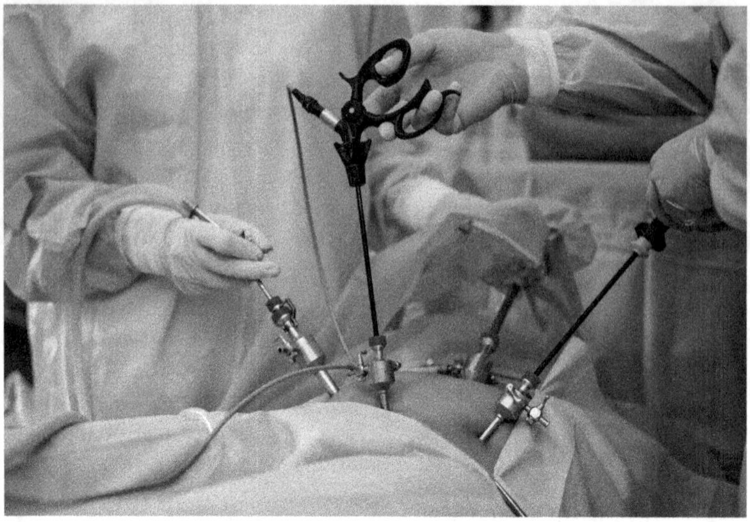

FIGURE 23.4 Laparoscopy.

most commonly used type of polymeric formulas. Even so, milk-based formulas usually have a better taste than lactose-free formulas. A patient with lactose intolerance may tolerate milk-based formulas if they are given slowly by continuous infusion.

Specialized formulas are used for patients that have problems digesting complex proteins. They include **hydrolyzed protein**, and amino acid formulas. These formulas are expensive, and usually not required. The majority of patients with pancreatic insufficiency, if they are given enzymes, and most patients with malabsorption, are able to digest complex proteins. Calorie-dense and protein-dense formulas (for patients that must have fluid restriction) and fiber-enriched formulas (for patients that are constipated) may be successful for therapy.

For tube feeding, the patient should sit upright at a 30° to 45° angle, and remain in the same position for one to two hours after feeding. This minimizes the likelihood of **nosocomial** aspiration pneumonia as gravity aides in propelling the food downward. Tube feedings are administered in **boluses**, several times per day, or via continuous infusion. Bolus feeding is better on a physiologic basis, and may be preferred if the patient has diabetes mellitus. Continuous infusion is required if boluses cause the patient to be nauseous. For bolus feeding, total daily volume is separated into four to six feedings, injected through the tube with a syringe, or infused via gravity from an elevated bag. The tube is flushed with water after feedings, to prevent it from becoming clogged.

Initially, nasogastric, gastrostomy, or nasoduodenal tube feeding often causes diarrhea. Therefore, feedings are usually begun with small amounts of diluted preparations, then increased as tolerated. In most cases, formulas contain 0.5, 1, or 2 kcal/mL. Formulas that have a higher caloric concentration, meaning less water per calorie, may result in decreased gastric emptying, and therefore higher gastric residuals, compared to when more dilute formulas are used that have the same number of calories. At the start, a 1-kcal/mL commercially prepared solution may be administered undiluted at 50 mL/hour. If the patient has not been fed for a while, it may be administered at 25 mL/hour. These solutions do not usually supply enough water – especially if vomiting, diarrhea, sweating, or fever has increased water loss. Therefore, extra water is administered in boluses through the feeding tube or via IV. Once a few days pass, the rate or concentration can be increased as required to meet caloric and hydration needs.

Jejunostomy tube feeding requires more dilution and smaller volumes. Feeding usually starts with a concentration of up to 0.5 kcal/mL, at a rate of 25 mL/h. After a few days pass, the concentrations and volumes can be gradually increased, eventually meeting the patient's caloric and hydration needs. In most cases, the maximum that can be tolerated is 0.8 kcal/mL, at 125 mL/h, which provides 2,400 kcal per day.

Complications of enteral tube feeding are unfortunately common and sometimes serious. They include the following problems, effects, and descriptions:

- *Tube-related complications:*
  - *Presence of the tube* – damage to the esophagus, nose, or pharynx, or sinusitis. If the tube is large, it is more likely to irritate tissues and cause them to erode. With sinusitis, the sinus ostia can become blocked.
  - *Blockage of the tube lumen* – inadequate feeding. Thick feedings or pills sometimes block the lumen (mostly of small tubes). Blockages are sometimes dissolved by instilling a solution of pancreatic enzymes or other commercially available products.
  - *Misplacement of a nasogastric tube intracranially* – brain trauma or an infection. A

tube can be misplaced intracranially if the cribriform plate is disrupted by severe facial trauma.
    - *Misplacement of a nasogastric or orogastric tube in the tracheobronchial tree* – pneumonia. A responsive patient will immediately cough and gag. An obtunded patient will have few immediate symptoms. If the misplacement is not discovered, feedings can enter the lungs (and cause pneumonia).
    - *Dislodgement of a gastrostomy or jejunostomy tube* – peritonitis. Once dislodge, a tube can be replaced into the peritoneal cavity. If a tube was originally placed with an invasive technique, replacement is more difficult to achieve, and more likely to cause complications.

- *Formula-related complications:*
    - *Intolerance of one of the main nutrient components of the formula* – diarrhea, GI discomfort, nausea, vomiting, and occasional mesenteric ischemia. Intolerance occurs in about one of every five patients, and half of all critically ill patients. It is more common with bolus feedings. GI discomfort may have other causes, which include reduced stomach compliance because of shrinkage caused by lack of feeding, distention due to volume of feedings, and decreased gastric emptying because of pyloric dysfunction.
    - *Osmotic diarrhea* – stools that are loose and frequent. Sorbitol, which is often a component of liquid drug preparations administered through feeding tubes, can worsen diarrhea.
    - *Nutrient imbalances* – electrolyte disturbances, hyperglycemia, volume overload, hyperosmolarity. The patient's body weight and blood levels of electrolytes, glucose, magnesium, and phosphate must be monitored frequently. During the first week, this is done daily.

- *Other complications:*
    - *Reflux of tube feedings, or difficulty with oropharyngeal secretions* – aspiration, which may occur even tough tubes are correctly placed, and the head of the bed is elevated if the patient has either of these problems.

Test Your Knowledge

1. What are the reasons that enteral nutrition is better than parenteral nutrition?
2. When is a jejunostomy tube indicated?
3. How does tube feeding occur?

FOCUS ON ENTERAL TUBE FEEDING VS PARENTERAL NUTRITION

In general, enteral nutrition is preferred to parenteral nutrition as it is more physiological, simpler, cheaper, and less complicated. However, even nasogastric feeding requires care, and the more complex types of enteral nutrition, such as gastrostomy and jejunostomy, need great care due to the possibility of becoming dislodged or skin irritation at the site of insertion.

TOTAL PARENTERAL NUTRITION

Total parenteral nutrition (TPN) is given by IV and supplies all of a patient's daily nutritional requirements. It is able to be used in hospitals or at home. Since TPN solutions are concentrated and able to cause **thrombosis** of the peripheral veins, a central venous catheter is usually required. This type of nutrition is not for routine use in a patient with an intact GI tract. In comparison with enteral nutrition, TPN causes more complications, does not preserve structure and function of the GI tract as well, and is more expensive. Another form, *partial parenteral nutrition*, supplies only part of the daily nutritional requirements, and is used to supplement oral intake. Many hospitalized patients receive dextrose or amino acid solutions via this method. TPN is sometimes the only realistic option if a patient does not have a functional GI tract, or has disorders that require total resting of the intestines. These include bowel obstruction, short bowel syndrome (because of surgery), some stages of ulcerative colitis, and in children, disorders such as congenital GI abnormalities and prolonged diarrhea (regardless of its cause). TPN requires the following components:

- *Water* – 30–40 mL/kg of body weight/day
- *Energy* – 30–35 kcal/kg of body weight/day based on energy expenditure (up to 45 kcal/kg/day for a critically ill patient) – medical patients usually need 30–35 kcal/kg/day; postoperative patients need 30–45 kcal/kg/day; and hypercatabolic patients need 45 kcal/kg/day – note that requirements for energy increase by 12% for every 1°C of fever
- *Amino acids* – 1–2 g/kg of body weight/day based on degree of catabolism – medical patients usually need 1 g/kg/day; postoperative patients need 2 g/kg/day; hypercatabolic patients may need 3 g/kg/day
- *Essential fatty acids* – commercially available lipid emulsions are often added to supply these essential fatty acids as well as triglycerides; 20%–30% of total calories are usually supplied as lipids; however, withholding lipids as well as their calories may help an obese patient mobilize endogenous fat stores, which increases insulin sensitivity

- *Vitamins* – ascorbic acid (100 mg), biotin (60 mcg), cobalamin (5 mcg), folate (folic acid, 400 mcg), niacin (40 mg), pantothenic acid (15 mg), pyridoxine (4 mg), riboflavin (3.6 mg), thiamin (3 mg), vitamin A (4,000 International units), vitamin D (10 mcg, or 400 units), vitamin E (15 mg), vitamin K (200 mcg)
- *Minerals* – acetate/gluconate (90 mEq), calcium (15 mEq), chloride (130 mEq), chromium (15 mcg), copper (1.5 mg), iodine (120 mcg), magnesium (20 mEq), manganese (2 mg), phosphorus (300 mg), potassium (100 mEq), selenium (100 mcg), sodium (100 mEq), zinc (5 mg)

Children that require TPN may have different fluid requirements, and need more energy and amino acids. They may require up to 120 kcal/kg/day of energy and up to 2.5 or 3.5 g/kg/day of amino acids.

Basic TPN solutions require sterile techniques for their preparation, which is often done in liter batch sizes based on standard formulas. Usually, 2 liters per day of the standard TPN solution is required. Solutions are modified based on laboratory test results, underlying conditions, hypermetabolism, and a variety of other factors. Most calories are supplied as carbohydrate. Usually, 4–5 mg/kg/minute of dextrose is administered. Standard solutions contain as much as 25% dextrose. However, the amount and concentration are based on the patient's metabolic needs and the proportion of caloric needs supplied by lipids.

Many TPN solutions are quite commonly used. Electrolytes can be added based on the patient's requirements. TPN solutions are adjusted based on other present disorders and the age of the patient. For a patient with renal insufficiency who is not being treated with dialysis, or if a patient has liver failure, the TPN solution contains reduced protein content and has a high percentage of essential amino acids. For a patient with heart or kidney failure, there is a limited volume of liquid intake. For a patient with respiratory failure, there is a lipid emulsion that will provide most non-protein calories, to reduce carbon dioxide production via carbohydrate metabolism. For neonates, dextrose is present in lower concentrations, of 17%–18%.

Strict sterile technique is required during insertion and maintenance of the TPN line since the central venous catheter will remain in place for a long time. The TPN line is not to be used for any other purpose. External tubing must be changed every 24 hours, with the first bag of the day. In-line filters do not decrease complications. Dressings must be kept sterile. They are usually changed every 48 hours, with strict sterile techniques followed. If TPN is administered outside of a hospital, the patient must be taught to recognize infection symptoms. Qualified home nursing must be provided. The solution is started slowly, at 50% of the calculated needs, using 5% dextrose to provide the balance of fluid requirements. Energy and nitrogen are given simultaneously. The patient's plasma glucose level determines the amount of regular insulin that is given, which is added directly to the TPN solution. If the glucose level is normal and the final solution contains 25% dextrose, the usual starting dose will be 5–10 units of regular insulin per liter of TPN fluid.

The patient's progress with the TPN line is followed on a flowchart. For monitoring, an interdisciplinary nutrition team should be involved. A complete blood count should be obtained, and there is regular monitoring of the patient's weight, electrolytes, and **blood urea nitrogen** (BUN). This may be done daily for inpatients. The plasma glucose level should be monitored every 6 hours until the patient and the glucose level have stabilized. There must be continuous monitoring of fluid intake and output. When the patient is stable, blood tests can be done less regularly. Liver tests are required, with twice weekly measurement of **plasma proteins**, plasma, **prothrombin time**, urine osmolality, calcium, magnesium, and phosphate. The plasma proteins monitored include serum albumin, and sometimes **transthyretin**. When possible, blood tests should not be performing during glucose infusion. Full nutritional assessment that includes body mass index calculation and **anthropometric** measurements are to be repeated every two weeks.

Between 5% and 10% of patients with a TPN line experience complications related to central venous access. Catheter-related sepsis rates occur less often, since the introduction of guidelines emphasizing sterile techniques for catheter insertion and skin care in the area surrounding the insertion site. Infections have been reduced because dedicated healthcare terms that specialize in specific procedures, including catheter insertion, are common in today's healthcare systems.

It is important to note that hyperglycemia or hypoglycemia, or liver dysfunction, affect more than 90% of patients on TPN. Hyperglycemia can be avoided by monitoring plasma glucose often and adjusting the insulin dose in the TPN solution, plus by giving subcutaneous insulin when it is required. Hypoglycemia can be avoided by suddenly stopping constant concentrated infusions of dextrose. Treatment is based on the degree of hypoglycemia. Short-term hypoglycemia can be reversed with an IV of 50% dextrose. Extended hypoglycemia may require an infusion of 5% or 10% dextrose for 24 hours before TPN via the central venous catheter can be resumed.

Liver complications include dysfunction, painful hepatomegaly, and hyperammonemia. These can occur at any age, but are usually seen in infants – especially those delivered prematurely. Liver dysfunction can be transient, indicated by increased transaminases, bilirubin, and alkaline phosphatase. It usually occurs when TPN is started. Any delayed or persistent elevations may be due to excess amino acids. The pathogenesis is unknown, but **cholestasis** and inflammatory may be involved. Sometimes, progressive fibrosis develops, so reducing delivery of proteins may be helpful. Painful hepatomegaly suggests an accumulation of fat, so carbohydrate delivery should be reduced. In infants, **hyperammonemia** can develop, resulting in lethargy, twitching, and generalized seizures. This can be corrected by arginine supplementation, at 0.5–1 mmol/kg/day. If any liver complication develops in an infant, the amino acids may need to be limited to 1 g/kg/day.

Abnormalities of serum electrolytes and minerals can be corrected by modifying the additional infusions, or if correction must occur quickly, by starting appropriate infusions into the peripheral veins. When TPN solutions are correctly administered, vitamin and mineral deficiencies are rare. If there is elevated BUN, this may indicate dehydration, which is correctable with administration of free water as 5% dextrose into a peripheral vein. Any volume overload, suggested by more than 1 kg/day of weight gain, can occur if the patient has high daily energy requirements and requires large fluid volumes.

Osteoporosis or osteomalacia sometimes develops in patients on TPN for more than three months, and is not fully understood. Advanced disease may cause severe pain that can be periarticular, in the legs, or in the back. Adverse reactions to lipid emulsions are not common, but can occur early, especially if the lipids are given as more than 1 kcal/kg/hour. The reactions may include cutaneous allergic reactions, dyspnea, headache, back pain, nausea, sweating, and dizziness. Temporary hyperlipidemia can occur, especially in patients with kidney or liver failure, but treatment is usually not needed. Delayed adverse reactions to lipid emulsions include hepatomegaly, slight elevation of liver enzymes, splenomegaly, leukopenia, thrombocytopenia, and (mostly in premature infants that have respiratory distress syndrome), abnormalities of pulmonary function. These adverse reactions can be prevented or reduced by temporarily or permanently slowing or stopping infusion of lipid emulsions.

Gallbladder complications may include **cholelithiasis**, **cholecystitis**, and gallbladder sludge (see Figure 23.5). The complications can be caused or exacerbated by chronic gallbladder stasis. Stimulating gallbladder contraction by providing 20%–30% of calories as fat, and stopping glucose infusion for several hours per day, is helpful, as is oral or enteral intake. For some patients with cholestasis, metronidazole, ursodeoxycholic acid, phenobarbital, or **cholecystokinin** is helpful.

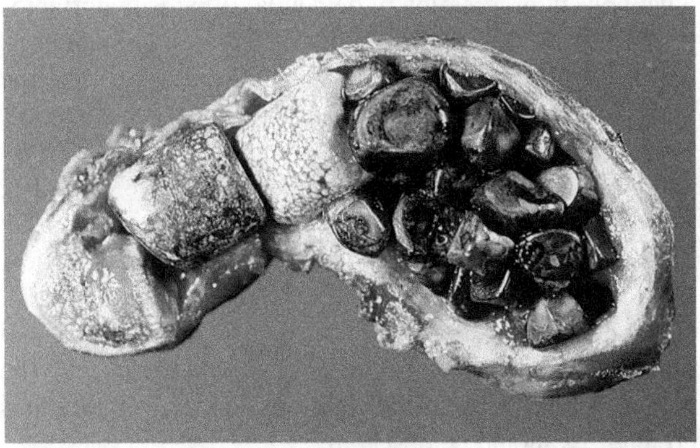

FIGURE 23.5 Resected gallbladder with cholelithiasis (gallstones).

Test Your Knowledge

1. When is total parenteral nutrition the only realistic option for feeding a patient?
2. What components are present in total parenteral nutrition?
3. What conditions affect most patients who are on TPN?

NUTRITIONAL THERAPY FOR DYING PATIENTS

A terminally ill patient eventually loses all appetite, and tube feeding or IV feeding methods may be required – this is often a concern for family members. Even so, for a dying patient, nutritional support appears not to have any benefit since it does not really prolong life or improve quality of life. Many healthcare professionals believe that in the days before death, the patient may actually made less comfortable if given nutritional support, or made to eat more than they want. Dying patients are usually not distressed by feeling hungry and are mostly more comfortable to eat and drink as they want to. As the body starts to shut down, the person may lose all desire to eat or drink. When death is not expected to occur within hours or days, nutritional support may be attempted for a limited time to see if the patient's comfort, energy, or mental clarity improves – this is often not the case. There should be an explicit agreement between the patient, family members, and healthcare team about when to try nutritional support and when to stop it. An *advance directive* is used for this purpose.

Regardless, family members and caregivers may offer food to the dying patient slowly, in small portions. The patient's favorite foods, strongly flavored foods, or easy-to-swallow foods are suggested. Even a small amount of a preferred alcoholic drink can be offered 30 minutes before meals. It is most important to allow the dying patient to make all food or drink choices. Sometimes, appetite stimulants or antidepressants such as megestrol or dronabinol are helpful. Comforting care to the dying patient may include brushing the teeth, moistening the mouth with wet cloths as needed, giving the patient ice chips, or applying lip balm. Hospice care personnel are trained in providing these types of support (see Figure 23.6). Sometimes, family members need counseling to understand the use or stoppage of nutritional support.

NUTRITIONAL THERAPY FOR ANOREXIA NERVOSA

For patients with **anorexia nervosa**, nutritional supplementation is often used along with behavioral therapy. Supplementation begins by providing 30–40 kcal/kg/day, and can result in weight gains of up to 1.5 kg/week in inpatient care, and 0.5 kg/week in outpatient care. Oral feedings with solid foods are preferred, but many weight restoration plans also include liquid supplements. Resistant undernourished patients may require nasogastric tube feedings. For

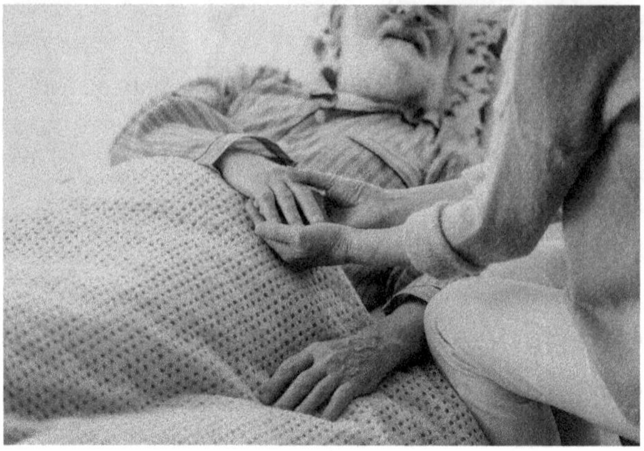

FIGURE 23.6 A patient in hospice care.

bone loss, elemental calcium at 1,200–1,500 mg/day and vitamin D at 600–800 International units per day are often prescribed. Long-term treatment begins only after nutritional, fluid, and electrolyte status are stabilized, with psychotherapy being highly important. Treatments continue for one year after weight has been restored. For adolescents, family members are taught correct feeding techniques with supervised family meals. Nutritionists can provide specific meal plans or information about calories to restore weight to a normal level. Some patients also require medications such as olanzapine to aid weight gain.

For a person with anorexia nervosa, the long periods of starvation may have caused biochemical abnormalities, including deficiencies in proteins, micronutrients, and fatty acids. Therefore, special dietary plans must be created so that additional problems are not caused as the imbalances are corrected. Weight should not be gained until deficiencies are corrected. Aggressive attempts to boost weight gain in the early stages of treatment may be very hazardous. The patient may find nutritional therapy challenging and upsetting because of the altered connection they have with food. If weight loss symptoms are severe and health is critical, the patient is admitted to a special recovery unit in a hospital. Forced nutritional therapy is only done if the patient is likely to die without medical help. For patients discharged from inpatient treatment that still require support and monitoring, daycare treatment is beneficial. It is usually recommended if an outpatient suffers a slight relapse.

For recovery, patients should start by eating very small amounts of food, increasing intake gradually over time. It is important to develop a routine, eating food regularly a certain times each day, consisting of three well-balanced meals. There should be a target weight set, providing a goal for the patient. A weight gain of just 0.5–1 kg per week is widely recommended, achieved by eating 3,500–7,000 extra calories per week. Daily intake of foods containing protein of high biological value is recommended, such as whey, casein, and egg white, which contain a high concentration of essential amino acids per gram and calorie density. Consuming these foods along with foods perceived by the patient to be less "challenging" – usually vegetables – help gain a quicker restoration of nutrient status even when the body is still underweight. A variety of protein sources, including fleshy fish and poultry, should be encouraged. Recommended Daily Allowances for vitamins and minerals are varied by age and gender. They can be met by use of multivitamin and multimineral tablets or liquids. Placing emphasis on nutrient intake opposed to caloric intake can help reduce anxiety and resistance to refeeding.

Test Your Knowledge

1. What type of agreement should be drawn up regarding nutritional therapy for a dying patient?
2. What biochemical abnormalities does anorexia nervosa cause?
3. For recovery, what food regimen is used for a patient with anorexia nervosa?

NUTRITIONAL THERAPY FOR DEMENTIA

People with dementia experience forgetfulness, memory loss, personality changes, and impaired thinking. Many are unable to follow a special diet, and dementia patients often struggle with their body weight. Weight loss is common and usually worsens as the condition progresses. Some individuals forget to eat. Other reasons for weight loss in the dementia patient include faulty appetite triggers in the brain, medications that reduce appetite, reduced senses of smell and taste, difficulty focusing on eating resulting in less food consumed, reduced coordination that impairs eating, and chewing or swallowing problems. Some patients are prescribed diets that include softer foods to encourage intake, or thickened liquids for easier swallowing. With severe dementia, the individual may not be able to distinguish food from non-food objects, causing intake of items that are not digestible, or that have toxic properties.

Supplements may be required for vitamin or mineral deficiencies. The Mediterranean diet, dietary approaches to stop hypertension (DASH) diet, and Mediterranean-DASH dietary intervention for neurodegenerative delay (MIND) diet have been studied in reference to abilities that somewhat prevent progression of dementia. What is important is that the individual eats a variety of foods to provide good nutrition. Increased calories may be needed because the individual starts to move around more due to the dementia. Oral nutrition supplements are often recommended to get sufficient calories and nutrients to maintain weight. Also, thirst sensation decreases with age, leading to increased risks for dehydration. Fluid intake should be encouraged, and foods rich in water (fruits and vegetables) are helpful. Many dementia patients cannot shop or prepare food and require assistance from a caregiver. Foods enjoyed by the patient should be selected, and any cultural or religious preferences should be observed.

Mealtimes are an important part of the process, with meals served at a table to help the individual focus on eating.

Distractions should be minimized so that the individual can focus. A family-style setting is preferred since it may encourage the person to eat more as part of the group. With increased memory loss, verbal prompts may be needed to encourage the individual to eat. Bite-sized finger foods may be helpful since utensils are not required. Modified food textures are often prescribed since they are easier to chew and swallow.

With progression of dementia, other forms of assistance may be needed. Changes in eating or drinking habits should be discussed with healthcare providers. Registered dietitian nutritionists, speech language pathologists, and occupational therapists are skilled at helping dementia patients and their caregivers. The patient's nutritional needs are discussed and an individualized eating plan is developed, taking into account personal food preferences and abilities for self-feeding.

FOCUS ON MIND DIET FOR DEMENTIA PATIENTS

The MIND diet can significantly lower risks for developing Alzheimer's disease. It is also known as the *Mediterranean-DASH Intervention for Neurodegenerative Delay diet.* It lowers risks for AD as much as 53% in individuals that adhere to it rigorously, and by about 35% in those that follow it moderately well. The 15 dietary components of the MIND diet are 10 brain-healthy food groups (green leafy vegetables, other vegetables, nuts, berries, beans, whole grains, fish, poultry, olive oil, and wine) and five unhealthy groups (red meats, butter and stick margarine, cheese, pastries and sweets, and fried or fast food).

NUTRITIONAL THERAPY FOR HEAD AND NECK CANCER

Most head and neck cancers are **squamous cell carcinomas**. This type of cancer begins in the flat squamous cells that make up the thin layer of tissue on the surface of structures in the head and neck, including the nasal cavity, mouth, oral cavity, tongue, salivary glands, throat, and larynx. Head and neck cancer starts in this region and does not metastasize from another body area. Mouth cancer is the most common type of head and neck cancer. *Laryngeal cancer* is a throat cancer that is also very common. People being treated for head and neck cancer have unique and sometimes difficult challenges with eating and maintaining healthy nutrition. Treatments can cause weight loss, fatigue, diarrhea, nausea, constipation, low white blood cells count, and increased risks for infection. Therefore, the ability to stay nourished can be inhibited, which may impact treatment. Some patients experience discomfort and pain while chewing and swallowing, as well as loss of taste sensation. Eating many soft and moist foods can help alleviate painful side effects of eating as treatment is continuing, and afterwards. A blender can be used to puree fruits and vegetables as well as to create soups. It is very important to drink plenty of water and liquids to minimize symptoms of dry mouth.

More protein should be added to the diet. Shakes and smoothies can be made out of protein powder, low-fat milk, soy milk, or rice milk, and fruits can be added to improve the flavor. Cancer-fighting foods should be consumed as much as possible. High levels of *phytochemicals* from plants strengthen the immune system and fight infections, so plenty of fruits and vegetables are beneficial. Red berries and green tea are also recommended. Fish oils are excellent additions to nutritional therapy for head and neck cancer. They contain fatty acids that are needed as part of this therapy, are available in liquid or capsule forms, contain natural anti-inflammatory properties, promote healing, and help maintain weight. Foods that cause discomfort should be avoided. Sharp or crunchy foods should be avoided, as well as those that require a lot of chewing. Spicy or acidic foods should be also limited since they can cause mouth pain. Drinks or food products that contain alcohol (such as rum cake) should be avoided. Patients should discuss nutritional supplements with their physicians. Vitamin supplements are important – especially vitamins B and D. Zinc may stimulate taste sensations, so it is important as well.

As part of monitoring patients undergoing therapy for head and neck cancer, tracking the weight helps assess that nutritional efforts are on course. Patients should weigh themselves every three to five days, or as often as the clinical dietitian nutritionist asks them to, and always around the same time each weighing day. The same amount of clothes should be worn each time the patient steps on the scale, and the same scale should always be used. It is normal to lose weight during therapy for head and neck cancer, but the nutritionist can help keep excessive weight loss from occurring. The dietary needs will probably need to be adjusted based on the common side effects of therapy, which occur generally in the following schedule:

- Weeks 1–3 – taste changes or lack of taste, mouth sores, fatigue, decreased appetite
- Weeks 4–6 – taste changes or lack of taste, mouth sores, painful swallowing, fatigue, decreased appetite, thick mucus or phlegm, dry mouth, nausea
- Two weeks after treatment ends – same as for weeks 4–6
- One month after treatment ends – taste changes or lack of taste, painful swallowing, thick mucus or phlegm, dry mouth

For taste changes or lack of taste, marinades, herbs, or spices can be added to food – however, these should not be added if there are mouth sores or painful swallowing. If the patient has a metallic taste sensation, plastic utensils should be used instead of metal utensils, and drinking out of cans should be avoided. Some previously favored foods may need to be limited or avoided because they may not taste the same. This helps prevents the creation of negative thoughts about the "new" flavors of these foods, so that in the future, when treatment is done, the patient will be able to once again enjoy foods that were previously favored.

For mouth sores and painful swallowing, soft and bland foods should be eaten. Extremely hot foods and drinks should be avoided. Acidic fruits or fruit juices, spicy foods should be avoided. Patients should rinse their mouths every 4–6 hours, or more often if needed for comfort. The following options can be used for rinsing:

- One quart of water mixed with one teaspoon of salt and one teaspoon of baking soda
- One quart of water mixed with one teaspoon of salt
- One quart of water mixed with one teaspoon of baking soda
- Plain water
- A mouthwash with no alcohol or sugar

To rinse, the liquid should be swished around and gargled for 15–30 seconds, then spit out. If mouth pain or painful swallowing still continue, a prescription medication may be needed. There may also be a need for a referral to a swallowing specialist, who can recommended foods and liquids that are safe and easy to swallow.

For fatigued patients, ready-made or quickly cooked foods may be helpful. Single-serving items such as cottage cheese, yogurt, hard boiled eggs, canned creamy soups, tuna salad, or pre-cooked rotisserie chicken may be good options. For decreased appetite, eat small meals often and avoid large, heavy meals (such as six smaller meals during the day instead of three large ones). Foods that are high in calories and protein are emphasized. Eating should occur in a pleasant environment, and with family and friends if they are comforting. For thick mucus in the throat, clear liquids should be sipped on during the day, such as water, non-acidic fruit juice, sports drinks, broth, or nutrition drinks designed to reduce mucus. Another option is to drink warm water or warm tea with honey. If there are no mouth sores, gargling with club soda may be helpful.

For dry mouth, soft and moist foods should be chosen, such as pudding, yogurt, and watermelon. Ice pops or popsicles are a good option. To moisten foods, add liquids such as gravies, sauces, or applesauce. While eating, drink a spoonful of warm soup or other liquid between mouthfuls of solid foods. Foods made with gelatin are usually helpful. Carry bottled water on a regular basis. Also, spray bottles full of water may be helpful to assist with dry mouth. Sugar-free mints or lemon drops, or sugar-free gum can help create more saliva. Fruit nectars are suggested, such as apricot, peach, or pear. There are also over-the-counter (OTC) saliva supplements for dry mouth. Avoid alcoholic drinks, beverages with caffeine, mouthwashes that contain alcohol, and dry or starchy foods.

For nausea, avoid spicy foods, high-fat and fried foods, and do not lay down immediately after eating. If food odors cause nausea, try eating food at room temperature or cold instead of hot foods. Smaller, frequent meals help fight off nausea more than larger, less frequent meals. It is important to eat and chew slowly so that it is better digested. Drinking large amounts of liquids at once should be avoided because getting too full can worsen nausea. Products that contain ginger are helpful, including ginger tea, **ginger ale**, non-alcoholic ginger beer, and candies that contain real ginger. Low-fat, starchy foods can often be tolerated well, such as rice, white toast, crackers, whole grain oat cereals, melba toast, or angel food cake. Salty foods such as pretzels or saltine crackers may also be tolerated well. If adverse effects of head and neck cancer therapy are making it too difficult to eat, a feeding tube may be required.

For patients that are still able to eat normally, choose foods that are high in protein in all meals and snacks, including poultry, meat, eggs, beans, nuts, nut butters, and dairy products. Adding good sources of calories is also important, including nuts and nut butters, avocados, olive or canola oils, and whole fat dairy products. If more calories are needed, choose drinks that have calories instead of water, such as fruit juices or nectars, and liquid nutritional supplements. However, diabetic patients should discuss these options with a physician or clinical dietitian nutritionist before using them in order to help control blood glucose. Hydration is important, so many fluids need to be consumed during and after treatment for head and neck cancer.

Homemade nutritional shakes or smoothies are also recommended, and for some patients, become the only food options that can be tolerated near the end of cancer treatment. Bases for these shakes or smoothies can consist of commercially available nutritional liquids. Mix-in products that can be added include whole or almond milk, heavy cream, cream of coconut, banana, full-fat ice cream, 2% plain Greek yogurt, vegetable oil, **Benecalorie**, whey protein powder, plant-based protein powder, peanut butter, powdered peanut butter, milk powder, and mixed berries.

Soft and bland foods include milk and dairy products such as whole milk, plain or well-blended yogurt without fruit pieces, pasteurized eggnog, cottage cheese, thin ricotta cheese, and mild or processed cheese that is melted into a sauce. For vegetables, carrot and other vegetable juices are good choices, plus well-cooked diced vegetables (carrots, green beans, peas, beets, butternut squash, wax beans), and chopped or creamed spinach. For fruits, non-acidic fruits juices and nectars (apple and pear), smooth applesauce, any canned fruits that can be tolerated, any cooked fruits without the skin, and ripe bananas are all good options. Choices of starches include cooked cereals, cream of wheat, farina, cream of rice, oatmeal, hominy grits, whipped or smooth masked white or sweet potatoes, well-cooked paste, white or brown rice, soft whole grains such as barley and farro, soft rolls, soft muffins, soft French toast, pancakes, and dry cereal soaked in a small amount of milk. For fats and oils, choices include butter, margarine, sour cream, cooking fats or oils, gravy, whipped toppings or heavy cream, cream-style salad dressings (with acidic dressings avoided), and avocado. For meats and meat substitutes, try tender cooked meat, fish, and poultry, chicken salad, tuna salad, egg salad without celery or onion, meatloaf, meatballs, salmon loaf or croquettes, casseroles, baked or broiled fish (filet of sole, roughy, flounder, salmon), scrambled eggs or souffle, plain cheese quiche, hummus, well-cooked beans, and tofu. For soups, excellent choices include broth, bouillon, soups with pureed or strained vegetables, cream soups, chicken noodle, and chicken rice soup. Sweets and desserts may include plain custards or puddings, sherbet, ice cream, frozen yogurt, milkshakes, gelatin desserts, flavored fruit ices, popsicles, fruit whips, seedless jelly, honey, maple syrup, sugar or sugar substitutes, chocolate syrup, pies without crust, pastries and cakes without seeds or nuts, and soft cookies. Drinks may need to be watered down. Miscellaneous options include herbs, syrups, and gravies.

One month after treatment has finished, pureed or soft solid foods can become a regular part of the diet, such as ¼ cup per meal, at least three times per day. Nutritional supplements are also indicated, as needed. It is advisable to keep a daily food and drink log, or to use a phone app such as *MyFitnessPal*.

FOCUS ON RISK FACTORS FOR HEAD AND NECK CANCER

The primary risk factors associated with head and neck cancer include tobacco use, alcohol consumption, human papillomavirus (HPV) infection (for oropharyngeal cancer), and Epstein-Barr virus (EBV) infection (for nasopharyngeal cancer). Worldwide, head and neck cancer accounts for approximately 900,000 cases and over 400,000 deaths annually. In the United States, head and neck cancer accounts for 3% of malignancies, with approximately 66,000 cases annually and 15,000 deaths.

Test Your Knowledge

1. How is loss of thirst sensation combated in older patients with dementia?
2. How do phytochemicals assist in the treatment of patients with head and neck cancer?
3. What dietary elements should be used for a patient with head and neck cancer that is experiencing nausea?

NUTRITIONAL THERAPY FOR ESOPHAGEAL CANCER

Esophageal cancer develops in the esophagus, which is the tube that connects the oropharynges to the stomach. Tumors arise in the mucosa, which is the inner lining of the esophagus (see Figure 23.7). There are two types of esophageal cancer, each with different risk factors: adenocarcinoma and squamous cell carcinoma. **Adenocarcinoma** starts in gland cells at the bottom of the esophagus. It is the most common esophageal cancer and usually occurs closer to the stomach. Chronic acid reflux, gastroesophageal reflux disease, **Barrett's esophagus**, and chronic heartburn can increase the risk of developing esophageal cancer. Squamous cell carcinoma arises from squamous cells that are primarily located in the upper esophagus. They are associated with heavy alcohol consumption, smoking, and organ transplants. Difficulty swallowing is the first symptom, followed by pain in throat or behind the sternum, vomiting, hematemesis, and unintentional weight loss.

For esophageal cancer, there is usually difficulty eating and weight loss. Therefore, good nutrition is an important part of the treatment plan. Treatments such as surgery, chemotherapy, radiation therapy, and others can all affect the ability to eat and get adequate nutrition. Esophageal cancer narrows the esophagus and makes it painful to swallow. A diet of soft and high-protein foods may be helpful. Tube feeding may be required for some patients. Parenteral nutrition is also sometimes required. For overweight patients, there should be a consultation with a physician or dietitian before calories are added to the diet during treatment for esophageal cancer. Otherwise, patients can add foods high in calories and protein. If swallowing is still difficult, there may be a need to soften foods with gravies or sauces. Some foods may need to be chopped up into small pieces. After surgery for esophageal cancer, the stomach may be smaller and fill up quickly, so smaller meals can be eaten more often during the day. Fluids before meals should be avoided so that they don't fill up the stomach and take the place of the higher nutrition found in the actual meals themselves. Snacks can be eaten in between meals, such as calorie-dense choices (cheese with crackers, toast with peanut butter, hummus with crackers, yogurt with fruit, and cereal with whole milk and fruit). Sipping fluids while eating may help make swallowing easier and help food pass through the esophagus. Butter, margarine, or oil should be added to foods whenever possible.

During and after therapy, patients are provided with enteral nutrition because the upper GI tract can no longer receive full nutrition. Parenteral nutrition is only recommended if the small intestine is not functional or enteral nutrition is not possible. Many patients rely on tube feeding for most of their nutritional needs during treatment. Some of them find that swallowing function improves within weeks of starting chemoradiation due to tumor shrinkage, and they regain the ability to eat. Jejunostomy tubes are often placed before chemotherapy and radiation, or during an **esophagectomy** procedure. These tubes allow for early postoperative feeding beyond the area of surgical **anastomosis**, and are preferred to gastrostomy tubes, since a gastrostomy could complicate surgical use of the stomach to form a new esophagus.

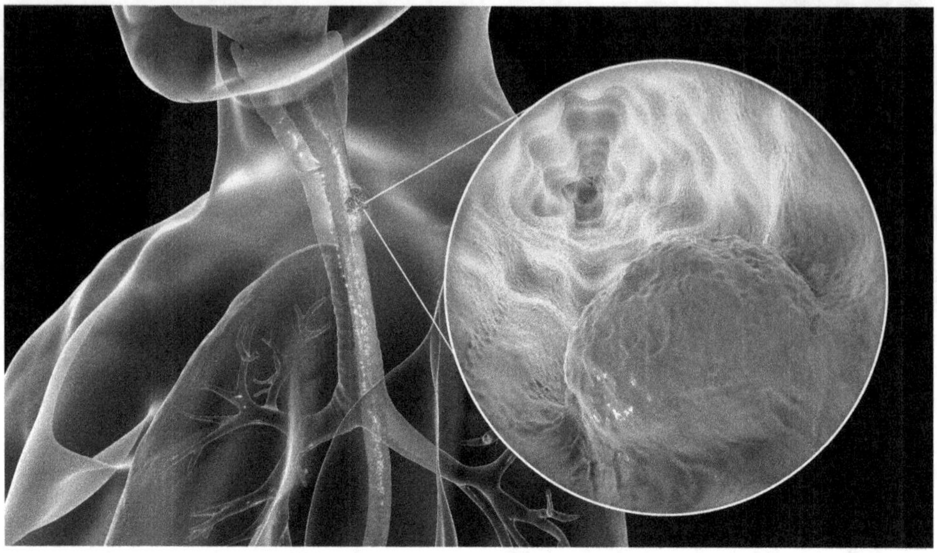

FIGURE 23.7 Esophageal cancer.

A high-protein formula is fed through a pump at a low rate, with feeding gradually advanced over several days. A 1.5 kcal/mL product offers more nutrition when the rate is low during the early postoperative period. Once enteral nutrition tolerance is established, patients are transitioned to nocturnal feeding cycles. Most patients at home prefer to receive enteral nutrition at night to be free of the feeding pump, and to have less fullness as they advance to an oral diet during the day. **Refeeding syndrome** is risk for patients that have lost a large amount of body weight, for those with little to no nutritional intake for at least seven days, or for those who have used alcohol excessively. These highly malnourished patients should be underfed for several days to prevent dangerous intercellular shifts in phosphorus, potassium, and magnesium levels. Caloric intake is adjusted gradually over three to five days if serum electrolyte levels are normal. Extra vitamin supplementation should be supplied. For weight maintenance, 25–30 kcal/kg is usually enough. If the patient must gain weight, energy needs can be as high as 35–40 kcal/kg. Protein requirements are usually 1.5 g/kg. Sufficient water is 30 mL/kg, though more may be needed if the patient has diarrhea, chest tube drainage, or extreme thirst.

When **chylothorax** occurs after surgery, dietary fat must be limited to minimize chyle flow and promote healing. If closure doesn't occur on its own, additional surgery may be needed. Most patients tolerate a nearly fat-free diet high in protein and carbohydrate. The enteral nutrition product used must be a low-fat, elemental type formula, low in long-chain fatty acids, with a significant proportion of fat content in the form of medium-chain triglycerides.

For patients with **bloating**, fullness, or nausea, the enteral nutrition feeding rate can be decreased, two shorter feeding cycles can replace one longer cycle, a more concentrated formula can be used to decrease volume, the patient's upper body can be elevated, and antinausea medications can be given. Fiber-free formulas are sometimes helpful. Prune juice, stool softeners, or laxatives are sometimes indicated. For diarrhea, medications should first be reviewed, followed by tests for infections, followed by antidiarrheal medications. If maldigestion is suspected, soluble fiber can be added, the feeding rate can be slowed, smaller feeding cycles can be initiated, or elemental enteral nutrition formulas can be used.

After esophagectomy, nothing is given by mouth for one week. When anastomotic leak is ruled out, clear liquids and then full liquids are started. A week later, the postesophagectomy diet begins, with small and frequent meals of soft moist foods that do not become tough or thick. Carbonated beverages are avoided. If **dumping syndrome** occurs, sugars are avoided and fluids with meals are limited. The upper body of the patient must remain elevated at night to reduce reflux. The patient is closely monitored. Tube feedings are usually reduced to one per night for several days. If oral intake improves and weight is returning to normal, tube feedings are decreased by one can of enteral nutrition solution per night until completely weaned off of the tube. Other foods are reintroduced at the discretion of the surgeon.

Patients with esophageal cancer often have loss of muscle mass, muscle strength, or both. **Sarcopenia** and cachexia are prognostic factors for surgical complications, decreased survival, and poor response to chemotherapy. The surgical procedure of esophagectomy is one of the most invasive, time-consuming operations of all GI surgical procedures. Surgical advances have increased integrity of anastomoses, making early oral enteral feeding a feasible option. Supplemental parenteral nutrition after esophagectomy contributes to better coverage of the patient's calorie requirements since large amounts of enteral nutrition are not usually tolerated in the first postoperative days. The daily guidelines of postoperative care of patients with the popular *fast-track surgery pathway* are as follows:

- Day 1 – jejunostomy tube feeding 500 mL, starting at 20 mL per hour, early postoperative mobilization program, two or more hours out of bed, physical therapy and nebulizers, remove urine catheter, head of bed raised to 30°, supply albumin, chest tube to suction, promoted to lung recruitment
- Day 2 – jejunostomy tube feeding 1,000 mL (40 mL/hour), chest tube to suction, expand mobilization with four or more hours out of bed, continue physical therapy and nebulizers, continue to supply albumin
- Day 3 – jejunostomy tube feeding 1,500 mL (60–80 mL/hour), remove chest tube and epidural catheter, expand mobilization with six or more hours out of bed, continue physical therapy and nebulizers, continue to supply albumin
- Day 4 – **Gastrografin** opacification of upper gastrointestinal tract, if swallow shows no leak, then advance patient to oral drinking, jejunostomy tube feeding 1,500 mL (60–80 mL/hour), continue physical therapy and nebulizers, provide education on aspiration precautions, and on chewing and swallowing
- Day 5 – Jejunostomy tube feeding 1,500 mL (60–80 mL/h), advance patient to a full liquid diet, continue aspiration precautions, physical therapy, and nebulizers
- Day 6 – Increase liquid diet, decrease jejunostomy tube feeding (500 or 1,000 mL), continue aspiration precautions, physical therapy, and nebulizers
- Day 7 – Remove jejunostomy tube, full liquid diet, discharge home on soft and liquid diet, continue aspiration precautions

FOCUS ON OUTCOMES OF ESOPHAGEAL CANCER AND ITS TREATMENT

Esophageal cancer and its treatment can cause severe and complicated nutrition issues. However, early intervention and consistent nutritional follow-up throughout the treatment course can help patients transition to normalcy successfully.

Test Your Knowledge

1. What are the two types of esophageal cancer?
2. When a patient with esophageal cancer has problems swallowing, what are the options?
3. After esophagectomy, what does the patient receive for nourishment?

NUTRITIONAL THERAPY FOR PANCREATITIS

Pancreatitis is caused by inappropriate activation of the pancreatic enzymes. This results in autodigestion of pancreatic tissue. Acute pancreatitis is one of the most common GI reasons for hospital admission in the United States. Chronic pancreatitis greatly impairs quality of life. For both, nutrition is an important factor in treatment and management. Pancreatitis can lead to life threatening complications. In most (40%–70%) cases, gallstones are the primary cause. They can cause inflammation as they pass through a bile or pancreatic duct and get lodged there. Many cases, 25%–35%, are due to heavy alcohol use of more than 50 g per day for over five years. Acute pancreatitis also occurs in people with triglyceride levels over 1 g/dL, or if they have benign or malignant pancreatic tumors. Recurrent episodes of acute pancreatitis can lead to chronic pancreatitis. This can then lead to permanent damage. Symptoms include abdominal pain that can become constant, and often worsens after eating. The pain in the upper abdomen that may spread to the back, chest, or sides of the abdomen (flanks). Fever, nausea, and vomiting can also be present. For unknown reasons, as chronic pancreatitis progresses, the pain may be lessened. The signs and symptoms for chronic pancreatitis may include diarrhea, oily and foul-smelling stools, and weight loss.

Treatments for pancreatitis include pain medications, alcohol and smoking cessation, pancreatic enzyme replacement therapy, **proton pump inhibitors**, insulin-sensitizing medications, IV fluids, antibiotics, surgical interventions and rarely, removal of the pancreas or gallbladder.

Nutritional therapy for acute pancreatitis generally begins with avoiding all foods by mouth for an individually determined period of time. TPN can provide nutrition during this time, but must be monitored closely since intestinal resting is linked to atrophy of the intestinal mucosa and worsening of small intestinal barrier function in about 60% of patients, which can lead to serious complications. There is also a risk of infections from the central venous catheter. Enteral nutrition can be used to protect the intestinal mucosa and prevents bacterial overgrowth by stimulating gut motility. It can reduce systemic infections, multiorgan failure, and death. Enteral nutrition started within 48 hours of admission reduces the rate of major infections, and sometimes, death. The nasojejunal route is preferred because it greatly reduces stimulation of the pancreas will still prompting gut motility, but nasojejunal tubes are relatively difficult to place and require specialized staff members. Therefore, the nasogastric tube feeding method is just as often recommended. In more recent studies, oral feeding (after 72 hours following hospitalization) has not caused any major problems.

Nutritional therapy for chronic pancreatitis is different. Ongoing management includes nutrition, supplemental digestive enzymes, and cessation of tobacco and alcohol use. Malnutrition is common due to increased energy expenditure plus pain-related loss of appetite or a fear of eating, pancreatic enzyme insufficiency, delayed gastric emptying, and continued alcohol abuse. Therefore, high-protein, high-calorie foods are recommended to be consumed in five to six small meals per day. High-fiber diets are avoided. Protein intake of 1–1.5 g/kg is usually sufficient and well tolerated. Usually, foods supplemented with pancreatic enzymes before each meal or snack works well, but 10%–15% of patients need oral nutritional supplements and 5% need enteral nutrition. Based on what is tolerated, whole protein based or peptide based oral nutritional supplements can be given. Patients at risk of unintended weight loss may supplement with MCT oil. This is absorbed directly into the bloodstream without a need for pancreatic enzymes. This oil is found in coconut and **palm kernel oils** and is also available as a supplement.

Supplements may include multivitamins, calcium, folate, iron, and vitamins A, B12, D, and E. Chronic pancreatitis causes the pancreas to eventually lose endocrine function, putting the individual at risk for type 1 diabetes mellitus. Refined sugars and simple carbohydrates must therefore be avoided. If pancreatic enzymes are prescribed, they must be taken regularly in order to prevent flare-ups.

FOCUS ON COMPLICATIONS OF CHRONIC PANCREATITIS

Persistent abdominal pain, pancreatic scarring, diabetes mellitus, and pancreatic cancer are all complications of chronic pancreatitis. Maldigestion, malnutrition, and malabsorption may occur, and can lead to osteopenia and osteoporosis, leading to bone fractures.

FOCUS ON PALM KERNEL OILS

Palm oil is used for preventing vitamin A deficiency, cancer, brain disease, skin aging, and in the treatment of treating malaria, high blood pressure, high cholesterol, and cyanide poisoning. Palm oil is used for weight loss and increasing the body's metabolism. As a food product, palm oil is used for frying.

Test Your Knowledge

1. What is the primary cause of pancreatitis?
2. How does nutritional therapy for acute pancreatitis usually begin?
3. How is nutritional therapy for chronic pancreatitis different?

NUTRITIONAL THERAPY FOR BONE MARROW TRANSPLANTATION

Bone marrow transplantation may use healthy blood stem cells from a patient's own body (**autologous** transplant) or from a donor (**allogeneic** transplant). It consists of administration of high-dose chemoradiotherapy, followed by IV infusion of **hemopoietic stem cells** to reestablish function of damaged or defective marrow. It is used in the treatment of solid tumors, acute and chronic leukemias, **multiple myeloma**, immune deficiencies, **hemoglobinopathies**, and **aplastic anemia** (see Figure 23.8). Newer techniques include peripheral blood progenitor cell transplants, with autologous or allogenic infusion of hemopoietic stem cells collected from peripheral blood after administration of **hemopoietic growth factors**, or cord blood transplantation, using infusion of hemopoietic stem cells harvested from cord and placental blood immediately after delivery.

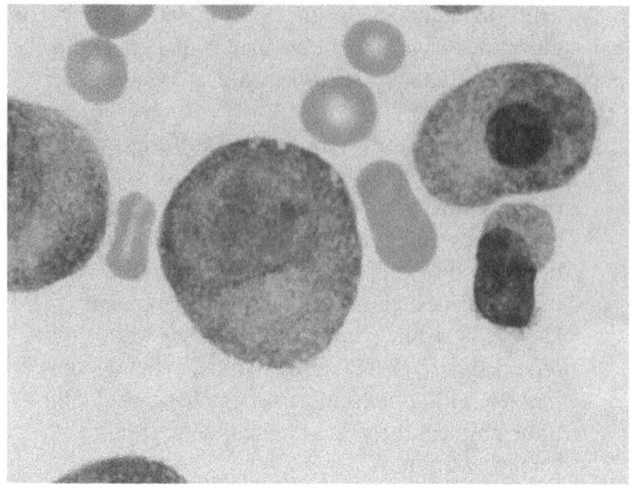

FIGURE 23.8 Multiple myeloma cells shown via Wright staining.

After bone marrow transplant, the patient may need to adjust the diet to stay healthy and to prevent excessive weight gain. A dietitian and other members of transplant team will work with the patient to create a healthy eating plan that meets the needs and complements of lifestyle. The dietitian can also give food suggestions to control side effects of chemotherapy and radiation, such as nausea. Some of the dietitian's recommendations may include:

- Following food safety guidelines to prevent foodborne infections
- Eating a wide variety of healthy foods, including vegetables, fruits, whole grains, lean meats, poultry, fish, legumes, and healthy fats such as olive oil
- Limiting salt intake
- Restricting alcohol
- Avoiding grapefruit and grapefruit juice due to their effect on a group of immunosuppressive medications

FOCUS ON NUTRITIONAL COMPLICATIONS

Bone marrow transplantation often results in nutritional complications. Common conditions that affect dietary intake include mucosal membrane injuries, nausea, vomiting, and anorexia. Most often, patients receive a sterile, low-microbial, modified, or normal diet.

NUTRITIONAL THERAPY FOR CHEMOTHERAPY AND RADIOTHERAPY

The effects of chemotherapy and radiotherapy upon cancer patients have been well documented for many years. Chemotherapy agents can be single agents or those used in combination, based on the type of cancer and the patient's overall health status. There are several functional categories of chemotherapy agents, which is a systemic treatment that affects the whole body. More potential adverse effects may occur in chemotherapy than radiotherapy. Common nutrition-related adverse effects include anorexia, early satiety, taste changes, nausea, vomiting, diarrhea, mucositis or esophagitis, and constipation. Since cancer and the adverse effects of chemotherapy can greatly impact nutrition status, health care providers must anticipate possible problems and design a plan along with the patient, to prevent malnutrition and weight loss. Malnutrition and weight loss can affect a patient's ability to regain normal health and acceptable blood counts between cycles of chemotherapy. This can directly affect the ability to follow the treatment schedule, which is essential for achieving a positive outcome.

Radiation therapy can cause nutrition-related adverse effects such as changes in taste or the ability to swallow, nausea, vomiting, diarrhea. Effects of radiation therapy are based on the area that is irradiated, total dose, **fractionation**, duration, and the volume irradiated. Most effects are acute and begin around the second or third week of treatment. They usually reduce about two or three weeks after the completion of radiation therapy. Some effects are chronic, continuing or occurring after treatment is done. Nutrition support during radiation therapy is essential, since there can be changes in normal physiologic function that can diminish the nutrition status via interference with ingestion, digestion, or absorption of nutrients. Aside from the effects of radiation therapy to areas within the head and neck, it may cause dysphagia, **odynophagia**, esophagitis, nausea, vomiting, loss of appetite, esophageal stenosis, fibrosis, or necrosis, diarrhea, chronic enteritis or colitis, and intestinal stricture or obstruction. The adverse effects of chemotherapy and nutritional therapies that may combat them are described as follows:

- *Constipation* – gradually increase intake of foods higher in dietary fiber by including them in meals and snacks, drink plenty of water
- *Nausea without vomiting* – eating the right foods at the right times may help (small, more frequent meals, foods containing ginger, cool and light foods instead of greasy and high-fat foods)
- *Diarrhea* – eat small and frequent meals, eat easy-to-digest foods that are lower in fiber, slowly sip non-caffeinated fluids throughout the day, limit beverages and foods with sugar alcohols
- *Sore or dry mouth and throat* – though prescribed medications may be required, tips to reduce irritation include soft and liquid foods, softening foods with milk, broth, sauces, or gravy, regular sipping of water, frozen fruits, avoiding acidic, crunchy, dry, or hot food sources, avoiding alcohol and foods with small seeds
- *Lack of appetite* – eating smaller and more frequent meals, keeping healthy snacks nearby, eating favored foods any time of the day, discussing fiber intake with a dietitian since higher fiber foods can promote fullness, drinking fat-free or low-fat milk, 100% fruit juice, or smoothies
- *Weight gain or increased appetite* – choose healthy snacks, ask for help managing anxiety and stress, avoid fatigue with light to moderate physical activity such as walking

Radiation therapy often causes cancer patients to lose weight, so maintaining proper nutrition can increase chances for successful outcomes, and improve quality of life. Getting the right amount of protein during radiation therapy is very important, so every meal or snack should have some source of protein. This helps to spare lean muscle mass while repairing damage from the radiation. Good protein-rich foods include eggs, nuts and nut butters, seeds, soy and tofu, dairy products, meats, poultry, and fish. Meal replacement drinks containing protein may be good if there is difficulty eating solid foods. Hydration helps make adverse effects of radiation therapy less severe and reduces chances of missing or delaying cancer treatments. Avoiding dehydration during treatment protects body organs from long-term damage. All non-alcoholic beverages count toward keeping the body hydrated. Flavored waters or waters infused with fruits or vegetables can be used to replace regular water. For radiation therapy patients, 8–12 cups are recommended per day. Caffeinated drinks such as tea or coffee should be reduced to no more than one to two glasses per day, since they worsen dry mouth, a common adverse effect of treatment. Alcoholic beverages are best to avoid during radiation therapy – this should be discussed with a physician. Antioxidant supplements must be avoided during radiation therapy since they can actually protect the cancer cells – discuss all supplements with a physician or dietitian/nutritionist.

FOCUS ON RADIATION THERAPY

Radiotherapy may be used in the early stages of cancer, or after it has started to spread. It can be used to try to cure the cancer completely (curative radiotherapy), or to make other treatments more effective. For example, it can be combined with chemotherapy or used before surgery.

Test Your Knowledge

1. What is the difference between autologous and allogenic bone marrow transplantation?
2. If chemotherapy causes a lack of appetite, what can be done?
3. During radiation therapy, why must dehydration be prevented?

KEY TERMS

Acesulfame K

Adenocarcinoma

Allogeneic

Anastomosis

Anorexia nervosa

Anthropometric

Aplastic anemia

Autologous

Barrett's esophagus

Benecalorie

Bloating

Blood urea nitrogen

Chia seeds

Cholecystitis

Cholelithiasis

Cholestasis

Chylothorax

Daisy

Depressed sensorium

Dumping syndrome

Dysphagia

Enteral tube nutrition

Esophagectomy

Fractionation

Gastrografin

Ginger ale

Guar gum

Hemoglobinopathies

Hemopoietic growth factors

Hemopoietic stem cells

Hydrolyzed protein

Hyperammonemia

Hyperosmolar

Inulin

Laparoscopic techniques

Medium-chain triglyceride

Multiple myeloma

Nosocomial

Odynophagia

Orogastric

Pancreatitis

Plasma proteins

Polymeric formulas

Prothrombin time

Proton pump inhibitors

Psyllium husk

Refeeding syndrome

Sarcopenia

Short bowel syndrome

Squamous cell carcinomas

Tapioca dextrin

Thrombosis

Transthyretin

CLINICAL CASE STUDIES

Clinical Case Study 1

An 83-year-old woman, living in a 24-hour care facility, had been diagnosed with Alzheimer's disease eight years ago. Over the last few weeks, her food intake was decreased by half. She sometimes struggles with constipation. The patient coughs a lot when she drinks beverages during meals. The healthcare team believes that worsening of her AD is impacting her food intake. Their goals are to improve the patient's nutritional status, prevent further weight loss, achieve and maintain adequate hydration as well as food intake.

CRITICAL THINKING QUESTIONS

1. What are the reasons for weight loss in dementia patients?
2. What type of foods may be prescribed for this patient?
3. Which diets may be able to somewhat prevent the progression of dementia?

Clinical Case Study 2

A 37-year-old man was hospitalized because of severe abdominal discomfort, nausea, vomiting, fever, and chills. His past history included hyperlipidemia, gastroesophageal reflux, alcoholism, anxiety, and depression. His family had a history of diabetes mellitus and coronary disease. The patient's body mass index was 31.4, putting him into stage 1 obesity. Tests result in a diagnosis of acute pancreatitis. Treatments begin, which include fasting, fluid and electrolyte support, antibiotics, and pain medications. Due to the severity of the patient's condition, he is eventually placed onto enteral nutrition. He is educated about the dangerous of excessive alcohol in relation to pancreatitis.

CRITICAL THINKING QUESTIONS

1. What is the cause of pancreatitis?
2. How prevalent is the connection between heavy alcohol use and gallstones, resulting in pancreatitis?
3. How is enteral nutrition used to treat acute pancreatitis?

Clinical Case Study 3

A 52-year-old woman had been diagnosed with ovarian cancer. Her symptoms included pelvic discomfort, reduced appetite, weight loss, abdominal distension, reflux, and worsening shortness of breath. Though being ambulatory and capable of self-care, she no longer had the ability to work at her job. Imaging revealed a large pelvic mass, which biopsy confirmed as ovarian cancer. Chemotherapy was initiated. Upon first meeting her dietitian, the patient's diet consisted only of soups, clear fluids, and milk. She was given oral nutritional supplements, which she tolerated well, and encouraged to add small amounts of semi-solid foods, which she did. Over time, the patient began to improve and was able to add some solid foods to her diet. She underwent a total abdominal hysterectomy, bilateral salpingo-oophorectomy, total omentectomy, and excision of bulky paracaval nodes. The patient had additional chemotherapy, and remains cancer-free and well-nourished over several months of follow-up as a result of the combined types of treatments.

CRITICAL THINKING QUESTIONS

1. What are the common nutrition-related adverse effects of chemotherapy?
2. What considerations are required for cancer patients receiving chemotherapy?
3. How important is it to prevent chemotherapy-related malnutrition and weight loss in cancer patients?

STUDY QUESTIONS

1. All of the following are protein sources in oral nutritional supplements, EXCEPT:
   A. Soybeans
   B. Fish oil
   C. Daisy flower
   D. Pea protein

2. Which of the following conditions is NOT an indication for the use of oral nutritional supplements?
   A. Dysphagia
   B. Total gastrectomy
   C. Hypertension
   D. Short bowel syndrome

3. Laparoscopic techniques can be used for which of the following types of tube feeding?
   A. Enteral nutrition
   B. Jejunostomy
   C. Nasogastric feeding
   D. Oral nutritional supplements

4. Which of the following positions is most appropriate for tube feeding?
   A. Sit upright at a 45° angle
   B. Sit upright at a 60° angle
   C. Sit upright at a 90° angle
   D. Sit upright at a 15° angle

5. Which of the following may be caused by nasogastric tube feeding?
   A. Diarrhea
   B. Urine retention
   C. Hypertension
   D. Sinusitis

6. Which of the following may be caused by total parenteral nutrition?
   A. Vomiting
   B. Hypotension
   C. Aplastic anemia
   D. Thrombosis

7. How many milliliters per day is required for a standard TPN solution?
   A. 300 mL
   B. 500 mL
   C. 1,000 mL
   D. 2,000 mL

8. All of the following affect patients on TPN, EXCEPT:
   A. Liver dysfunction
   B. Urine retention
   C. Hypoglycemia
   D. Hyperglycemia

9. Nutritional supplementation is often used for anorexia nervosa along with which of the following?
   A. Chemotherapy
   B. Enzyme replacement therapy
   C. Behavioral therapy
   D. Radiation therapy

10. Squamous cell carcinoma is caused by all of the following, EXCEPT:
   A. Smoking
   B. Drinking coffee
   C. Organ transplantation
   D. Alcohol consumption

11. Refeeding syndrome is a risk for patients with all of the following, EXCEPT:
   A. Loss of a large amount of body weight
   B. Excessive use of alcohol
   C. Use of antidiuretic medications
   D. No nutritional intake for at least one week

12. Which of the following is the primary cause of pancreatitis?
   A. Gallstones
   B. Stomach cancer
   C. Multiple myeloma
   D. Hemoglobinopathy

13. All of the following are common nutrition-related adverse effects of chemotherapy, EXCEPT:
   A. Vomiting
   B. Hyperthyroidism
   C. Mucositis
   D. Anorexia

14. Which of the following is NOT a factor that affects radiation therapy?
   A. Total dose
   B. The area that is irradiated
   C. The weight of the patient
   D. The volume that is irradiated

15. Bone marrow transplantation is used for all of the following conditions, EXCEPT:
   A. Multiple myeloma
   B. Iron deficiency anemia
   C. Aplastic anemia
   D. Hemoglobinopathies

FURTHER READING

1. Aadhaar O'Gormon, E. (2012). *Complete Tubefeeding: Everything You Need to Know about Tubefeeding, Tube Nutrition, and Blended Diets.* CreateSpace Independent Publishing Platform.
2. American Cancer Society, Besser, J., and Grant, B. (2018). *What To Eat During Cancer Treatment*, 2nd Edition. American Cancer Society.
3. Balch, P.A. (2010). *Prescription for Nutritional Healing: A-To-Z Guide to Supplements.* Avery.
4. Creagan, E.T., and Wendel, S. (2018). *Farewell: Vial End-of-Life Questions with Candid Answers from a Leading Palliative and Hospice Physician.* Write On Ink Publishing.
5. Douglas, D. (2022). *Pancreatitis Diet for Beginnings: Comprehensive Guide on Pancreatitis Control, Management, and Treatment with Healthy Recipes, Food List, and Meal Plan for Healthier Lifestyle.* Douglas.
6. Douglas, W. (2022). *Recent Advances in Stem Cell and Bone Marrow Transplantation.* States Academic Press.
7. Garcia, M.C. (2023). *The Dental Nutritional Therapy – The Amazing Connection Between your Teeth, Real Nourishment, and Life Changing Natural Health.* Garcia.
8. Jeejeebhoy, K.N. (2018). *Total Parenteral Nutrition in the Hospital and at Home.* CRC Press / Taylor & Francis Group.
9. Kalamian, M., and Seyfried, T.N. (2017). *Keto for Cancer – Ketogenic Metabolic Therapy as a Targeted Nutritional Therapy.* Chelsea Green Publishing.
10. Kane, K., and Prelack, K. (2018). *Advanced Medical Nutrition Therapy.* Jones & Bartlett Learning.
11. Lazarides, L. (2011). *Principles of Nutritional Therapy.* Naturostudy.
12. Leigh, I. (2022). *A Guidebook to Nutrition – A Comprehensive Guide to Essential Vitamins, Minerals, and Omega Oils.* Inara Leigh.
13. Lock, J., and Le Grange, D. (2015). *Treatment Manual for Anorexia Nervosa: A Family-Based Approach.* The Guilford Press.
14. McKay, J., and Schacher, T. (2009). *The Chemotherapy Survival Guide: Everything You Need to Know to Get Through Treatment*, 3rd Edition. New Harbinger Publications.
15. Nelms, M., and Sucher, K.P. (2019). *Nutrition Therapy and Pathophysiology*, 4th Edition. Cengage Learning.
16. Nelms, M., and Roberts, K. (2021). *Medical Nutrition Therapy – A Case Study Approach*, 6th Edition. Cengage Learning.
17. Ouren, M. (2022). *Cancer Treatments: Good Nutrition for Cancer Patients.* Ouren.
18. Plaskett, L. (2018). *The Nutritional Therapy of Cancer.* Lulu.com.
19. Schlenker, E., and Gilbert, J.A. (2018). *Williams' Essentials of Nutrition and Diet Therapy.* Elsevier.
20. Stephen, N. (2022). *Nutritional Therapy on High Fiber Diet – A Complete Guide with Benefit, Delicious and Healthy Recipes for the Diet.* Stephen.
21. Viola, S., and Evans, N. (2021). *When Waves Rise: Navigating Difficult Moments Associated with Dementia.* SV Grace LLC.

24 The Global Burden of Nutritional Problems

OUTLINE

LEARNING OBJECTIVES

After study of this chapter, readers should be able to:

1. Identify the risk factors for stunted growth.
2. Explain ready-to-use therapeutic food.
3. Describe undernutrition and overnutrition.
4. Explain the role of WHO in relation to global malnutrition.
5. Discuss sustainable development goals of the UN.
6. Explain food safety regulations.
7. Compare the differences between stunted growth and wasting.
8. Describe the labeling requirements and advertising restrictions of food products.
9. Explain the financial impact on common nutrition-related chronic diseases.
10. Describe steps to end global nutritional problems.

OVERVIEW

Malnutrition is one of most serious but least-addressed development challenges in the world today. Its human and economic costs are enormous, greatly impacting the poor, women, and children. In 2020, 149 million children under five years old were stunted, which indicates a failure to achieve a person's own genetic potential for height, and also predicts developmental problems. These include cognitive deficits and future economic opportunities, which impede populations' abilities to survive. Poor diets and resulting malnutrition creates one of the planet's most extreme societal challenges. More coordinated actions are required to address this situation. The global nutrition crisis has been worsened by factors such as wars and other conflicts, environmental crises, and the COVID-19 pandemic. Food security and availability has become very prevalent in many countries. International and public resources have been impacted due to economic downturns. As a result, populations in the poorest countries are experiencing a reduction in crucial support.

STUNTED GROWTH

Stunted growth occurs in children because of poor nutrition, chronic infections, and poor psychosocial stimulation. A child is defined as "stunted" when the height-for-age is more than two **standard deviations** below the World Health Organization's *Child Growth Standards* median (see Figure 24.1). Stunting that occurs in early life, especially up until age two, results in serious functional problems such as poor cognition, poor educational performance, and in adulthood, lower wages, lost productivity, and if accompanied by later excessive weight gain, increased risks for nutrition-related chronic disease. In early childhood, **linear growth** is the most important marker of healthy growth, in relation to its association with morbidity and mortality risks, as well as later noncommunicable diseases, learning capacity, and productivity. Linear growth is closely linked with child development in cognitive, language, and sensory-motor functions.

Almost one-third of children below the age of five years are stunted in developing regions of the world. Furthermore, stunting is the cause of 14% of childhood deaths. Today, it affects 22% of children. Though progress has been made, there are still large inequalities between and within many countries, and much more work is needed to improve the situation. Stunted children are two to four times more likely to die before age five than non-stunted children. Stunting is related to delayed cognitive development and as much as an 11-point reduction in expected intelligence quotient (IQ). It reflects limitations in a country's ability to compete and is related to costs of as much as 13% of expected gross domestic product per year. Multiplied by millions of children across many countries, stunted growth contributes to reduced economic productivity and national growth, plus increased health costs. The top 25 countries with the most stunted growth during childhood include Burundi, Eritrea, Timor-Leste, Papua New Guinea, Niger, Guatemala, Yemen, Mozambique, Democratic Republic of the Congo, Madagascar, Malawi, Central African Republic, Sudan, Afghanistan, Libya, Chad, Pakistan, Angola, Ethiopia,

DOI: 10.1201/b22969-28

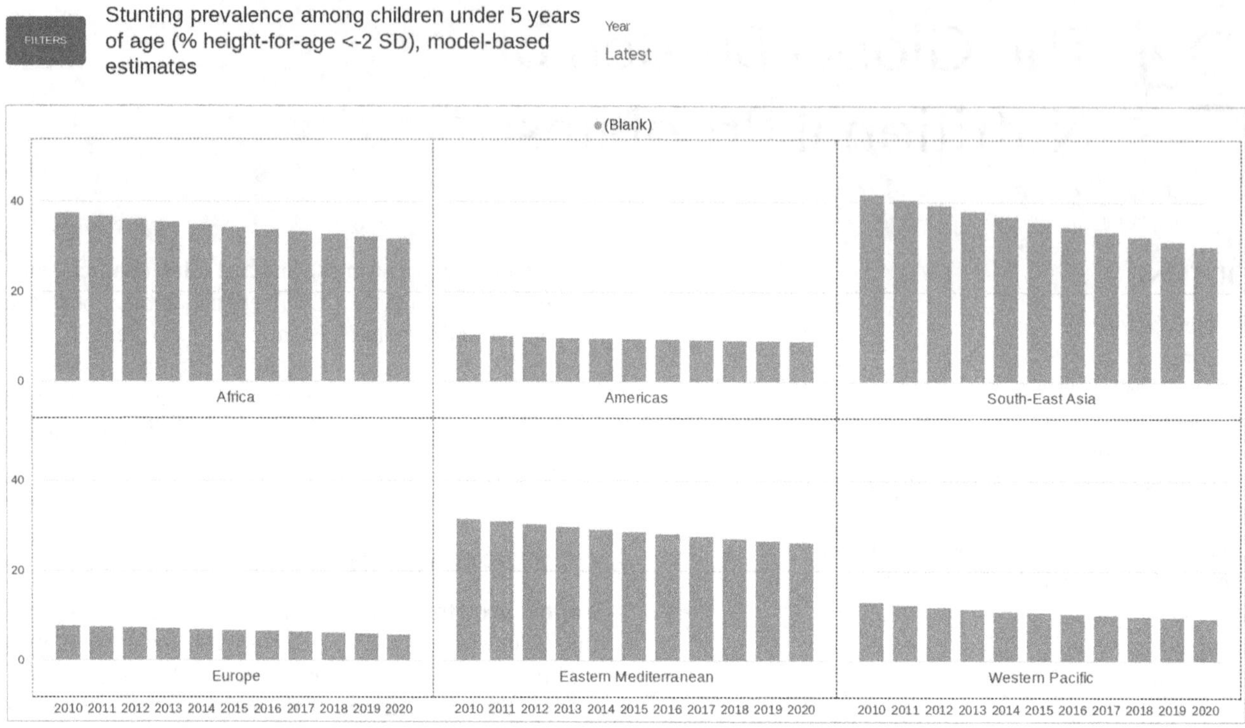

FIGURE 24.1 Graph showing the standard deviations (plus or minus 2%) used as part of the World Health Organization's "Child Growth Standards" median.

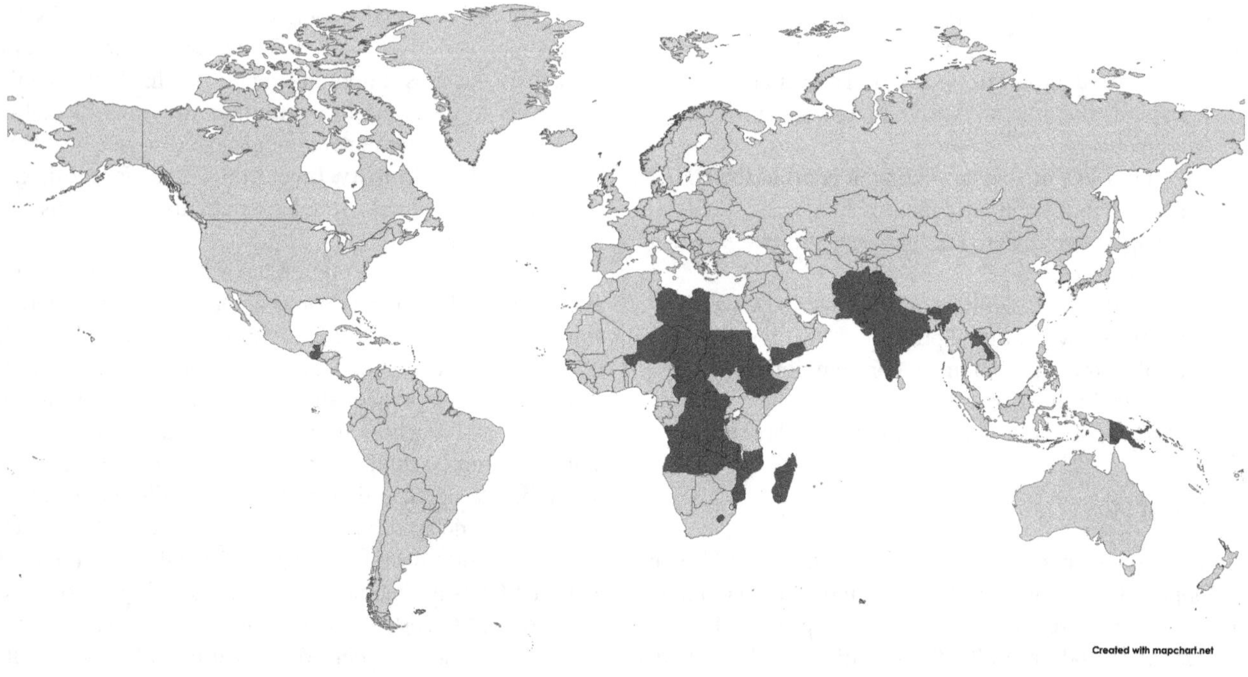

FIGURE 24.2 Countries with the most stunted growth during childhood.

India, Lesotho, Zambia, Bhutan, Djibouti, and Lao People's Democratic Republic (see Figure 24.2).

Causes of stunted growth include poor nutrition, recurrent infections, and chronic diseases which result in poor nutrient intake, absorption, or utilization. Lack of access to diverse foods, poor sanitation, no access to clean drinking water, lack of proper healthcare for children as well as their mothers, inadequate psychosocial stimulation or parent-infant bonding. Other contributing factors include gender equality, the father's participation in parenting, and conflicts. Along with income opportunity, food pricing, and environmental factors, conflicts can affect food availability and contribute to undernutrition or malnutrition. Stunted growth is often intergenerational, since stunted children are more likely, once becoming adults, to have stunted children themselves. A stunted child is more likely to become overweight as an adult, leading to additional health risks. The primary symptom that may indicate a growth problem is when a child grows less than 2 inches a year after the second birthday. Other symptoms may include slow development of physical skills, such as rolling over, sitting up, standing, and walking. Also, there may be delayed social and mental skills.

FOCUS ON RISK FACTORS FOR STUNTED GROWTH

In relation to nutrition, specific risk factors for stunted growth include premature births, zinc deficiency, and maternal malaria. Another important consideration is maternal malnutrition, with a body mass index less than 18.5, anemia, and height less than 62.9 inches (160 cm). Teenage pregnancies and periods between births less than 24 months also increase the risk for stunted growth.

Test Your Knowledge

1. How is stunted growth defined?
2. What are the causes of stunted growth?
3. What are the signs and symptoms of stunted growth?

WASTING

The term **wasting** is a key indicator used to assess childhood malnutrition. A child is *wasted* when the weight is too low in comparison to the height. Wasting is also called acute malnutrition. Short periods of undernutrition result in extreme wastage of muscle and fat tissue (see Figure 24.3). Wasting can be caused by severe periods of food shortage, disease, or both. This is often related to severe food insecurity, such as during famine, or regularly poor crop harvests. Wasting can also be due to infections, in which a child's energy requirements may be higher while their ability to absorb and retain nutrients is only limited. A child whose weight falls two standard deviations below the expected weight-for-height is defined as wasted. The prevalence of a population's wasting is defined as the share of children under five years old that fall two standard deviations below the expected weight-for-height. The deviations are set forth in the *child growth standards* of the WHO.

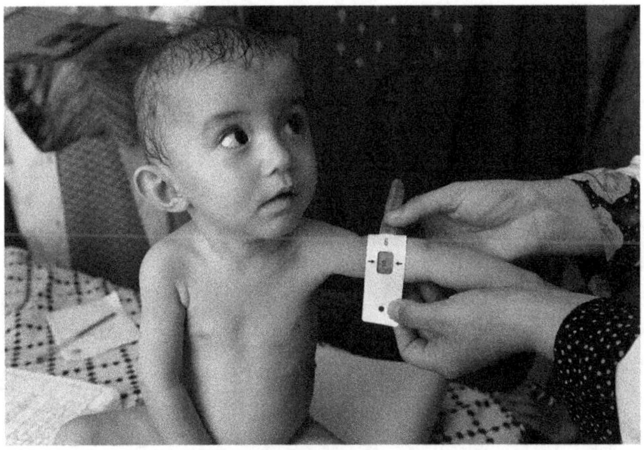

FIGURE 24.3 A child with wasting of muscle and fat tissue.

Wasting is the most immediate, visible, and life-threatening form of malnutrition, caused by a failure in preventing malnutrition among children considered to be the most vulnerable. Affected children also have weak immune systems, and some have *nutritional edema*, with swelling of the face, feet, and limbs. Wasting is the result of maternal malnutrition, low birthweight, poor feeding and care, and infections linked to food insecurity, limited access to clean drinking water, and poverty. Wasting, like stunted growth, occurs very early in life and mostly affects children under two years of age. The same causes and risk factors are present for wasting as well as stunted growth. However, 66% of affected children live in places that are not facing emergency conditions. Unfortunately, only one in three children with severe wasting receive timely treatment and care.

In most cases, children with wasting can be treated with *ready-to-use therapeutic food (RUTF)* and recover in their own homes instead of hospitals (Figure 24.4). This is an energy-dense micronutrient paste that is made using peanuts,

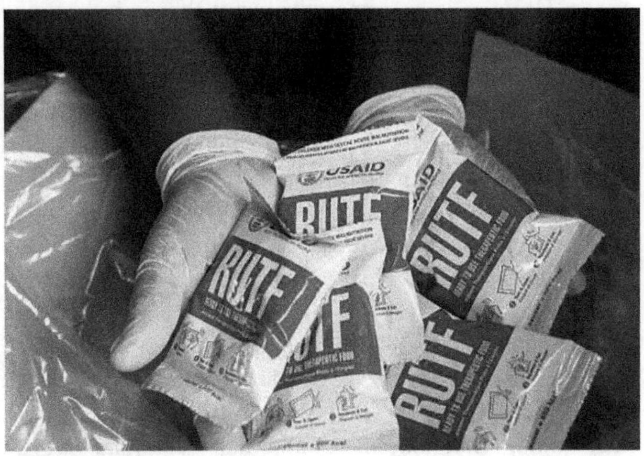

FIGURE 24.4 A container of ready-to-use therapeutic food, commonly known as RUTF.

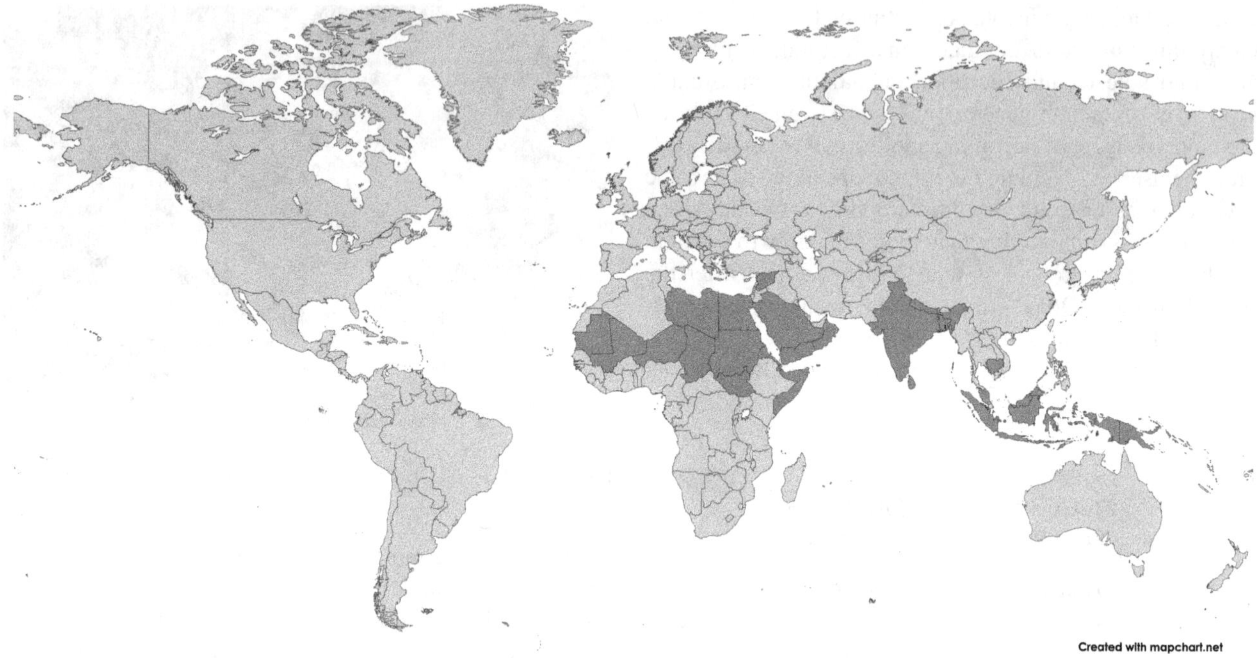

FIGURE 24.5 Countries with the most childhood wasting.

sugar, milk powder, oil, vitamins, and minerals. It is available in a one-dose container made of aluminum foil, lasts on the shelf for up to two years, and does not have to be refrigerated at any time. There is no preparation or mixing required, and it can be eaten right out of the container.

Severe wasting is the most lethal form of malnutrition. About one of every five childhood deaths before age five are attributed to severe wasting. It is caused by a lack of nutritious food and repeated bouts of diseases such as diarrhea, measles, and malaria. It is also called *severe acute malnutrition*, and affects about 13.6 million children around the world. Severe wasting is likely to increase because of ongoing conflicts and environment-related emergencies. The war in Ukraine is an important factor that is influencing the increase in severe wasting. The price of RUTF is projected to increase greatly over the near future, meaning that even more children are at risk for severe wasting. Affected children often die from normal childhood diseases that become life threatening because their bodies have no way to fight against pathogens. A severely wasted child is up to 11 times more likely to die of common childhood diseases than a healthy child. The countries with the most childhood wasting are shown in Figure 24.5. They include South Sudan, India, Yemen, Sudan, Mauritius, Sri Lanka, Eritrea, Somalia, Papua New Guinea, Nepal, Saudi Arabia, Syria, Niger, Comoros, Indonesia, Libya, Chad, Djibouti, Mauritania, Bangladesh, Cambodia, Malaysia, Egypt, Mali, and Oman.

Test Your Knowledge

1. What factors influence the development of wasting in a child?
2. What can be used to treat most children that have wasting?
3. How lethal is severe wasting?

EXCESSIVE WEIGHT

The epidemic of excessive weight is worldwide, and more than four million people die every year due to being overweight or obese, according to the WHO *global burden of disease* reports. Rates of excessive weight continue to increase in adults as well as children. Between 1975 and 2016, there were over four times as many children and adolescents (5–17 years of age) that were overweight or obese. Obesity is more common than being underweight in all regions of the world except for sub-Saharan Africa and Asia. While excessive weight used to be a problem only in high-income countries, it is now rising quickly in low- and middle-income countries as well, mostly in urban settings. The great majority of overweight or obese children live in developing countries. The rate of increase has been over 30% higher than the increase in developed countries.

The global presence of obesity has quadrupled in men over the past four decades (3%–12%), and more than doubled in women (7%–16%). Combined with population growth, this change resulted in greater than a six-times increase in the number of obese adults (100 million to 671 million). The largest absolute increase in obesity occurred in men and boys in high-income Western countries, and in women and girls in Central Asia, the Middle East, and North Africa. Changes in the global food system are largely to blame, since it promotes energy-dense foods that are poor in nutrients, along with fewer opportunities for physical activity. This serious problem is linked with potentially life-threatening conditions. This situation is expected to increase along with increases in being overweight or obese. Obesity and its complications were discussed in Chapters 8 and 9 in detail.

FOCUS ON UNDERNUTRITION AND OVERNUTRITION

Undernutrition is characterized by a lack of nutrients and insufficient energy supply. Overnutrition is characterized by excessive nutrient and energy intake, and can result in obesity, a significantly serious global health threat. Together, they comprise the *double burden of malnutrition.*

AREAS OF GREATEST MALNUTRITION

It is estimated that up to 811 million people around the world often go to bed hungry. Conflicts, drought, and disease are contributing factors. As of 2020, about 928 million people had severe food insecurity. The number of hungry people in Africa represents over 33% of undernourished individuals in the world. This is more than double the proportion, by population, of any other region. The five regions with the most undernourished people include the following (also see Figure 24.6):

- Middle Africa – 31.8%
- East Africa – 28.1%
- Western Africa – 18.7%
- Caribbean – 16.1%
- Southern Asia – 15.8%

The countries that are most affected by hunger and malnutrition, according to the Global Hunger Index in 2022, are shown in Figure 24.7. They include Yemen, Central African Republic, Madagascar, the Democratic Republic of the Congo, Chad, Liberia, Haiti, Niger, Lesotho, Sierra Leone, Guinea-Bissau, Timor-Leste, Afghanistan, Zambia, India, Sudan, Republic of the Congo, Ethiopia, Nigeria, Rwanda, Comoros, Papua New Guinea, Afghanistan, Pakistan, Angola, and the Democratic People's Republic of Korea (North Korea).

Ethiopia, Nigeria, South Sudan, and Yemen are at risk for catastrophic degrees of hunger, malnutrition, and starvation. Countries facing critical levels of food insecurity include Afghanistan, the Central African Republic, the Democratic Republic of the Congo, Haiti, Honduras, Sudan, and Syria. Since many people in developing countries engage in farming activities to provide their own food, global organizations are providing them with access to agricultural tools. These include seeds that are able to resist drought conditions, training in crop diversity and crop rotation, livestock farming, and water retention and irrigation. They teach adults about proper nutrition with locally-available foods and better preparation techniques.

Haiti's food problem is the worst in the world, with about 45% of the population in 2022 facing acute food insecurity. About 1.3 million people are projected to fall into the food security category that is just above *famine.* Two of every three Haitians survive on about the equivalent of $2.00 or less per day. Even though agriculture is a large part of Haitian society, extremely poor crop yields require the country to import 80% of its staple food (rice). The agricultural system is almost totally dependent upon rain, since only 10% of the agricultural lands are irrigated. One of every three children in Haiti are stunted, and about 100,000 suffer from acute malnutrition. Also, 33% of women and children suffer from anemia. Throughout the world, Haiti has the lowest food availability of all, at just 1,976 calories per person per day.

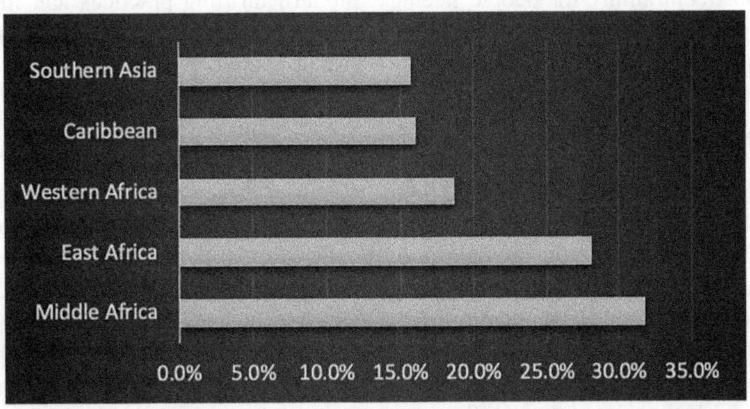

FIGURE 24.6 The five world regions with the most undernourished people.

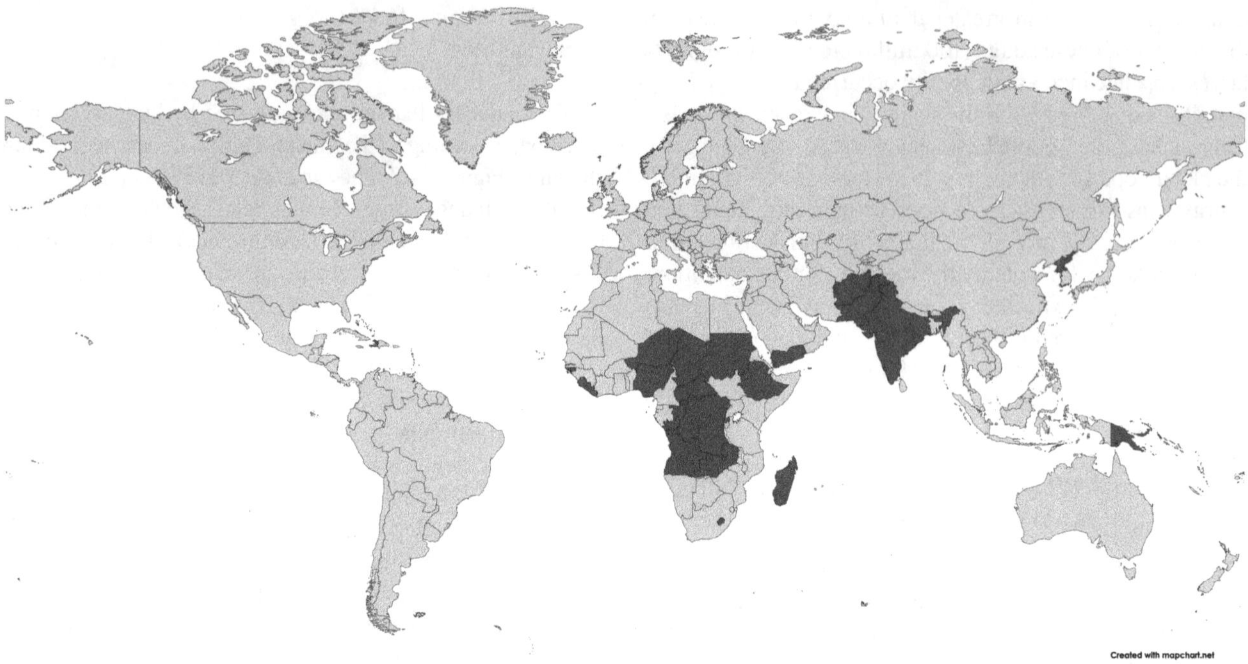

FIGURE 24.7 The countries most affected by hunger and malnutrition in 2022.

Democratic Republic of the Congo has 72% of its population at poverty levels, largely because of armed conflicts, population displacement, and widespread corruption. Even with plentiful resources and crop lands, there is still a severe food crisis. In over 50% of the republic, the acute malnutrition rate is above 10%. The chronic malnutrition rate of children between six months and five years is 43.4%, which is described as *critical* by WHO. The COVID-19 epidemic hit the country hard, with 20% more of the population facing hunger issues between 2020 and 2021. Food availability is 2,056 calories per person per day.

The country of Chad is extremely vulnerable to food scarcity because of a lack of proper healthcare facilities and safe drinking water, compounded by drought conditions. Nearly 800,000 people require emergency food assistance. Chad has the highest rate of malnutrition in Western Africa. The child malnutrition rate is between 6.8% and 13.3%. Chad is also a major host community for people fleeing conflict and instability in neighboring countries. There are over 500,000 refugees now living in areas of the country that have the poorest climate. Childhood stunting is either remaining at the same levels or increasing in certain areas. Food availability is at 2,074 calories per person per day.

In Kenya, over one million people suffer from food insecurity. About 240,000 children have moderate acute malnutrition while 2,600 have severe acute malnutrition. Internal conflicts regularly displace populations, including those related to the **El Niño** weather phenomenon, infectious diseases, refugee crises, and high rates of HIV/AIDS. This all means that Kenyans are extremely susceptible to food crises and undernourishment. Food availability is at 2,092 calories per person per day.

Ethiopia has widespread low food availability due to severe droughts, soil erosion, a lack of infrastructure, and poor farming methods. About 28% of child deaths are due to undernutrition. Nearly 81% of cases of child malnutrition are untreated, and two of every five children suffer from stunting. Economic consequences are serious. The high death rate related to stunting has reduced the adult workforce by 8%. Approximately 16.5% of the country's gross domestic product is spent on reversing malnutrition. Food availability is at 2,097 calories per person per day.

Approximately 40% of the population of Mozambique is undernourished, and citizens have a life expectancy at birth of only 48 years. Nearly 64% of the population is food insecure. Poverty and malnutrition are also aggravated by a significant HIV/AIDS prevalence. There is a high susceptibility to natural disasters, including frequent crop infections, **cyclones**, droughts, and floods. Along with a lack of modern farming practices and financial support, agricultural yields are very low. Food availability is at 2,112 calories per person per day.

Yemen is at the center of one of the worst humanitarian crises in the world, with conflict within the country as well as experiencing the effects of conflicts in surrounding countries. Since the start of the Yemeni Civil War in 2014, the economy was destroyed and poverty increased dramatically. Ruined public health and water systems, along with sanitation systems, have led to increased cases of cholera, measles, and polio. Malnutrition, as a result, has become even more deadly. The country has a high dependence upon food imports, and with the war in Ukraine, costs have increased even more quickly. Many people cannot afford basic foods any longer.

A widespread humanitarian crisis has plagued the Central African Republic since 2012. One out of four people have been displaced by violence, increasing rates of hunger and malnutrition. Farmers have lost crops because of this displacement, returning to find them decimated due to lack of maintenance. Since most of them grow foods for their own families, they are likely to starve.

About 25% of the population of Madagascar live in areas that often have natural disasters such as cyclones, droughts, and floods. Along with large-scale deforestation and poor land management, there is a resultant high prevalence of food insecurity. About 35.8% of the rural population suffers from food insecurity, and almost two million children are stunted because of chronic malnutrition. Poor farming practices, gender inequality, and a lack of economic support and education combine to cause a low agricultural output. About 48.5% of the country's population was undernourished between 2019 and 2021. Approximately 40% of the children are stunted and 7.7% are experiencing wasting. The child mortality rate is at 5%. At the beginning of 2022, the country was also hit by two cyclones that devastated many farmlands and crops. Food availability is at 2,117 calories per person per day.

About 42% of the children under age five in the country of Tanzania are stunted. There are areas that suffer from acute malnutrition, such as Zanzibar, in which 12% of the children do not receive proper nutrition. About 33% of Tanzania's children between ages six months and five years have iron and vitamin A deficiencies. Over 18 million Tanzanians do not receive sufficient amounts of dietary iodine. Adolescent girls and young women are often severely malnourished. Food availability is at 2,137 calories per person per day.

The country of Niger has seen slowed progress in addressing malnutrition compared to previous years. Desert areas are expanding, the economy is struggling, and armed conflict is a regular factor. Outside groups are attempting to help address the poor food system in the country, providing nutritionally-fortified flour at affordable prices that is of high quality, and also identifying the most important areas of action that need to be improved by the government.

Liberia had a 14-year-long civil war, followed by the largest Ebola epidemic of any country. Hunger and malnutrition are prevalent. Though many farms have good conditions and soil for growing crops, there is a limited availability of equipment and farming supplies. Therefore, the country depends on important staple foods, which have become more expensive due to the COVID-19 pandemic. More than 50% of the population live under the poverty line, at the equivalent of $1.90 per day.

Lesotho is a country that is completely surrounded by South Africa, and combats extremes in climate and poor agriculture. The country is mountainous, so only 10% of its land can be farmed. Even so, about 45% of the people work in agriculture and in rural areas, up to 70% of the people work in farming just for their own families' needs. Poor rain and frequent droughts, combined with some flash flooding, has deprived people of food sources, lowered incomes, and increased food prices. The rural population spends about 45% of their income on food.

Sierra Leone, though rich in natural resources, has been devastated by over 11 years of civil war. About 40% of the country's children are chronically undernourished, and about one in four children die before reaching five years of age. Nearly 25% of the rural population has insufficient or borderline food consumption. The country was also at the epicenter of the 2014 to 2016 Ebola virus epidemic, and in 2017 had the highest maternal mortality rates in the world. The COVID-19 pandemic shrunk the country's economy to –2% in 2020. The conflict in Ukraine led to increased inflation that affected Sierra Leone, impacting costs of basic necessities. Food availability is at 2,162 calories per person per day.

Guatemala also has a low level of food availability due to frequent floods, droughts, soil erosion due to deforestation and poor farming practices, and a lack of good economic policies for agricultural management. Nearly 50% of children under five years of age are undernourished. The most vulnerable people include women and children that live in the country's "dry corridor". More than half of Guatemalans live below the poverty line. Food availability is at 2,244 calories per person per day.

Zambia, though a beautiful country, suffers from poverty and malnutrition that is widespread. Chronic malnutrition affects many children. About 50% of the population has no work opportunities and over 85% live below the poverty line. Crop infestations, dry spells, and flooding compound the situation even more. Zambians also have certain belief systems, such as boys not being allowed to eat round foods because this will harm their future ability to father children. Therefore, many healthy foods such as eggs, potatoes, guavas, oranges, and watermelons are not eaten by boys.

The country of Malawi faces recurrent hunger issues. Droughts have caused major food shortages and degraded the already-fragile agricultural system. Fortunately, global organizations are assisting farmers to increase crop yields through irrigation farming, rainwater harvesting, resource management, and the use of drought-resistant seeds. Farmers have been taught to raise dairy animals to provide new sources of nutrition and income.

The Republic of Burundi is one of the smallest countries in Africa, and most of the population lives in extreme poverty and hunger. After a 12-year civil war, the country took a long time to start to recover. About 58% of children under age 5 are stunted. Most families can only afford to eat one meal per day. Global organizations are teaching the population the importance of breastfeeding infants, how to prepare nutritious meals, and how to cultivate household gardens to increase and diversify crops.

Timor-Leste is an island just north of Australia that only became a nation in 2002. Though rich in oil and gas reserves, it is still the poorest nation in Asia. There is little food variety and children lack necessary nutrients. About

58% of children under age five have stunted growth. Global organizations are offering seeds to help the country vary its crops, and are training farmers in new cultivation methods.

In India, the 2nd most populated country in the world (behind China), over 80% of the population lives on the equivalent of less than $1.25 per day. Even though the economy is growing quickly, India's nutritional growth is not. About 48% of children under age five are stunted. Supplementary feeding programs are being implemented to help prevent malnutrition.

In Afghanistan, one of the most dangerous places in the world, political turmoil, war, drought, and severe winters impact the people's chances of survival. Chronically malnourished children and widespread stunting are everywhere. About 60% of Afghan children are stunted, often developing brain impairments, a reduced ability to be employed, and weakened immune systems. However, attempts are being made by outside organizations to train Afghans about better care for pregnant women and children, farming techniques, more balanced diets, and support is given with agricultural tools and drought-resistant seeds.

FOCUS ON THE IMPACTS OF GLOBAL MALNUTRITION

Globally, malnutrition affects many children under the age of five years. Chronic undernutrition can lead to stunting or wasting, which can have long-term effects upon children and their later physical and cognitive development. On the other side of the situation, being overweight or obese can increase risks for diet-related noncommunicable diseases, including diabetes, heart disease, and cancers with a significant global impact.

Test Your Knowledge

1. What are the five regions with the most undernourished people in the world?
2. Which country has the worst food problem in the world, and what are its impacts?
3. Where does the majority of overweight or obese children live?

THE ROLES OF THE UNITED NATIONS

The United Nations Global Nutrition Agenda (UNGNA) provides a framework for aligning work of its agencies in the support of future global and national nutrition goals.

Sustainable development goals of the UN include all of the following:

- Ending poverty in all its forms, everywhere
- Ending hunger while achieving food security and improved nutrition, promoting sustainable agriculture
- Ensuring healthy lives and promoting wellbeing for all ages
- Ensuring inclusive, equitable quality education while promoting life-long learning
- Achieving gender equality and empowering all women and girls
- Ensuring availability and sustainable management of water and sanitation for all
- Ensuring access to affordable, reliable, sustainable, and modern energy for all
- Promoting sustained, inclusive, and sustainable growth, full and productive employment, and decent work for all
- Building a resilient infrastructure, promoting inclusive industrialization and fostering innovation
- Reducing inequality within countries
- Making cities and human settlements inclusive, safe, resilient, and sustainable
- Ensuring sustainable production
- Acting urgently to combat environmental changes and their impacts
- Conserving and using the ocean, sea, and marine resources sustainably
- Protecting, restoring, and promoting sustainable use of terrestrial ecosystems
- Promoting peaceful, inclusive societies with access to justice for all, and building effective, accountable institutions
- Strengthening and revitalizing global partnerships for sustainable development

The United Nations is a key role player for taking responsibility and being accountable for realizing nutrition goals. Nutrition is embedded in policies and governance systems at all levels. Adequate support systems are in place: evidence, data, human, and financial resources. Quality programs that are nutrition-specific and nutrition-sensitive are implemented.

THE ROLES OF THE WORLD HEALTH ORGANIZATION

The WHO strives to stop malnutrition throughout the world. The organization works with many partners to support member status in order to develop, implement, and monitor effective strategies and plans, advocate for supportive regulatory actions and policies, and monitor progress. The WHO is providing scientific advice and decision-making tools that can help countries address all forms of malnutrition to support and wellbeing for all people. Essential nutrition actions to achieve optimal health and nutritional wellbeing are identified for people of all ages. The *Sustainable Development Goals* and the *United Nations Decade of Action on Nutrition* focus on ending hunger and eradicating all forms of global malnutrition. There is a potential of double-duty actions to effectively and simultaneously address the global challenge of the double burden of malnutrition (undernutrition and overnutrition). Double-duty actions, through integrated interventions, programs, and policies have the ability to improve nutrition outcomes across the entire spectrum of malnutrition.

Appropriate investments in nutrition could save 3.7 million lives by year 2025. The WHO's report entitled *Essential Nutrition Actions: Mainstreaming Nutrition Throughout the Life-Course* argues that primary health care is a "whole-society" approach to health and wellbeing centered on the needs and preferences of individuals, families, and communities. Key nutrition intervention recommendations include the following:

- Providing iron and folic acid supplements as part of antenatal care
- Delaying umbilical cord clamping to ensure that babies receive important nutrients required after birth
- Promoting, protecting, and supporting breast feeding
- Providing advice on diet, such as limiting intake of free sugars
- Limiting salt intake to reduce risks for heart disease and stroke

The WHO's commitments include supporting countries as they formulate good public health policies, especially in reference to the promotion and protection of breastfeeding and adequate complementary feeding, and to strengthen monitoring systems for nutrition. Specifically, the WHO is working on further expansion of the guidance on chronic undernutrition and maternal nutrition. The organization will also complete development of a monitoring framework, and produces reports on the achievement of global targets.

FOCUS ON WORKING TOGETHER TO COMBAT MALNUTRITION

The UN and the WHO regularly work together to combat malnutrition, along with the World Food Programme, and a variety of other organizations. The Coalition of Action for Healthy Diets from Sustainable Food Systems brings together all of these entities to align, mobilize, and support collective action toward getting people access to nutritional food sources, to prevent nutritional disorders.

POLICIES AND POLITICS

Even with the unprecedented rise in diet-related chronic diseases, government policies have continued to emphasize agricultural production of staple products and support for the food industry that is motivated by conventional views on food security, economics, and trade. Governments have tended to use educational policy measures directed at individuals in response to the rise in chronic diseases. These measures aim to influence diet quality by emphasizing personal responsibility and choice through dietary guidelines, food labels, menu labeling, and clinical counseling. Multiple, complex factors beyond personal decisions strongly influence dietary choices and patterns. Governments can use many policies, from voluntary to mandatory, including bills, laws, acts, statutes, agency implementations, court decisions, guidelines, and directives to shape future policies.

Classifications of policy interventions include the level, target, domain, and mechanism, which are described as follows:

- *Level* – city, state, or national government; international agencies; organizations such as schools, workplaces, healthcare facilities; local neighborhoods and communities
- *Target* – consumers, organizations such as schools and worksites, health systems, farming and other agricultural production sites, industries that include manufacturing, retail, and restaurants
- *Domain* – population education such as dietary guidelines and the mass media, point-of-purchase information, fiscal policies, food quality standards, built environment changes, research, and innovation
- *Mechanism* – changing consumer preferences or choices, food formulations, or food availability and accessibility

Fiscal incentives and **fiscal disincentives** aimed at consumers, producers, and retailers, have had consistent evidence of effectiveness. Disincentives include sales taxes on unhealthy items such as sugar-sweetened beverages and junk food, or removal of industry tax benefits for development and marketing of unhealthy products. Disincentives on specific foods can be politically difficult, though this approach is becoming more widely accepted. To increase the health effect, tax revenues can be used for other health promotion strategies that include retail, manufacturing, or agricultural incentives, to reduce the price of healthier food products. Instead of being **punitive**, economic incentives and disincentives help to normalize the market, party by bringing the prices of different foods closer to their true societal cost.

Limitations or standards on trans-fat and sodium have been implemented in many countries. Similar standards are being implemented for free or added sugars. Nutrition procurement standards should be set for all governmental food purchases across agencies and programs. In schools, after-school programs, and early childcare programs, governments should promote nutrition standards for onsite meals and competitive foods as low cost, sustainable interventions. Free or low price provision of fruits and vegetables, farm-to-school programs, and school gardens are also promising strategies. Workplace wellness programs do not only improve health, but also lower costs and increase productivity. Governments should invest in employee workplace wellness programming and pursue policies such as guidelines and tax incentives to promote the implementation and evaluation by private employers of workplace efforts for healthier eating.

Governments should also promote policies that support implementation of evidence-informed action in the healthcare system, and with relevant partners such as community health workers, pharmacies, and other community-based organizations. Important strategies include multidisciplinary lifestyle programs for conditions such as prediabetes, medically-tailored meals for patients with complex chronic diseases, prescriptions for fruits and vegetables for health promotion and disease prevention, and nutrition counseling during pregnancy and early childhood. Additional actions include educating healthcare providers on food and nutrition, systematic introduction of these new ideas through national reform of medical and specialty licensing exams plus continuing medical education, expansion of nutrition counseling services through new reimbursement strategies with task sharing between community partners, and inclusion of standardized clinic and mobile assessments of diet quality and food insecurity in electronic health records.

Some countries currently limit advertising and use of cartoon characters to market products to children that do not meet standards for added sugar, added saturated fats, and sodium. Strong government funding for basic nutrition and applied research and innovation is required to develop evidence-based priorities for dietary policies. Government funding should make applied research a priority, including new technologies for nutritional assessment and behavior change, and policy implementation and evaluation. Government should also promote the food industry's shift toward healthier foods, taking advantage of the rapidly rising consumer demand. Tax incentives and other policies should promote research, development, and marketing of healthier foods in the food industry, combined with disincentives for marketing and promoting sugar-sweetened beverages and junk foods. A program of government funding and transparent public-private partnerships for nutrition research is needed to help reduce conflicts of interest and biases (both perceived and real).

Actions should be coordinated between ministries, agencies, and at local, national, and international levels. Strong government leadership is required to help deliver a comprehensive, sustained, multitargeted, and multilevel approach. Unclear or unevenly enforced government provisions concerning conflicts of interest can increase the influences of the food industry upon consumers. Certain food companies have actively opposed governmental policies about healthier foods, especially in low- and middle-income countries. The food industry must be a facilitator and not a barrier to healthy food policies, using their knowledge, scale, innovation, and marketing to develop, distribute, and market healthier foods. There are many examples of companies that produce sugar-sweetened beverages and junk food putting up strong resistance and lobbying to counter national policy actions tarted at obesity prevention. They have shifted the blame for obesity and chronic diseases away from specific products and toward physical inactivity and energy balance. Governments have a duty to ensure that interests that are not in the public good do not influence individuals or institutions responsible for public decision making, and preserving integrity and public trust.

Strong regulations on transparency and activities are required to maintain effective and unbiased policy making. Governance of public-private partnerships is important to ensure that efforts to improve food and nutrition line up with ethical, transparency, and accountability principles. The food and beverage industry must not participate in decision making about the design, implementation, or evaluation of obesity prevention policies. Additional government regulation and standards are important to enforce the implementation of health-related food and nutrition policies. Strong government policy is essential for achieving a healthy, profitable, equitable, and sustainable food system that benefits everyone. There are six major ideas about how governments can incentivize food and nutrition policies, which are described as follows:

- *Subsidize fruits, vegetables, nuts, and sustainably produced meat* – these products must be made more affordable. Since taxpayers already fund agriculture, that money needs to be redirected.
- *Terminate subsidies to big agribusiness and food corporations* – the largest growers should not be receiving the largest farm subsidies, especially when they produce unsustainable and inedible crops for fuel or animal feed instead of nourishing humans. Corn and soy monocultures degrade landscapes while producing raw materials that become unrecognizable after ending up as additives in fast foods and in most items on store shelves.
- *Incentivize consumers to purchase affordable produce* – programs that make fresh produce more affordable need to be expanded. This could be done by offering dollar-for-dollar matching programs – if a consumer spends a certain amount on "double up food dollars", the receive an identical amount good for local produce at participating stores and farmers' markets. More programs would encourage consumption of healthy produce from local producers.
- *Raise taxes on the marketing and sale of unhealthy foods* – though taxes on soda are already high, they should be expanded to include other low-nutrient, high-calorie foods. The tax money can then be used toward nutrition education, urban gardening, and other educational programs.
- *Imperfect produce can be discounted* – currently, produce that is too small or large, or abnormal in shape is usually thrown away. This is a huge waste of food. Instead, it should be sold at discounted prices, reducing food waste, and making produce more affordable. There also needs to be a shift in consumer preferences about "imperfect" produce.

- *Pass zoning laws that encourage urban gardens* – highly essential in food deserts and areas with low-income and minority populations, the ability to grow food allows people to taste fresh produce, gain confidence and responsibility in their abilities, and to not always go to the food industry to get nutritious food.

The Food and Nutrition Service (FNS) Center for Nutrition Policy and Promotion (CNPP) works to improve the health and wellbeing of Americans by developing and promoting dietary guidance that links scientific research to consumers' nutrition needs. The CNPP was created within the U.S. Department of Agriculture in 1994. It is made up mostly of nutritionists that specialize in nutrition science, analytics, nutrition evaluation, education, and communication. Many of them are Registered Dietitian Nutritionists. The organization is also made up of economists, public health experts, policy advisers, graphic designers, and librarians. The CNPP serves as the Federal authority on evidence-based food, nutrition, and economic analyses to inform policies and programs. The organization translates science into actionable food and nutrition guidance for all Americans. It also leads national communication initiatives that apply science-based messages to advance consumers' dietary and economic knowledge and behaviors. The Nutrition Guidance and Analysis Division provides national leadership, technical expertise, and cooperation for development of the *Dietary Guidelines for Americans*, and Federal nutrition and economic initiatives. The Nutrition Education and Innovation Division designs, leads, and implements a wide range of nutrition education and communication projects. It created and manages *MyPlate.gov*, *DietaryGuidelines.gov*, and *NESR.usda.gov*.

Regulations can affect varieties and qualities of foods available for purchase, prices that consumers must pay, information consumers receive about products, and consumer confidence in the food supply. There are four categories, as follows:

- **Farm assistance programs** – include Federal price and income support programs plus producer-funded marketing orders, and research and promotion agreements. Some marketing orders set quality standards for marketed supplies of foods. Promotion programs attempt to influence demand for commodities through generic advertising. Federal and state price support programs for wheat, rice, feed grains, oilseeds, milk, peanuts, and sugar are intended to stabilize or support prices, and sometimes, producer incomes for these products. Also, producers of milk, fruits, vegetables, and specialty crops are allowed to organize marketing orders to achieve orderly marketing. Several commodities are also covered by federally authorized research and promotion agreements. Programs include:
  - *Federal price and income support programs*
  - *Marketing orders for fruits, vegetables, and specialty crops*
  - *National research and promotion programs*
- **Food safety regulations** – include inspections of processing plants and food products, approval of food additives, and restrictions on pesticide use and animal drugs. Programs include:
  - *Food inspections by the Food and Drug Administration (FDA) and the Food Safety and Inspection Service (FSIS)*
  - *Food safety technology approval*
  - *Food additive approval*
  - *Pesticide regulations*
  - *Animal drug approval*
- **Information regulations** – include labeling requirements and advertising restrictions, standards of identity, and product grades. Programs include:
  - *Food labels and advertising including nutrition labeling and non-health information, plus safe handling labels*
  - *Standards of identity*
  - *Quality grades*
- **Regulations covering sectors other than agriculture** – include environmental requirements and worker safety, restrictions on mergers, and trade policies. Programs include:
  - *Environmental controls*
  - *Worker safety*
  - *Protection of competition*
  - *Trade policy*

These regulations have been shown to affect some individual foods or population groups significantly.

FOCUS ON NUTRITION AND FOOD POLICIES

Nutrition policy is a statement by a government or other authoritative body of its intent to act in order to maintain or alter the food supply, nutritional status, or some other indicator. It is distinct from food policy, since food policy does not explicitly incorporate public health concerns. Another term, "food and nutrition policy" incorporates both public health concerns and intersecting actions with food policy.

Test Your Knowledge

1. What key nutrition interventions are recommended by the WHO?
2. What disincentives can governments use to improve global nutrition?
3. How do some food companies oppose governmental policies about healthier foods?

FINANCIAL IMPACT OF NUTRITIONAL PROBLEMS

The financial impacts of nutritional problems are mostly lost wages, higher employment costs, and reduced government revenue. The four most common nutrition-related chronic diseases are heart disease, obesity, type 2 diabetes mellitus, and cancer. The total financial impact of these diseases in the United States between 2011 and 2020 was estimated at $16 trillion, which was almost 9% of the gross domestic product (GDP) per year. This does not account for premature death or reduced lifetime earnings, which are likely to significantly increase this cost. It also does not account for comorbidities associated with these diseases, which include depression and chronic pain, also known to greatly decrease productivity. Between 2021 and 2022, the four primary diseases are estimated to cost an estimated additional $2.9 trillion per year.

It is estimated that, based on an average of 54.9 hours of reduced productivity per year, cancer is the disease that impacts productivity the most, followed by heart disease (11.2 hours lost), diabetes mellitus (11.1 hours lost), and obesity (7 hours lost). Based on average annual prevalence over the past ten years, assuming an 8-hour workday, this totals 113.5 million days of lost productivity as a result of these four diseases, *per year*. After considering average annual compensation costs, this productivity loss cost employers $295.9 billion between 2011 and 2020, and employers will likely lose another $114.4 billion from 2021 to 2023. In 2020 alone, the total cost due to treatment and lost productivity, in billions of dollars, is illustrated in Figure 24.8.

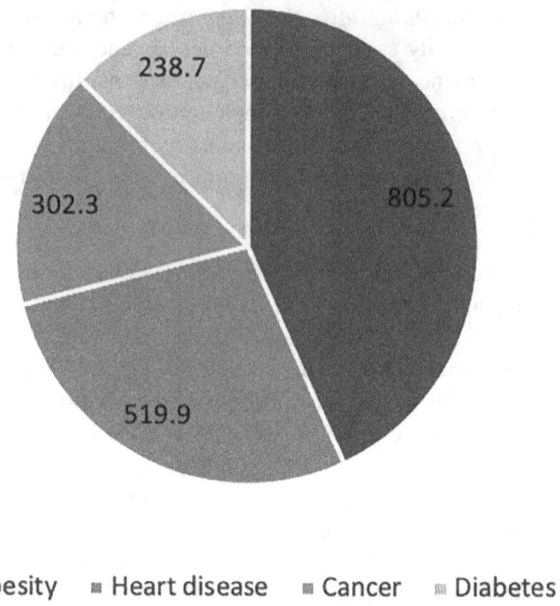

FIGURE 24.8 Total cost due to treatment and lost productivity, 2020, in billions of dollars.

The National Heart, Lung, and Blood Institute reported that Americans spend more than $50 billion per year on care for diabetes, and cardiometabolic diseases, which include heart attack or stroke. While the period of "healthy years" is elevated, with increased disease due to nutritional disorders, healthcare spending is also steadily increasing. The increase in disease rates has seen the rise of healthcare spending to reach 17.7% of the GDP in 2019, which was $3.8 trillion. According to the Economic Commission for Latin America and the Caribbean, economic losses for 13 countries across the region, due to undernutrition, reached the equivalent of $17 billion, or up to 4% of the GDP on average. Lobbyists for big food companies do not help the situation, since in the United States alone, they donate a fortune to politicians. Nearly $34 million was spent on this type of Federal political lobbying in 2015 alone. Table 24.1 summarizes the financial impact of improved health behaviors, in terms of weekly and annual savings.

The cost of malnutrition to the global economy, in lost productivity and health care expenses, is overwhelming. It exists in all regions and socio-economic classes. Investing in solution to malnutrition can improve nutritional outcomes over the long term. Research shows that for every billion dollars invested annually in micronutrient supplements, food fortification, and biofortification of staple crops over five years, this would generate annual benefits of nearly 13 times the expense, and result in better health, fewer deaths, and increased future earnings.

For obesity alone, if trends continue, obesity-related medical costs in the United States alone could reach $66 billion per year, contributing to a global total of approximately $500 billion annually, imposing huge burdens on the health budgets of emerging countries. If African countries most affected by stunting could achieve a 40%

TABLE 24.1
Financial Impact of Improved Health Behaviors

Improved Health/Nutrition Practice	Weekly Savings	Annual Savings
Getting two meals from one by eating smaller servings	$9	$468
Reducing the number of meals eaten away from home by two	$10	$520
Substituting pasta, beans, soups, for meat two to three times per week	$15	$780
Saving $3.00 per day currently spent on junk food, fast food, or alcohol	$21	$1,092
Quitting smoking (one pack per day)	$35	$1,820

reduction by 2025, there could be a gain in over $83 billion between 2035 and 2060, which is when the 40% fewer undernourished children would enter the labor force at 18 years of age. For Ethiopia alone, the reward would be about $15 billion. If Cambodia were to achieve the same goal, their government could prevent a yearly loss of about $50 million.

FOCUS ON WEIGHT LOSS AND RELATED REDUCTION IN MEDICAL COSTS

According to the CDC, a 10% weight loss could reduce an overweight person's lifetime medical costs by $2,200–$5,300. Delaying the onset of diabetes mellitus can save thousands of dollars per year in increased medical costs. Inactivity alone is estimated to cost between $670 and $1,125 per person, per year.

Test Your Knowledge

1. What are the four most common nutrition-related chronic diseases, and how big is their financial impact?
2. How much money could a 10% weight loss save an average adult?

STEPS TO END GLOBAL NUTRITIONAL PROBLEMS

In the United States, the *Global Malnutrition Prevention and Treatment Act (GMPTA)* was approved in 2022, directly targeting the problem by providing the United States Agency for International Development with resources that were needed to increase their efforts. The GMPTA is expected to strengthen crucial coordination efforts across governments and non-profit entities, to ensure that women and children receive comprehensive nutritional resources where and when they are most needed. In order to end global nutrition problems, there are many factors that first need to be addressed. These include the following:

- Nutrition policies do not sufficiently respond to challenges that countries and regions are facing today – especially the double burden of malnutrition
- Nutrition policies often do not include evidence-based interventions in a comprehensive manner – including interventions such as complementary feeding, iron and folic acid supplementation, food fortification, and those addressing adult obesity
- Many nutrition policies do not sufficiently consider or address the underlying and basic causes of malnutrition – food insecurity, inadequate health service, and inadequate care for women and children
- Nutrition policies are often not officially adopted – for example, those in the region of the Americas are the least often officially adopted, while those in the Eastern Mediterranean Region are the most often officially adopted
- Food security strategies do not comprehensively address malnutrition in all forms – including the serious circle of malnutrition with foodborne and other infectious diseases
- National development plans and poverty reduction strategy papers are often not considered as important policy documents for improving nutrition – especially in countries with a high burden of stunting
- Policies do not clearly state plans and programs of work – they may not have clear goals, targets, timelines, or deliverables; may not specify roles and responsibilities; may not identify the capacity and areas of competence required of the workforce; may not include process-and-outcome evaluation with appropriate indicators; and may not have the needed or adequate budget for implementation

Countries have inadequate coordination mechanisms to address existing nutrition challenges. There is poor or insufficient coordination with and between ministries, as well as with United Nations agencies and other partners. Coordination mechanisms are rarely included in high-level policymaking structures or frameworks. There are often inconsistencies between policies at the national level and programs being implemented at lower levels.

Regarding implementation of programs, a comprehensive set of interventions addressing the life course is not being implemented. Nutrition interventions, including many key interventions for maternal, infant, and young child nutrition are seldom implemented well. The International Code of Marketing of Breast-milk Substitutes, subsequent World Health Assembly resolutions, and the Global Strategy on Infant and Young Child Feeding are not being implemented sufficiently. Vitamin and mineral supplementation and fortification programs are inconsistent, and usually inadequate in terms of nutrient mix, target groups, and coverage. Women are not reached with important interventions prior to becoming pregnant. Implementation of programs that address obesity and diet-related noncommunicable diseases varies widely by region. There is low implementation in regions where the double burden of malnutrition is worsening. Schools and workplaces are not sufficiently used to reach and deliver nutrition interventions. When they are not cover the entire spectrum of nutritional problems. The national capacity for public health nutrition is limited, especially in community health workers that primarily work with delivery of nutrition programs. Financial resources for nutrition are also lacking.

The way forward toward ending the global burden of nutritional deficiencies is via evidence-informed, effective nutrition interventions, which need to be increased widely. Global malnutrition is being improved through the combined efforts of the *Zero Hunger Initiative, Global Strategy for Women's and Children's Health,* and the *Comprehensive Framework for Action of the High Level Task Force on the Global Food Security Crisis.* Great progress has been made in nutrition policy development and implementation since the first intergovernmental conference on nutrition was held in 1992 (the International Conference on Nutrition). Even so, nutrition considerations need to be integrated into sectoral plans in order to be effective and generate long-lasting change.

The *World Food Programme (WFP)* brings lifesaving food and nutrition assistance to people trapped or displaced by fighting. The organization reaches out to those in need, even in the most remote areas, by using all-terrain vehicles and dropping food from planes. This work is contributing to improving prospects for peach as well, by increasing access to contested natural resources, boosting social cohesion, and resolving grievances within and between communities. The WFP also increases opportunities and trust between people and governments by strengthening state accountability and the delivery of services. Extreme achievements have been made already in El Salvador, Iraq, Kyrgyzstan, and Mali. The WFP's forecast-based financing uses improved early warning based on weather forecasts, so that communities can be alerted to climate shocks 15 days in advance, and provide with insurance mechanisms to prepare. The WFP provides access to modern cooking solutions such as gas stoves, mini-gasifiers, and electronic pressure cookers. The organization strives to empower small farmers through sustainable distribution of energy equipment and services for productive use, to boost agricultural market development. The WFP provides coordination and information management in the response to large-scale disaster, and leads the Emergency Telecommunications Cluster. Their Fast Information Technology and Telecommunications Emergency and Support Team of responders is ready to deploy anywhere, to establish and restore communications and information technology (IT) networks. The organization helps restore unproductive land, connects small farmers to markets, helps farms diversify crops and increase business potential, provides cash assistance, supports governments in protecting citizens from poverty, inequality, and hunger; and works to enhance these systems in their response to disasters or mass population displacements. The WFP also teaches small farmers how to use improved post-harvest handling methods, using hermetic storage equipment to protect against animals, mold, and moisture. The organization set up global passenger and cargo movement services so that health supplies can reach vulnerable people around the world. In relation to COVID-19, the WFP increased its cash as well as food assistance programs, supporting governments in their attempts to assist their citizens. As described by *Concern Worldwide U.S.,* there are nine hunger solutions described in order to meet goals set for the year 2030. These include the following:

- *Embracing climate smart agriculture* – to allow farmers to adapt and become more resilient against unpredictable climates, including diversifying crop varieties, conservation agriculture, and low-water sack gardens
- *Responding to the refugee crisis* – by finding new ways to generate income; for example, Syrian refugee women and their Lebanese neighbors have learned to make staples like cheese and yogurt, and to sell them at market for a profit
- *Advocating for gender equality* – giving female farmers equal access to resources as their male counterparts could increase farm production by 20%–30%, potentially reducing the number of hungry people in the world by up to 150 million; also, by better prioritizing women's health and nutrition, complications for them and their future children can be prevented, continuing through pregnancy, breastfeeding, and the remainder of life
- *Reducing food waste* – this type of reduction also reduces the waste of other natural resources including water; it is important to ask political representatives to commit to policies that reduce waste so that the entire food system benefits
- *Investing in disaster risk reduction* – this is most important in vulnerable communities such as subsistence agriculture (growing what they eat); it involves protecting and diversifying crops as well as homesteads and livestock
- *Supporting hygiene and sanitation* – to prevent diarrhea, other waterborne illnesses, and to facilitate proper absorption of nutrients; uncontaminated drinking and washing water can save lives in multiple ways
- *Controlling infestations and crop infections* – pest or fungus invasions can decimate crops, which in recent years has occurred in countries such as Kenya, Ethiopia, Somalia, South Sudan, Yemen, Iraq, and Iran, resulting in over 13 million people going hungry; aerial sprays are used to curb insect swarms; other agricultural practices can combat smaller invasions or deadly fungi; disaster preparedness utilizes cash transfers, new seeds, and needed supplies
- *Enhancing crops with biofortification* – biofortified crops include iron-enriched beans, pearl millet, and sweet potatoes, which are high in vitamin A; these crops allow families to greatly increase intake of critical micronutrients, and can be saved by farmers for future replanting without losing the biofortified traits
- *Improving food storage systems* – this may require building or rehabilitating grain storage areas, use of solar dryers for the sun-drying of vegetables; these eco-friendly devices accelerate the process while reducing contamination and nutrient loss

Test Your Knowledge

1. What are the underlying and basic causes of malnutrition that are not sufficiently considered by many nutrition policies?
2. How is the World Food Programme reaching out to those in need?

KEY TERMS

Cyclones

El Niño

Fiscal disincentives

Fiscal incentives

Linear growth

Punitive

Standard deviations

Stunted growth

Wasting

CLINICAL CASE STUDIES

Clinical Case Study 1

A seven-year-old girl from Syria fled with her family because of wartime bombing near their home, ending up in a refugee camp in another part of the country that was safer. The girl had previously had a fever that was not sufficiently treated, which left her with hearing and speech impairments. Without enough work, her parents can only afford meat in their diet about once per month, and though they can regularly get fruits and vegetables, these food items are expensive. Therefore, everyone in the family doesn't eat enough and are very thin. A physician diagnoses the girl with malnutrition, and she is put into a supplemental food program that is sponsored by charity organizations. Slowly, her health and nutritional status begin to improve.

CRITICAL THINKING QUESTIONS

1. Are wars and other conflicts related to malnutrition?
2. Can infections be related to wasting?
3. Which organizations are working together to combat global malnutrition?

Clinical Case Study 2

A nine-year-old Ethiopian patient was assessed because of severe malnourishment. His family was very poor and could not afford proper food for all of them. The boy is placed on treatments that included vitamin A, folic acid, and medicines to treat an infection that he had. After about one week, food supplements had begun to stabilize his condition, but he was not gaining enough weight. Testing revealed that he had tuberculosis, which was not anticipated by the physicians treating him. Treatments began and he slowly began to return to normal as the tuberculosis resolved and his nutrition improved.

CRITICAL THINKING QUESTIONS

1. How significant is undernutrition in Africa?
2. What are the causes of the malnutrition situation in Ethiopia?
3. How much are Ethiopian children being affected by the malnutrition situation?

Clinical Case Study 3

In India, a one-year-old child with severe acute malnutrition was put into a nutrition rehabilitation center. She was given small meals of fresh food every few hours, which included supplementary nutrition packets. After three months, the girl regained normal weight and nutritional status.

CRITICAL THINKING QUESTIONS

1. What is severe acute malnutrition, and what is its prevalence?
2. What is ready-to-use therapeutic food that is used to treat malnutrition?
3. What is the nutritional situation in India?

STUDY QUESTIONS

1. In early childhood, which of the following is the most important marker of healthy growth?
   A. Bone growth
   B. Linear growth
   C. Weight growth
   D. Fetal growth

2. Which of the following is the most immediate, visible, and life-threatening form of malnutrition?
   A. Wasting
   B. Stunting
   C. Prematurity
   D. Obesity

3. All of the following are among the largest absolute increases in obesity, EXCEPT:
   A. In men in high-income Western countries
   B. In women in the Middle East
   C. In men in North Africa
   D. In women in Central Asia

4. Severe wasting is the most lethal form of which of the following?
   A. Infection
   B. Iron deficiency anemia
   C. Hyperlipidemia
   D. Malnutrition

5. Which of the following countries is at risk for a catastrophic degree of hunger?
   A. Iran
   B. South Africa
   C. Ethiopia
   D. Mexico

6. Which of the following countries has the worst food problem?
   A. Haiti
   B. India
   C. Libya
   D. Australia

7. Which of the following organizations or agencies provides a framework for future global and national goals in relation to nutritional problems?
   A. WHO
   B. CDC
   C. UNGNA
   D. FNS

8. Strong governmental policies are essential for achieving all of the following, EXCEPT:
   A. Healthy food
   B. Disincentives
   C. Equitability
   D. Profitability

9. Strong regulations on transparency and activity are required for all of the following, EXCEPT:
   A. Unbiased policymaking
   B. Maintaining effective policymaking
   C. Controlling prices
   D. Accountability

10. Which of the following is NOT a major idea about how governments can incentivize food and nutrition policies?
   A. Encourage consumers to purchase affordable produce
   B. Subsidize food corporations
   C. Discount imperfect produce
   D. Raise taxes on the marketing of unhealthy goods

11. All of the following are programs that concern food safety regulation, EXCEPT:
   A. Food inspections by the FDA
   B. Food additive approval
   C. Food cost regulations
   D. Pesticide regulations

12. Which of the following is NOT one of the four most common nutrition-related chronic diseases?
   A. Chronic meningitis
   B. Diabetes mellitus type 2
   C. Heart disease
   D. Cancer

13. Which of the following is NOT a factor relating of the financial impact of nutritional problems?
   A. Lost wages
   B. Higher employment costs
   C. Reduced government revenue
   D. Increased government revenue

14. Food additive approval includes which of the following categories of regulation on quality of foods?
   A. Food safety regulation
   B. Information regulations
   C. Farm assistance programs
   D. Regulations covering sectors other than agriculture

15. Limitations or standards exist concerning which of the following dietary components in many countries?
   A. High-calorie soft drinks
   B. Total protein
   C. Trans-fats
   D. Fruit juices

FURTHER READING

1. Adams, F. (2021). *The Right to Food: The Global Campaign to End Hunger and Malnutrition*. Palgrave Macmillan.
2. Apt Russell, S. (2021). *Within Our Grasp: Childhood Malnutrition Worldwide and the Revolution Taking Place to End It*. Random House.
3. Barth, M.M., Bell, R.A., and Grimmer, K. (2020). *Public Health Nutrition – Rural, Urban, and Global Community-Based Practice*. Springer.
4. Boyle, M.A. (2022). *Personal Nutrition*, 11th Edition. Cengage Learning.

5. Butterly, J.R., and Shepherd, J. (2010). *Hunger: The Biology and Politics of Starvation (Geisel Series in Global Health and Medicine).* Dartmouth College Press.
6. Cheo, A.E., and Tapiwa, K.A. (2021). *SDG2 – Zero Hunger: Food Security, Improved Nutrition and Sustainable Agriculture (Concise Guides to the United Nations Sustainable Development Goals).* Emerald Publishing Ltd.
7. De Pee, S., Taren, D., and Bloem, M.W. (2017). *Nutrition and Health in a Developing World, 3rd Edition (Nutrition and Health).* Humana Press.
8. Fanzo, J., and Davis, C. (2021). *Global Food Systems, Diets, and Nutrition – Linking Science, Economics, and Policy.* Palgrave Macmillan.
9. Food and Agriculture Organization of the United Nations, International Fund for Agricultural Development, World Food Programme, World Health Organization, and United Nations International Children's Emergency Fund. (2020). *The State of Food Security and Nutrition in the World 2020: Transforming Food Systems for Affordable Healthy Diets.* Food and Agriculture Organization of the United States.
10. Garoma Berra, W. (2012). *Common Nutritional Problems of Public Health Importance in Ethiopia – Community Nutrition.* Lap Lambert Academic Publishing.
11. Hyman, M. (2020). *Food Fix: How to Save Our Health, Our Economy, Our Communities, and Our Planet – One Bite at a Time.* Little, Brown Spark.
12. McLaren, S.W. (2022). *Nutrition and Global Health.* Wiley Blackwell.
13. Parker, C. (2014). *Nutrition and Science (Nutrition – A Global View).* Village Earth Press.
14. Shekar, M., Kakietek, J., Dayton Eberwein, J., and Walters, D. (2017). *An Investment Framework for Nutrition – Reaching the Global Targets for Stunting, Anemia, Breastfeeding, and Wasting. (Directions in Development – Human Development).* World Bank Group.
15. Simone, J. (2014). *Nutrition and Politics (Nutrition – A Global View).* Village Earth Press.
16. Simons, R. (2014). *Nutrition and Poverty (Nutrition – A Global View).* Village Earth Press.
17. Sirohi, M. (2018). *Nutritional Status and Health Problems of Middle Aged Women.* Lap Lambert Academic Publishing.
18. Stein, N. (2014). *Public Health Nutrition – Principles and Practice in Community and Global Health.* Jones & Bartlett Learning.
19. Tappan, J. (2017). *The Riddle of Malnutrition: The Long Arc of Biomedical and Public Health Interventions in Uganda (Perspectives on Global Health).* Ohio University Press.
20. Walker, I. (2016). *Nutrition and You (Nutrition – A Global View).* Village Earth Press.

Answer Key to Clinical Case Studies

CHAPTER 1: NUTRITION AND HEALTH

Clinical Case Study 1

1. In the intensive care unit, it if is available, indirect calorimetry is used. It is estimated based on 25 kcal per kg of body weight per day.
2. Enteral nutrition in the ICU is preferred initially unless it is contraindicated. It is started within 48 hours at 30 mL per hour, then escalated in most cases.
3. A well-nourished patient in the ICU can actually wait for seven days without enteral nutrition or total parenteral nutrition.

Clinical Case Study 2

1. Trauma causes a cardiovascular response (hemorrhage, tissue damage, pain, anxiety), an inflammatory response (cytokine production, swelling), and a metabolic response (hypermetabolism, insulin resistance, hyperglycemia, increased protein breakdown, wound healing).
2. A trauma patient's nutritional state is highly influential upon wound healing. Moderate-to-severe protein energy malnutrition impairs or delays this. Protein deficiency interferes with formation of new capillaries, proliferation of fibroblasts, proteoglycan production, and synthesis of collagen. Of the amino acids, arginine is known to improve wound healing and immune function. Other needed nutrients include vitamins A, C, and E, plus zinc, copper, selenium, and manganese. Iron also plays a part in wound healing.
3. Early nutritional support, within 72 hours, is more beneficial than delayed feeding if the patient has blunt or penetrating trauma, since it leads to three times lower chances for sepsis. Total enteral nutrition is preferred over total parenteral nutrition since it allows for better use of nutrients, prevents atrophy of the GI mucosa, preserves GI flora, reduces stress response, and maintains immunocompetence.

Clinical Case Study 3

1. The prominent clinical features in adults are weight loss and in children, growth failure, with excluding any endocrine disorders. Related features include anorexia, inflammation, and increased muscle protein breakdown.
2. With cachexia, over an extended period of time there is significant weight loss as well as the loss of lean body mass. Wound healing slows since the body has insufficient energy and nutritional substrate. To build new tissue, proteins must be available to fuel anabolism. The patient with cachexia does not have these proteins available.
3. For patients with any form of cachexia, diet intervention focuses on providing 55%–60% of total calories as complex carbohydrates, 20%–25% of total calories as protein, and 20%–25% of total calories as fat (which should not exceed 2 g per kg of body weight per day, since amounts higher than this may affect lipid levels).

Clinical Case Study 4

1. Nutrition after surgery, protein is extremely essential. Protein helps repair body tissues, form antibodies to fight infections, and synthesize collagen so that scars can form. Good protein sources include fish, lean poultry, seafood, legumes, nuts, and seeds. Fatty red meats should be limited since they may trigger inflammation.
2. Foods that help reduce pain and inflammation after surgery include canola oil, extra virgin olive oil, soybean oil, dark-colored fruits, fatty fish, flaxseed meal or oil, green and black tea, onion, garlic, green leafy vegetables, soy products, turmeric, walnuts, almonds, and peanuts.
3. Vitamins that reduce inflammation and accelerate wound healing include vitamin A, vitamin C, and vitamin D. The mineral calcium is essential for bone repair,

soft tissue healing, normal blood clotting, muscle contraction, and normal heartbeat. The minerals zinc and copper are also important.

Clinical Case Study 5

1. Severe burns cause significant metabolic abnormalities, making nutritional support extremely important and challenging. They cause a continuing hypermetabolic state and increased catabolism, resulting in increased muscle wasting and cachexia. The metabolic rates of burn patients can be more than twice the normal rates.
2. Carbohydrates are the preferred energy source for burn patients since high carbohydrate diets promote wound healing and result in a protein-sparing effect. Care is needed, since glucose given in excess of what the patient can utilize leads to hyperglycemia, conversion of glucose to fat, glucosuria, and dehydration. Many patients need supplemental insulin in order to maintain satisfactory blood glucose.
3. Healthy eating for burn patients means eating small meals, five to six times per day. High-protein foods include meat, eggs, beans, milk, yogurt, cheese, nuts, peanut butter, and tofu.

CHAPTER 2: GLOBAL ISSUES WITH NUTRITION

Clinical Case Study 1

1. The risk factors of obesity may be modifiable, nonmodifiable, or environmental. Modifiable energy input risk factors include excess calories, while modifiable energy output risk factors include a sedentary lifestyle. Nonmodifiable risk factors include aging, ethnicity, gender, genetics, menopause, prenatal and postnatal effects, physiologic factors, and psychological factors. Environmental energy input risk factors include a built environment, motorized transportation, automation, and mechanization. Environmental energy output risk factors include food policy, access, availability, cost, marketing, and quality.
2. Our built environments usually discourage physical activity. In urban settings, people usually rely more on cars and other motorized methods of transportation. People often drive for long distances to get to and from work. Automatic and mechanization have reduced physical activity requirements at work. These requirements in school have declined from about 45% of the school day to about 25%. Out behaviors have increased in their sedentary qualities, such as the use of computers, video games, and television.
3. In men, obesity has different prevalence based on age group (40.3% of men aged 20–39 are obese; this is 46.4% in men 40–59, and 42.2% in men 60 and over).

Clinical Case Study 2

1. Food insecurity means a lack of food availability, access, and utilization.
2. Wasting is defined as "low weight-for-height" and often indicates recent, severe weight loss. However, wasting can also last for a long time, usually because of poor quality of food, or insufficient quantities of food, sometimes accompanied by frequent or chronic illnesses. Without adequate treatment, wasting in children is linked to a higher risk of death. Wasting affected about 7.3% (49 million) children under five years of age in 2018 throughout the world.
3. Though the global prevalence of moderate-to-severe food insecurity has been increasing since 2014, in 2020, the increase was so large that it equaled the increase of the previous five years combined. Almost one in three people throughout the world (2.37 billion) did not have access to adequate food in 2020. This is an increase of nearly 320 million people within one year.

CHAPTER 3: NEWBORNS AND PREMATURE INFANTS

Clinical Case Study 1

1. Breastfeeding should continue for a minimum of six months, with solid foods being introduced from that time up to one year. After one year, breastfeeding can continue for as long as the mother and infant desire, but it should be a complement to a full diet of solid foods and fluids.
2. Breast milk has a variety of important features, including high lactose content, large amounts of vitamin E, twice the amount of calcium compared to phosphorus, protection against bacterial diarrhea, transfer of protective antibodies from mother to infant, cholesterol, taurine, and omega-3 plus omega-6 fatty acids.
3. For infants, the first solid food is usually an iron-fortified rice cereal. It is non-allergenic, easy to digest, and supplies a good amount of iron. Pureed meat can follow, which is a good source of iron and zinc. If the parents are vegetarian, sufficient iron and zinc can be supplied via iron-fortified cereals and grains, green leafy vegetables, dried beans, and yeast-fermented whole-grain breads.

Clinical Case Study 2

1. Any baby that is born before 37 weeks of gestation is considered premature. Prematurity is defined by the gestational age at birth. About 10% of births are premature. In the case of Amy (in this clinical case), she would be classified as extremely preterm because she was born at less than 28 weeks of gestation.
2. Common feeding problems during infancy include difficulty swallowing, aspiration, refusal to drink or eat, arching the back or stiffening while feeding, crying or fussiness while feeding, taking more than 30 minutes for each feeding, lack of alertness or falling asleep while feeding, avoiding foods with certain textures, extreme drooling, coughing or gagging while feeding, difficulty breathing while feeding, frequent spitting up or vomiting, or vocal hoarseness during or after feeding.
3. Switching from breastfeeding to formula too early is bad for an infant and can also cause painful breast engorgement in the mother. Making a switch such as this quickly without a slow transition is not suggested by medical professionals. It can take from two to six weeks for an infant to fully transition to formula.

Clinical Case Study 3

1. Failure to thrive is a term used to describe an infant or child's weight being consistently below the third to fifth percentile for age and gender, a progressive weight decrease to below the third to fifth percentile, or a decrease in two major growth percentiles over a short period of time.
2. With the organic form of failure to thrive, growth failure is caused by an acute or chronic disorder, interfering with intake of nutrients, absorption, metabolism, or excretion. There may also be a disorder present that increases energy requirements, including illness of any organ system.
3. An infant's basal metabolic rates are high, partly because their body surface area is large compared to their overall size. Limited physical activity means that their total expenditure of energy is rather low. Over the first few months, the activities of an infant are primarily eating and sleeping.

CHAPTER 4: CHILDREN AND ADOLESCENTS

Clinical Case Study 1

1. For children between 4 and 8 years of age, the recommended daily allowances of various nutrients include 0.95 g/kg of body weight per day of proteins, 130 g per day of carbohydrates, no RDA for fats, 400 mcg per day of vitamin A, 25 mg per day of vitamin C, 7 mg per day of vitamin E, 1,000 mg per day of calcium, 10 mg per day of iron, 5 mg per day of zinc, and 1.7 L per day of fluids.
2. Attending school often requires busy morning schedules, but children should never skip breakfast or eat insufficient quantities of food. Hunger during school increases risks for behavioral and learning problems. In school, many children eat whatever they want, or in excessive amounts. They often trade items in home-packed lunches that they don't really like for other items that are preferred, even though they may be poorer in nutritional value. Sometimes, a proper lunch is not consumed in order to have more time for recess with friends.
3. Common nutrient deficiencies related to neurodevelopmental disorders in children include vitamins B1, B3, B5, B6, B12, C, folic acid/folate, biotin, selenium, magnesium, taurine, essential fatty acids, and the fat-soluble vitamins A, D, E, and K. The deficiencies are caused by low intake of nutrients, inability to digest and assimilate nutrients, and the inability to convert them to the active form at the cellular level.

Clinical Case Study 2

1. Vitamin B12 is found in high levels in dairy products, eggs, and vitamin-fortified breads, cereals, milk alternatives, and nutritional yeast.
2. The best choice of vegetarian diet for growing teens is a lacto-ovo diet, which includes dairy products and eggs. This and other vegetarian diets can be excellent choices since they prompt adolescents to eat more fruits and vegetables. Today many schools offer vegetarian meal choices. It is important for parents to discuss healthy eating with their children, especially if they consume a vegetarian diet.
3. Adolescents often greatly reduce calories or cut out all fats or carbohydrates, saying they are on a "vegetarian diet", but this indicates an eating disorder. It is important that parents monitor any self-imposed, restrictive diets. Preteens or teenagers must be instructed about understanding nutrients that may be missing from their diets. A good way to help monitor the situation is for the entire family to have at least one vegetarian meal together every week.

Clinical Case Study 3

1. Avoidant/restrictive food intake disorder is an eating disorder. In children, it results in extremely choosy food intake and often, little interest in eating. By eating only a limited variety of the foods they will accept, poor growth and nutrition can result.
2. Children with ARFID may not feel hungry, or are repelled by food odors, tastes, textures, or colors. Some affected children have a fear of choking, pain, or vomiting while they eat.

3. Children that have ARFID are more likely to have anxiety, obsessive-compulsive disorder, ADHD, autism spectrum disorder, and problems at home or school because of their eating habits.

CHAPTER 5: OLDER ADULTS

Clinical Case Study 1

1. Cortical atrophy progresses as we age, with a 6%–11% loss of brain weight once a person passes the age of 80. There are decreases in cerebral hemisphere volume, the frontal region, the temporoparietal region, and the parieto-occipital region, along with increased lateral ventricle and third ventricle volume.
2. In patients with Alzheimer's disease, there is a 20%–25% greater cortical atrophy than in patients of the same age that do not have the disease. Cerebral blood flow and oxygen consumption decrease, especially in areas with decreased gray and white matter.
3. The shrinkage rate of the brain increases even more than in previous decades by the age of 60. The frontal lobe and hippocampus experience the most shrinkage. As the cerebral cortex becomes thinner, its lower density leads to fewer connections, which may contribute to worsened cognitive processing.

Clinical Case Study 2

1. In the elderly, nerves in the airways that trigger coughing become less sensitive to foreign particles, so when the particles increase in the lungs, they can damage the tissues.
2. Simple methods to protect the respiratory system and maintain better function throughout life include avoiding or quitting smoking, avoiding air pollution, regular exercise, maintaining a healthy weight so that excess abdominal fat does not accumulate, not sleeping excessively, having regular healthcare checkups, and getting annual vaccinations.
3. After age 35, the function of the lungs begins to decline. Breathing can slowly become more difficult year by year. The alveoli can lose their shape and become "baggy". The diaphragm may weaken, decreasing the ability to inhale and exhale. However, this change is only significant while exercising.

Clinical Case Study 3

1. With aging, there are many changes that affect the digestive system, beginning with a reduction in the senses of smell and taste. The gums recede, there may be difficulty swallowing, peristalsis in the esophagus decreases, the esophageal sphincters lose tension, the stomach walls lose elasticity, there is decreased production of bicarbonate and gastromucosal protection, there is delayed gastric emptying, the liver shrinks (affecting is function), and the pancreas and intestines also decline in functionality.
2. About 50% of people aged 65–80 and about 75% of those over age 80 have a significant loss of the sense of smell. Accompanying this are age-related changes in taste cell membranes, which reduce the sense of taste. Diminished food intake can lead to weight loss and malnutrition, while the inability to taste and enjoy food can lead to anxiety. The ability to taste salty foods is reduced, and can lead to overconsumption of sodium-rich meals, aggravating hypertension and other conditions.
3. Age-related shrinkage of the maxillary and mandibular bones, and reduction in bone calcium causes the tooth sockets to slowly erode, leading to gum recession and a higher risk for tooth decay. People that are missing teeth or have poorly fitting dentures may find chewing difficult, resulting in them eating less, and the development of malnutrition.

CHAPTER 6: PREGNANT WOMEN

Clinical Case Study 1

1. A pregnant woman that does not gain enough weight during pregnancy has a greater chance of giving birth to a low-birthweight baby, which is what happened in this case.
2. Low-birthweight babies have an increased chance of developing infections, learning disabilities, and experiencing poor physical development. Some die within the first year of life.
3. If underweight before pregnancy (BMI less than 18.5), a woman should gain 28–40 pounds during pregnancy.

Clinical Case Study 2

1. Gestational diabetes is becoming more common and is diagnosed in up to 10% of pregnancies. It is usually temporary, with the pregnant woman being unable to produce enough insulin or becoming insulin resistant, with raised levels of blood glucose.
2. Gestational diabetes is more common in women that are obese, over age 35, or from the Native American, African-American, or Hispanic racial or ethnic groups.
3. A healthy diet and regular physical activities will reduce risks for developing gestational diabetes. Treatment includes special meal plans, scheduled physical activity, and sometimes, daily blood glucose tests and insulin injections.

Clinical Case Study 3

1. When obese women become pregnant, they are more at risk for serious health problems such as preeclampsia, gestational diabetes, and obstructive sleep apnea.
2. Children of obese woman have higher rates of childhood obesity and metabolic abnormalities.
3. When an obese woman develops polycystic ovary syndrome, she is three to four times more likely to develop pregnancy-related forms of hypertension and diabetes than in healthy women. There is also twice the risk for preterm birth.

CHAPTER 7: UNDERNUTRITION AND EATING DISORDERS

Clinical Case Study 1

1. Primary carnitine deficiency is a rare condition caused by an abnormal gene, sometimes leading to only low carnitine levels in muscles. The body cannot utilize certain fats for energy, especially while fasting. When the liver and heart are affected, the condition may be called systemic carnitine deficiency. Primary carnitine deficiency is also known as carnitine uptake defect.
2. The symptoms of primary carnitine deficiency are more severe than with the secondary form of the disease. Affected children usually have symptoms beginning in the first few years of life, though symptoms can also appear in adulthood.
3. If carnitine deficiency is familial, couples are advised to see a genetic specialist before having children, to assess risks of passing the disease on. If the abnormal gene is present, in vitro fertilization can be done, and the embryos can be tested for the deficiency. Amniocentesis also helps test for it during early pregnancy.

Clinical Case Study 2

1. With vitamin A deficiency, eye abnormalities begin that lead to conjunctival xerosis, followed by Bitot's spots, which often progress to keratomalacia and scarring. These sequential eye changes are collectively known as xerophthalmia, which causes irreversible blindness in millions of people throughout the world.
2. Conditions related to impaired absorption, storage, or transport of vitamin A that can cause keratomalacia include celiac disease, ulcerative colitis, cystic fibrosis, liver disease, or conditions affecting absorption of the fat-soluble vitamins. Also, intestinal bypass surgery can be implicated as a cause.
3. Primary vitamin A deficiency and keratomalacia are common in areas where rice is a major dietary component, such as Southeast Asia, since rice lacks beta-carotene, which is converted into vitamin A.

Clinical Case Study 3

1. Anorexia nervosa involves extreme weight loss, distortions of body image, and an irrational fear of weight gain and obesity. The affected person often denies his or her appetite and hates looking in a mirror. Anorexics believe they are fat no matter what the truth is and what others tell them. Some people focus on body areas, such as the stomach, thighs, and buttocks, which they believe to be excessively fat.
2. Family conflict is a common underlying factor of anorexia nervosa. If a family's expectations are very high, including expectations about body weight, frustration results in arguments. Anorexic individuals often feel hopeless about human relationships and become socially isolated by family dysfunction.
3. Anorexics have very low body weights and fear gaining any amount of weight. They have a distorted view of their weight and their self-worth is nearly entirely based on it. There are continual thoughts about controlling food, eating, and weight, while human relationships are reduced.

CHAPTER 8: OBESITY AND METABOLIC SYNDROME

Clinical Case Study 1

1. At 5 feet, 10 inches tall, with a weight of 370 pounds, this patient's body mass index (BMI) would be at more than 3471.8 lb/square inches, classifying him in the "extreme obesity" class of III. If measured in kg/square meters, his BMI would be above 40.
2. Gastric bypass surgery can improve or resolve heart disease, hypertension, obstructive sleep apnea, type 2 diabetes, nonalcoholic fatty liver disease (NAFLD), nonalcoholic steatohepatitis (NASH), gastroesophageal reflux disease (GERD), and osteoarthritis.
3. Gastric bypass may work by altering the incretins that drive insulin secretion and sensitivity.

Clinical Case Study 2

1. Type 2 diabetes mellitus eventually leads to circulatory, nervous, and immune system disorders.
2. In the treatment of obesity, diets should not be done temporarily, stopping once desired weight is lost. When diets are short-term, most people regain the lost weight, returning to being obese. The emphasis should be on healthy and active lifestyles, with lifelong dietary modifications. Weight loss must be slow and steady in order to promote lasting weight control. A goal of one or two pounds of weight loss per week is suggested.
3. For women between 30 and 55, without cardiovascular disease or cancer, one large study revealed them to have a 90% higher total mortality because of obesity. This was over four times higher for cardiovascular mortality and more than twice as high for cancer mortality compared to non-obese women. About 53% of deaths among women with a BMI over 29 were because of their obesity. Gaining 10 kg or more of weight after age 18 and a BMI of more than 22 at age 18 predicted death from cardiovascular disease in middle adulthood.

Clinical Case Study 3

1. Risk factors of metabolic syndrome that increase risks for type 2 diabetes mellitus and cardiovascular disease include obesity (especially abdominal obesity), insulin resistance or glucose intolerance, which results in high blood glucose, high blood triglycerides and LDL cholesterol, low HDL cholesterol, hypertension, increased inflammatory blood proteins such as C-reactive protein, and increased concentrations of oxidized LDL cholesterol.
2. According to the American Heart Association and National Heart, Lung, and Blood Institute, three (or more) of the following must be present in order to diagnose metabolic syndrome: waist circumference greater than 40 inches (for men) and 35 inches (for women), fasting triglyceride levels above 150 mg/dL, blood HDL cholesterol below 40 mg/dL (for men) and below 50 mg/dL (for women), elevated BP above 130/85 mm Hg, and fasting blood glucose above 100 mg/dL.
3. The Mediterranean diet emphasizes foods that were commonly consumed around the Mediterranean region in the 20th century and earlier, including many vegetables, fruits, fish, poultry, whole grains, legumes, dairy products, and extra virgin olive oil. It is especially effective in preventing heart disease.

CHAPTER 9: COMPLICATIONS OF OBESITY

Clinical Case Study 1

1. Obesity is related to an increased risk of developing cardiovascular disorders. IT changes the composition of the body, affecting hemodynamics and altering heart structure. Adipose tissue produces pro-inflammatory cytokines, which can cause cardiac dysfunction as well as promote the formation of atherosclerotic plaques.
2. The cardiovascular disorders that are complications of obesity include atherosclerosis, dyslipidemia, hypertension, stroke, and pulmonary embolism.
3. Obesity is a risk factor for the development of postoperative complications. Obese patients experience more concomitant diseases, increased risks of wound infection, more intraoperative blood loss, and longer operation times.

Clinical Case Study 2

1. Obstructive sleep apnea is the most common form of sleep apnea, and is characterized by partial or complete obstructions of the upper airway. There is also an uncommon condition referred to as obstructive sleep apnea syndrome that occurs between the ages of 30 and 60.
2. Just a 10% increase in body weight had an average of a 32% increase in the apnea-hypopnea index, and a six times higher risk of developing moderate-to-severe obstructive sleep apnea. A 10% decrease in

body weight was associated with a 26% decrease in the apnea-hypopnea index.

3. The causes of obstructive sleep apnea are a natural relaxation of throat muscles as sleeping begins. There may be additional complicating factors, such as being overweight or obese, a smaller than normal jaw, enlarged tonsils or adenoids that partially block breathing passages, or having a large tongue.

Clinical Case Study 3

1. Breast cancer is the second most common cancer in women in the United States, and worldwide, it is the most common invasive cancer in women. Breast cancer usually involves the glandular cells of the ducts or lobules.
2. Breast cancer is the second leading cause of cancer death in Caucasian, African-American, Asian/Pacific Islander, and American Indian/Alaska Native women. However, in Hispanic women, it is the leading cause of cancer death.
3. Having a first-degree relative (mother, sister, or daughter) with breast cancer doubles or triples the risks. However, breast cancer in more distant relatives only increases risk slightly. If two or more first-degree relatives have breast cancer, the risk may be five to six times higher.

CHAPTER 10: VITAMIN DEFICIENCY, DEPENDENCY, AND TOXICITY

Clinical Case Study 1

1. The top three food sources for vitamin A are beef liver, sweet potato, and carrots.
2. More than 90% of the vitamin A stores are in the liver. Smaller amounts are in the adipose tissue, bone marrow, kidneys, eyes, and testicles.
3. Eye changes are common with vitamin A deficiency. If blood retinol is lacking, the retinal lost in the visual cycle cannot be replaced. The rods regenerate rhodopsin slower than normal and night blindness results. Without sufficient retinoic acid, mucous-forming cells deteriorate and mucus cannot be synthesized. The cornea and other parts of the eyes are affected since mucus helps keep them moist and washes away dirt particles. As a result, conjunctival xerosis develops. Often, keratomalacia and scarring occur. These changes (xerophthalmia) result in irreversible blindness on a global scale, affecting millions of individuals.

Clinical Case Study 2

1. Darker-skinned people have more melanin, which can block ultraviolet light and prevent sufficient synthesis of vitamin D3. Use of sunscreens with a sun protection factor of 8 or higher decreases risks for skin cancer, but also prevent sufficient synthesis of vitamin D3. It is often recommended that people expose their hands, face, and arms to UV light for two to three times per week, for 10–15 minutes each time. Darker-skinned people may require sun exposure of 30 minutes or more, or supplementation with vitamin D. Those with insufficient UV-light exposure should take steps to ensure correct amounts of vitamin D in the diet.
2. Foods that have percentages of vitamin D that are over 20% include cod liver oil, eel, salmon, herring, and tuna.
3. Osteomalacia occurs in adults because of insufficient calcium and phosphorus, resulting in the bones becoming soft and deformed. It is usually caused by low levels of vitamin D in the diet, but also by not getting enough sunlight, or a problem with the way the body uses vitamin D. There is poor calcification of newly synthesized bone, so fractures of the hips or spine are common. Osteomalacia is most common with kidney or liver disease, which impair calcitriol synthesis, or intestinal diseases that impair fat absorption, such as Crohn's disease.

Clinical Case Study 3

1. Folate is actually the generic name of vitamin B9, and refers to various subtypes found in food sources. Folic acid refers to the synthetic form present in supplements and fortified foods.
2. Pregnancy increases needs for vitamin B9 greatly (the RDA is 600 mcg per day) due to increased rates of cell division and DNA synthesis. Prenatal multivitamin and mineral supplements are fortified with folate to compensate for these extra needs during pregnancy.
3. When a pregnant woman is deficient in folate, neural tube defects in the fetus are much more likely. The most common defects are spina bifida, and anencephaly, the lack of brain development. Spina bifida may cause incontinence, paralysis, and learning disabilities. Anencephaly is fatal.

CHAPTER 11: MINERAL DEFICIENCY AND TOXICITY

Clinical Case Study 1

1. Hypernatremia means excessive sodium intake has occurred. This condition is well understood to be related to hypertension and cardiovascular disease. Blood pressure and deaths from cardiovascular disease can often be reduced by decreasing sodium intake.
2. Though 2,300 mg per day is the upper level and daily value for adult sodium consumption, less than 33% of adults consume less than this. For most people, reducing sodium to less than the upper daily level will required that sodium levels – primarily in processed and restaurant foods – must be reduced.
3. The possible complications of hypertension for this patient include arterial damage, aneurysm, heart disease, brain damage, stroke, dementia, poor vision, kidney damage, sexual dysfunction, and hypertensive crisis.

Clinical Case Study 2

1. Hypokalemia can be life-threatening. Symptoms include fatigue, weakness, muscle spasms, nausea, loss of appetite, and arrhythmia. If severe, muscle paralysis can occur and the arrhythmias can be fatal. Hypokalemia also raises risks for bone loss and kidney stones.
2. Hypocalcemia results in abnormal muscle function and increased likelihood of osteoporosis and osteopenia.
3. The signs and symptoms of magnesium deficiency include arrhythmias that may be accompanied by muscle spasms, weakness, disorientation, nausea, vomiting, and seizures. There may be abnormal nerve cell function due to impaired sodium/potassium pumping. Deficiency can also cause a decrease in parathyroid hormone release that results in low blood calcium.

Clinical Case Study 3

1. Just a mild to moderate iron deficiency can affect immune function and the ability to perform well while working. As the deficiency progresses and the body's stores are depleted, a lack of iron needed for heme and hemoglobin synthesis causes iron deficiency anemia to develop. Oxygen transport in the blood is impaired, resulting in fatigue and a lower ability to enjoy normal activities. Immune function, energy metabolism, and cognitive development are all affected.
2. Pregnant women are at high risk of iron deficiency because more iron is needed as the blood volume and numbers and red blood cells increase, both in the mother's bloodstream and in the fetus.
3. Iron deficiency is one of the most prevalent forms of malnutrition. Iron deficiency anemia accounts for several hundred millions of cases of anemia. Africa and parts of Asia make up 71% of the global mortality burden, while North America bears only 1.4% of the global burden.

Clinical Case Study 4

1. When hyperkalemia is severe, symptoms such as difficulty breathing, heart palpitations, chest pain, arrhythmia, and sudden collapse may occur.
2. Potassium occurs naturally in a variety of food sources, with unprocessed foods being the best sources – including kidney beans (73%), fruits and vegetables (20%), milk and milk drinks (11%), whole grains and grain-based dishes (10%), meats including poultry (10%), coffee and tea (7%), and fruit or vegetable juices (5%).
3. Hyperkalemia is extremely rare in healthy persons since excess potassium is easily excreted in the urine. However, if kidney function is poor, potassium can quickly increase in the blood to cause arrythmias or cardiac arrest. In these cases, dietary potassium must be carefully controlled.

Clinical Case Study 5

1. Symptoms of zinc deficiency include delayed growth and sexual maturation, loss of appetite, dermatitis, alopecia, impaired vitamin A function, decreased taste sensitivity, immune dysfunction, poor wound healing, birth defects, severe diarrhea, and higher occurrence of infant mortality.
2. When the body's zinc status is compromised, the integrity of structural proteins that contain zinc is impaired in cell membranes, protein receptors, and zinc fingers. The proteins become unable to perform normal functions.
3. There are mild zinc deficiencies seen in people with Crohn's disease or other malabsorption conditions, young children, patients undergoing kidney dialysis, and in those that restrict intake of animal-based foods.

CHAPTER 12: ELECTROLYTE AND ACID-BASE IMBALANCE

Clinical Case Study 1

1. Hypernatremia is usually caused by insufficient water consumption, severe dehydration, excessive loss of body fluids (from vomiting, diarrhea, sweating, or respiratory illnesses), and use of corticosteroids.
2. Sodium helps control body fluids and impacts blood pressure. It is also necessary for muscle and nerve function.
3. Sodium is the main extracellular cation. The extracellular sodium concentration is at an average of 140 milliequivalents per liter (140 millimoles per liter). The intracellular sodium concentration is only at 12 mEq/L (12 mmol/L).

Clinical Case Study 2

1. The heart is especially sensitive to potassium levels, and hypokalemia (or hyperkalemia) can disrupt its electrical conduction and lead to sudden death.
2. Hypomagnesemia is usually caused by alcohol use disorder, malnutrition, malabsorption, chronic diarrhea, excessive sweating, heart failure, and use of certain diuretics or antibiotics.
3. The neurologic outcomes of alkalemia include delirium, lethargy, seizures, stupor, and tetany. The respiratory outcomes include compensatory hypoventilation with hypercapnia and hypoxemia.

Clinical Case Study 3

1. Dehydration can be caused by diarrhea, vomiting, sweating, urine abnormalities, fever, an inability to consume enough fluid (such as through unconsciousness), burns, poorly controlled diabetes mellitus, and diabetes insipidus, due to a deficiency of ADH.
2. When dehydration is severe, fluid replacement requires medical supervision. Without replenishment, severe progression will lead to death.
3. Hypotonic dehydration refers to a decrease of electrolyte concentration in the extracellular fluid. In hypotonic dehydration, the cells expand as water in the extracellular fluid moves toward the higher sodium concentration inside the cells. Reducing ECF osmolality inhibits ADH release. Less water is reabsorbed. Excess water is flushed quickly out of the body via the urine. Hypotonic dehydration results in severe metabolic disturbances.

Clinical Case Study 4

1. Pedal edema is an abnormal accumulation of fluid in the interstitial space. The tissues swell, but the cells do not. There is an increase in volume of the interstitial fluid. The extra fluid can harm tissue function since it decreases the distance over which oxygen and nutrients must diffuse between the blood and cells.
2. The signs and symptoms of edema depend on the underlying cause, but in peripheral edema swelling, tightness, and pain are common. The skin may retain a "dimple" after a few seconds of pressure, with visible anomalies. There may be puffiness of the affected area.
3. Complications of untreated peripheral edema include painful swelling, with pain that gets worse, stiffness and difficulty walking, stretched and itchy skin, infection in the area of swelling, scarring between the layers of tissue, poor blood circulation, loss of elasticity (in arteries, veins, and joints), and ulcerations on the skin.

Clinical Case Study 5

1. Metabolic alkalosis is caused by acid loss or retention of bicarbonate. Respiratory alkalosis is caused by hyperventilation.
2. The pH establishes whether acidosis or alkalosis is the primary process occurring, but it will move toward the normal range as compensatory efforts occur. However, complex or mixed acid-base imbalances involve several primary processes.
3. The first step in interpreting an acid-base imbalance is to check the pH, followed by considering bicarbonate concentrations relative to the normal reference range. The third step is to measure the partial pressure of carbon dioxide to determine if the condition is respiratory or metabolic. The last step is to assess the anion gap, paying the most attention to bicarbonate, sodium, potassium, and chloride.

CHAPTER 13: NUTRITIONAL EFFECTS ON THE NERVOUS SYSTEM

Clinical Case Study 1

1. Wernicke encephalopathy involves an acute onset of confusion, nystagmus, ataxia, and partial ophthalmoplegia that is linked to a thiamin deficiency. There may be insufficient intake or absorption of thiamin. The condition is also linked to continuous ingestion of carbohydrates. Severe alcoholism is often an underlying condition.
2. Many patients with Wernicke encephalopathy have severe autonomic dysfunction with signs of sympathetic hyperactivity, such as agitation and tremor. In some, hypoactivity may be present, signified by hypothermia, postural hypotension, and syncope.
3. With Wernicke encephalopathy, the patient must stop drinking alcoholic beverages. This is because the effects of alcohol can lead to permanent damage to the Wernicke area of the brain, which are irreversible.

Clinical Case Study 2

1. The psychosis caused by niacin deficiency is described as being characterized by disorientation, memory impairment, confusion, and confabulation. The main symptoms may be depression, excitement, delirium, mania, or paranoia.
2. Before niacin deficiency-related encephalopathy develops, cerebral manifestations include headache, irritability, confusion, fatigue, apathy, and insomnia. Mental changes include delirium, depression, and irritability. Additional symptoms include loss of appetite, nausea, tiredness, weight loss, a coated tongue, mouth sores, anemia, and forgetfulness.

Clinical Case Study 3

1. Peripheral neuropathy is dysfunction of the peripheral nerves, which are the parts of the nerves distal to the root and plexus. There are varying degrees of pain, sensory disturbances, diminished deep tendon reflexes, muscle weakness and atrophy, and vasomotor symptoms. All of these can occur singularly or in various combinations.
2. Vitamin B12 deficiency may result in demyelination, which is damage to the myelin sheath. Nerve conduction is slowed down. Demyelination mostly affects heavily myelinated fibers to cause large-fiber sensory dysfunction.
3. Dietary vitamin B12 deficiency usually occurs from inadequate absorption, but vegans that do not take vitamin supplements can also develop it. Deficiency of vitamin B12 causes damage to the white matter of the CNS, peripheral neuropathy, and megaloblastic anemia. Subacute combined degeneration of the nervous system may result in demyelinating or axonal peripheral neuropathies. Later on, spasticity, extensor plantar responses, increased loss of position and vibratory sensation in the legs, and ataxia will appear. Some patients develop irritability and slight depression.

Clinical Case Study 4

1. The toxic accumulation of copper in the body, known as hypercupremia, is a feature of Wilson's disease. It can be inherited, or acquired. Wilson's disease results in accumulation of copper in the brain and liver. Copper diffuses out of the liver into the bloodstream and accumulates in the brain. It seriously damages the brain, liver, and kidneys.
2. Initial signs and symptoms of Wilson's disease in children may reflect CNS involvement. Dystonia, tremors, dysarthria, dysphagia, chorea, incoordination, and drooling are developed. The clinical manifestations also include abdominal pain, fatigue, jaundice, aseities, and edema.
3. Wilson's disease is suspected in people under age 40 if they have an unexplained liver, neurologic, or psychiatric disorder; an unexplained chronic elevation of hepatic transaminases; fulminant hepatitis; or a parent, sibling, or cousin with Wilson's disease.

CHAPTER 14: NUTRITIONAL EFFECTS ON THE CARDIOVASCULAR SYSTEM

Clinical Case Study 1

1. Avoidable risk factors for atherosclerosis as well as cardiovascular disease include obesity, high cholesterol, smoking, and hypertension.
2. Statins are used as preventive therapy for atherosclerotic cardiovascular disease, LDL cholesterol that is 190 mg/dL or higher, patients aged 40–75 with diabetes and LDL cholesterol of 70–189 mg/dL, and for patients aged 40–75 with LDL cholesterol of 70–189 mg/dL, and an estimated ten-year risk of arteriosclerotic cardiovascular disease at 7.5% or higher.
3. Treatment for cardiovascular disease involves aggressive modification of risk factors to slow the disease progression and aid in plaque regression. The lower that LDL levels become, the more the patient's condition

will improve. Statins basically work by lowering LDL, and enhance endothelial nitric oxide production. They stabilize and regress plaques while reducing lipid accumulation in artery walls.

Clinical Case Study 2

1. High triglyceride levels can cause acute pancreatitis. If the levels of LDL become extremely high, they can cause confusion, hepatosplenomegaly, dyspnea, and paresthesia. High levels of LDL can cause arcus senilis and tendinous xanthomas of the phalangeal joints, or near the elbow, knee, and Achilles tendons. Other findings with high LDL, such as familial hypercholesterolemia, include xanthelasma.
2. Hypertension involves activation of the sympathetic nervous system and renin-angiotensin system, sodium retention, and various abnormalities. Obesity increases the risk for hypertension, and is associated with increased blood flow, vasodilation, cardiac output, and glomerular filtration rate.
3. The five leading causes of a stroke include hypertension, hypercholesterolemia, smoking, obesity, and diabetes. The patient in this scenario has four out of these five risk factors.

Clinical Case Study 3

1. Diabetes mellitus is a highly significant secondary cause of dyslipidemia, since patients usually have a combination of high triglycerides, high LDL, and low HDL. This is known as diabetic dyslipidemia. Patients with type 2 diabetes are at the highest risk. This may be related to obesity, poor diabetic control, or both, increasing circulating free fatty acids.
2. By losing weight, getting more exercise, and eating healthier foods, there are many positive changes. These include better elasticity of blood vessels, lower blood pressure, higher HDL cholesterol, lower LDL cholesterol, and a reduced chance of developing type 2 diabetes.
3. Symptoms of myocardial infarction (and conditions such as unstable angina, ischemic stroke, or resting limb pain) may develop if unstable plaques rupture and block a major artery, with the addition of thrombosis or embolism.

Clinical Case Study 4

1. Adult hypertension is most common in African-Americans (56%) compared to Caucasians (48%) or Hispanics (39%). Morbidity and mortality are also greater in African-Americans.
2. Hypertension is classified as primary (essential) in over 90% of cases and as secondary in the remainder. In primary hypertension, there are multiple factors, and heredity is a predisposing factor. The exact causative mechanism is not clear. Environmental factors include obesity, dietary sodium, and stress. These appear to affect only genetically susceptible individuals, at younger ages.
3. The prevention of hypertension requires a healthy lifestyle. A healthy diet is required, with limited amounts of sodium and increased amounts of potassium. Foods should be lower in fat and include many fruits, vegetables, and whole grains. Regular exercise, including aerobic exercise, is very important. Stress management is also important to improve emotional and physical health, and lower blood pressure.

Clinical Case Study 5

1. An ischemic stroke is caused by a blockage cutting off the blood supply to the brain, and is the most common type of stroke. Of the forms of stroke, 80% are ischemic and 20% are hemorrhagic. The five leading causes of a stroke include hypertension, hypercholesterolemia, smoking, obesity, and diabetes.
2. Stroke occurs suddenly with numbness, weakness, or paralysis of the contralateral limbs and face, aphasia, confusion, visual disturbances, headache, dizziness, and loss of balance and coordination.
3. Complications of strokes include aphasia, spasticity, confusion, depression, sleep problems, incontinence, pneumonia, and swallowing dysfunction, which can lead to aspiration, dehydration, or undernutrition.

CHAPTER 15: NUTRITIONAL EFFECTS ON THE ENDOCRINE SYSTEM

Clinical Case Study 1

1. Growth hormone is essential for normal growth, muscle and bone strength, and distribution of body fat. It helps control glucose and lipid levels in the body. Without enough GH, a child is likely to grow slowly and be much shorter than other children of the same age and gender.
2. Growth hormone deficiency (GHD) can be present at birth or develop later. It can be the result of genetic defects, severe brain injury, or being born without a pituitary gland. Sometimes, GHD can be associated with lower levels of other hormones, such as vasopressin, gonadotropin hormone, thyrotropin hormone, or adrenocorticotrophic hormone.
3. Children who are malnourished often do not produce enough growth hormone and fail to reach normal height for their age group. Foods that increase GH include pumpkin seeds, quinoa, black beans, cheese, chicken, broccoli, brown rice, whole milk, mushrooms, beef, oats, cottage cheese, fish oil, kale, spinach, yogurt, lentil beans, cornmeal, wheat germ, and soy (in moderation).

Clinical Case Study 2

1. People living far away from oceans or at higher altitudes have a higher risk for iodine deficiency. In the environment, iodine is present as iodide in seawater. Small amounts enter the atmosphere, then fall back to earth in rain, entering ground water and soil near oceans. Iodine deficiency is uncommon in areas where iodized salt is used, yet it is relatively common worldwide.
2. If a severe iodine deficiency causes hypothyroidism, it can decrease fertility, and increase risks for stillbirth, spontaneous abortion, and prenatal or infant mortality.
3. In areas of iodine deficiency, methods that reverse the condition include iodine supplementation of salt, oral administration of iodized oil, annual intramuscular administration of iodized oil, and iodination of water, crops, or animal fodder. Any goitrogens that are being eaten should be removed from the diet. Sometimes, suppression of the hypothalamic-pituitary axis with thyroid hormone will block TSH production, stimulating the thyroid.

Clinical Case Study 3

1. Primary hypothyroidism is caused by thyroid disease, while secondary hypothyroidism is caused by disease of the hypothalamus or pituitary gland.
2. Though signs and symptoms of primary hypothyroidism are often slight, the most common manifestations are fluid retention and puffiness of the eyes, cold intolerance, tiredness, and mental fogginess. Organ system manifestations may be metabolic, neurologic, psychiatric, dermatologic, ocular, gastrointestinal, gynecologic, cardiovascular, or described as "other" (pleural or abdominal effusions, hoarse voice, and slow speech).
3. In females that have hypothyroidism, signs and symptoms of secondary hypothyroidism include history of amenorrhea instead of menorrhagia, and some suggestive physical differences. Secondary hypothyroidism involves the skin and hair being dry but not very coarse, skin depigmentation, macroglossia, atrophic breasts, and hypotension. The heart is smaller than normal, and serous pericardial effusions are not seen.

Clinical Case Study 4

1. Parathyroid hormone controls the levels of calcium and phosphorus, so insufficient parathyroid hormone causes abnormal levels of calcium.
2. Signs and symptoms of hypoparathyroidism include tingling of the lips, fingers, and toes; muscle cramps, tetany, confusion, dry hair, scaly skin, cataracts, brittle nails, and arrhythmias.
3. Treatment for hypoparathyroidism usually includes parathyroid hormone. calcium supplements, high doses of vitamin D, magnesium supplements, and thiazide diuretics.

CHAPTER 16: NUTRITIONAL EFFECTS ON THE GASTROINTESTINAL SYSTEM

Clinical Case Study 1

1. Stomach cancer (gastric) mostly affects older people. The average age of diagnosis is 68. About six of every ten people diagnosed with stomach cancer each year are age 65 or older.
2. Stomach cancer incidence and mortality are highly variable by region and significantly depend on diet and *Helicobacter pylori* infection. It is caused by a variety of factors, which include *pernicious anemia*, *H. pylori* infection, smoking, being overweight or obese, a diet high in certain foods (pickled, salty, or smoked), chronic alcohol use, surgery for a stomach ulcer, having type A blood, and family history of the disease.
3. Red and processed meats, sugar-sweetened beverages, and highly processed foods should be limited, to possibly prevent stomach cancer. Avoiding or limiting alcohol also lowers risks.

Clinical Case Study 2

1. Crohn's disease, in most cases, the distal ileum and colon are affected, though effects can occur anywhere in the GI tract. The disease starts with crypt inflammation and abscesses that can progress to tiny focal aphthoid ulcers. These lesions of the mucosa may form deep longitudinal and transverse ulcers along with mucosal edema. This is followed by a cobblestone appearance of the intestine, spreading inflammation, lymphedema, thickening of the bowel wall and mesentery, hypertrophy, strictures, and bowel obstruction.
2. The causes of Crohn's disease are not yet well understood, but recent research suggests that deficiencies of the *immune system, as well as hereditary, genetic, and environmental causes* must be considered. The disease can occur at any age, it is most prevalent in adolescents and adults between the ages of 15 and 35.
3. When symptoms of Crohn's disease are not present, patients can eat whole grains and a variety of fruits and vegetables. It is important to start new foods one at a time, in small amounts. When symptoms are present, such as diarrhea or abdominal pain, it is important to avoid high-fiber foods, raw and gas-producing vegetables, most raw fruits, and beverages that contain caffeine.

Clinical Case Study 3

1. Colorectal cancers are extremely common, making up nearly 148,000 cases and over 53,000 deaths annually in the United State alone. Incidence rises sharply at ages 40–50. More than 50% of cases occur in the rectum and sigmoid, with 95% of cases being adenocarcinomas. Colorectal cancer is slightly more common in men than in women.
2. The diagnosis of colorectal cancer is based on colonoscopy, fecal occult blood testing, and sometimes, flexible sigmoidoscopy, fecal DNA testing, or CT colonography.
3. For colorectal cancers, it is important to eat small, frequent meals throughout the day. Protein-rich foods help the body to repair cells and tissues and support the immune system. These include lean meats, eggs, low-fat dairy products, nuts, nut butters, beans, and soy foods. Whole-grain foods provide great sources of carbohydrates and fiber, and include oatmeal, whole wheat breads, brown rice, and whole-grain pastas. A variety of fruits and vegetables are indicated, and patients should try to eat at least five servings per day. Healthy fats include olive oil, avocados, nuts, and seeds.

Clinical Case Study 4

1. The risk factors for pancreatic cancer include smoking, a history of chronic pancreatitis, the male gender, obesity, and the African-American race. Heredity is also implicated.
2. The signs and symptoms of pancreatic cancer include abdominal pain and weight loss, but these are nonspecific to the disease, until it is later diagnosed because of metastasis.
3. For pancreatic cancers, it is important to monitor and maintain a healthy weight. Patients must remain hydrated with at least 64 ounces of fluids per day. Small, frequent meals are indicated. High-protein meals are important. It is important to choose foods that are easy to digest. Essential whole grains are excellent. Whole fruits and vegetables are high in antioxidants, so at least five servings should be consumed per day. Sweets and added sugars must be limited. There may be other needed dietary alterations or supplemental pancreatic enzymes.

Clinical Case Study 5

1. Primary liver cancer is usually discovered to be hepatocellular carcinoma, with other types being uncommon or rare. They include fibrolamellar carcinoma, cholangiocarcinoma, hepatoblastoma, and angiosarcoma.
2. The most common symptoms of liver cancer include abdominal pain, weight loss, right upper quadrant mass, and unexplainable deterioration.
3. Options for treatment of liver cancer include liver transplantation, surgical resection, ablative treatments, radiofrequency ablation, and medications (sorafenib, levatinib, regorafenib, and nivolumab). Systemic immunotherapies are quickly evolving, and include atezolizumab and bevacizumab.

CHAPTER 17: NUTRITIONAL EFFECTS ON THE INTEGUMENTARY SYSTEM

Clinical Case Study 1

1. The dermatitis involves a localized, pigmented rash. The diarrhea develops from gastroenteritis. The dementia is part of widespread neurologic deficits that include cognitive decline.
2. Insufficient dietary niacin can be compensated for by eating foods that are rich in tryptophan (such as dairy

products), since dietary tryptophan is metabolized to niacin.
3. Nicotinamide is used for the treatment of pellagra, since it does not cause burning, flushing, itching, or tingling the way that nicotinic acid dose. Nicotinamide is given in daily oral doses.

Clinical Case Study 2

1. The most common form of skin hyperpigmentation is melasma, which involves dark brown or grayish patches on the face, and is due to a deficiency of folic acid.
2. Melasma is most common during pregnancy or when a woman is taking birth control pills.
3. Melasma is usually temporary, and can be reduced by increasing consumption of folic acid. While the problem can be embarrassing, the appearance of dark patches of skin does not usually indicate a serious medical condition.

Clinical Case Study 3

1. Insufficient exposure to sunlight can lead to a vitamin D deficiency. This impairs bone mineralization and can result in rickets (osteomalacia). Vitamin D deficiency is relatively common worldwide.
2. In the diet, vitamin D is mostly found in fish liver oils and salt water fish. IN some developed countries, milk and other types of foods are fortified with vitamin D.
3. Vitamin D deficiency may be suspected based on known history of insufficient sunlight exposure or dietary intake, signs and symptoms of bone or muscle conditions, and characteristic bone changes discovered in x-rays and blood tests.

Clinical Case Study 4

1. When omega-6 fatty acids are deficient in the body, the skin may be severely dry, scaly, flaky, cracked, peeling, lacking in a normal healthy appearance, bumpy, dull in certain patches, oily, irregular, thick, or callused.
2. Omega-6 fatty acid deficiency may also cause the fingernails to be soft, frayed, split, brittle, dull, or slow-growing. The eyes, mouth, and throat may often be dry. There may be excessive ear wax, excessive thirst, asthma, hay fever, stiff or painful joints, cravings for fatty foods, and in women, a lack of vaginal lubrication, menstrual-like cramps, and premenstrual breast aches or tenderness.
3. Omega-6 fatty acids must be taken in the correct quantities because overconsumption can result in increased risks for heart disease, cancer, bronchial asthma, arthritis, and depression.

CHAPTER 18: NUTRITIONAL EFFECTS ON THE MUSCULOSKELETAL SYSTEM

Clinical Case Study 1

1. Rhabdomyolysis is the breakdown of skeletal muscle fibers. It is a rare condition that requires emergency medical treatment, and can be fatal, or result in permanent disability.
2. Rhabdomyolysis occurs when muscle fibers die and release a damaging type of protein into the bloodstream, potentially harming the kidneys and heart. It largely affects people who routinely perform intense physical activity and work in hot environments – construction workers, firefighters, first responders, professional athletes, and farmers.
3. Factors that can cause rhabdomyolysis include extremes of body temperature, ischemia of muscle tissue, low phosphate levels, long surgical procedures, seizures, muscle tremors, severe physical exertion, severe dehydration, trauma, crush injuries, and use of cocaine, amphetamines, statins, or heroin.

Clinical Case Study 2

1. To reduce or prevent frailty and the likelihood of sarcopenia, exercise and a healthy diet are recommended. Older adults that engage in regular aerobic exercise, via walking, running, or swimming, have increased life expectancy and less functional decline, compared to sedentary adults. Weight training is able to help increase bone mass, and reduce risks for falling and bone fractures. A healthy diet can prevent or reduce risks for contributing diseases that make an individual become frail.
2. The best treatment for sarcopenia is exercise – primarily, resistance training or strength training, which increase strength and endurance. Resistance training uses resistance bands, and can help the neuromuscular system and hormones, improving the ability to convert protein to energy in only two weeks.
3. Medications being studied for sarcopenia include urocortin II, testosterone supplements, growth hormone supplements, and medications for treating metabolic syndrome (insulin resistance, obesity, and hypertension).

Clinical Case Study 3

1. Most osteoporotic fractures occur in the thoracic and lumbar spine, wrist, and hip, where they are known as fragility fractures.
2. Fragility fractures often occur with much less trauma than a person would expect would be needed. They include falls while standing or kneeling, and falls out of bed.
3. Over 95% of cases of osteoporosis in women and about 80% in men are classified as primary, with no identified cause. Most cases occur in postmenopausal women and older men. The primary mechanism of bone loss is increased resorption of bone, causing decreased bone mass and microarchitectural deterioration.

Clinical Case Study 4

1. Osteomalacia is primarily caused by vitamin D deficiency, worsened by inadequate exposure to sunlight. Other causes include chronic kidney disease, rental tubular disorders, familial vitamin D-resistant (hypophosphatemic) rickets, chronic metabolic acidosis, hyperparathyroidism or hypoparathyroidism, disorders or medications that impair bone matrix mineralization, and insufficient dietary calcium.
2. Osteomalacia predisposes all adults to fractures. Elderly people may have hip fractures from only slight trauma.
3. Patients with osteomalacia can be cured by administration of 1,600 units vitamin D3 orally once per day. By the third week of treatment, sufficient calcium and phosphate have been deposited in the bones so that they appear on x-rays. After about one month, doses can usually be slowly reduced to the common maintenance levels of 600 units daily.

Clinical Case Study 5

1. A greenstick fracture occurs when a bone bends and cracks, instead of breaking completely into separate pieces. They occur in children younger than ten years of age.
2. The most common cause of a greenstick fracture is a fall. The majority of greenstick fractures occur in the arms, when children attempt to catch themselves as they fall.
3. A greenstick fracture is not a type of compound fracture, which is an open fracture, in which there is an open wound or break in the skin near the site of the broken bone. Compound fractures are extremely painful, and a very serious injury.

CHAPTER 19: NUTRITIONAL EFFECTS ON CANCER

Clinical Case Study 1

1. The prevention of colon cancer is based on reduced caloric intake, regular exercise, avoiding tobacco products, limiting alcohol intake, good amounts of calcium from dairy products, vitamin D, fruits, vegetables, whole grains, fish, low-dose aspirin, and regular colon cancer screening tests based on age, family history, and risk factors.
2. There are nearly 148,000 cases of colon cancer in the United States annually, and over 53,000 deaths – mostly in people between 40 and 50 years of age. IN elderly people, the incidence of colon cancer is increased.
3. The five-year survival rates for colon cancer are nearly 90% (if limited to the mucosa), 70%–80% (if there is extension through the colon wall), 30%–50% (if there are positive lymph nodes), and less than 20% (if there is metastatic disease).

Clinical Case Study 2

1. Large amounts of salt infuses foods in the preservation process, resulting in damage to the stomach lining and the development of lesions that may lead to stomach cancer. Also, much dietary salt is hidden in foods, so people may be unaware of just how much they are consuming.
2. Gastric adenocarcinoma makes up 95% of malignant stomach tumors, with less common forms including localized gastric lymphomas and leiomyosarcomas.
3. Symptoms of stomach cancer include dyspepsia, early satiety, dysphagia, weight loss, reduced strength, massive hematemesis, melena, secondary anemia from occult blood loss, jaundice, ascites, heme-positive stools, epigastric masses, lymph node enlargement, and hepatomegaly. There may be pulmonary, central nervous system, or bone metastasis.

Clinical Case Study 3

1. Adenocarcinoma of the prostate gland is the most common cancer in men age 50 and older. In the United States, there are nearly 249,000 cases and over 34,000 deaths per year. Incidence increases with each decade of age, and autopsies reveal this cancer to be present in 15%–60% of men between 60 and 90 years of age. About one of every six men is diagnosed with prostate cancer.
2. Once symptoms of prostate cancer appear, they include hematuria, straining, hesitancy, weak or intermittent urine stream, incomplete emptying, terminal dribbling, renal colic, flank pain, renal dysfunction, bone pain, pathologic fractures, or spinal cord compression.
3. Treatments for prostate cancer are guided by PSA levels, grade and stage of the tumor, patient age, any coexisting disorders, life expectancy, and patient preferences. Radical prostatectomy is considered best for patients less than 75 years of age with a tumor that is only within the prostate. Other treatments include cryotherapy, standard external beam radiation therapy, hypofractionation, and brachytherapy.

CHAPTER 20: NUTRITIONAL EFFECTS ON HEREDITARY METABOLIC DISORDERS

Clinical Case Study 1

1. The main signs of untreated phenylketonuria (PKU) are severe intellectual disability and behavioral problems. There are also psychoses, an unpleasant "mousy" body odor, eczema, microcephaly, and light skin, hair, and eyes.
2. Treatment of PKU started after two to three years may only help to control the extreme hyperactivity and seizures. Treatment of PKU is with lifelong dietary phenylalanine restriction.
3. This child will need a diet that is low-protein, and includes natural fruits, vegetables, and certain cereals. There are a variety of commercially-available products designed specifically for the age of each patient with PKU.

Clinical Case Study 2

1. If treatment is started after the first ten days of life, the majority of infants with severe or classic galactosemia will die because of a systemic infection. If they do survive the first month of life untreated, they are likely to develop cirrhosis.
2. Even if children receive treatment at an early age, delays in learning and development, as well as speech defects, are common. The specific issues and level of delay varies from child to child, but may include learning disabilities, neurological impairments, and ovarian failure in females.
3. Galactose is found in breast milk, cow's milk, and other dairy foods. When galactose cannot be changed to glucose, the byproducts such as galactose-1-phosphate, build up in tissues and blood, affecting many parts of the body.

Clinical Case Study 3

1. Type B Niemann-Pick disease does not include the motor difficulty commonly found in type A.
2. The other signs and symptoms of type B Niemann-Pick disease include low blood platelets, psychiatric disorders, peripheral nerve problems, lung problems, high lipids in the blood, short stature, and eye abnormalities.
3. Niemann-Pick disease affects the body's ability to metabolize cholesterol and lipids within the cells.

Clinical Case Study 4

1. Medium-chain acyl-CoA dehydrogenase deficiency is the most common fatty acid oxidation disorder.
2. An individual with medium-chain acyl-CoA dehydrogenase deficiency will become extremely ill if energy demands exceed energy intake, such as during infections or repeated vomiting. Affected children are unable to fast for very long without developing hypoglycemia.
3. Fatty acid oxidation disorders are a group of inherited metabolic conditions that lead to an accumulation of fatty acids, and a decrease in cell energy metabolism. These disorders result from an inability of the body to produce or utilize an enzyme required to oxidize fatty acids. The enzyme can be missing or incorrectly structured. Therefore, the body is unable to produce energy in the liver and muscles from fatty acid sources.

Clinical Case Study 5

1. Lesch-Nyhan syndrome is classified as a purine salvage disorder. These disorders also include the condition known as adenine phosphoribosyltransferase deficiency. Lesch-Nyhan syndrome is a rare, X-linked recessive disorder.
2. Lesch-Nyhan syndrome progresses to central nervous system involvement with intellectual disability, spastic cerebral palsy, involuntary movements, and self-mutilating behavior (particularly biting). Later, chronic hyperuricemia causes symptoms of gout.

3. The enzyme deficiencies of Lesch-Nyhan syndrome result in failure of the salvage pathway for hypoxanthine and guanine. These purines are instead degraded to uric acid.

CHAPTER 21: ENVIRONMENTAL EFFECTS ON NUTRITION

Clinical Case Study 1

1. *E. coli* is usually found in undercooked meat and raw vegetables.
2. *E. coli* bacteria produces a toxin that irritates your small intestine. The Shiga toxin is what causes food-borne illness.
3. Some people, particularly young children and older adults, may develop a life-threatening form of kidney failure called hemolytic uremic syndrome (HUS), which causes destruction of red blood cells, leading to kidney failure.

Clinical Case Study 2

1. Acute mercury compound poisoning causes burning mouth pain, salivation, severe gastroenteritis, abdominal pain, colitis, vomiting, anuria, nephrosis, and uremia.
2. Elemental mercury poisoning may occur via a liquid form (ingestion or skin contact) and through mercury vapors. For ingestion of the liquid form, there may be no symptoms. If it is injected intravenously, pulmonary emboli may develop. Severe pneumonitis occurs because of mercury vapor inhalation.
3. Mercury poisoning is signified by tremors, insomnia, memory loss, neuromuscular effects, headaches, and cognitive and motor dysfunction.

Clinical Case Study 3

1. Cadmium is a metal that is soft, malleable, and bluish-white in its elemental form. While it is a relatively widespread element, it is rarely found on its own as a pure metal. Most often, it forms complex compounds in zinc ores.
2. Cadmium is most widely used today in nickel-cadmium rechargeable batteries. It is also found in plating on iron and steel products, plastic stabilizers, alloy elements (for lead, copper, and tin), cigarette smoke, and silver jewelry.
3. Cadmium toxicity occurs when high levels of cadmium are inhaled from the air, or when contaminated food or water is consumed. In the general population, exposure to cadmium occurs primarily by eating foods grown in contaminated soil.

CHAPTER 22: NUTRITIONAL CLINICAL MEDICINE

Clinical Case Study 1

1. Malabsorption that occurs because of celiac disease, Crohn's disease, tropical sprue, and damage from radiation treatments regularly causes nutritional deficiencies. Many patients, especially those that are older and in acute hospitalization situations, have unsuspected nutritional deficiencies.
2. Nutritional status should be regularly evaluated as part of clinical examinations for infants, children, older adults such as this patient, those taking multiple medications, those with psychiatric disorders, and those with systemic disorders lasting more than a few days.
3. Treatment of undernutrition at home involves discussions with diet planners and advisers, gradual increase of nutrients, dietary supplements, use of protein bars, regular monitoring of body mass index (BMI), occupational therapists, various medical specialists, and sometimes, soft or pureed foods.

Clinical Case Study 2

1. If there are problems swallowing, options include nasogastric tubes, percutaneous endoscopic gastrostomy tubes, and parenteral nutrition. These treatments usually begin in a hospital, but can be continued in the patient's home if the individual is healthy enough.
2. Dietary counselors can teach patients how their bodies respond to food choices. Meal plans are created the promote either weight loss or weight gain, as needed, plus wellness. Eating habits are carefully evaluated so that the plan that is created results in positive and lasting changes. Dietary counseling succeeds, with greater long-term results, than when patients try to accomplish the same thing on their own.
3. A severe negative energy balance can reduce metabolism by bone mass, thyroid hormones, and testosterone level concentration. It leads to weight loss as the body detects an energy deficit and fat reserves are used to make up the difference.

Clinical Case Study 3

1. The basal metabolic rate (BMR) is influenced by physical activity levels, body growth, pregnancy, hormones, fever, hyperthyroidism, epinephrine, leptin, climate, illness, and tissue damage.
2. It is important that therapy for undernutrition begins as soon as possible in order to avoid the immune system shutting down, which increases chances for illness, infection, and reduced healing.
3. Undernutrition is what most people think of when the term "malnutrition" is used. It is a deficiency of nutrients due to an inadequate diet or problems absorbing nutrients from foods. Undernutrition may cause visible wasting of muscle and fat, but it can also be unseen.

CHAPTER 23: NUTRITIONAL THERAPY

Clinical Case Study 1

1. Dementia patients often struggle with their body weight. Weight loss is common and usually worsens as the condition progresses. Some individuals forget to eat. Other reasons for weight loss include faulty appetite triggers in the brain, medications that reduce appetite, reduced senses of smell and taste, difficulty focusing on eating (resulting in less food consumed), reduced coordination that impairs eating, and chewing or swallowing problems.
2. Some patients are prescribed diets that include softer foods to encourage intake, or thickened liquids for easier swallowing. Supplements may be required for vitamin or mineral deficiencies.
3. The Mediterranean diet, DASH diet, and MIND diet have been studied in reference to abilities that somewhat prevent progression of dementia. The MIND diet can significantly lower risks for developing Alzheimer's disease. It is also known as the Mediterranean-DASH Intervention for Neurodegenerative Delay diet. It lowers risks for AD as much as 53% in individuals that adhere to it rigorously, and by about 35% in those that follow it moderately well.

Clinical Case Study 2

1. Pancreatitis is caused by inappropriate activation of the pancreatic enzymes. This results in autodigestion of pancreatic tissue.
2. In 40%–70% of cases, gallstones are the primary cause of pancreatitis. Many cases (25%–35%) are due to heavy alcohol use of more than 50 g per day for over five years.
3. Enteral nutrition can be used to protect the intestinal mucosa and prevents bacterial overgrowth by stimulating gut motility. It can reduce systemic infections, multiorgan failure, and death. Enteral nutrition started within 48 hours of admission reduces the rate of major infections, and sometimes, death.

Clinical Case Study 3

1. Common nutrition-related adverse effects of chemotherapy include anorexia, early satiety, taste changes, nausea, vomiting, diarrhea, mucositis or esophagitis, and constipation.
2. Since cancer and the adverse effects of chemotherapy can greatly impact nutrition status, health care providers must anticipate possible problems and design a plan along with the patient, to prevent malnutrition and weight loss.
3. Malnutrition and weight loss can affect a cancer patient's ability to regain normal health and acceptable blood counts between cycles of chemotherapy. This can directly affect the ability to follow the treatment schedule, which is essential for achieving a positive outcome.

CHAPTER 24: THE GLOBAL BURDEN OF NUTRITIONAL PROBLEMS

Clinical Case Study 1

1. Along with income opportunity, food pricing, and environmental factors, conflicts can affect food availability and contribute to undernutrition or malnutrition.
2. Wasting can also be due to infections, in which a child's energy requirements may be higher while their ability to absorb and retain nutrients is only limited. Affected children also have weak immune systems, and some have nutritional edema, with swelling of the face, feet, and limbs. Wasting is the result of maternal malnutrition, low birthweight, poor feeding and care, and infections linked to food insecurity, limited access to clean drinking water, and poverty.
3. The UN and WHO regularly work together to combat malnutrition, along with the World Food Programme, and a variety of other organizations.

Clinical Case Study 2

1. The number of hungry people in Africa represent over 33% of undernourished individuals in the world. This is more than double the proportion, by population, of any other region.
2. Ethiopia has widespread low food availability due to severe droughts, soil erosion, a lack of infrastructure, and poor farming methods.
3. About 28% of child deaths are due to undernutrition. Nearly 81% of cases of child malnutrition are untreated, and two of every five children suffer from stunting. The high death rate related to stunting has reduced the adult workforce by 8%.

Clinical Case Study 3

1. Severe acute malnutrition, also called severe wasting, is the most lethal form of malnutrition. About one of every five childhood deaths before age five are attributed to severe wasting, which affects about 13.6 million children around the world.
2. *Ready-to-use therapeutic food (RUTF)* is an energy-dense micronutrient paste that is made using peanuts, sugar, milk powder, oil, vitamins, and minerals. It is available in a one-dose container made of aluminum foil, lasts on the shelf for up to two years, and does not have to be refrigerated at any time. There is no preparation or mixing required, and it can be eaten right out of the container.
3. In India, the 2nd most populated country in the world, over 80% of the population lives on the equivalent of less than $1.25 per day. Even though the economy is growing quickly, India's nutritional growth is not. About 48% of children under age five are stunted. Supplementary feeding programs are being implemented to help prevent malnutrition.

Answer Key to Study Questions at Ends of the Chapters

CHAPTER 1: NUTRITION AND HEALTH

1. A
2. C
3. D
4. A
5. B
6. C
7. B
8. A
9. D
10. B
11. A
12. C
13. B
14. C
15. A

CHAPTER 2: GLOBAL ISSUES WITH NUTRITION

1. C
2. D
3. B
4. C
5. A
6. C
7. D
8. B
9. A
10. C
11. B
12. D
13. A
14. A
15. D

CHAPTER 3: NEWBORNS AND PREMATURE INFANTS

1. B
2. D
3. A
4. C
5. B
6. D
7. A
8. D
9. B
10. A
11. B
12. A
13. A
14. D
15. B

CHAPTER 4: CHILDREN AND ADOLESCENTS

1. D
2. B
3. B
4. C
5. A
6. A
7. C
8. A
9. D
10. A
11. C
12. A
13. C
14. A
15. B

CHAPTER 5: OLDER ADULTS

1. B
2. A
3. B
4. A
5. B
6. C
7. D
8. D
9. B
10. D

11. C
12. D
13. B
14. B
15. A

CHAPTER 6: PREGNANT WOMEN

1. B
2. C
3. A
4. C
5. A
6. C
7. A
8. C
9. D
10. A
11. C
12. D
13. A
14. D
15. B

CHAPTER 7: UNDERNUTRITION AND EATING DISORDERS

1. C
2. B
3. D
4. A
5. B
6. C
7. A
8. D
9. B
10. D
11. C
12. C
13. A
14. C
15. D

CHAPTER 8: OBESITY AND METABOLIC SYNDROME

1. C
2. A
3. D
4. D
5. A
6. D
7. B
8. A
9. C
10. B
11. A
12. C
13. C
14. B
15. A

CHAPTER 9: COMPLICATIONS OF OBESITY

1. C
2. A
3. D
4. B
5. C
6. A
7. C
8. C
9. A
10. D
11. B
12. C
13. A
14. D
15. D

CHAPTER 10: VITAMIN DEFICIENCY, DEPENDENCY, AND TOXICITY

1. C
2. B
3. C
4. A
5. B
6. D
7. A
8. B
9. C
10. B
11. A
12. C
13. B
14. A
15. D

CHAPTER 11: MINERAL DEFICIENCY AND TOXICITY

1. C
2. B
3. C
4. A
5. C
6. B
7. A
8. C
9. D
10. A
11. D
12. B
13. C
14. A
15. C

CHAPTER 12: ELECTROLYTE AND ACID–BASE IMBALANCE

1. D
2. C
3. B
4. C
5. A
6. C
7. A
8. B
9. A
10. D
11. B
12. C
13. A
14. C
15. A

CHAPTER 13: NUTRITIONAL EFFECTS ON THE NERVOUS SYSTEM

1. C
2. B
3. D
4. A
5. C
6. B
7. D
8. A
9. B
10. C
11. A
12. C
13. B
14. D
15. A

CHAPTER 14: NUTRITIONAL EFFECTS ON THE CARDIOVASCULAR SYSTEM

1. C
2. A
3. D
4. B
5. A
6. B
7. A
8. C
9. C
10. D
11. B
12. D
13. C
14. A
15. C

CHAPTER 15: NUTRITIONAL EFFECTS ON THE ENDOCRINE SYSTEM

1. D
2. A
3. B
4. C
5. D
6. C
7. B
8. C
9. A
10. C
11. B
12. C
13. A
14. D
15. A

CHAPTER 16: NUTRITIONAL EFFECTS ON THE GASTROINTESTINAL SYSTEM

1. A
2. D
3. C

4. A
5. C
6. A
7. D
8. D
9. B
10. A
11. C
12. B
13. C
14. D
15. A

CHAPTER 17: NUTRITIONAL EFFECTS ON THE INTEGUMENTARY SYSTEM

1. B
2. C
3. A
4. C
5. A
6. D
7. A
8. C
9. D
10. C
11. B
12. A
13. C
14. C
15. B

CHAPTER 18: NUTRITIONAL EFFECTS ON THE MUSCULOSKELETAL SYSTEM

1. C
2. B
3. D
4. C
5. A
6. C
7. C
8. B
9. C
10. A
11. C
12. D
13. B
14. C
15. A

CHAPTER 19: NUTRITIONAL EFFECTS ON CANCER

1. C
2. D
3. B
4. A
5. C
6. B
7. A
8. C
9. B
10. D
11. C
12. A
13. C
14. B
15. A

CHAPTER 20: NUTRITIONAL EFFECTS ON HEREDITARY METABOLIC DISORDERS

1. B
2. D
3. A
4. C
5. B
6. A
7. C
8. B
9. D
10. A
11. D
12. A
13. D
14. D
15. B

CHAPTER 21: ENVIRONMENTAL EFFECTS ON NUTRITION

1. B
2. D
3. C
4. A
5. B
6. C
7. D
8. B
9. A
10. C

11. A
12. B
13. D
14. C
15. A

CHAPTER 22: NUTRITIONAL CLINICAL MEDICINE

1. B
2. B
3. D
4. C
5. A
6. D
7. D
8. C
9. A
10. B
11. C
12. A
13. C
14. B
15. C

CHAPTER 23: NUTRITIONAL THERAPY

1. B
2. C
3. B
4. A
5. A
6. D
7. D
8. B
9. C
10. B
11. C
12. A
13. B
14. C
15. B

CHAPTER 24: THE GLOBAL BURDEN OF NUTRITIONAL PROBLEMS

1. B
2. A
3. C
4. D
5. C
6. A
7. C
8. B
9. C
10. B
11. C
12. A
13. D
14. A
15. C

Glossary

Abrasion – a lesion caused by scraping or wearing away.

Absence seizures – generalized onset seizures, beginning in both sides of the brain simultaneously, involving brief, sudden lapses of consciousness.

Acesulfame K – a calorie-free sweetener that has somewhat sour taste as well.

Acetaldehyde – a colorless liquid or gas produced by partial oxidation of ethanol by the liver enzyme called alcohol dehydrogenase.

Achalasia – a rare disorder that makes it difficult for food and liquids to pass from the esophagus into the stomach.

Achilles tendon – the strong fiber that connects the muscles in the back of the calf to the heel bone.

Achlorhydria – insufficient production of hydrochloric acid by the stomach.

Acidosis – a condition of acid buildup or loss of bicarbonate in the body; it may be respiratory or metabolic.

Acinar cells – pancreatic cells highly specialized to produce large amounts of digestive enzymes.

Acne – a skin condition that occurs when hair follicles become plugged with oil and dead skin cells.

Acrodermatitis enteropathica – a disorder of zinc metabolism that occurs either as a congenital form or one of two acquired forms.

Acromegaly – a rare condition, in which the body produces too much growth hormone, causing tissues and bones to grow more quickly than normal.

Actinic keratosis – a rough, scaly patch on the skin, from chronic sun exposure.

Addison's disease – adrenal insufficiency; an uncommon illness occurring when the body does not manufacture certain hormones, usually cortisol or aldosterone.

Adenocarcinoma – cancer that forms in glandular tissue.

Adenoma – a benign tumor that starts in gland-like cells of the epithelial tissue.

Adenosylmethionine – a natural compound in most body tissues and fluids, with roles in immunity, cell membranes, and breakdown of brain chemicals.

Adenotonsillar hypertrophy – abnormal growth of the pharyngeal and palatine tonsils.

Adhesins – cell surface components or appendages of bacteria that facilitate adhesion or adherence to other cells or to surfaces, primarily in the host they are infecting or living in.

Adipocytes – lipocytes (fat cells); those that mostly compose adipose tissue, specialized in storing energy as fat.

Adipokine – a cytokine secreted by adipose tissue, such as leptin; it is implicated in obesity-related low-grade inflammation or development of metabolic syndrome.

Adipose – related to (primarily) body tissue used for the storage of fat.

Adolescence – the period following onset of puberty, in which a young person develops from a child into an adult.

Adrenal fatigue syndrome – nonspecific symptoms that include aches, fatigue, nervousness, sleep disturbances, and digestive problems.

Adrenocorticotrophic hormone – produced in the pituitary gland, a hormone that stimulates production and release of cortisol; it interacts with responses to stress.

Aflatoxin – a poisonous carcinogen or mutagen produced by certain molds.

Afterload – the amount of pressure the heart needs to eject blood during ventricular contraction; it is recorded as the systolic pressure.

Ageusia – loss of the sense of taste.

Albuminuria – excessive albumin in the urine, signifying kidney disease.

Alcohol dehydrogenase – the liver enzyme that defends against the effects of alcohol.

Aldosterone – a steroid hormone from the adrenal cortex that helps control water and salt balance in the kidneys.

Alkaline phosphatase – an isoenzyme on the outer layer of cell membranes that catalyzes hydrolysis of organic phosphate esters in the extracellular space; testing of this isoenzyme is done to diagnose liver damage or bone disorders.

Alkalosis – excessive blood alkalinity due to excessive bicarbonate in the blood or a loss of acid from the blood; like acidosis, it also may be respiratory or metabolic.

Allergen – a substance that causes an allergic reaction.

Allogeneic – related to tissues or cells that are genetically dissimilar and immunologically incompatible, even though they come from individuals of the same species.

Alopecia – baldness.

Alpha-fetoprotein – a protein that develops in the fetal liver; it is measured to assess genetic disorders or neural tube defects.

Alpha1-antitrypsin – a liver protein that protects tissue from damaged caused by infection-fighting agents.

Alzheimer's disease – the most common type of dementia, involving areas of the brain that control thought, memory, and language.

Amenorrhea – absence of menstruation.

Amyloid beta – a peptide that appears to play a central role in the pathology of Alzheimer's disease.

Amyloidosis – a rare disease that occurs when the protein called amyloid builds up in orangs, affecting their function.

Amyotrophic lateral sclerosis – a progressive neurodegenerative disease that affects nerve cells in the brain and spinal cord; also called "Lou Gehrig's Disease".

Anabolism – constructive metabolism; synthesis of complex molecules from simpler ones along with the storage of energy.

Anastomosis – a cross-connection between adjacent channels, tubes, fibers, or other parts of a network; or a connection made surgically between adjacent structures.

Andropause – a condition associated with a decreased in testosterone due to aging.

Anemia – a condition of insufficient healthy red blood cells, resulting in inadequate delivery of oxygen to body tissues.

Anencephaly – a serious birth defect, with an infant born without parts of the brain and skull; it is a type of neural tube defect.

Aneurysm – an abnormal bulge or ballooning of a blood vessel wall.

Angina pectoris – chest pain or discomfort that recurs; it may be a symptom of coronary artery disease.

Angiokeratomas – hard skin lesions that are benign, occurring when capillaries enlarge or break open near the skin surface, which then thickens.

Angioplasty – a procedure used to open blocked coronary arteries caused by coronary artery disease.

Angiotensin II – a peptide endocrine hormone that is an important part of the renin-angiotensin-aldosterone system.

Animal fodder – any food source manufactured specifically for animals.

Anion – a negatively charged ion.

Anion gap – a measurement of the difference between negatively and positively charged electrolytes in the blood.

Anorexia nervosa – an eating disorder characterized by low body weight, fear of gaining weight, and a distorted perception of body image.

Antenatal testing – occurring before birth, it evaluates normal conditions of the fetus as well as good placental function.

Anthropometric – related to the study of human body measurements and proportions.

Antibodies – blood proteins produced in response to specific antigens; they combine chemically with substances the body recognizes as "foreign".

Antidiuretic hormone – a hormone that helps control blood pressure by affecting the kidneys and the blood vessels.

Antigens – toxins or other foreign substances that induce an immune response, especially the production of antibodies.

Antioxidants – substances that protect cells from damaged caused by free radicals.

Apathy – lack of interest, enthusiasm, or concern.

Aphasia – loss of the ability to understand or express speech, caused by brain damage.

Aphthous ulcers – common ulcerations of the oral mucosa or genital mucosa.

Aplastic anemia – a condition occurring when the body stops producing enough new blood cells, resulting in fatigue, infections, and uncontrolled bleeding.

Apnea – breathing that stops from any cause.

Apoenzymes – protein portions of enzymes.

Apoprotein – a protein of a lipoprotein.

Apoptosis – the death of cells, which is a normal, controlled part of growth and development.

Apraxia – the loss of ability to execute or carry out skilled movement and gestures, despite having the physical ability and desire to perform them.

Arcus senilis – a white, light gray, or blueish ring around the edge of the cornea, formed from lipids (mostly cholesterol).

Areola – a small circular area; especially, the ring of pigmented skin around a nipple.

Ariboflavinosis – riboflavin deficiency.

Arrhythmia – irregular heartbeat or one that beats too quickly or too slowly.

Arsenicosis – a chronic illness resulting from drinking water with high levels of arsenic over 5–20 years; arsenic poisoning.

Ascites – a condition in which fluid collects in the abdomen.

Asherman syndrome – a rare condition where scar tissue, also called adhesions or intrauterine adhesions, inside the uterus.

Assimilation – the absorption and digestion of food or nutrients; or the process of fully understanding information.

Asthma – a lung disease that causes repeated episodes of wheezing, breathlessness, chest tightness, and coughing.

Ataxia – poor muscle control, causing clumsy voluntary movements.

Atheromas – plaques; fatty materials that build up inside of arteries.

Atherosclerosis – the buildup of fats, cholesterol, and other substances in and upon artery walls; the buildup is called plaque.

Atrial gallop – a fourth heart sound, occurring during late diastole.

Atrial natriuretic peptide – a hormone secreted from the right atrium in response to atrial stretch from hypervolemia, and also in response to hypertension.

Atrophic gastritis – chronic inflammation and thinning of the stomach lining, with changes in the lining cells to mimic intestinal cells.

Atrophy – wasting away of tissues or organs.

Attention deficit disorder – a common neurodevelopmental disorder of childhood, involving trouble paying attention, and lack of impulse control, without hyperactivity.

Autism – also called autism spectrum disorder, a developmental disability caused by brain differences, causing problems with social communication and interaction, plus restricted or repetitive behaviors or interests.

Autoantibodies – antibodies made against substances formed by the host; they can directly destroy cells that have the substances on them or make it easier for other white blood cells to destroy them.

Autoimmune disorders – conditions in which the immune system mistakenly attacks the body, including rheumatoid arthritis, Crohn's disease, and certain thyroid conditions.

Autoimmune polyglandular syndrome – an inherited disease in which the immune system attacks healthy cells, especially those of the glands that produce hormones.

Autologous – related to cells or tissues obtained from the same individual.

Automation – technology applications where human input is minimized.

Autosomal recessive – a disorder that needs two copies of an abnormal gene to be present in order to develop.

Avidin – a biotin-binding protein, believed to function as an antibiotic.

Avulsion fracture – one that occurs when a small chunk of bone attached to a tendon or ligament is pulled away from the main part of the bone.

Baby boomers – people born between 1946 and 1964.

Baby bottle syndrome – a pattern of caries where the deciduous upper incisors and molars are severely affected, while the lower incisors are less affected.

Bacteroidetes – Gram-negative anaerobes that colonize the gastrointestinal tract.

Bariatric surgery – gastric bypass and other weight-loss surgeries in which parts of the digestive system are altered so that weight loss can occur.

Baroreceptors – sensory in the cardiac sinus and aortic arch that sense blood pressure so that it can be maintained.

Barrett's esophagus – a condition in which tissue similar to the intestinal lining replaces the lining of the esophagus.

Basal cell carcinoma – the most common form of skin cancer; it begins in the basal cells, usually in areas that are most exposed to the sun.

Benecalorie – an unflavored supplement that can increase the calorie and protein content of most foods and beverages.

Benign prostatic hyperplasia – enlargement of the prostate gland, most commonly in older men.

Beta-oxidation cycle – a process in which acyl-CoAs are shortened, and the two carboxy-terminal carbon atoms are released as acetyl-CoA units.

Biliary cirrhosis – a rare form of liver cirrhosis caused by disease or defects of the bile ducts.

Binge-eating disorder – earing large quantities of foods, with shameful feelings as a result, but with no purging behaviors.

Bioaccumulative – related to bioaccumulation, the gradual accumulation of substances.

Bioavailability – the proportion of a drug or other substance that enters the circulation when introduced into the body, causing an active effect.

Biocytin – an amide formed from biotin and the amino acid L-lysine.

Biofilms – groupings of surface-associated microbial cells within an extracellular polymeric substance matrix.

Biomarkers – measurable substances in the body that indicate disease, infection, or an environmental exposure.

Bisphenol A – a chemical produced in large quantities, mostly in the production of polycarbonate plastics.

Bitot's spots – collections of keratin, located superficially in the conjunctiva of the eyes.

Blind loop syndrome – when food does not follow the normal route of digestion and bypasses a section of the intestine.

Bloating – a condition in which the abdomen feels full and tight, often due to gas.

Blood urea nitrogen – a waste product that the kidneys remove from the blood.

Body mass index – a measure of body fat based on height and weight, in adults.

Bone density – the amount of bone minerals, such as calcium, present in the bones.

Bone marrow – the substance in the center of most bones that contains many blood vessels; it may be red or yellow in color.

Borborygmi – a rumbling or gurgling nose, made by movement of fluid and gas in the intestines.

Brachytherapy – a type of internal radiation therapy, often used to treat cancers.

Bradycardia – a slow heart rate, with the heart beating less than 60 times per minute.

Brain waves – oscillating electrical voltages in the brain measuring just a few millionths of one volt; they include alpha, beta, gamma, delta, and theta waves.

Bronchopulmonary dysplasia – a chronic lung disease that affects newborns, usually those born prematurely or needing oxygen therapy; with tissue destruction of the alveoli.

Bulimia nervosa – an eating disorder characterized by overeating, then self-induced vomiting or purging, strict dieting, or extreme exercise.

Burton's line – a very thin, black, blue or purple line on the gums because of chronic lead poisoning.

C-reactive protein – a liver protein that increases due to inflammation.

Cachexia – a wasting syndrome that leads to loss of skeletal muscle and fat.

Calcitonin – a hormone formed by the C cells of the thyroid that helps maintain healthy levels of blood calcium.

Calcitriol – a form of vitamin D used to treat and prevent low levels of calcium and bone disease in patients with abnormal kidney or parathyroid gland function.

Calorimetry – the process of measuring the amount of heat released or absorbed during a chemical reaction.

Candida albicans – a naturally occurring fungus within the body; it may cause disease when there is unmanaged diabetes, poor immunity, poor diet, and because of antibiotics, steroids, hormones, or oral contraceptives.

Candidiasis – a fungal infection caused by a yeast called *Candida*; it is signified by itching and irritation.

Carbohydrates – sugar molecules, which are the body's main fuel source.

Carcinoid tumor – a type of neuroendocrine tumor that grows from neuroendocrine cells.

Cardiomegaly – enlargement of the heart due to an underlying condition.

Carotenemia – a clinical condition characterized by yellow skin pigmentation and increased beta-carotene levels in the blood.

Carotenoids – yellow, orange, or red pigments, including carotene, that are antioxidants, protecting against disease, and enhancing the immune system.

Carpal tunnel syndrome – a common neurological disorder occurring when the median nerve becomes pressed or squeezed at the wrist.

Carpopedal spasm – a painful cramp or contraction that usually occurs in the muscles of the hands and feet.

Casal necklace – a hyperpigmented scaly rash in the shape of a necklace that occurs as part of the disease known as pellagra.

Catabolism – the breakdown of complex molecules to form simpler ones along with the release of energy.

Cataracts – cloudy areas in the lenses of the eyes, which are more common with aging.

Catechins – natural polyphenolic phytochemicals in food and medicinal plants; they have strong antioxidant activity.

Catecholamine – a type of neurohormone that is important in stress responses.

Cation – a positively charged ion.

Celiac disease – an immune reaction to eating gluten, a protein found in wheat, barley, and rye.

Cellulitis – a common bacterial skin infection that causes redness, swelling, and pain.

Cerebral atrophy – loss of neurons and the connections that help them communicate in brain tissues, such as occurs with stroke, Alzheimer's disease, and traumatic brain injury.

Cerebral edema – excess accumulation in the intracellular or extracellular spaces of the brain.

Cerebral palsy – a group of disorders affecting the ability to move and maintain balance and posture; the most common motor disability of childhood.

Ceruloplasmin – a liver protein that stores and carries copper to the bloodstream and body tissues.

Chaperone therapy – a new molecular therapeutic approach, mostly for lysosomal diseases; the misfolded mutant enzyme is digested quickly or aggregated, to induce endoplasmic reticulum stress and loss of catalytic activity.

Cheilitis – an acute or chronic inflammation of the lips.

Chemical buffer systems – aqueous solutions of weak acids and their conjugate bases, or weak bases and their conjugate acids.

Cherry angiomas – small, pinhead-like skin lesions that mostly appear on the torso, arms, and legs.

Chia seeds – the seeds of the chia plant that are rich in minerals, omega-3 fat, antioxidants, and fiber.

Chlorophyll – a natural compound in green plants that gives them their color.

Cholangiocarcinomas – cancers of the bile ducts.

Cholecalciferol – vitamin D3; essential for the deposition of calcium in the bones; it is formed by the action of sunlight upon dehydrocholesterol in the skin.

Cholecystitis – inflammation of the gallbladder, often due to gallstones.

Cholecystokinin – a hormone secreted by cells in the duodenum that stimulates release of bile into the intestine and secretion of pancreatic enzymes.

Cholelithiasis – gallbladder; hardened deposits of digestive fluid that can form in the gallbladder.

Cholestasis – reduced or stopped bile flow.

Cholestatic hepatobiliary disease – an impairment of bile formation or flow due to gradual destruction of bile ducts, accumulation of bile acids, or inflammation.

Cholesterol – a waxy, fat-like substance found in all body cells, used to build cells and manufacture vitamins and other hormones; excessive amounts can lead to heart disease and stroke.

Choline – an essential nutrient, naturally present in some foods; it is also available as a dietary supplement.

Chondrocytes – cells responsible for cartilage formation and endochondral ossification.

Chylomicrons – large triglyceride-rich lipoproteins produced in enterocytes from dietary lipids – primarily fatty acids and cholesterol.

Chylothorax – a rare, serious condition in which lymph forms in the digestive system and accumulates in the chest cavity.

Chymotrypsin – a serine protease produced by the pancreas that hydrolyzes peptide bonds of tryptophan, leucine, tyrosine, and phenylalanine.

Cirrhosis – late stage scarring of the liver, often due to hepatitis or alcoholism.

Citric acid cycle – the Krebs cycle or tricarboxylic acid cycle; a series of chemical reactions to release stored energy through oxidation of acetyl-CoA.

Claudication – pain in the arms or legs that occurs while walking or using the arms.

Claw hand – bending in of the fingers toward the wrist; ulnar nerve palsy.

Cleft palate – an opening or split in the roof of the mouth occurring when tissue does not fuse together during development in the uterus.

Clubbing – changes in the areas under and around the nails that may result from chronic low blood oxygen levels.

Coagulopathy – a condition in which the blood's ability to form clots is impaired.

Coarctation of the aorta – constriction in part of the aorta of the heart.

Coccidioidomycosis – "valley fever"; an infection caused by the fungus Coccidioides.

Coenzymes – nonprotein compounds necessary for enzyme function.

Cofactors – nonprotein chemical compounds or metallic ions required for an enzyme to function as a catalyst, to increase the rate of a chemical reaction.

Cognitive – related to cognition (conscious mental activities), such as thinking, reasoning, remembering, imagining, learning words, and using language.

Colic – extended crying, for no obvious reason, in a healthy infant; most common during the first six weeks of life, affecting up to one of every four newborns.

Collagen – a protein in connective tissue, skin, tendons, bones, and cartilage that provides structural support.

Collagenous sprue – a small bowel mucosal lesion associated with chronic diarrhea, weight loss, and severe malabsorption.

Colostrum – the first milk produced by a woman's body during pregnancy.

Comminuted fracture – one in which a bone is broken in at least two places.

Comorbidity – the simultaneous presence of two or more medical conditions in a patient.

Complement proteins – those that opsonize pathogens and induce inflammatory responses that help immune cells fight infection and maintain homeostasis.

Compound fracture – open fracture, in which there is an open wound or break in the skin near the site of the broken bone.

Cones – photoreceptors cells in the retina that give humans color vision.

Confabulation – production or creation of false or erroneous memories without meaning to deceive; or a false memory by someone that believes the truth is being remembered.

Conjunctival xerosis – a dull, dry appearance of the conjunctiva, with slight wrinkling.

Contralateral – relating to the opposite side of the body.

Corneal verticillata – a whorl-like pattern of golden brown or gray opacities in the corneal epithelium.

Corneal xerosis – a dry, hazy appearance of the cornea that can lead to more damage.

Covalent bonds – chemical bonds that involve the sharing of electrons to form electron pairs between atoms.

Cradle cap – crusty or oily, scaly patches on the scalp; seborrheic dermatitis.

Creatine kinase – an enzyme mostly found in the skeletal muscles and heart.

Creatinine – a waste product produced from normal wear and tear on the muscles; when tested, it measures kidney function in regards to filtering the blood.

Creatures – animals, aside from human beings.

Cretinism – a condition of abnormal mental and physical development, due to a deficiency of thyroid hormone in fetal or early life.

Crohn's disease – a form of inflammatory bowel disease that causes inflammation in the digestive tract, leading to pain, diarrhea, fatigue, weight loss, and malnutrition.

Cryotherapy – the use of freezing or near-freezing temperatures to remove abnormal tissue.

Crypt – a small tubular gland, pit, or recess.

Cryptorchidism – one or both testes failing to descend from the abdomen into the scrotum.

Cushing's syndrome – a disorder caused by insufficient cortisol production, causing a fatty hump between the shoulders, a rounded face, and stretch marks on the skin.

Cyclones – large air masses that rotate around a strong center of low atmospheric pressure.

Cystathionine – an amino acid derivative used in the synthesis of cysteine.

Cystic fibrosis – a genetic disorder that affects breathing and digestion.

Cytokine – a protein made by certain immune and nonimmune cells, which has an effect on the immune system.

Cytoplasmic enzymes – those that are within the cytoplasm; the most important are L-lactate-dehydrogenase, aminoacyl-t-RNA-synthase, and the enzymes of glycolysis.

Cytosol – the aqueous component of cell cytoplasm that suspends various organelles and particles.

Daisy – a flowering plant that is part of the aster family (Asteraceae).

Deconjugation – any reaction that disrupts a system of conjugated double bonds, leading to loss of conjugation.

Decubitus ulcers – bedsores, caused by lying in one position for too long a time.

Delirium – a temporary mental state characterized by confusion, anxiety, incoherent speech, and hallucinations.

Delta gap – a difference between the change in anion gap and bicarbonate, used to determine if there is a normal anion gap metabolic acidosis present.

Dementia – an impaired ability to remember, think, or make decisions that interferes with everyday activities; it mostly affects older adults and is not part of normal aging.
Dental caries – tooth decay; cavities.
Dentin – the part of a tooth beneath the enamel and cementum.
Depressed fracture – a break in a cranial bone with depression of the bone in toward the brain.
Depressed sensorium – a condition characterized by the inability to think clearly or concentrate.
Dermatomyositis – a rare disease causing muscle weakness and skin rash.
Dermis – the thick layer of tissue below the epidermis that forms the true skin.
Diabetic dyslipidemia – elevated fasting and postprandial triglycerides, low HDL cholesterol, elevated LDL cholesterol, and a predominance of small, dense LDL particles.
Diaminoaciduria – an increased urine level of any amino acid carrying two amino groups (asparagine, glutamine and lysine, cystine, ornithine).
Diaphragm paralysis – a condition caused by pressure on the phrenic nerve or damage to the nerve.
Diaphyseal fracture – a fracture of the shaft of the tibia, resulting from a direct blow or a rotational force.
DiGeorge syndrome – a condition present from birth that can cause a range of chronic conditions including heart defects and learning difficulties.
Dihydroxylation – the process by which an alkene hydrocarbon is converted into a vicinal diol, in which two hydroxy functional groups are attached to adjacent carbon atoms.
Diverticula – small, bulging pouches that can form in the lining of the digestive system, usually in the lower part of the large intestine.
Diverticuli – outpouchings of the wall of the G.I. tract that form sacs, from the esophagus to the colon.
Docosahexaenoic acid – an omega-3 fatty acid found in cold water, fatty fish such as salmon, as well as fish oil supplements.
Dopamine – a chemical released in the brain that results in pleasurable feelings.
Down syndrome – a chromosomal disorder that causes mental retardation, distinctive facial features, and an increased risk for heart defects and digestive problems.
Drooling – when excess saliva flows out of the mouth involuntarily.
Ductal carcinoma in situ – the presence of abnormal cells inside a milk duct of the breast.
Dumping syndrome – a condition in which food (usually when high in sugar) moves from the stomach to the small intestine too quickly.
Dwarfism – short stature that results from a genetic or medical condition; generally defined as an adult height of 4 feet 10 inches or less.
Dynorphin – a neuropeptide involved in pain, addiction, and mood regulation.
Dysarthria – difficulty speaking due to brain damage.
Dysgeusia – a taste disorder that makes foods taste sour, sweet, bitter, or metallic.
Dyslipidemia – an imbalance of lipids (cholesterol, LDL cholesterol, triglycerides, and HDL cholesterol).
Dysmenorrhea – menstrual cramps.
Dyspepsia – indigestion.
Dysphagia – difficulty swallowing.
Dystonias – movement disorders that cause muscles to contract involuntarily.
Ecchymoses – a skin discoloration due to bleeding underneath, usually from bruising.
Eclampsia – a severe complication of preeclampsia, which hypertension causes seizures during pregnancy.
Eczema – atopic dermatitis, which causes dry, itchy, inflamed skin.
Ehlers-Danlos syndrome – a group of inherited disorders that affect the connective tissues – mostly the skin, joints, and blood vessel walls.
Eicosapentaenoic acid – an omega-3 fatty acid, found in cold water, fatty fish, that (along with docosahexaenoic acid) helps lower risks for heart disease.
El Niño – the warm phase of the El Niño-Southern Oscillation, associated with a band or warm ocean water that develops in the Pacific Ocean.
Elastosis – degenerative changes in dermal tissue, with increased deposition of elastin material.
Electrolytes – substances containing ions that is electrically conducting through the ions' movements, but no conducting electrons.
Electron – a negatively charged subatomic particle, either bound to an atom or unbound.
Embolism – a blocked artery caused by a foreign body, such as a blood clot or an air bubble.
Emphysema – a lung condition that causes shortness of breath due to destruction and dilatation of the alveoli.
Enamel – the thin outer covering over the crown of a tooth.
Endemic goiter – an adaptive disease produced by persistent stimulation of the thyroid gland because of an iodine deficiency.
Endogenous – having an internal cause or origin.
Endometrioid adenocarcinoma – the formation of malignant cells in the tissues of the endometrium; this form is the most common type of endometrial cancer.
Endometriosis – a condition in which cells similar to the endometrium grow outside of the uterus.
Endotoxins – primary components of the outer membranes of cells walls of Gram-negative bacteria.
Engorgement – a condition that occurs when breast milk is not fully removed, usually as the milk is transitioning from colostrum to mature milk.
Enteral tube nutrition – tube feeding; a way of delivering nutrition directly to the stomach or small intestine.

Enterocytes – cells of the intestinal lining.
Enterokinase – a protease of the intestinal bush border that cleaves the acidic propeptide from trypsinogen, to yield active trypsin.
Epidermis – the surface epithelium of the skin that overlies the dermis.
Epididymis – a narrow, coiled tube attached to the testicles, where sperm cells finish maturing and are stored.
Epigenetic – the study of how behavior and environment can cause genetic function changes; the changes are reversible.
Epigenetic marker – a marking that determines the exact section of a gene to be "switched off".
Epigenetic tags – marks that record a cell's experiences upon DNA, which helps to stabilize gene expression.
Epiphyseal plates – growth plates; thin layers of cartilage lying between the epiphyses ad metaphyses, where growth of long bones occurs.
Epiphyses – the end parts of long bones, initially growing separately from the shaft.
Epistaxis – nosebleed.
Ergocalciferol – one of a class of vitamin D analogs, also called vitamin D2.
Erythema – superficial skin reddening, usually in patches, due to injury or irritation that causes dilatation of blood capillaries.
Erythrasma – a superficial skin infection caused by Corynebacterium minutissimum, a gram-positive, non-spore-forming bacillus.
Erythrocytosis – a high concentration of red blood cells.
Esophagectomy – a surgical procedure to remove some or all of the esophagus and reconstruct it using part of the stomach or another organ.
Esophagitis – inflammation of the esophagus.
Estrogens – a sex hormone responsible for development and regulation of the female reproductive system and secondary sex characteristics.
Euthyroid – having a normally functioning thyroid gland.
Exogenous – having an external cause or origin.
Exposure medium – a chemical exposure occurring as part of breathing, eating, and contacting soil, water, food, or air.
Extracellular fluid compartment – all body fluid outside the cells of the body; the main component is the interstitial (tissue) fluid that surrounds the cells.
Fabry disease – alpha-galactosidase-A deficiency; an inherited neurological disorder in which lipids cannot be efficiently broken down in order to provide energy.
Facilitated diffusion – the passive movement of molecules along a concentration gradient.
Fad diets – plans that promote results such as fast weight loss without proven evidence to support such claims.
Famine – widespread scarcity of food, caused by factors such as war, natural disasters, crop failure, population imbalance, poverty, economic catastrophes, or government policies.
Fatty liver – storage of extra liver fat that may lead to liver damage.
Fatty liver disease – steatosis; a common condition caused by excessive fat buildup in the liver.
Fatty streak – the first visible lesion in the development of atherosclerosis.
Female athlete triad – abnormal menstruation, weight loss or loss body mass index, and stress fractures.
Fenton growth chart – a tool designed for growth monitoring of preterm infants with birth gestational age less than 37 weeks.
Ferritin – a blood protein that contains iron.
Fetal alcohol effects – less severe than those of fetal alcohol syndrome, they include hyperactivity, attention deficit, or impaired learning.
Fetal alcohol syndrome – a serious set of impairments caused by maternal alcohol consumption, including physical defects, CNS problems, and social and behavioral issues.
Fibroblasts – cells that contribute to formation of connective tissue.
Fibromyalgia – a chronic disorder causing widespread pain and tenderness, plus fatigue and difficulty sleeping.
Fibrosis – overgrowth, hardening, or scarring of various tissues; due to excessive deposition of collagen or other extracellular matrix components.
Fight-or-flight – a response that is an automatic physiological reaction to a stressful or frightening event.
Firmicutes – bacteria of the G.I. tract that can produce resistant endospores, which maintain viability and germinate in the intestine to facilitate transmission.
Fiscal disincentives – percentages of earnings lost to higher taxes or lower benefits when jobseekers return to work after two months of unemployment.
Fiscal incentives – tax holidays or allowances, exemptions from customs duties, or local indirect taxes.
Fish gills – branching organs through which fish breathe.
Fistulae – abnormal connections between body parts, due to injuries, surgeries, infections, or inflammation.
Flaccid – soft, hanging loosely or limply.
Floppy muscle tone – hypotonia, sometimes called "floppy muscle syndrome".
Fluid compartments – primarily, the intracellular and extracellular fluid compartments.
Fluorosis – a condition that causes changes in the appearance of tooth enamel.
Foam cells – a type of macrophage that localizes to fatty deposits on blood vessel walls.
Folacin – folic acid or folate (vitamin B9).
Follicle cells – the functional units of the hair follicles.
Follicular hyperkeratosis – a skin condition, with excessive keratin development in hair follicles, causing rough, elevated papules due to closure of the follicles with white plugs of sebum.

Food aversions – intense dislikes of specific foods, including unpleasant reactions.

Fractionation – a separation process in which a certain amount of a mixture is divided into small quantities, in which the composition changes according to a gradient.

Fragile X syndrome – a genetic disorder causing many developmental problems including learning disabilities and cognitive impairment.

Frailty – the condition of being weak and delicate.

Free radicals – highly reactive, unstable molecules made during normal cell metabolism; if they build up, they can damage DNA, lipids, and proteins.

Friction rub – a liver condition described in those with liver tumors or abscesses, syphilitic hepatitis, gonococcal perihepatitis, or after biopsy.

Fulminant – severe and sudden in onset.

Funduscopic examination – a routine part of an eye examination in which the retina is visualized with an ophthalmoscope.

G cells – neuroendocrine cells responsible for the synthesis and secretion of gastrin.

Gait training – a form of physical therapy to improve standing or walking.

Galactocerebrosidase – an enzyme that removes galactose from ceramide derivatives.

Galactosemia – a rare, hereditary disorder of carbohydrate metabolism that affects the ability to convert galactose to glucose.

Gangliosides – molecules composed of glycosphingolipids that are very important in immunology, and may become therapeutics for neurodegenerative disorders.

Gastrectomy – surgery to remove all or part of the stomach.

Gastric cardia – the portion of the stomach closest to the esophagus.

Gastric lavage – stomach pumping; an invasive procedure that involves cleaning and removing stomach contents via a tube inserted through the mouth or nose.

Gastric plication – a minimally invasive endoscopic procedure, in which the stomach is folded in on itself and sutured, to make it smaller and shorter.

Gastrin – a hormone that stimulates secretion of gastric juice.

Gastrografin – a liquid radiocontrast agent that contains iodine.

Gaucher disease – the result of a buildup of fatty substances in organs such as the spleen and liver, as well as bone tissue, causing changes in function and weak structures.

Generalized seizures – loss of consciousness, sometimes with spasms, stiffening, shaking, muscle contractions, or loss of muscle tone; these seizures include absence, atonic, tonic, clonic, tonic-clonic, myoclonic, and febrile seizures.

Geophagia – deliberate consumption of earth, soil, or clay.

Geropsychology – a specialty that applies knowledge and methods of psychology to understanding and helping older adults.

Gestational age – the length of a pregnancy, measured in weeks, from the date of the last menstrual period.

Gestational diabetes – a type of diabetes diagnosed initially during pregnancy.

Ghrelin – a hormone produced and released by the stomach that signals the brain when an individual is hungry.

Ginger ale – a carbonated soft drink flavored with ginger.

Gingivitis – a common, mild form or periodontal disease, causing irritation, redness, and inflammation of the gingiva around the base of the teeth.

Glasgow Coma Score – a number used to assess the level of a coma, with 3 being worst and 15 being highest.

Globotriaosylceramide – a glycosphingolipid that builds up in cells, especially those in blood vessels of the skin, plus cells of the kidneys, heart, and nervous system; this leads to signs and symptoms of Fabry disease.

Glomerulonephritis – inflammation of the glomeruli (filters) in the kidneys.

Glucagon – a hormone made by the pancreas that helps regulate blood glucose levels.

Glucocorticoids – corticosteroids involved in the metabolism of carbohydrates, proteins, and fats; they have anti-inflammatory activities.

Glucosuria – the presence of glucose in the urine.

Glutathione – a substance that is an important antioxidant, made from glycine, cystine, and glutamic acid; it is produced by the liver.

Gluteally – referring to the gluteal region (buttocks).

Gluten enteropathy – celiac disease; an autoimmune inflammatory disease of the small intestine precipitated by ingestion of gluten (part of wheat protein).

Gluten-free – an eating plan that excludes foods containing gluten, a protein found in wheat, barley, and rye.

Glycogen – the stored form of glucose made up of connected glucose molecules.

Glycogen phosphorylase – a phosphorylase enzyme that catalyzes sequential phosphorolysis of glycogen to release gluose-1-phosphate; it is the main enzyme in utilization of muscle and liver reserves of glycogen.

Glycogen storage diseases – rare metabolic disorders in which the body cannot store or breakdown glycogen, affecting the liver, muscles, and other body areas.

Glycolytic inhibitor – a substance used to treat cancer; it is highly effective against cancer cells with defective mitochondria, or if they are under hypoxic conditions.

Glycosaminoglycans – mucopolysaccharides; negatively charged polysaccharide compounds with widespread functions in the body.

Glycosylated hemoglobin A1c – a type of hemoglobin tested to diagnose diabetes mellitus.

Goblet cells – specialized epithelial cells that line mucosal surfaces and secrete mucus to provide a protective barrier.

Goiter – an irregular enlargement of the thyroid gland, most often due to lack of iodine.

Goitrogens – naturally occurring substances that may interfere with thyroid gland function.

Gonadotropin hormone – a glycoprotein hormone secreted by the anterior pituitary; it acts on the gonads to control gamete and sex hormone production.

Granulomas – small areas of inflammation; they are usually benign.

Greenstick fracture – one in which a bone bends and cracks instead of breaking completely into separate pieces; most common in children younger than age ten.

Growth landmarks – parameters measured in infants, children, and adolescents that help to gauge where they are on a continuum of normal growth and development.

Gruels – cereals such as ground oats, wheat, rye, or rice heated or boiled in water or milk.

Guar gum – a food additive used to thicken and bind food products.

Gut microbiota – the largest population of microorganisms in the human body, residing within the intestine.

Hair follicles – tube-like pores that surround the roots and strands of hairs.

Hallucinations – perceived sounds, sights, odors, tastes, or feelings that are not actually present.

Hartnup disease – a condition caused by an inability to absorb certain amino acids from the diet; vitamins and proteins can therefore not be produced.

Hashimoto thyroiditis – a disease that causes the thyroid to make less thyroid hormone than is needed, resulting in goiter, tiredness, weight gain, and muscle weakness.

Heat stroke – the most serious heat-related illness, occurring when the body's temperature control is lost.

Heberden nodes – small, pea-sized bony growths on the joint closest to the tip of the finger (the distal interphalangeal joint).

Helicobacter pylori – a type of bacteria that infects the stomach, usually in childhood.

Helminths – parasitic worms with elongated, flat, or round bodies.

Hematemesis – the presence of significant amounts of blood in the vomitus.

Hematocolpos – vaginal retention of menstrual blood at puberty.

Hematocrit – the percentage by volume of red blood cells in the blood.

Hematogenous – originating in or carried by the blood.

Hematoma – a pool of mostly clotted blood that forms in an organ, tissue, or body space.

Hematometra – a collection or retention of blood in the uterus, usually due to an imperforate hymen or transverse vaginal septum.

Hematuria – blood in the urine.

Heme – an iron-containing compound of the porphyrin class; it forms the nonprotein part of hemoglobin and other biological molecules.

Heme-positive stools – those that have occult blood in them, prompting a colonoscopy.

Hemiparesis – weakness or inability to move on one side of the body.

Hemochromatosis – a disorder in which the body can build up too much iron in the skin, heart, liver, pancreas, pituitary gland, and joints; leading to tissue and organ damage.

Hemodialysis – a treatment to filter wastes and water from the blood, to control blood pressure and mineral balance.

Hemodynamics – basic measures of cardiovascular function; how blood flows through the arteries and veins, and the forces that affect blood flow.

Hemoglobinopathies – a group of disorders passed down through families, in which there is abnormal production or structure of the hemoglobin molecule.

Hemolysis – destruction of red blood cells.

Hemolytic anemia – a disorder in which red blood cells are destroyed faster than they can be made.

Hemopoietic – related to the formation of blood or blood cells.

Hemopoietic growth factors – hormone-like substances that help bone marrow make new blood cells.

Hemopoietic stem cells – immature cells that can develop into white or red blood cells as well as platelets.

Hemorrhoid – a swollen vein in the anus and lower rectum, similar to a varicose vein.

Hepatic bruit – a sound coming from the liver that indicates alcoholic hepatitis, or primary or metastatic cancer.

Hepatic steatosis – fatty liver disease; the presence of extra fat in the liver.

Hepatocellular carcinoma – the most common type of primary liver cancer.

Hepatocytes – specialized epithelial cells that make up nearly 80% of the total liver mass; they have pivotal roles in metabolism, detoxification, and protein synthesis.

Hepatoma – a cancer of the cells of the liver.

Hepatomegaly – enlargement of the liver.

Hepatosplenomegaly – enlargement of both the liver and spleen.

Hepcidin – a peptide hormone from the liver that is vital for iron homeostasis.

Herbicides – chemicals used to manipulate or control undesirable vegetation (plants).

Heterocyclic amines – carcinogenic and mutagenic chemicals formed from cooking muscle meats such as beef, pork, fowl, and fish.

Heterogeneous diseases – medical conditions with several causes, such as hepatitis or diabetes mellitus.

Hippocampus – elongated ridges on the floor of each lateral ventricle of the brain.

Hodgkin lymphoma – a type of cancer that affects the lymphatic system; lymphocytes grow out of control, causing swollen lymph nodes and growths throughout the body.

Holoenzymes – biochemically active compounds formed by combinations of enzymes with coenzymes.

Homeostasis – a relatively stable equilibrium (balance) in the body.

Homocysteine – an amino acid broken down by vitamins B6, B9, and B12 to create other needed chemicals.

Homozygous – having two identical alleles of a gene or genes.

Hospitalism – the adverse effects of a prolonged stay in a hospital.

Human chorionic gonadotrophin – a hormone produced by the placenta during pregnancy, wherein the egg (ova) is nourished after fertilization and implantation.

Hurler syndrome – the most severe form of mucopolysaccharidosis type I, in which cells cannot breakdown glucose molecules, causing life-threatening symptoms.

Hydrogen phosphate – a phosphate ion that is the conjugate base of dihydrogen phosphate, which has roles as a metabolite and cofactor.

Hydrolyzed protein – a solution derived from hydrolysis of a protein into its component amino acids and peptides.

Hydrostatic – of or relating to fluids at rest, or to the pressures they exert or transmit.

Hyperammonemia – a condition that happens when there are high levels of ammonia in the blood; it is life-threatening and requires immediate medical treatment.

Hyperbilirubinemia – a condition in which there is too much bilirubin in the blood, which can build up and affect other tissues and fluids in the body.

Hypercapnia – the presence of excessively high carbon dioxide in the blood.

Hyperemesis gravidarum – severe or prolonged vomiting during pregnancy, leading to weight loss and dehydration.

Hyperglycemia – high blood glucose, occurring when there is insufficient insulin, or when the body cannot use insulin properly.

Hyperhomocysteinemia – a condition of abnormally high levels of homocysteine in the blood; it can trigger atherosclerosis and many related conditions.

Hyperkalemia – a high level of potassium in the blood.

Hypermetabolic – having hypermetabolism, with an elevated resting energy expenditure, often due to burns, hyperthyroidism, sepsis, and use of steroids.

Hyperosmolar – a serious complication of diabetes mellitus, occurring when blood glucose levels are too high for a long period, leading to severe dehydration and confusion.

Hyperplastic obesity – a condition that occurs when an adult eats or manufactures too much fat and the adipocytes fill with liquid.

Hypertrophic obesity – a condition associated mostly with adipose cell enlargement in adult men; adipose cell size, independent of body mass index, is negatively correlated with whole body insulin sensitivity.

Hypha – each of the branching filaments that form the mycelium of a fungus.

Hypocapnia – the presence of excessively low carbon dioxide in the blood.

Hypochromic microcytic anemia – a condition that impairs the normal transport of iron in cells.

Hypofractionation – a treatment schedule in which the total radiation dose is divided into large doses, with treatments given once a day or less often.

Hypokalemia – low blood potassium.

Hypolactasia – lactose malabsorption (either congenital, primary, or secondary).

Hyponatremia – a low level of sodium in the blood.

Hypoparathyroidism – a condition caused by insufficient production of parathyroid hormone by the parathyroid glands.

Hypopnea – a common symptom of obstructive or central sleep apnea, with 10 seconds or more of shallow breathing in which the airflow drops by 30% or more.

Hypoproteinemia – a low level of protein in the blood.

Hypothyroidism – underactive thyroid, resulting in insufficient production of thyroid hormone.

Hypotonia – decreased muscle tone.

Hypotonic hydration – adequate levels of water associated with effective osmolality of body fluids.

Hypouricemia – serum urate concentration of less than 2 mg/dL; it may be renal hypouricemia or xanthinuria.

Ileocecal valve – a sphincter muscle situated at the junction of the ileum and colon.

Immunoglobulin A – an antibody found in mucous membranes, saliva, tears, and breastmilk.

Indirect calorimetry – the method of measuring respiratory gas exchange to estimate energy expenditure.

Infantile beriberi – a potentially fatal disorder caused by a thiamine deficiency.

Infertility – an inability to conceive, or become pregnant, after one year or more of unprotected sex.

Inflammasome – an innate immune system receptor/sensor that regulates factors that induce inflammation in response to infectious microbes and molecules derived from host proteins.

Inflammatory bowel disease – a disorder involving chronic inflammation of tissues in the digestive tract, including ulcerative colitis and Crohn's disease.

Inhibin – a polypeptide secreted by cells in the gonads that inhibits synthesis and release of follicle-stimulating hormone and reduces luteinizing hormone-releasing hormone content.

Insensible water loss – the amount of body fluid lost daily that is difficult to measure, from the respiratory system, skin, and stool.

Insulinoma – a pancreatic tumor that manufactures extra insulin, resulting in hypoglycemia and sometimes, coma.

Intelligence quotient – a number representing a person's reasoning ability as compared to the statistical norm or average for their age.

Intermittent – occurring at irregular intervals.

Intermittent claudication – a waxing and waning condition in which cramping leg pain is induced by exercise, usually due to arterial obstruction.

Interstitial fluid – the fluid in the spaces around cells, from substances that leak out of blood capillaries.

Interstitial nephritis – a kidney disorder in which spaces between kidney tubules become inflamed, causing functional problems.

Intimal hyperplasia – an abnormal accumulation of cells in the vascular tunica intima.

Intracellular fluid compartment – the fluids contained inside the cells, consisting of cytosol and fluid in the cell nucleus.

Intrauterine insemination – a form of artificial insemination in which sperm is placed directly into the uterus using a small catheter.

Intrinsic factor – a protein, made by cells in the stomach lining, which helps the intestines absorb vitamin B12.

Intrusion – the entering of water into structures, causing a variety of problems.

Inulin – a type of prebiotic that remains in the bowel and helps certain beneficial bacteria to grow.

Invasins – proteins associated with the penetration of pathogens into host cells.

Irritable bowel syndrome – a common disorder that affects the stomach and intestines to cause cramping, pain, bloating, gas, diarrhea, and constipation.

Ischemia – an inadequate blood supply to an organ or body part (especially, the heart muscle).

Isolated systolic hypertension – a condition in which diastolic blood pressure is less than 80 mm Hg while the systolic BP is 130 mm Hg or higher; common in older adults.

Jaundice – a condition in which the skin, sclera, and mucous membranes turn yellow due to a high level of bilirubin, formed from the breakdown of red blood cells.

Jejunoileitis – a type of Crohn's disease that causes inflammation in the jejunum.

Jejunostomy – surgery to create an opening into the jejunum of the small intestine from outside of the body so that a feeding tube can be placed.

Juvenile diabetes – type 1 diabetes (usually diagnosed before age 40); in children, most diagnoses occur between ages 4 and 14.

Juxtaglomerular complex – a structure in the kidney that regulates the function of each nephron.

Kawasaki disease – an acute febrile illness of unknown cause that mostly affects children younger than five years of age.

Kayser-Fleischer rings – golden to greenish-brown annular deposition of copper in the periphery of the cornea.

Keratin – a protein that helps form hair, nails, and the epidermis.

Keratomalacia – drying and clouding of the cornea due to vitamin A deficiency.

Kernicterus – a type of brain damage that can result from high levels of bilirubin in an infant's blood, leading to athetoid cerebral palsy, hearing loss, vision problems, tooth abnormalities, and intellectual disabilities.

Keshan disease – an endemic, extremely lethal cardiomyopathy; it causes congestive or acute heart failure and cardiac arrhythmias.

Ketones – chemicals made in the liver when glucose is in short supply.

Ketonic odor – a sweet, fruity, or nail polish-like odor caused by chemicals the body creates during ketosis.

Ketosis – a metabolic state, when the body burns fat for energy instead of glucose.

Kilocalories – units of energy of 1,000 calories; the energy required to raise the temperature of 1 kg of water by 1 degree Celsius.

Klinefelter syndrome – a chromosomal disorder that results in taller than average stature, abnormal puberty, and later, less muscle or hair development.

Korsakoff psychosis – a late complication of Wernicke encephalopathy, causing memory deficits, confusion, and behavioral changes.

Krabbe disease – a rare, inherited metabolic disorder, with harmful amounts of lipids building up in various cells and tissues, and with destruction of brain cells.

Kupffer cells – phagocytic cells that form the lining of the liver sinusoids; they are involved in breakdown of red blood cells.

Kwashiorkor – a severe form of malnutrition signified by excessive tissue fluid that causes edema.

Lactose malabsorbers – individuals that lack complete hydrolysis of lactose due to a lactase deficiency.

Lanugo hair – fine, soft, unpigmented hair, often present in young children, or because of certain disease states.

Laparoscopic techniques – surgeries in which short, narrow tubes are inserted into the abdomen through incisions less than 1 cm in size.

Laparotomy – a surgical incision into the abdominal cavity to examine and often repair internal abnormalities.

Large-fiber sensory – a neurological problem seen with Sjogren's syndrome, usually causing numbness and paresthesia.

Lassitude – a state of physical or mental weariness; lack of energy.

Leavening – a substances used in dough or batter to make it rise, such as yeast or baking powder.

Leiomyosarcomas – a rare type of cancer that grows in the smooth muscles.

Leptin – a hormone that adipose tissue releases, which helps the body maintain normal weight on a long-term basis.

Lesch-Nyhan syndrome – a rare, inherited disorder caused by an enzyme deficiency, causing impaired kidney function, acute gouty arthritis, and self-mutilating behaviors.

Let-down reflex – a process that stimulates the flow of breastmilk; suckling by an infant stimulates nerves that cause prolactin and oxytocin to be released into the bloodstream.

Lethargy – a lack of energy and enthusiasm.

Leukemia – cancers of the blood cells, bone marrow, and lymphatic system.

Leukopenia – insufficient amounts of leukocytes in the blood, resulting in a higher risk for various diseases.

Leukotrienes – inflammatory molecules that are used in inflammatory states and allergic diseases.

Lewy body dementia – a disease associated with abnormal deposits of the protein called alpha-synuclein in the brain; the second most common type of progressive dementia.

Life expectancy – the number of years a person can expect to live.

Linear growth – the growth by a constant amount for each unit of time.

Lipids – fatty acids or their derivatives, which are insoluble in water but soluble in organic solvents, such as many natural oils, waxes, and steroids.

Lipocalin 2 – a protein that is encoded by the LCN2 gene; the protein plays a role in innate immunity by limiting bacterial growth.

Lipoproteins – soluble proteins that combine with and transport fat and other lipids in the blood plasma.

Liposuction – a surgical procedure that uses suction to remove fat from the abdomen, hips, thighs, buttocks, arms, or neck, and also contours these areas.

Liver spots – also called age spots; small, flat dark areas on the skin, usually in sun-exposed areas.

Locus ceruleus – part of the reticular activating system; it is the main source of the neurotransmitter noradrenaline (norepinephrine).

Longitudinal fractures – uncommon fractures in which a diaphyseal fracture line occurs parallel to the long axis of a bone in the absence of direct trauma.

Looser zones – cortical infractions, Milkman lines, or pseudofractures traversing partway through a bone, usually due to osteomalacia or rickets.

Lymphedema – inflammation caused by buildup of lymph fluid.

Lysosomal storage diseases – inherited metabolic diseases characterized by abnormal buildup of toxic materials in the cells.

Macrocytic anemia – a blood disorder caused by bone marrow production of abnormally large red blood cells.

Macroglossia – enlarged tongue; it occurs in children more than adults.

Macrominerals – minerals needed in larger quantities, including calcium, phosphorus, magnesium, sodium, potassium, and chloride.

Macronutrients – the nutrients used in the largest amounts (carbohydrates, fats, and proteins).

Macrophages – large phagocytic cells, in a stationary form in tissues, or as mobile white blood cells, mostly at sites of infection.

Macrosomia – growth beyond a specific threshold regardless of gestational age.

Macular degeneration – an eye disease that blurs central vision, due to aging.

Macular edema – a condition caused by blood vessels leaking into the macula of the retina.

Malabsorption syndromes – digestive disorders that prevent the body from effectively absorbing nutrients.

Malnutrition – lack of proper nutrition; it includes undernutrition and overnutrition.

Mamillary bodies – brainstem nuclei on the posteroinferior aspect of the hypothalamus.

Maple syrup urine disease – a rare, serious inherited condition in which some amino acids cannot be processed, causing their harmful buildup in the blood and urine.

Marasmus – a severe manifestation of protein-energy malnutrition, leading to an overt loss of adipose tissue and muscle.

Marfan syndrome – a genetic condition that affects connective tissue, damaging blood vessels, the heart, eyes, skin, lungs, and bones.

Marfanoid habitus – a group of symptoms resembling Marfan syndrome, including long limbs, crowded oral maxilla, high arch in the palate, arachnodactyly, and hyperlaxity.

Mastitis – inflammation of breast tissue that causes pain, swelling, warmth, and redness; it is most common in women that are breast-feeding an infant.

Mastocytosis – a rare condition caused by an excessive number of mast cells gathering in body tissues.

Meconium – the first bowel movement of an infant; it is sticky, thick, and dark green, made up of cells, protein, fats, and intestinal secretions such as bile.

Medium-chain triglyceride – a fat made in a laboratory from coconut and palm kernel oils.

Megaloblastic anemia – a form of anemia characterized by large red blood cells, with the inner contents being incompletely developed.

Megaloblasts – large nucleated red blood cell precursors with non-condensed chromatin.

Melanin – a substance that produces hair, eye, and skin pigmentation.

Melanocytes – cells in the skin and eyes that produce and contain the pigment called melanin; they lie within the layer of basal cells at the deepest part of the epidermis.

Melanoma – a disease in which malignant cells form in melanocytes.

Melasma – a skin condition of patches and spots, usually on the face, which are darker than the natural skin tone.

Melena – dark, sticky feces containing partly digested blood.

Menaquinone – the quinone used for electron transfer by many bacteria, alone or together with ubiquinone.

Menarche – the first occurrence of menstruation.

Menkes disease – lack of regulation of copper metabolism, mostly affecting male infants.

Menorrhagia – menstrual bleeding that lasts for more than seven days, or heavy menstrual bleeding.

Mesentery – a fold of membrane attaching the intestine to the abdominal wall.

Metabolic acidosis – the buildup of acid in the body due to kidney disease or failure.

Metabolic alkalosis – a disorder that elevates serum bicarbonate, mostly caused by use of diuretics and external loss of gastric secretions.

Metabolic syndrome – a cluster of conditions that increase risks of heart disease, stroke, and type 2 diabetes (including hypertension, hyperglycemia, excess abdominal fat, and abnormal cholesterol or triglyceride levels).

Metabolic traits – molecular phenotypes that can influence clinical phenotypes, and may predict disease progression.

Metabolic water – the water created through metabolism by oxidizing energy-containing substances in food.

Metabolism – the process by which the body changes nutrients into energy.

Metabolites – substances made or used when the body breaks down food, drugs, chemicals, or its own tissues.

Metalloenzymes – a broad group of enzymes that use a metal cation as a cofactor in the enzyme active site.

Metaplasia – a change of cells to a form that does not normally occur in the tissue in which they are found.

Metaplastic – a rare, aggressive form of breast cancer, usually fast-growing.

Methane – a hydrocarbon that is a primary component of natural gas.

Methylation – a chemical reaction in which a small methyl group gets added to DNA, proteins, or other molecules to affect function.

Micelles – aggregates of molecules in colloidal solutions, such as those formed by detergents.

Microbeads – a category of microplastics that are smaller than 5 mm in size.

Microbiome – the internal environment consisting of microbes that are both helpful and potentially harmful.

Microbiota – the range of microorganisms that may be commensal, symbiotic, or pathogenic.

Microcytic hypochromic anemia – an anemia in which circulating red blood cells are smaller than their usual size and have decreased red color.

Microminerals – minerals needed in smaller quantities, including manganese, copper, iodine, fluorine, selenium, chromium, iron, molybdenum, and zinc.

Micronutrients – the nutrients used in the smallest amounts (vitamins and minerals).

Microplastics – tiny plastic particles resulting from commercial product development and breakdown of larger plastics; they are harmful to the environment and animal health.

Milkman syndrome – a type of osteomalacia characterized by radiolucent zones or bands of decalcification, usually at right angles to the long axis of the bone.

Millet – one of a group of small-seeded grasses, grown around the world as cereal crops or grains.

Miscarriage – spontaneous loss of a pregnancy before the 20th week.

Mitochondria – an organelle in which respiration and energy production occur in cells.

Monomers – molecules that can be bonded to other identical molecules, to form polymers.

Morbidity – the condition of suffering from a disease or medical condition.

Morning sickness – nausea and vomiting in pregnancy, usually early in gestation.

Mortality – death, or the state of being subject to death.

Multiple myeloma – a cancer that forms in the type of white blood cell known as a plasma cell; cancerous cells accumulate in the bone marrow.

Myasthenia gravis – a chronic autoimmune, neuromuscular disease that causes weakness in the skeletal muscles; it worsens after periods of activity and improves after periods of rest.

Mycotoxins – naturally occurring toxins produced by certain fungi that sometimes are found in food.

Myelin – an insulating layer or sheath around nerves, including those of the brain and spinal cord.

Myocytes – muscle cells; the smallest subunits of muscular tissues and organs.

Myoglobin – a protein in striated muscles the primarily supplies oxygen to myocytes.

Myopathy – a clinical disorder of the skeletal muscles leading to weakness and dysfunction.

Myotonic dystrophy – a common multi-system disorder that affects the skeletal muscles, smooth muscles, and cardiac muscles.

Myxedema coma – severe hypothyroidism, leading to decreased mental status, hypothermia, and other symptoms related to slowed function in multiple organs; it is a medical emergency with a high mortality rate.

Myxedema madness – a severe, complicated form of psychosis because of significant hypothyroidism; it involves depression, lethargy, and psychosis.

Nail cuticles – made up of a thin layer of clear dead skin at the nail bed; cuticles form between the eponychium and nail plate.

Necrosis – the death of body tissue.

Necrotizing cellulitis – death of infected skin and tissues; there is redness, warmth, occasional inflammation, and gas bubbles under the skin.

Negative energy balance – energy intake being less than energy expenditure, usually resulting in weight loss.

Neoantigens – new proteins that form on cancer cells when certain mutations occur in tumor DNA.

Neonatal abstinence syndrome – a condition that affects newborns that receive addictive substances through the placenta during pregnancy; withdrawal is experienced during the first few days of life.

Nephrosis – kidney disease characterized by edema and loss of protein from the plasm into the urine; also called nephrotic syndrome.

Neural tube – the early developmental structure that forms the brain and spine.

Neurogenesis – the process by which new neurons are formed in the brain.

Neurotransmitter – a chemical substance released at the end of a nerve fiber by arrival of a nerve impulse; it diffuses across a synapse or junction to cause transfer of the impulse to another nerve fiber, muscle fiber, or another structure.

Neurotransmitters – chemical messengers that are essential for normal functions; they carry chemical signs from one neuron to the next target cell.

Neutropenia – a lack of neutrophils.

Neutrophils – leukocytes that act as the immune system's first line of defense.

Night blindness – nyctalopia; an inability to see well at night or in poor light.

Night eating syndrome – an eating disorder that causes awakening in order to eat several times a night in order to fall back asleep.

Nitrosamines – chemicals found in tobacco products and tobacco smoke as well as many foods; they sometimes have carcinogenic effects.

Nomograms – mathematical devices that show relationships between height and weight measurements.

Nonelectrolytes – compounds that do not have any distinct ionic form to exist in when dissolved in an aqueous solution.

Noonan syndrome – a genetic disorder that prevents normal development in the face and heart, also causing short stature, other physical problems, and developmental delays.

Nosocomial – originating in a hospital, such as when an infection develops there.

Nucleotide polymorphisms – a DNA variation that occurs when a single nucleotide in the genome sequence is altered; it is present in 1% or more of the population.

Nutrient density – being high in nutrients but relatively low in calories.

Nutrients – substances that provide nourishment essential for growth and life.

Nystagmus – a vision condition in which the eyes make repetitive, uncontrolled movements.

Obesity paradox – a condition in which obesity in older subjects or those with several chronic diseases may actually be protective, and associated with decreased mortality.

Obsessive-compulsive disorder – a common, chronic, long-lasting disorder in which a person has uncontrollable, reoccurring thoughts and/or behaviors that he or she feels the urge to continually repeat.

Odynophagia – the medical term for painful swallowing.

Oligomenorrhea – infrequent menstrual periods.

Oocyte – a cell in an ovary that may undergo meiotic division to form an ovum.

Ophthalmoplegia – paralysis or weakness of the eye muscles.

Ornithine – a non-proteinogenic amino acid involved in the urea cycle.

Orogastric – related to a tube placed through the mouth that ends in the stomach.

Orotic aciduria – a hereditary condition characterized by elevated levels of orotic acid in the urine, usually seen in the first months of life.

Osmolality – the concentration of dissolved particles in your blood.

Osmolarity – the concentration of a solution expressed as the total number of solute particles per liter.

Osmoreceptors – sensory receptors mostly found in the hypothalamus; they detect changes in osmotic pressure.

Osmotic – related to osmosis, the passage of a liquid through a membrane from a less concentrate solution to a more concentrated solution.

Osteoarthritis – the most common form of arthritis, usually occurring in the hands, hips, and knees; cartilage in joints breaks down and underlying bone changes occur.

Osteoblasts – bone cells primarily responsible for synthesizing bone matrix proteins and minerals during early bone formation, but also controlling bone formation and mineralization throughout life.

Osteoclasts – cells that degrade bone to start normal bone remodeling; they mediate bone loss in pathologic conditions by increasing their resorptive activity.

Osteoid – unmineralized bone tissue that is used to develop mature mineralized bone.

Osteomalacia – softening of the bones, usually due to a problem with vitamin D.

Osteopenia – a loss of bone mineral density that weakens bones, most common in women over age 50.

Osteoporosis – decreased bone mineral density and mass, or changes in the structure and strength of bones.

Overdilution – diluting of infant formula to make it last longer because of financial problems.

Oxalic acid – an organic acid found in many leafy greens, vegetables, fruits, cocoa, nuts, and seeds.

Oxidative stress – a condition caused by an imbalance between production and accumulation of oxygen reactive species in cells and tissue, and the ability of the biological system to detoxify them.

Oxyntic glands – those that have ghrelin-containing cells, histamine-containing enterochromaffin-like cells, and somatostatin-secreting D cells.

Ozone precursor – a chemical compound such as carbon monoxide, methane, or nitrogen oxide; in the presence of solar radiation, it reacts with other chemical compounds to form ozone.

Pacemaker cells – highly specialized myocardial cells with an intrinsic ability to depolarize rhythmically and initiate and action potential.

Paget disease – a condition that interferes with normal recycling processes, so that old bone tissue cannot be correctly replaced by new bone tissue.

Palmar erythema – a skin condition causing the palms of the hands to redden.

Pancreatitis – inflammation of the pancreas due to activation of digestive enzymes, which irritate the pancreatic cells.

Paranoia – thoughts or feelings of being threatened, without any real evidence.

Parathyroid hormone – a hormone released from the parathyroid glands that controls calcium levels in the blood.

Parenchymal – relating to or affecting the functional tissue of an organ.

Parenteral nutrition solutions – mixtures that provide complete nutrition, which are administered by injections, bypassing the digestive system.

Paresthesia – an abnormal sensation – usually tingling or pricking – due to pressure or damage upon the peripheral nerves.

Parietal cells – those responsible for gastric acid secretion.

Parkinson's disease – a brain disorder that causes unintended or uncontrollable movements, including shaking, stiffness, and difficulty with balance and coordination.

Paronychia – nail inflammation due to trauma, irritation, or infection.

Passive diffusion – the process by which molecules diffuse from a region of higher concentration to a region of lower concentration.

Patent ductus arteriosus – a persistent opening between the two major blood vessels leading from the heart; it is a congenital heart defect.

Pathologic bone fractures – those that occur through areas of weakened bone, due to primary malignant lesions, benign lesions, metastasis, or metabolic abnormalities.

Pectus excavatum – a condition in which the breastbone is sunken into the chest.

Pellagra – a systemic disease caused by a severe deficiency of niacin (vitamin B3).

Pellagrous glove – a characteristic hand rash that is part of pellagra, caused by a photosensitivity reaction plus niacin deficiency.

Peptic ulcer – a sore on the lining of the stomach, small intestine, or esophagus.

Peripheral neuropathy – weakness, numbness, and pain, usually in the hands and feet, due to damage of the nerves located outside of the brain and spinal cord.

Peristalsis – the involuntary constriction and relaxation of the muscles of the intestine, creating wave-like movements that push contents forward.

Peritonitis – redness and swelling of the peritoneum, the lining of the abdomen.

Pernicious anemia – a type of vitamin B12-deficiency anemia that is an autoimmune condition, manifesting as megaloblastic anemia.

Peroxidation – the chemical reaction between mainly unsaturated fatty acids and reactive forms of oxygen.

Perspiration – the process of sweating.

Petechiae – pinpointed round spots on the skin, caused by bleeding.

Phenylketones – substances excreted in the urine; when excessive phenylalanine is metabolized into these substances, the condition called phenylketonuria develops.

Phenylketonuria – a rare inherited disorder that causes the amino acid called phenylalanine to build up in the body.

Pheochromocytoma – a tumor of the adrenal medulla that causes irregular secretion of epinephrine and norepinephrine.

Phosphorylase kinase – a regulatory protein kinase that stimulates glycogen breakdown.

Phylloquinone – a form of vitamin K found in green leafy vegetables.

Phytic acid – the major storage form of phosphorus in cereals, legumes, oils, seeds, and nuts.

Phytochemicals – chemicals produced by plants that may affect health but are not essential nutrients.

Pica – an eating disorder in which non-food items are consumed.

Pick's disease – a type of frontotemporal dementia that includes behavior changes, speech difficulty, and problems with cognition.

Pigeon chest – a chest wall deformity where there is overgrowth of cartilage between the ribs and the sternum, causing the middle of the chest to stick out.

Plasma – the largest portion of blood; it carries white blood cells, red blood cells, platelets, water, salts, enzymes, nutrients, hormones, and proteins.

Plasma proteins – the proteins that help maintain colloidal osmotic pressure; they include albumin and globulin.

Pleural effusions – buildups of fluid between the layers of tissue that line the lungs and chest cavity.

Plumbism – lead poisoning.

Plummer-Vinson syndrome – anemia caused by iron deficiency, plus a web-like growth of membranes in the throat that makes swallowing difficult.

Pneumaturia – air bubbles in the urine, due to infections or fistulas.

Pneumonia – an infection of the lungs that can cause mild to severe illness.

Pneumonitis – inflammation of lung tissue.

Polycystic ovarian syndrome – a problem with hormones during the reproductive years, in which the ovaries produce an abnormal amount of androgens.

Polycystic ovary syndrome – a hormonal disorder involving multiple cysts, which causes abnormal periods and ovaries, excess body hair, weight gain, skin problems, thinning hair, and infertility.

Polycystic renal disease – an inherited disorder in which clusters of cysts develop mostly in the kidneys, causing enlargement and dysfunction.

Polymeric formulas – mixtures that contain whole proteins, complex carbohydrates, and long chain triglycerides.

Polymorphisms – the presence of two or more variant forms of a certain DNA sequence that can occur in different individuals or populations.

Polyols – organic compounds containing multiple hydroxyl groups.

Polyphenols – compounds found in many plant foods; they include flavonoids, phenolic acids, lignans, and stilbenes.

Polyps – extra pieces of tissue that grow and have the potential to become cancerous.

Pompe's disease – a condition in which the body cannot manufacture a protein that breaks down glycogen for energy, resulting in muscle weakness and difficulty breathing.

Porphyria – a group of disorders that result from a building of natural chemicals that produce porphyrin in the body, causing abnormal iron binding and insufficient oxygen carried to the organs and tissues.

Portal hypertension – elevated pressures in the portal venous system of the liver.

Positive energy balance – energy intake being more than energy expenditure, usually resulting in weight gain.

Postural hypotension – orthostatic hypotension; blood pressure drops when changing from lying down to sitting up, or from sitting up to standing.

Potency – the power of something to influence or make an impression.

Preeclampsia – a pregnancy complication, with hypertension, hyperproteinuria, and other signs of organ damage; it can lead to more serious complications.

Premenstrual syndrome – a common condition in women of reproductive age, with mood swings, breast tenderness, food cravings, fatigue, irritability, and depression.

Prevalence – the proportion of a population that is affected by a medical condition in a given time period.

Prick test – a puncture or scratch test that checks for immediate allergic reactions.

Primary hyperparathyroidism – a condition in which one or more of the parathyroid glands manufactures too much hormone, leading to a loss of bone tissue.

Primary hypothyroidism – low levels of blood thyroid hormone due to destruction of the thyroid gland.

Prioritize – designate or treat something as more important than other things.

Probiotics – a mixture of live bacteria, yeast, or both that normally live in the body.

Progesterone – a female hormone that is an endogenous steroid, involved in the menstrual cycle, pregnancy, and embryogenesis.

Prohormone – a precursor of a hormone, consisting of peptide hormones.

Prolactin – a pituitary hormone that causes the breasts to grow and make milk during pregnancy and after birth.

Prolapse – a condition in which muscles and ligaments supporting a woman's pelvic organs weaken and drop lower, creating a bulge in the vagina.

Prophylaxis – an action taken to prevent disease.

Propulsive – having the quality of driving or pushing forward.

Prostaglandin – a lipid with hormone-like actions that the body makes mostly at sites of tissue damage or infection.

Prostaglandins – lipids with hormone-like actions, mostly made at sites of tissue damage or infection.

Prostate-specific antigen – a protein produced by normal or malignant cells of the prostate gland.

Prostatic intraepithelial neoplasia – a condition defined by neoplastic growth of epithelial cells in preexisting benign prostatic acini or ducts.

Prostatitis – inflammation of the prostate gland.

Protein-calorie malnutrition – inadequate food intake, without significant inflammation, injury, or another condition that causes systemic inflammation.

Protein-energy malnutrition – an energy deficit due to deficiency of all macronutrients.

Proteins – large, complex molecules that are needed by the body; they handle most cellular activities and are required for structure, function, and regulation.

Proteinuria – abnormal levels of protein in the urine.

Proteoglycan – a protein that is heavily glycosylated; the term glycosylation means "to react with a sugar to form a glycoside".

Prothrombin time – a test to evaluate blood clotting.

Proton – a stable subatomic particle with a positive electric charge equal in magnitude to an electron, which has a negative charge.

Proton pump inhibitors – medicines that work by reducing the amount of stomach acid made by glands in the stomach lining.

Protozoa – a group of single-celled eukaryotes that feed on organic matter.

Provitamin D3 – a substance converted to provitamin D3 by the action of ultraviolet radiation on the skin.

Pseudofractures – bands of bone material of decreased density alongside the surface of a cortical bone, with thickening of the periosteum.

Pseudohypoglycemia – a condition where the measured glucose level is falsely lower than the actual level, due to impaired circulation or in vitro glycolysis.

Psoriasis – patches of thick red skin and silvery scales, mostly on the elbows, knees, scalp, lower back, face, palms, and soles.

Psyllium husk – psyllium fiber; a water-attracting substance from the outer layer of psyllium seeds.

Ptosis – drooping of the upper eyelid over the eye.

Puberty – the time in life when a child becomes sexually mature; it usually begins between ages 7 and 13 in girls and between ages 9 and 15 in boys.

Pulmonary emboli – clumps of material, usually blood clots, that get stuck in a lung artery and block the flow of blood.

Pulsatility – a function of maximum flow rate that implicates that pulsatile flow generates higher wall shear stress than equal continuous flow.

Pulse pressure – the systolic pressure minus the diastolic pressure; generally, it is considered unhealthy if it is greater than 40 mm Hg.

Punitive – inflicting or intended as punishment; or an extremely high tax or other charge.

Purine salvage – a pathway that involves production of purine nucleotides to recover bases and nucleosides formed during degradation of RNA and DNA.

Purines – chemical compounds in food that cause gout.

Purpura – a condition in which small blood vessels leak blood under the skin.

Pyelonephritis – a kidney infection that can cause permanent damage or a systemic infection.

Pyrimidinuria – the presence of pyrimidines in the urine; it may be familial or associated with severe fluorouracil toxicity.

Radioimmunoassay – a technique for determining antibody levels, by introducing an antigen labeled with a radioisotope, and measuring subsequent radioactivity of the antibody component.

Redox potential – the tendence of a chemical species to be reduced by accepting electrons, or oxidized by donating electrons.

Refeeding syndrome – potentially fatal shifts in fluids and electrolytes that may occur in malnourished patients receiving artificial refeeding.

Refractory disease – a disease or condition that does not respond to treatment.

Relaxin – a reproductive hormone of the ovaries and placenta that helps the body stretch.

Remethylation – methylation that is subsequent to demethylation; remethylation defects are rare inherited disorders that lead to accumulation of homocysteine, and many methylation reactions.

Renin – an enzyme secreted by and stored in the kidneys, which promotes production of angiotensin.

Renin-angiotensin system – the system that plays a crucial role in regulation of renal, cardiac, and vascular physiology.

Respiratory acidosis – an acid-base disturbance due to alveolar hypoventilation; the production of carbon dioxide occurs rapidly and failure of ventilation quickly increases the partial pressure of arterial carbon dioxide.

Respiratory alkalosis – a medical condition in which increased respiration elevates blood pH as arterial levels of carbon dioxide reduce.

Respiratory distress syndrome – a common breathing disorder in newborns, due to a lack of surfactant in the lungs.

Retinal – the intermediate step between retinoic acid and retinol.

Retinoic acid – a nutrient needed by the body, in small amounts, to function and stay healthy.

Retinoids – compounds derived from vitamin A that have many cosmetic uses.

Retinol – vitamin A1; found in foods and used as a dietary supplement.

Rhabdomyolysis – a breakdown of skeletal muscle, due to muscle injury; without immediate treatment, it can result in kidney damage.

Rhodopsin – a G-protein coupled receptor – the most abundant protein in rod cells of the retina.

Rickets – softening and weakening of bones in children, usually due to prolonged vitamin D deficiency.

Rods – photoreceptor cells of the retina that provide good vision in low light.

Rooting reflex – a basic survival instinct that helps an infant find and latch onto a breast or bottle to begin feeding.

Saphenous veins – blood vessels in the legs that send blood from the legs and feet back up to the heart.

Sarcopenia – an age-related involuntary loss of skeletal mass and strength.

Saturated – containing the greatest possible number of hydrogen atoms, and lacking carbon-carbon double or triple bonds.

Sclerotherapy – injecting a chemical solution directly into a varicose or spider vein.

Scoliosis – a sideways curvature of the spine, usually diagnosed in adolescents.

Scurvy – a disease caused by a vitamin C deficiency, characterized by swollen, bleeding gums, and opening of previously healed wounds.

Seborrheic dermatitis – a common skin condition that mostly affects the scalp, causing scaly patches, inflamed skin, and chronic dandruff.

Seborrheic keratoses – common, noncancerous skin growths that are more common with aging, appearing as waxy, scaly, slightly raised lesions.

Secondary hyperparathyroidism – a form of hyperparathyroidism occurring from another disease that initially causes low calcium levels.

Secondary hypothyroidism – decreased activity of the thyroid, caused by failure of the pituitary gland.

Selenosis – a condition resulting from chronic selenium intoxication, including fatigue, and hair and nail damage or loss.

Seminal vesicles – glands that produce fluids that will turn into semen.

Sensible water loss – via routes of excretion such as urination and defecation.

Sepsis – the body's extreme response to an infection, in which it triggers a chain reaction throughout the body.

Serotonin – a chemical that carries messages between nerve cells in the brain and throughout the body, important for mood, sleep, digestion, nausea, wound healing, bone health, blood clotting, and sexual desire.

Shiga toxin – a component of certain E. coli that results in severe diarrhea, stomach cramps, and vomiting.

Short bowel syndrome – a condition in which the body is unable to absorb enough nutrients from food due to lack of enough of the small intestine.

Sickle cell disease – a common inherited blood disorder in which blood flow to organs is blocked, damaging them as well as nerves; it is often fatal.

Silent coronary artery disease – also called silent myocardial ischemia; reduced oxygen-rich blood flow to the heart without chest discomfort or other angina signs.

Simple nontoxic goiter – noncancerous enlargement of the thyroid gland that does not involve altered production of thyroid hormones.

Skin tags – also called acrochordons; small benign growths that are usually the same color as the skin, mostly in areas of skin rubbing.

Sleep apnea – a common disorder that causes breathing to stop or become very shallow; pauses can last from seconds to minutes.

Smelting – the extraction of metal from its ore by heating and melting it.

Solutes – components of solutions that are dissolved by solvents.

Sphingolipidosis – a metabolic storage disorder characterized by accumulation of harmful quantities of glycosphingolipids and phosphosphingolipids.

Sphingosine – an 18-carbon amino alcohol that forms a primary part of sphingolipids, which are cell membrane lipids.

Spider angiomas – small red to purple marks on the skin caused by dilated capillaries.

Spina bifida – a type of neural tube defect that leaves part of the spinal cord and spinal nerves exposed.

Squamous cell carcinoma – the second most common skin cancer, developing in squamous cells, sometimes as a result of actinic keratosis.

Stable angina – a type of chest pain that occurs when the heart muscle needs more oxygen than usual; usually linked to heart disease, cold temperatures, or exercise.

Stamina – the ability to sustain prolonged physical or mental effort.

Standard deviations – measures of amounts of variations or dispersions of sets of values.

Steatorrhea – increased fat excretion in the stool.

Stellate cells – liver-specific mesenchymal cells that play vital roles in liver physiology and fibrogenesis.

Stent retriever – tiny mesh tubes that grab and extract blood clots in blocked arteries.

Steric acid – also spelled "stearic acid"; a saturated fatty acid with an 18-carbon chain.

Stocking-glove distribution – a characteristic pattern of numbness in which the distal portions of nerves are first affected.

Stoma – an opening in the abdomen that can be connected to the digestive or urinary system to allow waste to be diverted out of the body.

Strabismus – hypertropia or crossed eyes; a misalignment that causes one eye to deviate inward or outward.

Stratum corneum – the outermost layer of the epidermis.

Stress fracture – a tiny crack in a bone, caused by repetitive force, often from overuse.

Stroke – a condition in which there is a blockage of the brain's blood supply or when a brain blood vessel bursts, leading to severe disability or death.

Stroke volume – the volume of blood pumped out of the left ventricle during each systolic cardiac contraction.

Stunted growth – impaired growth and development due to poor nutrition, repeated infections, and insufficient psychosocial stimulation.

Subluxation – a partial dislocation.

Substrate – an underlying substance or layer, or upon which an enzyme acts.

Sucrase-isomaltase – an enzyme on the brush border of the small intestine that catalyzes hydrolysis of linkages in oligosaccharides produces from starch and glycogen, and in isomaltose.

Sudden infant death syndrome – the sudden, unexpected death of a baby less than one year old, from a cause that was not obvious.

Superior vena cava syndrome – a group of symptoms caused by blockage or compression of the superior vena cava.

Surfactant – a complex mixture of lipids, proteins, and carbohydrates that acts to decrease the surface tension at the air/liquid interface of the lung alveoli.

Surgical blind loops – blind loop syndrome; when food does not follow the normal digestion route and bypasses part of the intestine.

Synaptic delay – the time interval between peak of inward current through the presynaptic membrane and start of inward current through the postsynaptic membrane.

Synovitis – inflammation of the synovium (connective tissue lining the inside capsule) of a joint.

Systemic lupus erythematosus – the most common type of lupus; it causes inflammation that can damage the skin, joints, heart, lungs, kidneys, circulating blood cells, and brain.

Tachypnea – abnormally rapid breathing.

Tannins – bitter, astringent chemical compounds that are also classified as polyphenols; they are present in many types of plants, legumes, and fruits such as grapes.

Tapioca dextrin – an adhesive coating for candy, snack, vegetable, and meat substrates.

Taste buds – the structures that contain taste receptor cells (gustatory cells).

Tay-Sachs disease – a rare genetic disorder in which an enzyme is lacking that helps break down fatty substances; gangliosides build up to toxic levels in the CNS.

Tendinous xanthomas – cholesterol deposits in tendons that manifest as firm to hard subcutaneous nodules.

Tenesmus – the feeling of needing to pass stools, though the bowels are empty.

Teratogens – agents that cause embryonal malformations.

Tetany – a condition of intermittent muscle spasms, due to malfunction of the parathyroid glands that causes a deficiency of calcium.

Thermic effect – the amount of energy required for the body to digest, absorb, and metabolize food.

Thermogenesis – dissipation of energy through the production of heat.

Thigmotropism – turning or bending in response to a touch stimulus.

Thrombosis – a condition that occurs when blood clots block blood vessels.

Thymic deficiency – a lack of thymosin from the thymus gland, causing low T cell counts and a higher susceptibility to infections.

Thyroid-stimulating hormone – a glycoprotein hormone produced by the anterior pituitary that is the main stimulus for thyroid hormone production.

Thyrotropin hormone – a hormone produced by the pituitary gland in response to signals from the hypothalamus.

Thyroxine – a hormone secreted by the thyroid gland into the bloodstream; once reaching organs, it is converted to its active form, triiodothyronine.

Tissue plasminogen activator – a protein involved in the breakdown of blood clots.

Tocopherol – vitamin E; a nutrient found in every body cell that helps the nerves and muscles to function well, prevents blood clots, and boosts the immune system.

Tofu – bean curd; prepared from coagulated soybean milk.

Tonicity – muscle tone, or the state of a solution in respect of osmotic pressure.

Tonsillectomy – surgical removal of the tonsils.

Tophi – stone-like deposits of monosodium urate in soft or synovial tissues, or in bones near joints.

Total parenteral nutrition – a method of feeding that bypasses the gastrointestinal tract; a special formula is administered intravenously.

Toxic megacolon syndrome – a rare, life-threatening complication of severe colon disease or infection; it requires immediate treatment.

Trans fatty acids – manufactured fats created during hydrogenation; they are dangerous for heart health and may pose risks for certain cancers.

Transsulfuration – a metabolic process involving interconversion of cystine and homocysteine through an intermediate known as cystathionine.

Transthyretin – a transport protein in the plasma and cerebrospinal fluid that transports thyroxine and retinol to the liver.

Transverse fractures – those that occur when a bone is broken perpendicular to its length, mostly affecting longer bones after a fall or accident.

Triglyceride – a type of lipid in the blood; calories that are not needed for use immediately are converted into these.

Trophoblastic disease – abnormal trophoblast cells growing inside the uterus after conception.

Tropical pancreatitis – a juvenile form of chronic calcific non-alcoholic pancreatitis, usually occurring in developing tropical countries.

Tropical sprue – a condition occurring in people that live in or visit tropical areas for extended time periods; it impairs nutrients from being absorbed from the intestines.

Truncal obesity – abdominal (or central) obesity, in which there is excessive visceral fat around the stomach and abdomen.

Trypsin – an enzyme in the first section of the small intestine that begins digestion of proteins by cutting long chains of amino acids into smaller pieces.

Turgid – swollen and distended, or congested.

Tylosis – focal thickening of the skin of the hands and feet; it is also a high risk factor for squamous cell carcinoma of the esophagus.

Ulcerative colitis – an inflammatory bowel disease that causes inflammation and ulcers in the large intestine.

Universal solvent – water; it is called this because it can dissolve more substances than any other liquid.

Unleavened breads – those prepared without using rising agents such as yeast.

Unsaturated – having carbon-carbon double or triple bonds, and lacking the greatest possible number of hydrogen atoms for the number of carbons; this type of fat is healthier than saturated fat.

Unstable angina – a condition in which the heart does not get enough blood flow and oxygen, which may lead to a heart attack.

Urban heat islands – areas that occur when cities replace natural land cover with large concentrations of pavement, buildings, and other surfaces that absorb and retain heat.

Urea – a substance formed by the breakdown of protein in the liver; it is filtered out of the blood by the kidneys and eliminated in the urine.

Uremia – an increased level of urea in the blood, or an increase in other nitrogenous waste compounds that are usually eliminated by the kidneys.

Uricosuria – excretion of uric acid in the urine, usually in excessive amounts.

Urinary incontinence – accidental leaking of urine, most common in older women.

Uterine fibroids – leiomyomas or myomas; benign growths in the uterus made of uterine muscle.

Valences – molecular weights and charges, in relation to minerals.

Variant angina – vasospastic angina; characterized by episodes of resting angina that quickly respond to short-acting nitrates and are linked to coronary artery vasospasm.

Varicocele – an enlargement of the veins within the scrotum.

Vasoconstriction – constriction of blood vessels by small muscles in their walls.

Vasodilation – widening of blood vessels due to relaxation of their muscular walls.

Vasopressin – antidiuretic hormone (or arginine vasopressin), a nonapeptide synthesized in the hypothalamus, which plays essential roles in osmotic balance, blood pressure regulation, sodium homeostasis, and kidney functioning.

Vegan – a person who does not eat any food derived from animals.

Vessel bifurcations – points on vessel centerlines where vessels split into other vessels.

Visuomotor – relating to the coordination of movement and visual perception by the brain.

Visuospatial – relating to the visual perception of the spatial relationships of objects.

Vitreous humors – transparent, colorless, gel-like substances in the posterior chamber of the eye, which helps maintain its shape.

Von Gierke disease – a condition in which the body cannot break down glycogen; it is also called Type I glycogen storage disease.

Wasting – causing a person or part of the body to become progressively weaker and more emaciated.

Weigh-ins – measurements of a person's weight to assess changes.

Weighed ad libitum diet – one in which food is consumed when hungry, and stopped once the individual feels full; weighing is also done to assess weight gain or loss.

Weight cycling – losing weight and regaining it on a continual basis.

Wernicke area – a region of the brain that contains motor neurons involved in the comprehension of speech.

Wernicke encephalopathy – a degenerative brain disorder caused by lack of vitamin B1, which may result from alcohol abuse or dietary deficiencies.

Wheezing – a high-pitched whistling sound made while breathing.

Whipple's triad – symptoms of hypoglycemia, with blood glucose levels less than 50 mg per deciliter, and relief of symptoms after ingestion of glucose.

White scales – fine skin scales left behind due to shedding, as part of xerosis.

Wilson's disease – a rare, inherited disorder that causes copper to accumulate in the liver, brain, and other vital organs.

Wisdom – the quality of having experience, knowledge, and good judgment.

Xanthomas – lesions on the skin containing cholesterol and fats, often associated with inherited disorders of lipid metabolism.

Xerosis – dry skin.

Xerostomia – dry mouth, due to insufficient production of saliva.

Zinc finger proteins – those that interact with DNA, RNA, and other proteins; they are involved in regulation of cellular processes.

Zollinger-Ellison syndrome – a rare digestive disorder that causes excessive gastric acid.

Zoochemicals – compounds in animals believed to provide health benefits beyond traditional nutrients found in food.

Index

Note: Bold page numbers refer to tables; *italic* page numbers refer to figures.

For Product Safety Concerns and Information please contact our EU
representative GPSR@taylorandfrancis.com
Taylor & Francis Verlag GmbH, Kaufingerstraße 24, 80331 München, Germany

www.ingramcontent.com/pod-product-compliance
Lightning Source LLC
LaVergne TN
LVHW080119011026
849160LV00013B/1133